Nutrition, health and disease

A lifespan approach

Simon Langley-Evans, BSc, PhD, DSc, PGCHE

School of Biosciences
University of Nottingham, UK

THIRD EDITION

WILEY Blackwell

Registered Offices
John Wiley & Sons, Inc., 111 River Street, Hoboken, NJ 07030, USA
John Wiley & Sons Ltd, The Atrium, Southern Gate, Chichester, West Sussex, PO19 8SQ, UK

Editorial Office
9600 Garsington Road, Oxford, OX4 2DQ, UK

For details of our global editorial offices, customer services, and more information about Wiley products visit us at www.wiley.com.

Wiley also publishes its books in a variety of electronic formats and by print-on-demand. Some content that appears in standard print versions of this book may not be available in other formats.

Library of Congress Cataloging-in-Publication Data applied for

PB ISBN: 9781119717515

Cover Design: Wiley
Cover Images: © pondsaksit/Getty Images, © monkeybusinessimages/Getty Images, © Rouzes/Getty Images, © Jose Luis Pelaez Inc/Getty Images, © Catherine Delahaye/Getty Images, © SCIEPRO/Getty Images

Set in 8.5/11pt MeridienLTStd by Straive, Pondicherry, India
Printed and bound by CPI Group (UK) Ltd, Croydon, CR0 4YY

C9781119717515_290721

Contents

Preface

This is the third edition of this textbook, an enterprise that I began back in 2007. The third edition will be the final update of the original text as it is my intention to retire and focus on other things in the near future. Writing this edition has been curious process, as the bulk of the researching and drafting was done under the conditions of the 2020/21 coronavirus pandemic. These words therefore come from a makeshift setup in my home, where my influences have tended to be drawn from reading in isolation and the company of my family and cats rather than my work colleagues.

For all editions of this book, I have tried to embrace the challenge of translating the complex evidence base that links diet and nutrition to health and disease, into a balanced account. My aim has been to take on big topics across the human lifespan and generate accounts that will be informative and of interest to undergraduate and Master's level students and helpful to those in training to become health professionals. In finding that balance, I have tried to blend the basics of nutrition as a discipline with evidence that is at the cutting edge of the subject, and where knowledge is constantly shifting. As you read the text, I hope that you gain an insight into how nutrition research works and where the limitations of techniques impinge upon capacity to create public health policy.

In the 14 years since the first word of this book was written, much has changed in nutrition. The multidisciplinary nature of the subject has expanded and as such this book has had to encompass evidence from genetic and epigenetic studies with epidemiology, physiology and the qualitative findings of social science researchers. The rapid rate of change in technology, particularly in molecular biology, has meant that some speculative ideas that made it into the first edition, are now established facts for the third. Human nutrition has been the focus of my career across four decades and it has never been a more exciting time to be part of the nutrition profession.

My intention for you as a reader of this work is that you use it as a platform for developing your own understanding of the subject matter. I have considered a broad body of evidence and synthesized a text which inevitably reflects my view of the world. Use my text and the supporting bibliographies to expand that understanding and keep abreast of the evidence base, which can shift markedly over a few years. As this is my final update of the book I will take one last opportunity to exhort you to embrace a spirit of enquiry. There is so much that we still need to discover, so be curious; be open-minded; be collaborative and, most importantly of all, challenge and ask questions.

Simon Langley-Evans
University of Nottingham
February 2021

Acknowledgements

Writing a book, whether it is the third edition or the first, is a huge undertaking. I would like to show my appreciation to my family, Alison, Effie, Hugh, Felix and the Jizz, for their endless support as I've wrestled with the text. Thank you to Effie Langley-Evans and Sam Kearn for assistance with illustrations.

Abbreviations

11βHSD2	11β-hydroxysteroid dehydrogenase-2
ADHD	attention-deficit hyperactivity disorder
AGRP	agouti-related peptide
AIDS	acquired immune deficiency syndrome
ALSPAC	Avon Longitudinal Study of Parents and Children
AMDR	acceptable macronutrient distribution range
ART	anti-retroviral therapies
ATP	adenosine triphosphate
AZD	Alzheimer's disease
b(a)P	benzo(a)pyrene
Bax	Bcl2-associated X protein
BiZiFED	Biofortification with Zinc and Iron for Eliminating Deficiency
BFHI	Baby Friendly Hospital Initiative
BMD	bone mineral density
BMI	body mass index
CALERIE	Comparative Assessment of Long-term effects of Reducing Intake of Energy
CHD	coronary heart disease
CI	confidence interval
COMA	Committee on Medical Aspects of Food Policy
CRONies	Caloric Restriction Optimal Nutrition Society
CVD	cardiovascular disease
DBP	diastolic blood pressure
DEER	desirable estimated energy requirement
DHA	docosahexaenoic acid
DMFT	delayed, missing and filled teeth
DNA	deoxyribose nucleic acid
DNMT	DNA methyltransferase
DRV	dietary reference value
EAR	estimated average requirement
EERM	estimated energy requirement for maintenance
EFSA	European Food Safety Authority
EPA	eicosapentaenoic acid
EPIC	European Prospective Investigation into Cancer
ERβ	oestrogen receptor beta
FAO	Food and Agriculture Organization
FAS	fetal alcohol syndrome
FSH	follicle-stimulating hormone
GI	glycaemic index
GLUT	glucose transporter
GMC	General Medical Council
GnRH	gonadotrophin-releasing hormone
GPx	glutathione peroxidase
hCG	human chorionic gonadotrophin
HDL	high-density lipoprotein
HIV	human immunodeficiency virus
HR	hazard ratio
IGF	insulin-like growth factor
IL	interleukin
IQ	intelligence quotient
IRS	insulin receptor substrate
JAK	Janus kinase
LCPUFA	long chain polyunsaturated fatty acid
LDL	low-density lipoprotein
LH	luteinizing hormone
LRNI	lower reference nutrient intake
LTL	leucocyte telomere length
MNA	Mini Nutritional Assessment
MODY	maturity onset diabetes of the young
MTHFR	methylenetetrahydrofolate reductase
MUFA	monounsaturated fatty acid
NDNS	National Diet and Nutrition Surveys
NHANES	National Health and Nutrition Examination Study
NIA	National Institute on Aging
NTD	neural tube defect
NVP	nausea and vomiting of pregnancy
OR	odds ratio
PI3K	phosphoinositol-3 kinase
PCOS	polycystic ovary syndrome
PPAR-γ2	peroxisome proliferator-activated receptor γ2
PKU	phenylketonuria
PPAR	peroxisome proliferator-activated receptor
PPH	postpartum haemorrhage
PUFA	polyunsaturated fatty acid
RAE	retinol activity equivalent
RCT	randomized controlled trial
RDA	recommended daily amount
RNA	ribonucleic acid
RNI	reference nutrient intake
ROS	reactive oxygen species
RR	relative risk
SBP	systolic blood pressure
SFA	short-chain fatty acid
SIDS	sudden infant death syndrome
SMR	sexual maturity rating
SNP	single nucleotide polymorphism
SOCS3	suppressor of the cytokine signalling-3
STAT-3	signal transducer and activator of transcription-3
TNFα	tumour necrosis factor alpha
USDA	United States Department of Agriculture
VLDL	very low density lipoprotein
WHO	World Health Organization
WNPRC	Wisconsin National Primate Research Centre

Glossary of terms used in this book

Adipocyte: A fat-containing cell found in adipose tissue.

Adipokines: Cytokines secreted by the adipose tissue.

Adiponectin: A hormone secreted by adipose tissue. It enhances insulin sensitivity and promotes glucose uptake.

Adipose tissue: The site of body fat deposition. Cells within adipose tissue store and release fat.

Adiposity rebound: Body mass index rises rapidly in the first two years of life and then declines until a point between the ages of four and six years, when it starts to increase again. The point where the trend reverses is termed the 'adiposity rebound'.

Adrenal glands: Endocrine organs located above the kidneys. The adrenals are the sites for production and release of adrenaline, noradrenaline and steroid hormones such as cortisol and aldosterone.

Adrenarche: The maturation of the adrenal cortex into three distinct zones, resulting in secretion of androgenic hormones during adolescence.

Aflatoxins: Mycotoxins formed by fungi such as *Aspergillus*. Aflatoxins are important contaminants of peanuts and groundnuts stored in humid climates.

Alkaloids: Toxic compounds found in plant foods (e.g. potatoes) or as contaminants on cereals, produced by mildew.

Allergic sensitization: The process through which exposure to foreign materials, either through ingestion, inhalation or skin contact, elicits immune responses that will manifest as allergic symptoms (rash or asthma). Initial contact with allergens may not produce a response but instead primes (sensitizes) the body to produce responses at further contact.

Allergy: Adverse reaction to antigens (for example proteins in certain foodstuffs) that is mediated by the immune system (production of antibodies).

Allium: Plants of the onion family. Includes onions and garlic.

Alzheimer's disease: An irreversible and progressive neurodegenerative disorder leading to memory loss, altered behaviour and dementia. The disease is characterized by the formation of plaques of amyloid beta peptide in the brain.

Amenorrhea: The absence of a menstrual period in a woman of reproductive age.

Ames test: A test used to determine the potential carcinogenicity of chemicals. The test uses cultures of *Salmonella typhimurium*, which must undergo a mutation to be able to grow on a limiting medium. Presence of colonies in the medium indicates potential mutagenicity of test compounds.

Anaemia: Deficiency of red blood cells or haemoglobin.

Androgens: The male sex hormones. The main androgens are the steroid hormones, testosterone and dehydroepiandrosterone.

Anencephaly: A defect of the formation of the embryonic neural tube which results in the non-formation of the cerebral arches.

Angina pectoris: Chest pain caused by the partial occlusion of the coronary arteries due to atherosclerosis.

Angiogenesis: The process through which new blood vessels branch off from existing vessels.

Anorexia nervosa: An eating disorder characterized by body image distortion and fear of weight gain. Anorexics, who are typically underweight, may voluntarily starve, indulge in excessive exercise, vomit or purge after eating and abuse laxatives or anti-obesity drugs.

Anovulation: The absence of ovulation in women of reproductive age.

Anterior pituitary: One of two lobes of the pituitary gland. This endocrine tissue responds directly to signals from the hypothalamus and plays a key role in regulation of the production of hormones from the adrenals and reproductive organs.

Anthropometry: The measurement of the human body in terms of the dimensions of muscle, and adipose (fat) tissue. Simple measures of height and weight, supplemented with measurements of skinfold thicknesses, mid-upper arm circumference, waist and hip circumferences can be used to estimate body composition and distribution of body fat.

Anti-oncogenes: *see* Oncogenes

Antioxidants: Molecules that are capable of quenching the reactivity of free radicals and other oxidizing agents (e.g. hydrogen peroxide). Antioxidants may be scavenging antioxidants, which are destroyed in reactions with reactive oxygen species or enzymes that are capable of rapid metabolism of high quantities of reactive oxygen species.

Apoptosis: Programmed cell death which involves a coordinated series of biochemical events leading to the death of the cell and removal of resulting debris.

Arrhythmia: Condition in which the heart beat is irregular or excessively slow or fast. Arrhythmias are the product of damage to the heart during myocardial infarction.

Arterial intima: The innermost layer of the arterial wall.

Ataxia telangiectasia: An immunodeficiency disorder.

Atherosclerosis: The process through which the artery accumulates a plaque containing cholesterol, collagen and calcium. Atherosclerotic plaques cause stiffening and narrowing of the arteries and act as a focus for clots. Atherosclerosis is the basis of all cardiovascular disease (coronary heart disease, stroke, peripheral artery disease).

Atopy: A predisposition to allergic responses.

Attention deficit hyperactivity disorder: A neurological disturbance in children, which leads to inattention and impulsive behaviour.

Axillary hair: Hair in the underarm region.

B lymphocytes: Cells of the immune system responsible for the production of antibodies.

Bacteroides: One of the six main genera of bacteria which contribute to the human intestinal microflora.

Bariatric surgery: Surgery to promote weight loss through restriction of the stomach capacity in order to limit food intake.

Basal metabolic rate, resting metabolic rate: The energy cost associated with maintaining the basic physiological processes of the body at rest (i.e. respiration, circulation, nerve and muscle tone). Basal metabolic rate is in proportion to body size, since it is determined by the amount of metabolically active tissue.

Betel chewing: The habit of chewing betel quid. The quid is a mixture of areca nut and leaves. This habit is most common in Pacific communities and in some parts of Asia (e.g. Taiwan).

Bifidobacterium: One of the six main genera of bacteria which contribute to the human intestinal microflora.

Bioimpedance: The measurement of body fat content through determination of the resistance of the body to the flow of an electrical current.

Biomarker: A measurement used to assess the state of a biological system. In nutrition biomarkers may include measurements of nutrient concentrations in suitable samples (e.g. blood and urine), or measurements of nutrient-dependent physiological functions.

Bisphosphonates: A class of drugs used in the treatment of osteoporosis. Bisphosphonates inhibit the action of osteoclasts.

Blood pressure: The pressure generated within the arteries due to the pumping of the heart. Between beats the vessels are at rest and the pressure is at the lowest point (diastolic pressure). Maximum pressure occurs with ejection of blood from the left ventricle (systolic pressure).

Body mass index (BMI): A measure of weight in relation to height (weight in kg/height in m^2). BMI is widely used as a tool to determine whether an individual is of healthy weight (BMI between 20 and 25), underweight (BMI <20), overweight (BMI 25–30) or obese (BMI <30).

Bone mineral density: A measure of bone mass. Reduced bone mineral density is generally indicative of conditions such as osteoporosis, in which fracture risk is increased.

Bulimia nervosa: An eating disorder linked to body image distortion and fear of weight gain. Affected individuals periodically binge eat and then compensate for excessive intake through excessive exercise, vomiting and purging.

Cachexia: Severe loss of weight and muscle mass, often accompanied by loss of appetite.

Caffeine: A methyl xanthine compound found in tea, coffee, chocolate and over-the-counter medications. Caffeine is a central nervous system stimulant.

Cancer: Disease involving the uncontrolled growth of cells to form a tumour. Cancer cells can invade tissues and organs at the point where they are first formed (primary tumours), or can spread to other organs through the process of metastasis, forming secondary tumours.

Carcinogen: Any agent that is capable of directly initiating the formation of a tumour or can promote the development or spread of existing tumours.

Carcinogenesis: The process through which exposure of cells to carcinogens initiates the formation of tumours, leading to cancer.

Cardiac output: The volume of blood pumped by the blood in a given unit of time. Cardiac output is generally measured in litres per minute. Cardiac output is one of the determinants of blood pressure.

Cardiovascular disease: The term used to collectively describe the diseases that involve the heart or blood vessels. Most clinically significant cardiovascular disease (coronary heart disease, stroke, peripheral artery disease) is related to atherosclerosis.

Carotenoids: Organic pigments found primarily in plants. This group of tetraterpenoids includes α- and β-carotene, lutein, lycopene and zeaxanthin.

Carotid intima-media thickness: A clinical measurement of the extent of atherosclerosis in the carotid artery. Development of plaques results in increased thickness of the arterial wall.

Case–control study: An epidemiological study design in which characteristics of a group of individuals suffering from a disease (cases) are compared to those of a group of healthy individuals (controls).

Catabolism: The metabolic breakdown (degradation) of macromolecules to release energy.

Catch-up growth: Accelerated growth which follows a period of growth restriction.

Chondrocytes: Cells found in cartilaginous tissues responsible for secreting the characteristic proteins of cartilage.

Chorion: A membrane that surrounds the embryo and fetus during development. Processes formed in this membrane develop into the chorionic villi, which invade the uterine lining during placentation.

Claudication: Pain, usually in the lower legs, caused by poor circulation due to peripheral artery disease.

Clotting factors: Factors that promote the coagulation of blood. In humans, the major clotting factors are fibrinogen, factor VII, factor VIII, prothrombin and von Willebrand factor.

Coeliac disease: An autoimmune disorder of the bowel in which an inflammatory response occurs in response to the ingestion of the gliadin portion of gluten.

Cohort study: An epidemiological study in which a group of individuals is followed over a period of time to determine how characteristics observed early in the study might influence the later development of disease. Prospective cohort studies define the characteristics of the population as soon as individuals are recruited; participants are followed-up as the study progresses. Retrospective cohort studies assess population characteristics after the disease data have been collected.

Colonic microflora: The bacterial species that colonise the human digestive tract. The human colon is home to over 500 species of bacteria, some of which are pathogenic, while others have benefits for human health.

Colostrum: The first milk produced by the mammary glands after giving birth. Colostrum is a protein-rich, thick fluid that is an important source of immunoprotective factors.

Complement: An element of the immune system which involves a cascade of enzyme-mediated events that kill infected cells and pathogens.

Complementary feeding: Weaning. Complementary foods are foods added to the diet of breastfed infants during the transition from full breastfeeding to family foods.

Complex carbohydrates: Carbohydrates with a complex chemical structure. The complex carbohydrates include the soluble and insoluble starches and those components of the diet that are generally referred to as dietary fibre (cellulose, lignans, chitin).

Confidence interval: All measurements are subject to error and summary statistics such as odds ratios, relative risk or estimated means lie within a range of values for the estimate. They are in fact 'best estimates' of the true value. The level of confidence of the confidence interval indicates the probability that the confidence range includes the true value. This level of confidence is represented by a percentage. Ninety-five per cent confidence indicates that 95% of the observed confidence intervals will hold the true value of the measurement.

Confounding factor: A factor in an epidemiological study that can lead to a false conclusion regarding an apparently causal association between a risk factor and disease endpoint, unless controlled for statistically.

Constipation: Impaired bowel function in which small hard stools are formed that are difficult to egest.

Coronary heart disease: Disease of the coronary arteries caused by the formation of atherosclerotic plaques. Plaques and associated clots can prevent blood and oxygen from reaching the muscles of the heart. Cells of the heart subsequently die, leaving a damaged area called an infarct.

Corpus luteum: The remnant of the Graafian follicle after the release of an egg during mammalian ovulation. The corpus luteum becomes a temporary endocrine organ, producing progesterone to maintain the uterine wall should pregnancy occur.

Cortical bone: Bone with a dense structure. Also termed compact bone.

Cross-sectional study: An epidemiological approach in which the prevalence of disease (outcomes) or determinants of health (exposures) are measured in a population at the same point in time or over a short period.

Cruciferous vegetables: Vegetables of the plant family *Brassicaceae*, which includes cabbage, Brussels sprouts, kale, cauliflower and broccoli.

Cryptorchidism: A condition in which the testicles fail to descend during normal male reproductive development.

Cytochrome P450 system: A large and diverse superfamily of enzymes, which are largely responsible for the metabolism of xenobiotics. Most reactions catalyzed by cytochrome P450s involve the addition of a hydroxyl group from water, which facilitates the subsequent conjugation and excretion of the agent.

Cytokines: Chemical messengers that can be produced by almost all cell types (unlike hormones that are produced by specific endocrine cells). Cytokines are especially important in mediating inflammatory and immune responses.

Dementia: Progressive loss of cognitive functions including memory, language and problem-solving skills. Dementia represents extreme loss of these functions that goes beyond normal age-related declines.

Developed countries: The economically successful countries, in which the national income translates into

significant advantages for the health and education of the population. The developed nations include Japan, Canada, the United States, Australia, New Zealand and the nations of Western Europe, along with Singapore, Hong Kong, South Korea and Taiwan.

Developing countries: Countries with a low industrial base and lacking economic wealth to invest in the health, education and welfare of the population.

Diabetes mellitus: A metabolic disorder characterized by raised circulating glucose concentrations, attributable to defects of glucose homeostasis. Type 1 diabetes is due to insufficient insulin production, while Type 2 diabetes arises from impaired responses to insulin, which may be present in very high concentrations.

Diaphysis: The shaft portion of a long bone.

Diastolic blood pressure: *see* Blood pressure

Dietary fibre: One of several terms used to describe the nondigestible matter present in food. Cellulose, chitin and insoluble starches all pass through the digestive tract largely unchanged. Fibre is also referred to as non-starch polysaccharides and complex carbohydrates.

Dieting: The process of restricting food intake with the intention of losing weight. Dieting may involve a reduction of all foods consumed, or the exclusion of particular food items, or groups of nutrients.

Dietitian: A health professional who uses dietary change as a tool for the management and treatment of disease states in her/his patients.

Diuretic: A pharmacological agent which stimulates the excretion of water.

Diverticular disease: A condition of the large intestine whereby small sacs or pouches called diverticula form in the wall of the large intestine. Diverticula may become infected, leading to a condition known as diverticulitis.

Dizygotic twins: Non-identical twins.

DNA methylation: Chemical modification of DNA that can be inherited without changing the DNA sequence. DNA methylation plays an important role in the silencing of gene expression and is an element of epigenetic regulation.

Doubly labelled water: A method for measuring energy expenditure, in which subjects are administered water labelled with deuterium and ^{18}O. Elimination of the isotopes allows determination of CO_2 production, which is a marker for total energy expenditure.

Dual x-ray absorptiometry: An x-ray technique in which patients are subjected to x-ray scans in two different planes. The absorption of the x-ray energy by soft tissues and by bone allows accurate determination of bone mineral content and density. It can also be used to estimate the fat mass of the body.

Dyslipidaemia: Disruption of the normal concentrations of lipids (mostly triglycerides and cholesterol) in circulation. The most commonly noted dyslipidaemias involve increases in circulating lipid concentrations (hyperlipidaemia).

Dysphagia: Difficulty in swallowing.

Eclampsia: A life-threatening complication of pregnancy, characterized by uncontrolled hypertension and multiple organ failure.

Ecological study: A type of study design in nutritional epidemiology. Ecological studies use observations of the trends in disease prevalence either over time or between different populations/geographical areas and attempt to relate these trends to variation in nutritional markers or other risk factors. Ecological studies are the weakest and least discerning approaches to studying diet–disease relationships and should always be followed up with more robust methods.

Ectopic pregnancy: An abnormal pregnancy in which the embryo implants outside the uterus.

Eicosanoids: Components of the inflammatory and immune responses that are synthesized from the long-chain fatty acids of the n-3 and n-6 series.

Embryogenesis: The process through which an embryo forms and develops through mitotic divisions.

Emetic: An agent that stimulates vomiting.

Endocrine disruptors: Chemical agents that have the capacity to interfere with normal hormone action, either by mimicking the action of particular hormones (e.g. oestrogen mimics) or antagonizing the action of hormones (e.g. anti-androgens).

Endometriosis: Condition in which the cells that normally line the uterus and slough off with each menstrual cycle, grow on the outside of the uterus. Endometriosis can be a cause of infertility and pelvic infections.

Endothelial dysfunction: Abnormal function of the cells that comprise the inner layer surrounding the lumen of arterial tissue. Altered function in terms of clotting, immune and inflammatory responses, production of nitric oxide and vasoconstriction or vasodilation to maintain normal blood pressure is a key step in the development of atherosclerosis and cardiovascular disease.

Enteral feeding: The provision of nutrients via a tube directly into the gastrointestinal tract. Enteral tube feeding can be directed to the stomach or, if necessary, to lower levels of the digestive tract.

Epigenetic regulation: The expression of genes can be modified by the environment to produce different phenotypes. Epigenetic gene regulation is the process through which patterns of gene expression can be modified through methylation of DNA or by altering chromosome packing rather than by differences in DNA sequence.

Epiphysis: The end portion of a long bone, for example the head of the femur.

Erectile dysfunction: Impotence. The inability for a man to develop or maintain an erection.

Erythropoiesis: The process through which the red blood cells are formed from stem cells in the bone marrow.

Escherichia coli: One of the bacterial species which contribute to the human intestinal microflora.

Essential amino acids: The amino acids required within the diet as they cannot be synthesized within the human body. Some amino acids are conditionally essential as the ability to synthesize enough to meet demand cannot be sustained in circumstances such as pregnancy.

Essential fatty acids: The fatty acids that cannot be synthesized within the human body and which are therefore required within the diet. The essential fatty acids are linoleic acid (n-6) and linolenic acid (n-3).

Estimated average requirement: One of the dietary reference value terms used in the UK. The estimated average requirement for a nutrient is the level of intake that should meet the requirements of 50% of individuals within a population.

Expressing milk: The process of drawing milk from the breast through manual stimulation of the let-down reflex. Many women express milk using specially designed breast pumps to leave breast milk for other individuals to feed to their infants via a cup, spoon or bottle and teat. Expressing milk may also be necessary to maintain lactation when mother or child are ill, or if the mother requires brief treatment with a drug that might be toxic to suckling infants.

Faddy eating: A common eating behaviour of young children, in which food is periodically refused or only a very narrow range of food items is habitually consumed.

Fast food: Food which is easily prepared and sold in quick service restaurants and snack bars as a meal or to be taken away.

Fatty acids: Organic acid molecules with long hydrocarbon tails. Fatty acids can be saturated or unsaturated (having double-bonded carbons within the hydrocarbon chain). The fatty acids are the basic building blocks of lipids within the body.

Fatty streak: The earliest stages of atherosclerosis are characterized by the appearance of deposits of macrophages bearing cholesterol and other fats in vesicles within the cytoplasm.

Foam cells: Foam cells are derived from macrophages within the intimal layer of arteries. Foam cells are the basic constituents of atherosclerotic plaques.

Follicle-stimulating hormone: A hormone of the anterior pituitary, which in both men and women regulates the production of sex steroids from the gonads. In women, it stimulates maturation of follicles. In men, it has a critical role in the production of spermatozoa.

Follicular phase: The early phase of the menstrual cycle in which the Graafian follicles mature in preparation for ovulation.

Food allergy: An adverse reaction to proteins in food. Allergies arise due to immune responses directed at allergenic proteins.

Food groups: Food groups are a means of classifying foods of similar types to simplify health promotion advice for the population. For example, within the UK Eatwell model, there are five food groups: fruits and vegetables; breads, cereals and potatoes; meat and alternatives; milk and dairy produce; foods containing fat and sugar.

Food intolerance: An adverse reaction to particular food items or components of food. Intolerance reactions are distinct from food allergies as there is no involvement of the immune system. Intolerances often arise due to a lack of digestive enzymes or secretions necessary to process particular items.

Food neophobia: A food behaviour often seen in children. Neophobia involves the rejection of foods that have not been previously encountered, often based purely on their appearance or aroma.

Food tables: Databases showing the macronutrient and micronutrient composition of foods.

Fortification: The process through which a nutrient is added to a staple foodstuff at the point of production to increase intakes of that nutrient within the whole population. In the UK, for example, margarines have been fortified with vitamin D to maintain intakes at similar levels to those associated with consumption of butter.

Fortifiers: Nutrient supplements that can be added to milk products used in infant nutrition. Fortifiers are mixed with human milk when feeding some premature infants to ensure that intakes of protein, micronutrients and energy are optimal.

Free radical: A free radical is any atom or molecule that has one or more unpaired electrons within its orbitals. The presence of unpaired electrons makes free radicals highly reactive, and they have the capacity to bond to or remove constituents from other molecules in their vicinity. In biological systems, this reactivity can be highly damaging to cells and is the basis of many major disease processes.

Functional food: A food developed to have ingredients that have health-promoting properties.

Galactosaemia: An inherited disorder in which sufferers lack the enzyme galactose-1-phosphate uridyl transferase, which prevents the normal metabolism of galactose. Unmanaged, this will lead to renal failure, enlarged liver and brain damage.

Gallstones: Solid, crystalline accretions of bile components that form within the gall bladder or bile duct. Also called choleliths.

Gastric parietal cells: Cells of the stomach epithelium which secrete intrinsic factor and hydrochloric acid.

Gastric reflux: Escape of acidic gastric secretions into the oesophagus. Also termed 'heartburn'.

Gastritis: Inflammation of the lining of the stomach.

Genomic imprinting: Process through which epigenetic marking of genes ensures that they are expressed in a specific manner. For example, certain genes in mammalian systems are expressed in a parent of origin-specific manner. This process allows paternally derived alleles that could be harmful to maternal health to be suppressed.

Genomic instability: Events associated with ageing and cancer. Genomic instability results in abnormalities in the chromosomal arrangement of DNA, often due to defects of DNA repair or high background levels of damage.

Glomerular filtration rate: The rate at which blood is filtered through the kidney.

Gluconeogenesis: The metabolic pathway leading to the generation of glucose from non-sugar substrates, including pyruvate, lactate, glycerol, and the glucogenic amino acids (e.g. glycine, serine, aspartate, glutamate).

Glucose homeostasis: Homeostasis is the regulation of metabolic and physiological systems to maintain a normal steady state function in response to environmental fluctuations. Glucose homeostasis describes the processes which maintain circulating and tissue glucose concentrations within optimal ranges.

Glucosinolates: Secondary products of plants of the Brassicaceae family. Glucosinolates are derivatives of glucose, with side chains containing sulphur and nitrogen.

Glutathione: A tripeptide synthesized from glycine, cysteine and glutamine. Glutathione is one of the most abundant compounds within the mammalian body and plays a key role in antioxidant defences and the metabolism of xenobiotics. The antioxidant capacity of glutathione is due to its role as a substrate for glutathione peroxidase.

Glycaemic control: A term used to describe the ability of patients with diabetes to maintain blood glucose concentrations within optimal ranges, either through dietary change or use of pharmacological agents.

Glycaemic index: A system used to rank foodstuffs in order of their ability to increase blood glucose concentrations following consumption. Foods with a high glycaemic index contain simple sugars that are rapidly absorbed and lead to a rapid peaking of blood glucose. Foods with a low glycaemic index contain complex carbohydrates which release glucose to the bloodstream more slowly.

Glycosylated haemoglobin: (HbA1c) A form of haemoglobin which is generated in the presence of excessive concentrations of blood glucose. Glucose binds to the haemoglobin and the glycosylated haemoglobin begins to accumulate on red blood cells. Measurement of HbA1c provides a good measure of the quality of habitual glycaemic control of diabetic individuals.

Gonadotrophin-releasing hormone: Peptide hormone released in a pulsatile manner by the hypothalamus. GnRH is the principal regulator of the reproductive axes in both males and females.

Growth hormone: A polypeptide hormone with largely anabolic functions. Growth hormone stimulates growth, increases muscle mass, promotes protein synthesis and hepatic glucose uptake and gluconeogenesis.

Haemochromatosis: An inherited disorder in which iron accumulates within organs, particularly the liver and pancreas.

Haemorrhoids: Blood-filled swellings around the anus, caused by dilation of varicose veins.

Hayflick limit: All differentiated cells have a limited capacity to divide. The number of divisions that can occur before cell death is termed the 'Hayflick limit'. In humans, the Hayflick limit is 52 divisions.

Height velocity: The rate at which height is increasing during growth, usually measured as centimetre gained per year.

Helicobacter pylori: A bacterial species that can colonize the human stomach and small intestine. *H. pylori* infection is associated with gastritis and peptic ulcers and is a major risk factor for stomach cancer.

Hepatic steatosis: Fatty liver.

Heterocyclic amines: Carcinogenic compounds that are generated during the cooking of meat.

High-density lipoprotein-cholesterol: One of the lipoprotein transporters that are required to carry cholesterol around the body. HDL transports cholesterol from peripheral tissues back to the liver for reutilization or excretion, and as such higher concentrations of HDL-cholesterol are associated with lower risk of atherosclerosis.

Hirsutism: Excessive growth of hair in women. Hirsutism generally occurs in response to increased production of androgens and is associated with growth of facial or chest hair, or increased growth of hair on the legs and arms.

Hyperemesis gravidarum: Intractable and excessive nausea and vomiting associated with pregnancy.

Hyperglycaemia: Circulating glucose concentrations that are above normal ranges. Blood glucose concentrations that are persistently over 126 mg/dl (7 mmol/l) are generally accepted as indicative of hyperglycaemia.

Hyperhomocysteinaemia: Elevated plasma homocysteine concentrations (in excess of 15 μmol/l). A risk factor for cardiovascular disease.

Hyperphagia: An abnormally increased appetite leading to habitually excessive consumption of food.

Hypertension: Raised blood pressure. In clinical settings hypertension is generally defined as a systolic pressure over 140 mmHg and diastolic pressure over 90 mmHg)

Hypertriglyceridaemia: Elevated plasma triglyceride concentrations (over 1.7 mmol/l).

Hypocalcaemia: Low circulating concentrations of calcium.

Hypospadias: A congenital defect of the penis in which the urethral opening is misplaced.

Hypothalamic–pituitary–adrenal axis: Hormonal cascade that regulates stress responses, the immune system, metabolism, appetite and sexual behaviour.

Hypothalamic–pituitary–gonadal axis: Hormonal cascade that regulates reproductive physiology. Elements of this axis also regulate skeletal development, body composition and immune functions.

Hypothalamus: A region of the brain seated above the pituitary gland. The hypothalamus is the central integrator of sensory input and responses to maintain homeostasis. The hypothalamus plays a critical role in the control of temperature, circadian cycles, thirst, appetite and reproductive functions.

Immunoglobulins: Immunoglobulins (Ig) are also known as antibodies. These globular proteins occur in several different classes (isotypes, IgG, IgA, IgM, IgE), all of which mediate specific functions within the immune system.

Inborn errors of metabolism: Genetic disorders in which a defect in the gene for an enzyme results in a failure of a metabolic pathway. This results in either accumulation of harmful metabolic intermediates, or a lack of substrates for further steps in the pathway and related pathways.

Incontinence: Involuntary leakage of urine or faeces.

Infertility: The inability of a man or woman to conceive a child. Infertility is clinically defined on the basis of failure to conceive within 12 months of attempting to do so. If a couple fail to conceive within one year of ending contraception, this is termed primary infertility. When a couple have previously had a pregnancy, but are unable to do so again, this is termed secondary infertility.

Inflammatory bowel disease: Chronic disease states involving inflammation of the small or large intestines. Crohn's disease generally impacts upon the ileum and parts of the large intestine, while ulcerative colitis affects the wall of the bowel within the colon and rectum.

Insulin resistance: The condition in which normal circulating concentrations of insulin are insufficient to allow normal responses to the hormone.

Intelligence quotient: IQ is a measure of performance in tests designed to assess intelligence. IQ tests are normalized against the typical performance of the population, with a score of 100 rated as average.

Intervention studies: Epidemiological studies in which the impact of limiting a potentially harmful exposure (e.g. reduction of red meat intake) or of increasing exposure to a potentially beneficial agent (e.g. increasing intake of dietary fibre) upon disease risk can be evaluated.

in vitro fertilization: The process through which eggs are fertilized to create embryos outside the body. in vitro fertilization is one of the techniques used in assisted reproduction.

Junk foods: Preprepared, foods which are high in sugar and fat, but which contain few micronutrients. Many nutritionists dislike the use of this term as it is a poor means of defining the composition of food and is only selectively applied to convenience foods. Also termed non-core foods.

Ketosis: The metabolic state in which the liver switches to the breakdown of fatty acids to ketones. This state is usually associated with the response to starvation, but can also be initiated by trauma and inflammation.

Kwashiorkor: A form of protein–energy malnutrition, characterized by oedematous swelling, fatty liver, bleaching of the hair and dermatitis. Classically defined as protein deficiency.

Lactation: The secretion of milk from the mammary glands.

Lactobacillus: One of the six main genera of bacteria which contribute to the human intestinal microflora.

Lactose intolerance: Condition in which a deficiency of lactase prevents the digestion of lactose. Consumption of dairy produce will lead to abdominal distension and diarrhoea.

Laxative: A pharmacological agent that loosens stools and induces defecation.

Let-down reflex: Hormonal response to stimulation of the nipples in breastfeeding women. Stimulation of mechanoreceptors leads to release of oxytocin (stimulates milk release) and prolactin (stimulates milk synthesis).

Leydig cells: Cells of the testis which synthesise testosterone.

Life expectancy: The average number of years a human is expected to live. This figure is conventionally calculated from the time of birth and is highly dependent on infant mortality rates in the region of birth.

Lignans: Polyphenolic compounds formed in plants. In the human diet lignans are generally consumed via seeds and certain vegetables (broccoli and other Brassicaceae). Lignans are one of the major classes of phytoestrogens.

Lipid hydroperoxides: Stable forms of oxidized lipids that are formed via the peroxidation cascade following free radical activity.

Lipolysis: The breakdown of fat stores to release free fatty acids to the circulation.

Lipoproteins: Complexes of lipids and proteins which are primarily involved in the transport of cholesterol and other fats. Lipoproteins may also be structural proteins, adhesion molecules and transmembrane receptors.

Low-density lipoprotein: LDL is one of the lipoprotein transporters that are required to carry cholesterol around the body. LDL transports cholesterol from the liver to peripheral tissues. LDL cholesterol is vulnerable to oxidation within the arterial endothelium, and this process is one of the prerequisite events for the development of atherosclerotic plaques.

Lower reference nutrient intake: One of the dietary reference value terms used in the UK. The LRNI for a nutrient is the level of intake that should meet the requirements of just 2.5% of individuals within a population.

Luteal phase: The phase of the menstrual cycle which follows ovulation.

Luteinizing hormone: A hormone of the anterior pituitary, which in both men and women regulates the production of sex steroids from the gonads. In women, it promotes ovulation. In men, it has a critical role in the production of testosterone.

Lymphocyte: A class of white blood cell, operative within the mammalian immune system. There are three major types of lymphocyte: T cells, B cells and natural killer cells.

Macrophages: Phagocytes of the immune system. Macrophages are derived from monocytes.

Macrosomia: A term used to describe a baby that is large for their gestational age.

Malnutrition: State in which an individual is chronically deprived of the macro- and micronutrients required to maintain normal physiological functions at an optimal level.

Mammary alveoli: The glandular tissues of the breast, which are the sites of milk synthesis.

Marasmus: A form of protein–energy malnutrition characterized by hunger, weight loss, muscle wasting and loss of adipose tissue reserves. Classically defined as energy deficiency.

Maturity onset diabetes of the young: Rare hereditary forms of type 2 diabetes, caused by mutations of transcription factors and enzymes involved in the normal response to insulin. There are at least six identified defects.

Menarche: The onset of reproductive cycling in females. The first menstrual bleeding.

Menopause: The end of reproductive cycling in females triggered by the cessation of ovarian function.

Meta-analysis: A statistical approach which overcomes problems of small sample size in epidemiological studies by combining the results of several studies that all address a related research hypothesis.

Metabolic syndrome: Cluster of metabolic disorders (hyperinsulinaemia, hypertriglyceridaemia), cardiovascular disorders (hypertension) and obesity, driven by insulin resistance. Metabolic syndrome is a major risk factor for cardiovascular disease.

Metastasis: The spread of cancerous cells from the initial site of tumour formation to other parts of the body.

Metformin: A drug used in the control of type 2 diabetes. Metformin increases insulin sensitivity and delays the uptake of glucose from the digestive tract.

Methyl-tetrahydrofolate reductase: Enzyme responsible for generation of 5-methyltetrahydrofolate from 5,10-methylenetetrahydrofolate. This is an essential step in the removal of potentially harmful homocysteine. Polymorphisms of the enzyme play an important role in establishing an individual's risk of cardiovascular disease and certain cancers.

Microalbuminuria: The leakage of albumin into the urine. This is indicative of kidney damage, which increases the permeability of the glomeruli.

Microbiome: The microbial community that coexists with host cells within the body. This community comprises bacterial, viral and fungal species. In humans, the colonic microflora represent one microbial community in the body, but the microbiome in saliva, vagina, bladder, lung, eyes and on the skin also play an important role in maintaining the health of tissues.

Micronutrient deficiency: The micronutrients are the vitamins, minerals and trace elements required by the body. Where the supply of these nutrients is insufficient to meet demands over a sustained period, deficiency may result. True deficiencies of micronutrients will be associated with clinically important disorders, each being characteristic of the nutrient concerned (e.g. ascorbate deficiency leads to scurvy, niacin deficiency leads to pellagra).

Miscarriage: The spontaneous loss of an embryo or fetus at a time before it is capable of survival.

Mitogen: An agent that stimulates cell division.

Monocytes: An immature form of phagocytic white blood cell. Monocytes have the capacity to differentiate into macrophages as they mature.

Monozygotic twins: Genetically identical twins derived from a single fertilized egg which subsequently splits into two.

Morbidity: The state of being diseased.

Morphogenesis: The process through which the cells of the embryo become organised into specialist structures and organs, and by which it develops a human shape and form.

Myocardial infarction: A heart attack. Occlusion of the coronary arteries due to formation of blood clots at atherosclerotic plaques starves the heart muscle of oxygen. This causes damage to the heart tissue (infarction) and can lead to death.

n-3 fatty acids: The family of fatty acids with the shared property of having a double-bonded carbon at the ω-3 position. α-linolenic acid is the essential precursor of the n-3 series.

n-6 fatty acids: The family of fatty acids with the shared property of having a double-bonded carbon at the ω-6 position. Linoleic acid is the essential precursor of the n-6 series.

Negative feedback: A term used in endocrinology to describe the process through which a hormone switches off the processes that lead to its own synthesis or release.

Neural tube defects: Birth defects in which the embryonic neural tube, which is destined to become the spinal cord and brain, fails to close over. This means that the effected individual will either have exposed nerves in the spinal cord (spina bifida) or will lack the bone covering for the cerebral tissues (anencephaly).

Non-starch polysaccharides: An alternative term used to describe dietary fibre.

Nutrient density: A term used to describe the ratio of the content of specific nutrients to energy within a foodstuff.

Nutritional analysis software: Software developed to provide simple access to food table based databases. An important tool in the analysis of food records and food frequency questionnaires.

Nutritional epidemiology: The study of how nutrients and nutrition-related factors influence patterns of disease within human populations.

Nutritional status: The state of a person's health in relation to the nutrients in their diet and subsequently within their body.

Obesity: A state of excessive body fat storage. Obesity can be diagnosed using a variety of anthropometric measures, such as body mass index, and is associated with increased risk of death due to cardiovascular disease and cancer.

Occult bleeding: Loss of blood in the faeces. Occult bleeding is a symptom of gastrointestinal diseases including colon cancer, inflammatory bowel disease, oesophagitis or gastritis.

Odds ratio: A measure of association between an exposure (e.g. diet) and an outcome (disease). The odds ratio represents the odds that an outcome will occur given a particular exposure, compared to the odds of the outcome occurring in the absence of that exposure.

Oedema: The swelling of organs or the extremities due to movement of water from intracellular to extracellular compartments. Oedema is often a response to inflammation, as seen in protein–energy malnutrition.

Oesophagitis: Inflammation of the oesophagus, generally resulting from gastric reflux or injury to the oesophagus during radiotherapy.

Oligorrhoea: Defective menstrual cycling in which the normal 28-day cycle is extended for periods of up to 90 days.

Oncogenes: A gene, or mutated gene, that encodes a protein which promotes cancer. Proto-oncogenes are genes that have the potential to become oncogenes if mutated. Anti-oncogenes are genes that encode proteins that block development and progression of cancer.

Oral glucose tolerance test: A test used to diagnose diabetes mellitus. Patients are given an oral load of glucose and blood sampled at baseline and at intervals up to three hours. Failure to restore baseline glucose concentrations within this time is indicative of diabetes and/or insulin resistance.

Organic produce: Foodstuffs (animal and plant) produced without the use of synthetic pesticides, fertilizers or feed additives.

Ossification: The process through which cartilaginous tissue becomes mineralised and transformed to bone tissue.

Osteoblast: A cell responsible for bone formation through the production of collagen and deposition of bone mineral.

Osteoclast: A cell responsible for the removal of bone tissue during skeletal repair or remodelling.

Osteopenia: Low bone density. In children, osteopenia may be caused by a failure to deposit minerals such as calcium. In adults, it may be a precursor of osteoporosis, caused by loss of calcium and other minerals from bone.

Osteoporosis: Condition of bone in which loss of bone mineral leads to increased risk of fracture.

Overnutrition: Condition in which the supply of nutrients (usually nutrient intakes) exceeds the physiological requirement for those nutrients. Overnutrition may be associated with adverse health consequences.

Ovulation: The process through which a mature Graafian follicle ruptures to release an ovum during the menstrual cycle.

Oxidative damage: The cellular and tissue damage that is caused by free radicals and other reactive oxygen species. All components of cells are vulnerable to such damage, which may include peroxidation of lipids, protein strand scission or DNA mutation.

Oxidative phosphorylation: The metabolic pathway found within mitochondria, through which energy substrates generate ATP through the donation of electrons to the electron transport chain.

Paget's disease of bone: A chronic disease of the skeleton in which the bones become enlarged and weaker, creating an increased risk of fracture.

Palatability: The acceptability of a food to the senses. Aroma, taste and texture all determine palatability.

Pancreatitis: Inflammation of the pancreas, often caused by other conditions of the gastrointestinal tract, such as gallstones.

Parenteral nutrition: A form of nutritional support in which simple nutrients are delivered to the body intravenously.

Periodontal disease: Inflammatory disease of the gum caused by infection with bacterial species. Severe periodontitis will result in loss of teeth and has been linked to systemic inflammation and infection.

Peripheral resistance: The resistance of the arterial system to the flow of blood. Resistance is one of the determinants of blood pressure.

Pernicious anaemia: A consequence of vitamin B12 deficiency arising from the loss of gastric parietal cells and hence intrinsic factor.

Personalized nutrition: An approach to providing nutritional advice which is based on assessment of genetic background and how this will determine the response to nutrients, and of measures of biomarkers of risk of disease.

Phenylketonuria: An inherited disorder in which individuals lack the enzyme phenylalanine hydroxylase. Accumulation of phenylalanine can lead to mental retardation, so the condition requires restriction of the intake of this amino acid.

Phospholipids: Lipids comprising a hydrophilic head group (e.g. phosphatidyl choline, phosphatidylserine) and hydrophobic fatty acid tails. Phospholipids are the principle components of biological membranes.

Phytoestrogens: Plant-derived molecules that can mimic the actions of oestrogens.

Pica: The consumption of non-nutritive substances such as clay or laundry starch.

Placental abruption: A complication of pregnancy in which the placenta breaks away from the uterine wall.

Plasticity: The ability of an organism adapt in response to changes in the environment.

Polycystic ovary syndrome: Disease of the ovaries characterized by the formation of cysts, leading to disruption of normal menstrual cycling and infertility.

Polymorphisms: Polymorphisms are multiple variables of a gene within a population. Individuals with variant alleles may be at greater, or lesser, risk of disease depending upon interactions with environmental or dietary factors.

Polyphenolics: Plant products comprising two or more phenol rings. The polyphenolics include the flavonoids, tannins and lignin. Many polyphenolics are antioxidants and may have other bioactivities within the human body.

Ponderal index: An alternative to body mass index that is sometimes applied to infants. Calculated as weight (kg)/ length (m^3).

Positive feedback: A term used in endocrinology to describe the means through which a hormone stimulates the processes that drive its own production.

Posterior pituitary: One of two lobes of the pituitary gland. This endocrine tissue responds directly to nerve signals from the hypothalamus and has two main products: vasopressin and oxytocin.

Postpartum haemorrhage: Excessive maternal bleeding after the delivery of the baby and placenta.

Prebiotics: Substances added to food to induce the multiplication of beneficial bacterial species in the colon.

Pre-eclampsia: A hypertensive disorder of pregnancy, characterized by elevated blood pressure and proteinuria.

Premature infant: A baby born before full-term gestation. Full term is 40 weeks and prematurity is generally defined as birth before 38 weeks.

Prevalence rates: A measure of the level of a disease within a population. The prevalence rate is usually expressed as the number of disease cases per 100 000 people in the population. Prevalence rates should not be confused with incidence rates, which are defined as the number of new cases arising within a population over a given period of time.

Programming: The process through which exposure of the developing fetus to an insult during a critical period of development, permanently alters the structure and function of tissues and organs.

Protein–energy malnutrition: Chronic undernutrition arising through insufficient intakes of protein and energy to meet metabolic and physiological demands. Protein–energy malnutrition is the most common form of clinically significant malnutrition and may arise due to inadequate food supply (as in developing countries) or high nutrient requirements associated with trauma.

Proteolysis: The degradation of proteins through the actions of proteases.

Proto-oncogenes: see Oncogenes

Pseudotumour cerebri: A medical condition characterized by persistent headache. It is often caused by increased blood and cerebrospinal fluid pressure within the brain.

Pubarche: The first appearance of pubic hair during sexual maturation.

Puberty: The process of physical change that marks the transition from childhood to sexual maturity.

Publication bias: A form of bias in research reports which arises from the tendency for researchers and journal editors to highlight study results that are positive rather than those that are inconclusive.

Public health nutrition: The application of the science of nutrition for the benefit of the population. Public health nutritionists are involved in investigation of the links between human nutrition and disease states, and the development of suitable disease prevention and health promotion strategies.

Pulmonary thromboembolism: Blockage of the pulmonary artery due to a clot from another site becoming dislodged and transferring to the lungs.

Quartile: Populations may be divided into equally sized groups based on key characteristics such as their nutrient intake, body mass index, height or weight. Where the division is into four groups, each group is termed as a quartile.

Quiescence: A resting state or state of dormancy.

Quintile: Populations may be divided into equally sized groups based upon key characteristics such as their nutrient intake, body mass index, height or weight. Where the division is into five groups, each group is termed as a quintile.

Reactive oxygen species: Collective term used to describe free radicals and other oxidizing species that are formed in biological systems through the use of oxygen in metabolic processes, such as respiration.

Reference nutrient intake: One of the dietary reference value terms used in the UK. The RNI for a nutrient is the level of intake that should meet the requirements of 97.5% of individuals within a population.

Relative risk: A measure of association between an exposure (e.g. diet) and an outcome (disease). Relative risk is calculated as the ratio of the probability of an event occurring (developing a disease) in an exposed group compared to the probability of the event occurring in a non-exposed group.

Resting metabolic rate: see Basal metabolic rate

Retinol activity equivalents: As vitamin A exists in different forms (retinol, α-carotene, β-carotene) and as each form difference in biological potency, retinol activity equivalents are used to define the standard units of vitamin A intake.

Rooting reflex: The innate ability of the human infant to locate and grasp the breast in preparation for suckling.

Safe intake: One of the dietary reference value terms used in the UK. Safe intake is applied to certain nutrients, for which there is insufficient evidence to define more detailed references. The safe intake would represent an intake expected to meet demands without posing a risk associated with excess.

Sarcopenia: Age-related degeneration of muscle mass and strength.

Satiety: The sensation of fullness leading to the loss of desire to eat.

Sedentary: Inactive.

Senescence: The process of ageing. Senescence refers to the biological processes that are associated with advanced age.

Sertoli cells: Cells of the testes which are responsible for supporting spermatozoa as they differentiate from immature forms.

Shoulder dystocia: A complication of pregnancy, in which the shoulders of the baby cannot pass through the birth canal following delivery of the head. This can be life-threatening and often results in fractures of the clavicle and injury to the nerves which supply the shoulders and arms.

Single-locus mutation: Mutation of a single gene leading to disease consequences.

Single nucleotide polymorphism: Many genes exist in variant forms (alleles) which differ by the substitution of a single base pair. For example, one allele could include the sequence TTCGAC, with a variant sequence TTTGAC. This difference is called a single nucleotide polymorphism, some of which have been identified as having links to human disease states.

Skinfold thickness: Body composition can be estimated using a skinfold test in which a pinch of skin is precisely measured using callipers at standardized points on the body. This determines the subcutaneous fat layer thickness, which can then be included in equations that converted the measurements to an estimated body fat percentage. Typically measured sites are the triceps, subscapular, suprailiac and abdominal regions.

Spina bifida: A defect of the formation of the embryonic neural tube, which results in a lesion of the spinal cord. Spina bifida is one of the most common human birth defects.

Statins: Class of drugs which lower circulating cholesterol concentrations by inhibiting the enzyme, 3-hydroxy-3-methyl-glutaryl-CoA reductase.

Steatorrhoea: Production of non-solid, often foul-smelling faeces. Often an indicator of malabsorption of fats.

Stillbirth: The delivery of a dead baby.

Stools: Faeces.

Stroke: Cerebrovascular accident. Strokes may be haemorrhagic, in which blood leaks from blood vessels in the brain causing damage to local tissue, or thrombotic. Thrombotic strokes are caused by atherosclerosis in vessels supplying the brain. Blockage of vessels by clots starves the brain of oxygen and cause tissue damage.

Stroke volume: The volume of blood that is ejected in a single contraction of the left ventricle. It is a key determinant of the cardiac output.

Strontium ranelate: A drug used in the treatment of osteoporosis. It acts by stimulating the activity of osteoblasts and inhibiting action of osteoclasts.

Stunting: Growth-faltering in which the full stature (height) of a growing child is not achieved.

Subconjunctival haemorrhage: Damage to the blood vessels in the eye.

Subcutaneous fat: The layer of fat which lies beneath the skin.

Supplementation: Supplementation of the diet with a nutrient involves the consumption of that nutrient in a purified and artificial form; for example, a multivitamin pill, or a soluble fibre drink. Supplements usually deliver nutrients in high doses, for example, the equivalent of the requirement for a full day in a single dose.

Systematic review: A research approach in which a literature review is written to focus solely on a single question. The systematic review attempts to synthesize together the findings of all high-quality research evidence in the area in an unbiased manner.

Systolic blood pressure: *see* Blood pressure

Telomere: A region of repetitive, non-coding DNA found at the end of a linear chromosome.

Teratogen: An agent that interferes with normal processes of development during embryonic or foetal life, and hence promotes congenital malformations.

Terpenoids: Plant compounds that provide the distinctive aromas found in cinnamon and ginger.

Tertile: Populations may be divided into equally sized groups based upon key characteristics such as their nutrient intake, body mass index, height or weight. Where the division is into three groups, each group is termed a tertile.

Testosterone: The principal androgenic hormone of mammals. Testosterone is a steroid hormone.

Thelarche: The first stage of breast development during puberty.

Thermogenesis: The process of endogenous heat production. Most thermogenesis is the product of metabolism within the liver, which maintains a constant body temperature. There are also components of thermogenesis that are activated by cold exposure (shivering and non-shivering thermogenesis) and by diet. Consumption of food generates heat associated with the digestion and metabolism of nutrients. Thermogenesis is an important component of total energy expenditure.

Thirst centre: Region of the hypothalamus which senses fluid balance and stimulates the desire to drink.

Total energy expenditure: The total energy used by an organism in a given period of time (usually measured over 24 hours). The components of total energy expenditure in an adult are the resting metabolic rate, thermogenesis and physical activity.

Trabecular bone: Bone of low density comprising a lattice-type structure through which bone marrow, nerves and blood vessels pass. Also called cancellous or spongy bone.

Trans-fatty acids: Unsaturated fatty acids with double bonds in the trans configuration as opposed to the cis arrangement of these isomers which is more usually seen in nature. Most trans-fatty acids in the human diet are the product of hydrogenation of vegetable oils to make them solidify.

Transformed cell: A cell which has become immortal (i.e. it has unlimited capacity to divide) through the mutation of a proto- or anti-oncogene.

Transit time: The time taken for components of food to pass from the mouth to the anus. This essentially measures the speed of digestion and elimination of waste products. Transit time can be measured through ingestion of a coloured marker such as carmine, which will appear in the stools.

Trauma: Physiological stress to the body. Trauma includes surgery, burns, infections, fractures and other injuries. All trauma events trigger a common metabolic response mediated by pro- and anti-inflammatory cytokines.

Trimester: A period of time relating to approximately one third of pregnancy.

Tuberculosis: An infectious disease caused by *Mycobacterium tuberculosis*, which affects the lungs and, if untreated, is fatal in approximately 50% of cases.

Tumour suppressor gene: A gene which encodes a protein product that inhibits cell division.

Ultra-processed food: Food made from extracted ingredients in other foods, largely added sugar, fats, hydrogenated fat and starch.

Uracil misincorporation: DNA and RNA differ in their profile of bases. While DNA contains thymine, in RNA this is replaced with uracil. The term 'uracil misincorporation' describes faulty DNA repair in which a lack of thymine results in uracil being included within DNA strands. As this cannot be transcribed, the affected genes are effectively mutated.

Vascular smooth muscle cells: Cells of the outer layers of arteries which provide the blood vessels with contractile properties.

Vegans: Individuals who follow an exclusively vegetarian diet, excluding all animal produce.

Vegetarians: Individuals who predominantly follow a diet that is of plant origin. There are different classes of vegetarian with varying dietary patterns. Vegans for example, exclude all animal produce, whilst lacto-ovo vegetarians will include eggs and milk in their diet but will not eat meat.

Visceral fat: The fat that is stored around the organs of the peritoneal cavity.

Vital capacity: A marker of lung function. Vital capacity is the maximum volume of air that can be exhaled after maximum inhalation.

Waist circumference: The measurement of the waist circumference provides a proxy measure for the amount of fat stored within the abdomen. Men of healthy weight should have a waist circumference of less than 94 cm, while in women it should be less than 80 cm.

Waist–hip ratio: The waist circumference divided by the circumference measured around the hips provides a proxy measurement for body fatness. The adverse health consequences associated with overweight and obesity correlate closely with a waist hip ratio greater than in 0.9 men and 0.80 in women.

Wasting: Loss of weight due to utilization of fat and muscle reserves. In children wasting will manifest as a failure to increase weight during the period of growth.

Weaning: See Complementary feeding.

Xenobiotic metabolism: Xenobiotics are exogenous chemicals such as drugs, toxins and pollutants, which may be harmful to the body. These agents are removed in two steps. In phase I metabolism, the cytochrome P450 adds hydroxyl groups to xenobiotics, facilitating their removal in phase II metabolism. Xenobiotics can be readily conjugated to sulphonates or glucuronic acid, to yield soluble products that are excreted via the urine.

Xeroderma pigmentosa: An inherited disorder of DNA repair in which sensitivity to ultraviolet damage leads to early onset skin cancers.

About the companion website

Don't forget to visit the companion web site for this book:

www.wiley.com/go/langleyevans/lifespan3e

There you will find valuable materials, including:

- About the self-assessment questions
- All Figures from the book

Scan this QR code to visit the companion website

CHAPTER 1

Introduction to lifespan nutrition

LEARNING OBJECTIVES

This chapter will enable the reader to:
- Describe what is meant by a lifespan approach to the study of nutrition and health
- Discuss the meaning of the term 'nutritional status' and describe how optimal nutrition requires a balance of nutrient supply and demand for nutrients in physiological and metabolic processes
- Show an awareness of the factors that contribute to undernutrition, including limited food supply and increased demands due to trauma or chronic illness
- Discuss global strategies for the prevention of malnutrition
- Understand that the biological response to food and nutrients is highly individual and is strongly dependent upon non-modifiable factors such as genetics, age and sex
- Discuss the potential for personalized nutrition to be used as the basis for population-wide dietary guidelines and interventions
- Understand the importance of a robust evidence base for nutritional science
- Describe how nutritional status is influenced by the stage of life due to the variation in specific factors controlling nutrient availability and requirements as individuals develop from the fetal stage through to adulthood
- Show an appreciation of how anthropometry, dietary assessment, measurements of biomarkers and clinical examination can be used to study nutritional status in individuals and populations
- Describe approaches used in nutritional epidemiology to explore relationships between diet and disease
- Understand and interpret the findings of epidemiological studies and appreciate the power of systematic review and meta-analysis as a research tool
- Discuss the need for dietary standards in making assessments of the quality of diet or dietary provision in individuals or populations
- Describe the variation in the basis and usage of dietary reference value systems in different countries

1.1 The lifespan approach to nutrition

The principal aim of this book is to explore relationships between nutrition and health and the contribution of nutrition-related factors to disease. In tackling this subject, there are many different approaches that could be taken; for example, considering diet and cardiovascular disease, nutrition and diabetes, obesity or immune function as separate and discrete entities, each worthy of their own chapter. The view of this author is that the late adult years are effectively the products of events that occur through the full lifespan of an individual. Ageing is a continual, lifelong process of change and development from the moment of conception to the point of death. It is therefore inappropriate to consider how diet relates to chronic diseases that affect adults without allowance for how the earlier life experiences have shaped physiology and metabolism.

The lifespan approach that is used to organize the material in this book essentially asserts three main points:

1 All stages of life from the moment of conception through to the elderly years are associated with a series of specific requirements for nutrition.
2 The consequences of less than optimal nutrition at each stage of life will vary according to the life stage affected.
3 The nature of nutrition-related factors at earlier stages of life will determine how individuals grow and develop. As a result, the relationship between diet and health in later stages of adult life, to some extent, depends upon events earlier in life. As a result, the nature of this relationship may be highly individual.

Although we tend to divide the lifespan into a series of distinct stages, such as infancy, adolescence, early adulthood, middle age and older adulthood, few of these divisions have any real biological significance, and they are therefore simply markers of particular periods within a continuum. There are, however, key events within these life stages, such as weaning, the achievement of puberty or the menopause, which are significant milestones that mark profound physiological and endocrine changes and have implications for the nature of the nutrition and health relationship. On a continual basis, at each stage of life, individuals experience a series of biological challenges, such as infection, a change in the diet or exposure to carcinogens that threaten to disturb normal physiology and compromise health. Within a lifespan approach, it is implicit that the response of the system to each challenge will influence how the body responds at later life stages. Variation in the quality and quantity of nutrition is one of the major challenges to the maintenance of optimal physiological function and is also one of the main determinants of how the body responds to other insults.

In considering the contribution of nutrition-related factors to health and disease across the lifespan, it is necessary to evaluate the full range of influences upon quality and quantity of nutrition and upon physiological processes. This book therefore takes a broad approach and includes consideration of social or cultural influences on nutrition and health, the metabolic and biochemical basis of the diet–disease relationships and the influence of genetics and, where necessary, provides overviews of the main physiological and cellular processes that operate at each life stage. While the arbitrary distinctions of childhood, adolescence and adulthood have been used to divide the chapters, it is hoped that the reader will consider this work as a whole. For those requiring a primer in nutrition before engaging with specific chapters, the Appendix to the book describes the nutrients in simple terms. In this opening chapter, we consider some of the basic terms and definitions used in nutrition and lay the foundations for understanding more complex material in the following chapters.

1.2 The concept of balance

Balance is a term frequently used in nutrition, and, unfortunately, the precise meaning of the term may differ according to the context and the individual using it. It is common to hear the phrase 'a balanced diet' and, indeed, most health education literature that goes out to the general public urges the consumption of a diet that is 'balanced'. In this context, we refer to a diet that provides neither too much nor too little of the nutrients and other components of food that are required for normal functioning of the body. A balanced diet may also be viewed as a diet providing foods of a varied nature, in proportions such that consumption of foods rich in some nutrients does not limit intakes of foods rich in others.

1.2.1 A supply and demand model

There is another way of viewing the meaning of balance or a balanced diet, whereby the relationship between nutrient intake and function is the main consideration. A diet that is in balance is one where the supply of nutrients is equal to the requirement of the body for those nutrients. Essentially, balance could be viewed as equivalent to an economic market, in which supply of goods or services needs to be sufficient to meet demands for those goods or services. Figure 1.1 summarizes the supply and demand model of nutritional balance.

Whether or not the diet is in balance will be a key determinant of the nutritional status of an individual. Nutritional status describes the state of a person's health in relation to the nutrients in their diet and subsequently within their body. Good nutritional status would generally be associated with a dietary pattern that supplies nutrients at a level sufficient to meet requirements, without excessive storage. Poor nutritional status would generally (though not always) be associated with intakes that are insufficient to meet requirements.

The supply and demand model provides a useful framework for thinking about the relationship between diet and health. As shown in Figure 1.1, maintaining balance with respect to any given nutrient requires the supply of the nutrient to be equivalent to the overall demand for that nutrient. Demand comprises any physiological or metabolic process that uses the nutrient and may include use as an energy-releasing substrate, as an enzyme cofactor, as a structural component of tissues, as a substrate for the synthesis of macromolecules, as a transport element or as a component of cell–cell signalling apparatus. The supply side of the balance model comprises any means through which nutrients are made available to meet demand. This goes beyond delivery through food intake and includes stores of the nutrient that can be mobilized within the body and quantities of the nutrient that might be synthesized de novo (e.g. vitamin D synthesized in the skin through the action of sunlight).

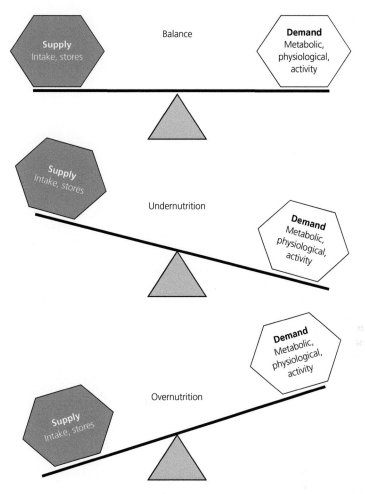

Figure 1.1 The concept of balance. The demands for nutrients comprise metabolic and physiological processes that use nutrients. Supply is determined by intakes of food, availability of nutrient stores and de novo production of nutrients.

1.2.2 Overnutrition

When supply does not match demand for a nutrient, the system is out of balance and this may have important consequences in terms of health and disease. Overnutrition (Figure 1.1) will generally arise because the supply of a nutrient is excessive relative to demand. This is either because intake of foods containing that nutrient increases, because the individual consumes supplements of that nutrient or because demand for that nutrient declines with no equivalent adjustment occurring within the diet. The latter scenario particularly applies to older adults, for whom energy requirements fall due to declining physical activity levels and resting metabolic rate (Folta *et al.*, 2015). Commonly, intakes of energy that were appropriate in earlier adulthood will be maintained, resulting in excessive energy intake.

The consequences of overnutrition are generally not widely considered in the context of health and disease unless the nutrient concerned is directly toxic or harmful when stored in high quantities. The obvious example here is, again, energy, where overnutrition will result in fat storage and obesity. For many nutrients, overnutrition within reasonable limits has no adverse effect, as the excess material will either be stored or excreted. At megadoses, however, most nutrients have some capacity to cause harm. Accidental consumption of iron supplements or iron overload associated with inherited disorders (haemochromatosis) is a cause of disease and death in children. At high doses, iron will impair oxidative phosphorylation and mitochondrial function, leading to cellular damage in the liver, heart, lungs and kidneys. Excess consumption of vitamin A has been linked to the development of birth defects in the unborn fetus (Ackermans *et al.*, 2011). Vitamin D intoxication, for example, can arise due to over-consumption of supplements (Conti *et al.*, 2014) and leads to the formation of kidney stones and neurological damage.

Overnutrition for one nutrient can also have effects upon nutritional status with respect to other nutrients and can impact on physiological processes involving a broader range of nutrients. For example, regular consumption of iron supplements can impact upon absorption of other metals such as zinc and copper by competing for gastrointestinal transporters and, hence, can promote undernutrition with respect to those trace elements. Having an excess of a particular nutrient within the body can also promote undernutrition with respect to another by increasing the demand associated with processing the excess. For example, a diet rich in the amino acid methionine will tend to increase circulating and tissue concentrations of homocysteine. The processing of this damaging intermediate increases the demand for B vitamins, folic acid, vitamin B6 and vitamin B12, which are all involved in pathways that convert homocysteine to less harmful forms (Lonn *et al.*, 2006; see Section 8.4.4.3.4).

1.2.3 Undernutrition

Undernutrition arises when the supply of the nutrient fails to meet demand. This can occur if intakes are poor or if demands are increased (Figure 1.1). In the short to medium term, low intakes are generally cushioned by the fact that the body has reserves of all nutrients that can be mobilized to meet demand. As such, for adults, it will usually require prolonged periods of low intake to have a significantly detrimental effect on nutritional status. Babies and infants lack such stores and are therefore more vulnerable to the impact of low intakes.

1.2.3.1 Increased demand

There are a number of situations that may arise to increase demand in such a way that undernutrition will arise if supply is not also increased accordingly. These include pregnancy, lactation and trauma. Trauma encompasses a wide range of physical insults to the body, including infection, bone fracture, burns, surgery and blood loss. Although diverse in nature, all these physiological insults lead to the same metabolic response. This acute phase response (Table 1.1) is largely orchestrated by the cytokines, including tumour necrosis factor alpha (TNF-α), interleukin-6 (IL-6) and interleukin-1 (IL-1; Grimble, 2001). Their net effect is to increase demand for protein and energy and yet paradoxically they have an anorectic effect. Thus, demand increases and supply will be impaired, together leading to protein–energy malnutrition. While in many developing countries, we associate protein–energy malnutrition with starvation in children, in developed countries such as the UK, protein–energy malnutrition is most commonly noted in surgical patients and patients recovering from major injuries (Wild *et al.*, 2010).

1.2.3.2 The metabolic response to trauma

The human body is able to adapt rates of metabolism and the nature of metabolic processes to ensure survival in response to adverse circumstances. The metabolic response to adverse challenges will depend upon the nature of the challenge. Starvation leads to increased metabolic efficiency, which allows reserves of fat and protein to be used at a controlled rate that prolongs survival time and hence maximizes the chances of the starved individual regaining access to food. In contrast, the physiological response to trauma generates a hypermetabolic state in which reserves of fat and protein are rapidly mobilized to fend off infection and promote tissue

Table 1.1 The acute phase inflammatory response to trauma or infection.

Acute phase response	Markers of the response
Metabolic change	Catabolism of protein, muscle wastage. Amino acids converted to glucose for energy or used to synthesize acute phase proteins. Catabolism of fat for energy
Fever	Body temperature rises to kill pathogens. Hypothalamic regulation of food intake disrupted, leading to loss of appetite
Hepatic protein synthesis	Acute phase proteins synthesized to combat infection (e.g. C-reactive protein, α1-proteinase inhibitor, caeruloplasmin). Liver reduces synthesis of other proteins, including transferrin and albumin
Sequestration of trace elements	Zinc and iron taken up by tissues to remove free elements that may be used by pathogens
Immune cell activation	B cells produce increased amounts of immunoglobulins. T cells release cytokines to orchestrate the inflammatory response
Cytokine production	Tumour necrosis factor-α and the interleukins 1, 2, 6, 8 and 10 work to produce a hypermetabolic state that favours production of substrates for immune function, but inhibits reproduction and spread of pathogens

repair (Table 1.1). Physiological stresses to the body, including infection, bone fracture, burns or other tissue injuries, elicit a common metabolic response regardless of their nature. Thus, a minor surgical procedure will produce the same pattern of metabolic response as a viral infection. It is the magnitude of the response that is variable, and this is largely determined by the severity of the trauma (Romijn, 2000).

The hypermetabolic response to trauma is driven by endocrine changes that promote the catabolism of protein and fat reserves. Following the initial physiological insult, there is an increase in circulating concentrations of the catecholamines, cortisol and glucagon. Increased cortisol and glucagon serve to stimulate rates of gluconeogenesis and hepatic glucose output, thereby maintaining high concentrations of plasma glucose. The breakdown of protein to amino acids provides gluconeogenic substrates and leads to greatly increased losses of nitrogen via the urine. Lipolysis is stimulated and circulating free fatty acid concentrations rise dramatically. These are used as energy substrates, together with glucose.

The response to trauma is essentially an inflammatory process and, as such, the same metabolic drives are noted in individuals suffering from long-term inflammatory diseases including cancer and inflammatory bowel disease (Richardson and Davidson, 2003). The inflammatory response serves two basic functions. First, it activates the immune system, raises body temperature and re-partitions micronutrients to create a hostile environment for invading pathogens (Table 1.1). Second, it allocates nutrients towards processes that will contribute to repair and healing.

The inflammatory response is orchestrated by the pro-inflammatory cytokines (e.g. TNF-α, IL-1 and -6) and the anti-inflammatory cytokines (e.g. IL-10). Whenever injury or infection occurs, the pro-inflammatory species are released by monocytes, macrophages and T helper cells. The level of cytokines produced is closely related to the severity of the trauma (Lenz *et al.*, 2007). The impact of pro-inflammatory cytokines is complex. On the one hand, they activate the immune system and protect the body from greater trauma. On the other, at the local level of any injury, they increase damage by stimulating the immune system to release damaging oxidants and other agents that indiscriminately destroy invading pathogens and the body's own cells. The production of pro-inflammatory cytokines therefore has to be counterbalanced, as an excessive response can lead to death (Grimble, 2001). This is the role of the anti-inflammatory cytokines and some of the acute phase response proteins, several of which inhibit the proteinases released during inflammation and therefore limit the breakdown of host tissues.

In addition to stimulating proteolysis and lipolysis within muscle and adipose tissue, the cytokines have a number of actions that impact upon nutritional status. First, they increase the basal metabolic rate. An element of creating a hostile environment for pathogens includes raising the core temperature of the body (fever). This greatly increases energy demands. The capacity to meet those demands through feeding is reduced, as cytokines also act upon the gut and the centres of the hypothalamus that regulate appetite, effectively switching off the desire to eat. As can be seen in Table 1.2, the increased metabolic rate associated with the response to trauma greatly increases the demands of the body for both energy and protein. In severe cases, requirements can be doubled, even though the critically ill patient will be immobilized and not expending energy through physical activity.

Table 1.2 The metabolic response to injury and infection increases requirements for energy and protein.

Nature and severity of trauma	Increase in energy requirement (x basal)	Increase in protein requirement (x basal)
Minor surgery or infection	1.1	1.0–1.5
Major surgery or moderate infection	1.3–1.4	1.5–2.3
Severe infection, multiple or head injuries	1.8	2.0–2.8
Burns:		
Up to 20% body surface area burned	1.5	—
20–40% body surface area burned	1.8	2.0–2.8*

* Dependent upon level of nitrogen losses in tissue exudates and age of patient. Children with burns have higher requirements.

Table 1.3 Causes of unintended weight loss.

Weight loss	Body composition change	Associated with
Anorexia (inadequate energy intake)	Mobilization of fat reserves precedes muscle wastage Infection Eating disorders	Food insecurity
Cachexia	Hypermetabolic response breaks down muscle and protein for energy	Cancer
Age-related sarcopenia	Muscle wastage associated with age-related metabolic changes	Aging AIDS Motor neuron disease Multiple sclerosis Crohn's disease Coeliac disease Advanced cystic fibrosis

This can pose major challenges for clinicians managing such cases, as the injured patient may be unable to feed normally and, due to the anorectic influences of pro-inflammatory cytokines, the capacity to ingest sufficient energy, protein and other nutrients is greatly reduced. Enteral or parenteral feeding is therefore a mainstay of managing major injuries.

With more severe trauma, the mobilization of reserves can produce marked changes in body composition. Muscle wasting may occur as the calcium-dependent calpains and ubiquitin–proteasome break down proteins rapidly to make amino acids available for gluconeogenesis and the synthesis of important antioxidants such as glutathione (Grimble, 2001). Body composition changes are beneficial to the injured patient as they primarily generate glucose. This is the optimal energy substrate for these circumstances, not least because it can be metabolized anaerobically to produce ATP in tissues where blood flow may be compromised and oxygen delivery impaired.

In the short term, the hypermetabolic response and the accompanying anorexia of illness are unlikely to impact significantly upon the nutritional status of an individual, although nutritional status prior to the onset of trauma would be an important consideration. For example, the nutritional consequences of a fractured hip in a young, fit adult male may be dramatically different to those in a frail elderly woman. Prolonged periods of disease accompanied by inflammatory responses that drive hypermetabolism will promote states of protein–energy malnutrition, such as kwashiorkor, or can produce the emaciated state of cachexia (Table 1.3). Nutritional support (i.e. supplemental feeding) of

chronically ill individuals or those who have suffered more acute trauma can limit the impact of the hypermetabolic response upon body composition and overall nutritional status. However, the catabolic metabolism cannot be reversed until the injury or illness is resolved, so the priority in these scenarios is limiting weight loss and loss of muscle mass, rather than achieving weight gain.

1.2.3.3 Compromised supply and deficiency

Clearly, there is a direct relationship between the supply of a nutrient to the body and the capacity of the body to carry out the physiological functions that depend upon the supply of that nutrient. As can be seen in Figure 1.2, the range of nutrient intakes over which optimal function is maintained is likely to be very broad, and there are a number of stages before functionality is lost. It is only when function can no longer be maintained that the term 'nutritional deficiency' can be accurately used.

A nutrient deficiency arises when the supply of a nutrient through food intake is compromised to the extent that clinical or metabolic symptoms appear. The simplest example to think of here relates to iron deficiency anaemia, in which low intakes of iron result in a failure to maintain effective concentrations of red blood cell haemoglobin, leading to compromised oxygen transport and hence the clinical symptoms of deficiency that include fatigue, irritability, dizziness, weakness and shortness of breath. Iron deficiency anaemia, like all deficiency disorders, reflects only the late stage of the process that begins with a failure of supply through intake to meet demands (Table 1.4). Once the body can no longer maintain function using nutrient supply directly from

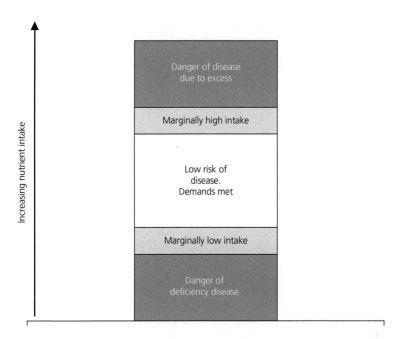

Figure 1.2 The association between nutrition and health. The requirements of the body for nutrients will be met by a broad range of intakes. Very low and very high intakes of any nutrient will be associated with ill health. The transition from intakes that are meeting demands and at which risk of disease is low to intakes that would be associated with disease is not abrupt.

Table 1.4 The three stages of iron deficiency.

Stage	Biochemical indicators and reference ranges
Normal iron status	Haemoglobin 14–18 g/dl (men) and 12–16 g/dl (women) Serum ferritin 40–280 µg/l Transferrin saturation 31–60%
Depleted iron stores	Falling serum ferritin Normal ranges for haemoglobin and transferrin saturation Ferritin 13–20 µg/l
Iron deficiency	Transferrin saturation falls as transport of iron declines Haemoglobin normal Serum ferritin <12 µg/l Transferrin saturation < 16%
Iron deficiency anaemia	Haemoglobin synthesis cannot be maintained and declines to <13.5 g/dl (men) and <12 g/dl (women) Serum ferritin <10 µg/l Transferrin saturation <15%

the diet, it will mobilize stores. In the case of iron, this will involve the release of iron bound to the protein ferritin to maintain haemoglobin concentrations. No change in function will occur at this stage, but the individual will now be in a state of greater vulnerability to deficiency. A further decline in supply through intake may not be matched through mobilization of stores, so full deficiency becomes more likely. This situation in which intakes are sufficiently low that, although there are no signs of deficiency, biochemical indicators show that nutrition is subnormal, is generally referred to as marginal nutrition or subclinical malnutrition.

1.2.3.4 Malnutrition

Malnutrition describes the state where the level of nutrient supply has declined to the point of deficiency and normal physiological functions can no longer be maintained. The manifestations of malnutrition will vary depending on the type of nutrient deficiencies involved and the stage of life of the malnourished individual. In adults, malnutrition is often observed as unintentional weight loss or as clinical signs of specific deficiency. In children, it is more likely to manifest as growth faltering, with the affected child being either underweight for their age (termed wasted) or of short stature for their age (termed stunted; see Section 6.2.2.1). Specific patterns of growth are indicative of different forms of protein–energy malnutrition. Wasting is associated with marasmus, where a weight less than 60% of standard for age is used as a cut-off. Oedema with a weight less than 80% of standard for age is indicative of kwashiorkor.

From a clinical perspective, protein–energy malnutrition is the most serious undernutrition-related syndrome. Marasmus and kwashiorkor are the classical definitions of this form of malnutrition. Historically, marasmus was considered to be a pure energy deficiency and kwashiorkor to be protein deficiency, but it is now clear that the two are different manifestations of the same nutritional problems. Marasmic wasting is a sign of a successful and effective physiological adaptation to long-term undernutrition. It is characterized by a depletion of fat reserves and muscle protein, together with adaptations to reduce energy expenditure. Children who become wasted in this way, if untreated, will generally die from infection as their immune functions cannot be maintained during the period of starvation. Kwashiorkor is a more rapid process, often triggered by infection alongside malnutrition. The metabolic changes with kwashiorkor are strikingly different to marasmus, as the adaptation to starvation is ineffective. Fat accumulates in the liver, and expansion of extracellular fluid volume, driven by low serum albumin concentrations, leads to oedema. Micronutrient deficiencies often occur alongside protein–energy malnutrition and may partly explain why individuals with kwashiorkor, unlike those with marasmus, are unable to adapt successfully to malnutrition.

The causes of malnutrition are complex and are not simply related to a limited food intake. Where intake is reduced, this is often due to food insecurity associated with famine, poverty, war or natural disasters. Reduced food intake can also arise due to chronic illness leading to loss of appetite or feeding difficulties. Malnutrition will also arise from malabsorption of nutrients from the digestive tract. This, again, could be a consequence of chronic disease or be driven by infection of the tract. Losses of nutrients are an important consequence of repeated diarrhoeal infections in areas where there is no access to clean water and adequate sanitation. Malnutrition may also be driven by situations that increase the demand for nutrients including trauma (as described earlier), pregnancy and lactation, if those increased demands cannot be matched by intake.

Malnutrition is most common and most deadly in the developing countries, where it is the major cause of death in children (Figure 1.3). Stunting is commonplace in some regions of the world, impacting on up to a third of children (Table 1.5). Stunting and wasting among malnourished children have long-term consequences too, as often the reduction in stature is not recovered, leading to reduced physical strength and capacity to work in adult life. As poverty is the most frequent cause of malnutrition, a self-perpetuating cycle can be established, as the stunted child becomes the adult with reduced earning capacity, whose children will live in poverty. Stunted, underweight women will also have children who are at risk due to lower weight at birth. Pregnancy is a time of high risk for malnutrition in women living in developing countries. Stunting is commonplace among women in South and Southeast Asia and is often accompanied by underweight. For example, in India and Bangladesh, up to 40% of women of childbearing age have a body mass index (BMI) of less than 18.5 kg/m^2 (Black et al., 2008). The prevalence of zinc deficiency among women is as high as 85% among women in rural Malawi (Lowe

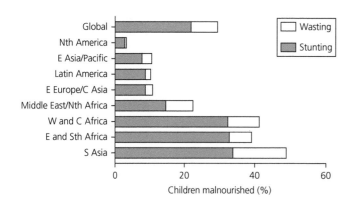

Figure 1.3 Prevalence of stunting and wasting in children under the age of five years. The global prevalence of stunting is 22%, with substantial variation between affluent and under-developed regions. The global prevalence of wasting is 7.8%. *Source:* data from Unicef (2019).

Table 1.5 Global mortality attributable to malnutrition in selected countries, grouped by high (> 10.5 per 100 000), moderate (0.5–10.5 per 100 000) and low (< 0.5 per 100 000) incidence.

Country	Deaths/100 000 population
High risk	
Somalia	33.03
Sierra Leone	30.12
Burkina Faso	30.03
Central African Republic	30.00
Mali	29.12
Angola	28.24
Burundi	27.27
Moderate risk	
Congo	9.11
Mozambique	8.97
Mexico	7.50
Namibia	7.23
Belize	7.06
Guyana	6.91
Peru	6.15
Low risk	
Slovakia	0.30
Israel	0.30
Romania	0.30
Canada	0.30
Portugal	0.28
Jordan	0.27
United Kingdom	0.08

Globally, malnutrition is responsible for 45% of all deaths among children under the age of 5 years. *Source:* data from World Health Organization (2017).

et al., 2020). Iron deficiency anaemia is endemic among pregnant women in developing countries, with prevalence of 60–87% in the countries of southern Asia (Seshadri, 2001). Maternal and childhood malnutrition are believed to cause 3.1 million deaths among the under fives every year (Black *et al.*, 2013).

Developed countries also have a burden of malnutrition among vulnerable groups. At greatest risk are older adults, who may develop protein–energy malnutrition or micronutrient deficiencies due to specific medical conditions or through low intakes associated with frailty or loneliness (see Section 9.5.1). Surgical patients are at risk of protein–energy malnutrition as a result of the inflammatory response to trauma. As in the developing countries, poverty increases the risk of malnutrition among children and immigrant groups. There are many ways of targeting these at-risk groups, for example, monitoring the growth of infants or including regular weighing and nutritional assessments of hospital patients.

Malnutrition is easily treated through appropriate nutritional support.

The prevention of malnutrition is a major public health priority on a global scale. While a lack of food security and the risk of protein–energy malnutrition remain a major issue for many populations, there have been a number of success stories in the battle to prevent clinically significant malnutrition. The basic approaches that can be used to prevent nutrient deficiency are diet diversification, supplementation of at-risk individuals and fortification (Table 1.6). All three approaches have, for example, been used to address the global problem of vitamin A deficiency. Vitamin A deficiency is one of the most common forms of malnutrition on a global scale (West, 2003), with greatest prevalence in Africa, Central and South America, and South and Southeast Asia. Subclinical vitamin A deficiency affects up to 200 million children every year and is a causal factor in up to half a million cases of childhood blindness and up to a million deaths of children under the age of five years. Vitamin A deficiency is also responsible for stunted growth in children and may cause blindness in women because of increased demands for vitamin A during pregnancy or lactation. In countries where rice is a staple crop, biofortification has had some success (Mayer, 2007; see Research Highlight 1.1), while in other countries diet diversification through promoting home gardening (Faber *et al.*, 2002), or including vitamin A-rich red palm oil in cooking (Zagré *et al.*, 2003) has been effective in improving population vitamin A status. The World Health Organization (WHO) promotes a vitamin A supplementation programme which provides high-dose supplements for children aged 6–59 months.

Iodine deficiency is an important issue for populations in all continents. Availability of iodine is essentially limited by the iodine content of the soil and hence its uptake by plants and animals. Iodine deficiency disorders, including cretinism and goitre, are a major manifestation of malnutrition, with approximately 740 million affected individuals worldwide. Fortification has been the cornerstone of the fight against iodine deficiency, with the universal salt iodization programme providing iodized salt (20–40 mg iodine/kg salt) to 70% of households in affected areas. These areas include countries from both developing (e.g. Pakistan) and developed (e.g. Australia) countries. Where the iodized salt is consumed, marked improvements in iodine status of the population are rapidly noted (Sebotsa *et al.*, 2005; Kapil *et al.*, 2007). There are still significant numbers of individuals at

Table 1.6 Strategies for the prevention of micronutrient deficiency.

Approach	Definition	Advantages	Disadvantages	Examples of application
Dietary diversification	Use of health education programmes and promotion of consumption of a greater range of foodstuffs to the diet. May include home gardening projects or rearing livestock.	Encourages changes in behaviour of population, which are long-term. Sustainable solution. Can tackle multiple micronutrient deficiencies.	Depends on population having secure access to land for cropping. Requires an element of knowledge for successful use. Requires resource to purchase animals or alternative seed stocks.	Encouraging greater use of cereal or nut crops to accompany green leafy vegetables and fruit increases intakes of zinc, protein, iron, thiamine and folate. Introducing poultry for meat and eggs increases intake of protein and all micronutrients.
Supplementation	Provision of micronutrients in an artificial form to provide a daily or regular dose to at-risk populations.	Ensures that at-risk populations receive specific micronutrient in a highly bioavailable form, at a dose which is safe and meets requirements.	Expensive. Challenging to deliver supplements in hard to reach regions. Population may choose not to take supplement.	World Health Organization vitamin A supplementation programme. Folic acid supplementation of women planning a pregnancy.
Fortification	The addition of nutrients to staple foods at the point of their production, thereby increasing the amount of nutrient delivered to all consumers of that foodstuff.	Everyone in population who consumes staple food will receive adequate supply of nutrient. Inexpensive as carried out at point of production.	Some in population could overconsume the nutrient. Possibility of harmful effects among some in the population. Poor populations may not consume the commercially available fortified foods. Removal of consumer choice.	Universal salt iodization programme. Fortification of wheat-based flours by 50 countries to prevent neural tube defects.
Biofortification	Improvement of plant nutrient content to increase micronutrient density available to human consumers. May be done through selective plant breeding, genetic modification or by enriching soil micronutrient content using fertilizers.	Costs are low if approach is to provide alternative seed stocks. New varieties are likely to have other desirable traits such as pest or drought resistance. Sustainable solution.	Loss of biodiversity when genetically modified crops are released. Cultural suspicion and preferences may limit use of the new crops. Poor rural populations may not be able to afford new crop varieties.	Golden rice genetically engineered to produce beta-carotene. Adding selenium and zinc to soil to increase mineral content of maize.

Research Highlight 1.1 Biofortification as a strategy to combat mineral deficiency.

Micronutrient deficiencies are endemic to large parts of the world and are often referred to as 'hidden hunger'. Some deficiency is driven by food insecurity, but for many minerals the issue stems from geographical features, including the leaching of minerals out of highland regions by rainfall or variations in the geological composition of the region, which determines soil mineral content. Where soil mineral content is low, plants will take up less from the soil, therefore reducing supply to the population (Joy *et al.*, 2015). In countries such as Malawi or Pakistan, soil types have a strong influence on the prevalence and distribution of mineral deficiency in rural populations which rely on locally grown crops as opposed to commercially source foods (Hurst *et al.*, 2013; Lowe *et al.*, 2020).

Biofortification is the process through which the micronutrient content of crops can be enhanced as a strategy to tackle hidden hunger. Traditional plant breeding is one way of doing this. It involves the selection and crossing of varieties to produce hybrids which have desirable traits, such as better uptake of minerals from the soil or reduced content of phytates and other agents which will inhibit mineral uptake in the human gut. Traditional breeding is slow and it can take up to a decade to develop, characterize and distribute new crop varieties. The approach is effective though, and Hambidge *et al.* (2004) reported on a small trial showing improved bioavailability of zinc from flour made from plants selected for lower phytate. The BiZiFED trial is evaluating the effectiveness of a high zinc wheat variety in improving zinc status in a Pakistani population (Ohly *et al.*, 2019). Transgenic crops, which either take up more mineral from the soil or which contain fewer inhibitors of absorption from the human gut, can be developed much faster, making biofortification more effective. Crops such as rice, maize and wheat have been engineered for this purpose (Hefferon, 2015; Kumar *et al.*, 2019). However, there are environmental and ethical concerns and consumer acceptance is poor.

An alternative is agrofortification, in which minerals are added to fertilizers that are added to the soil or crop foliage, or encapsulated with the seed. The latter approach (nanofortification) is attractive as is reduces waste and environmental contamination. Zinc-fortified seed varieties of wheat have been released in China, India, Pakistan and Bolivia, and rice varieties in China and Bangladesh (Lowe *et al.*, 2020). Soil fortification with selenium has been identified as an optimal solution to combat selenium deficiency in Malawi. Maize is the staple crop, providing up to 60% of dietary energy for rural populations, so the AHHA trial will use a randomized controlled trial (RCT) design to evaluate whether consuming flour made from maize grown on selenium fortified soil improves selenium status in the population (Joy *et al.*, 2019). The protocol has been inspired by the experience of Finland, which brought in mandatory fortification of crop fertilizers in 1984. Over the ensuing 26 years, the selenium concentration of cereals increased 15-fold and mean plasma selenium concentration of Finnish adults increased from 70.1 µg/l to 110 µg/l (Alfthan *et al.*, 2015).

risk of iodine deficiency disorders, due to lack of full coverage of the universal salt iodization programme and regional variation within countries. For example in India, 78% of households are covered by the programme, but consumption of the fortified salt is lower in rural than in urban populations and some regions in the south of the country have much lower coverage (62%; Pandav *et al.*, 2018). It also seems likely that universal salt iodization does not provide sufficient iodine to meet the requirements of pregnant women. While it does not provide the universal coverage that the name suggests, this fortification approach is widely considered to be a public health nutrition success for the WHO.

1.2.4 Classical balance studies

Nutritional status with respect to a specific nutrient can be measured using balance studies. These studies have classically been used to determine requirements for some nutrients in humans. Essentially, the balance method involves the accurate measurement of nutrient intake for comparison with accurate measures of all possible outputs of that nutrient via the urine, faeces and other potential routes of loss (Figure 1.4). If there is a state of balance (i.e.

intake and output are at equilibrium), it can be assumed that the body is saturated with respect to that nutrient and has no need for either uptake or storage. This technique can be applied to almost any nutrient and, by repeating balance measures at different levels of intake, it is possible to determine estimates of requirements for specific nutrients. The balance model works on the assumption that in healthy individuals of stable weight, the body pool of a nutrient will remain constant. Day-to-day variation in intake can be compensated by equivalent variation in excretion. The highest level of intake at which balance can no longer be maintained will indicate the actual requirement of an individual for that nutrient.

Nitrogen balance studies were used to determine human requirements for protein (Millward *et al.*, 1997). Such studies involved experiments in which healthy subjects were recruited and allocated to consume dietary protein at specified levels of intake. After four to six days of habituation to these diets, urine and faeces were collected for determination of nitrogen losses over periods of two to three days. On this basis, it was possible to state dietary protein requirements for different stages of life as being the lowest level of protein intake that maintained

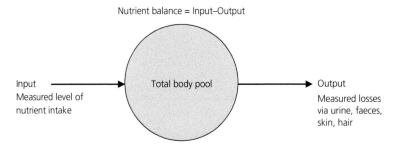

Nutrient balance = Input–Output

Input
Measured level of
nutrient intake

Total body pool

Output
Measured losses
via urine, faeces,
skin, hair

Balance = 0 indicates that there is no net storage or loss of
nutrient

Positive balance indicates that there is net deposition of
nutrient to the body pool

Negative balance indicates that there is net loss of nutrient

Figure 1.4 Determining nutrient requirements using the balance method. Precise measurements of nutrient intake and of output by all possible routes enable determination of nutrient requirements. The highest level of intake at which balance can no longer be maintained will indicate the actual requirement of an individual for that nutrient.

nitrogen balance in healthy individuals, maintaining body weight and engaging in modest levels of physical activity. Nitrogen balance studies are problematic in several respects, including the fact that 24-hour urine collections used in such studies are often incomplete, because studies may fail to allow sufficient time for subjects to habituate to their experimental diet and because factors such as unobserved infection, stress or exercise may increase demand for protein. It has also been impossible to use balance studies to examine protein requirements for all age groups and in all health situations, so requirements for pregnant and lactating women and for children are based on balance studies in young adults and make estimates of allowances for tissue deposition, growth and milk synthesis and secretion.

1.2.5 Overall nutritional status
The diet delivers a multitude of components rather than single nutrients, and it is unlikely that any individual will have a diet that perfectly achieves balance for all of them. For example, an individual can be in balance for protein while consuming more energy than is required and insufficient iron to meet demand. Hence, it is often not appropriate to discuss overall nutritional status of an individual without consideration of nutritional status with respect to specific nutrients.

Whether considering the overall nutritional status of an individual, examining nutritional status with respect to a specific nutrient or investigating the nutritional status of a population, it is important to take into account a broad range of factors. It should be clear from the previous discussions that

intake is just one component of the supply side of the balance model. Nutritional status is only partly determined by the food that is being consumed. It also depends upon the activities and health status of the individuals concerned.

Trauma and high levels of physical activity will increase demand, while a sedentary lifestyle will decrease demand. Most important, though, is the stage of life of the individuals under consideration. Physiological demands for nutrients vary to a wide degree, depending on age, body size and sex. The impact of variation within the diet upon health and wellbeing is largely, therefore, governed by age and sex.

1.3 The individual response to nutrition

The ingestion of food and nutrients is the beginning of a chain of events involving digestion and absorption, metabolic processing and physiological responses. For example, consumption of carbohydrate brings about an increase in blood glucose concentrations followed by insulin secretion and the uptake of glucose into cells and tissues for use in energy metabolism, which will drive muscle contraction, thermogenesis and a host of other processes. Ingestion of sodium will result in haemodynamic changes that impact upon blood pressure and kidney function. The nature of the metabolic and physiological changes that occur following ingestion means that the response to nutrients plays a fundamental role in determining health and disease. All individuals have unique characteristics that shape the nature of the response to nutrition. This poses a problem in establishing guidelines for healthy nutrition, as the desire is to provide general guidance on a 'one size fits all' basis, but the reality is that some guidance will be inappropriate for a significant proportion of any population. Many factors will contribute to the individual response to nutrition (Figure 1.5), but genetic background and lifespan-related factors are of major significance.

1.3.1 Stage of the lifespan
Nutritional status is determined by the balance between the supply of nutrients and the demand for those nutrients in physiological and metabolic processes. So far in this chapter, we have seen that both sides of the supply–demand balance equation can be perturbed by a variety of different factors. Intake, for example, can be reduced in circumstances of poverty, while demand is elevated by physiological trauma. The main determinants of demand are, however, shaped by other factors such as the level of habitual physical activity (which will increase energy requirements), by sex, by body size and by age. It is this last factor that provides the focus of this book.

The demand for nutrients to sustain function begins from the moment of conception. The embryonic and fetal stages of life are the least understood in terms of the precise requirements for nutrition, but it is clear that they are the life stages that are most vulnerable in the face of any imbalance. Demands for nutrients are high to sustain the rapid

growth and the process of development from a single-celled zygote to a fully formed human infant. An optimal balance of nutrients is essential, but the nature of what is truly optimal is difficult to dissect out from the competing demands of the maternal system and the capacity of the maternal system to deliver nutrients to the fetus. The embryo and fetus represent a unique life stage from a nutritional perspective, as there are no nutrient reserves and there is a total dependence on delivery of nutrients, initially by the yolk sac and later by the placenta. The consequences of undernutrition at this stage can be catastrophic, leading to miscarriage, failure of growth, premature birth, low weight at birth or birth defects (MRC Vitamin Study Group, 1991; Godfrey *et al.*, 1996; El-Bastawissi *et al.*, 2007). All of these are immediate threats to survival, but it is also becoming clear that less than optimal nutrition at this stage of life may increase risk of disease later on in life (Langley-Evans, 2015).

After birth, the newborn infant has incredibly high nutrient demands which, in proportion to body weight, may be two to three times greater than those of an adult. These demands are again related to growth and the maturation of organ systems as in fetal life. Growth rates in the first year of life are more rapid than at any other time, and the maturation of organs such as the brain and lung continues for the first three to eight years of life. Initially, the demands for nutrients are met by a single food source, milk, with reserves accrued from the mother towards the end of fetal life compensating for any shortfall in supply of

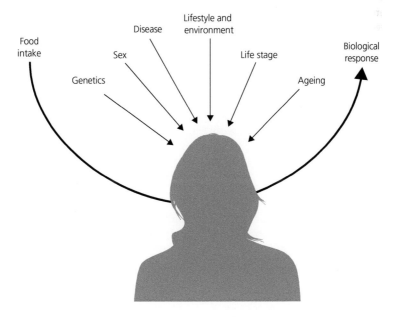

Figure 1.5 The individual response to food is complex and is determined by a range of modifiable and non-modifiable factors.

micronutrients. In later infancy, there is the challenge of the transition to a mixed diet of solids (weaning), which is a key stage of physiological and metabolic development. The consequences of imbalances in nutrition can be severe. Infants are very vulnerable to protein–energy malnutrition and to micronutrient deficiencies, which will contribute to stunting of growth and other disorders. Iodine deficiency disorders and iron deficiency anaemia can both impact upon brain development, producing irreversible impairment of the capacity to learn. Obesity is now recognized as a major threat to the health of children in the developed countries. In this age group, it is not simply a product of excessive energy intake and low energy expenditure. Increasingly, we are seeing that the type or form of foods consumed at this time can influence long-term weight gain, with breastfed infants showing a lower propensity for obesity than those who are fed artificial formula milks (Patro-Golab *et al.*, 2016). The nature of foods used at weaning is also important, and infants weaned on to high-protein foods at an early stage are also more likely to develop obesity (Pearce and Langley-Evans, 2013).

Beyond infancy, nutrient demands begin to fall relative to body weight but remain higher than those seen in adulthood through the requirement for growth and maturation. These demands are at their greatest at the time of puberty, when the adolescent growth spurt produces a dramatic increase in height and weight accompanied by a realignment of body composition. Proportions of body fat decline and patterns of fat deposition are altered in response to the metabolic influences of the sex hormones. Proportions of muscle increase and the skeleton increases in size and degree of mineralization. Nutrient supply must be of high quality to drive these processes, and in absolute terms (i.e. not considered in proportion to body size), the nutrient requirements of adolescence are the greatest of any life stage. However, adolescents normally have extensive nutrient stores and are therefore more tolerant of periods of undernutrition than preschool children (one to five years).

The adult years have the lowest nutrient demands of any stage of life. As growth is complete, nutrients are required solely for the maintenance of physiological functions. The supply is well buffered through stores that protect those functions against adverse effects of undernutrition in the short to medium term. In developed countries, and increasingly so in developing countries, the main nutritional threat is overweight and obesity, as it is difficult for adults to adjust energy intakes against declining physiological requirements and the usual fall in levels of physical activity that accompany ageing. Reducing energy intake while maintaining adequate intakes of micronutrients is a major challenge in older individuals. Chronic illnesses associated with ageing can promote undernutrition through increased nutrient demands, while limiting appetite and nutrient bioavailability.

For women, pregnancy and lactation represent special circumstances that may punctuate the adult years and increase demands for energy and nutrients. Nutrition is in itself an important determinant of fertility and the ability to reproduce (Hassan and Killick, 2004). In pregnancy, provision of nutrients must be increased for the growth and development of the fetus and to drive the deposition of maternal tissues. For example, there are requirements for an increase in size of the uterus, for the preparation of the breasts for lactation and for the formation of the placenta. To some extent, the mobilization of stores and adaptations that increase absorption of nutrients from the gut serve to meet these increased demands but, as described earlier, imbalances in nutrition may adversely impact the outcome of pregnancy. Lactation is incredibly demanding in terms of the energy, protein and micronutrient provision to the infant via the milk. As with pregnancy, not all the increase in supply for this process depends upon increased maternal intakes, and in fact, women can successfully maintain lactation even with subclinical malnutrition. Adaptations that support and maintain breastfeeding may impact upon maternal health. For example, calcium requirements for lactation may be met by mobilization of bone mineral and, if not replaced once lactation has ceased, could influence later bone health. However, although nutritionally challenging, most evidence suggests that lactation is of benefit for maternal health. A number of reports indicate that maintaining breastfeeding for more than one year can significantly lower risk of breast and ovarian cancers and type 2 diabetes (Chowdury *et al.*, 2015).

Lifespan factors clearly impact upon nutritional status, as they are a key determinant of both nutrient requirements and the processes that determine nutrient supply. In studying relationships between diet, health and disease, one of the major challenges is to assess the quality of nutrition in individuals and at the population level. Tools used for these nutritional assessments are described in the next section.

1.3.2 Genetics

Long-term disease states such as obesity, cancer or coronary heart disease are the products of a number of risk factors, working together, against a battery of protective factors. Disease is promoted by a poor diet, smoking, sedentary lifestyle and accumulated experiences across the lifespan. These factors all overlie the genetic background of the individual to determine how the body responds to nutrition and other environmental factors. The genotype of each individual comprises a complex set of traits that might be disease promoting (susceptibility genes) or disease suppressing (protective genes). For most disease states, more than one gene will be driving the components of risk.

Owing to the complexity of the genetic determinants of physiological function, individuals will respond to nutritional signals in different ways. For example, some individuals will have a genetic make-up that promotes high energy expenditure. This enables them to maintain a healthy weight at a level of energy intake that is sufficient to promote obesity in other individuals, who may instead carry obesity-promoting genes.

Some of the risk of chronic disease is determined by single nucleotide polymorphisms (SNPs, (pronounced 'snips'), which are variants in the sequences of genes that control specific aspects of physiological and metabolic function (Joost et al., 2007). SNPs are inherited sequences which differ from the most common sequence of a gene by just one base (e.g. a C replaced by a T; Figure 1.6).

Such a change may generate a protein product of altered tertiary structure and impact significantly upon physiological function. SNPs are now well characterized as having interactions with components of the diet, and some detailed examples are discussed in later chapters.

The C677T SNP in methylene tetrahydrofolate reductase (MTHFR) is one of the best studied examples of a genetic variant that impacts upon the variability of the individual response to diet. MTHFR is an enzyme that plays an important role in the metabolism of folates and effectively controls the availability of one-carbon donors in intermediary metabolism. Within the population, there will be three distinct populations based upon variants of C677T, namely, individuals carrying CC, CT or TT genotypes. For those carrying TT, circulating concentrations of the amino acid homocysteine will tend to be higher as activity of the enzyme is lower than with the CC variant (Figure 1.7). Hyperhomocysteinaemia is a known risk factor for cardiovascular disease, unless the diet delivers sufficient folate to offset this risk.

The contribution of a SNP to risk of disease should not be overestimated. Often, the influence of SNPs is miniscule compared with the impact of lifestyle factors. For example, a variant of the calpain-10 gene is associated with a 20% increase in risk of type 2 diabetes, which is dwarfed by the 4- to

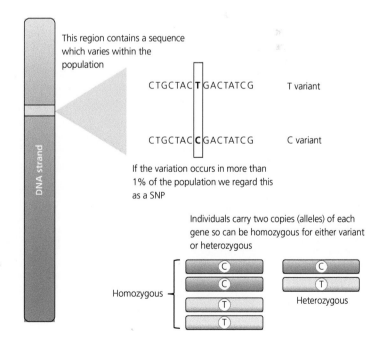

Figure 1.6 Single nucleotide polymorphisms arise when there are single base changes in the DNA sequence of a gene. As all individuals carry two copies of a gene, the polymorphism can result in individuals being homozygous or heterozygous for specific gene variants.

This region contains a sequence which varies within the population

CTGCTAC**T**GACTATCG   T variant

CTGCTAC**C**GACTATCG   C variant

If the variation occurs in more than 1% of the population we regard this as a SNP

Individuals carry two copies (alleles) of each gene so can be homozygous for either variant or heterozygous

DNA strand

Homozygous

C
C
T
T

C
T

Heterozygous

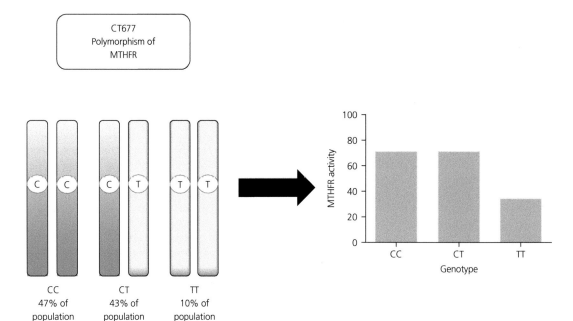

Figure 1.7 The CT677 SNP of methylenetetrahydrofolate reductase (MTHFR) influences the activity of the enzyme in tissues. This common variant of the gene can have significant impact on folate metabolism.

Research Highlight 1.2   Folate, polymorphisms of MTHFR and breast cancer.

Cancer is a cluster of separate diseases that share the feature of uncontrolled cell division following mutation of genes which regulate the normal processes of cell division and cell death. Diet impacts on cancer risk either by introducing compounds which cause mutation or by introducing agents which prevent mutation, allow abnormal cells to be eliminated or limit the speed of tumour growth. Folates are recognized as having a complex role in cancer as on the one hand they protect cells from tumour initiation, but on the other they promote the growth of established tumours.

There are key enzymes in folate metabolism which determine the availability of cellular folates. These are known to have SNPs that are related to the risk of breast cancer in women. Methyl tetrahydrofolate reductase (MTHFR) has three well-characterized SNPs: 677CT, 1298AC and 2756AG. Methionine reductase also has a common polymorphism (MTR2755AG). Generally speaking, the rarer forms of all of these polymorphisms result in lower enzyme activity and lower availability of folates to the cell.

Breast cancer is the most common cancer of women and is known to be associated with dietary factors, most notably obesity. Kakkoura *et al.* (2015) studied the three polymorphisms of MTHFR in a case–control study of breast cancer. This study reported on the adherence of the subjects to a healthy Mediterranean diet pattern. None of the polymorphisms were related to cancer risk until the diet pattern was taken into account. Interestingly, 677TT, 1298CC and 2756AA were all associated with lower breast cancer risk in women with high adherence to the healthier dietary pattern. This was in contrast to the report of Ericson *et al.* (2009), who found that risk was 1.86-fold higher in women with 677TT who had the highest intakes of folate, when compared with low folate consumers. Similarly Ma *et al.* (2009) reported that breast cancer risk was greater with high folate intake in women with 677TT or 677CT. Folate had no relation to cancer risk in women who were 677CC. Higher risk was also associated with high folate consumption in women with MTR2755AA.

These studies, although providing some conflicting results, illustrate that relationships between diet and disease are often complex and can be a result of interactions between variants in the genetic code, diet and other factors. While folate is widely seen as a 'healthy' nutrient, it is clear that for some in the population an excess may be detrimental. A one-size-fits-all approach to public health nutrition may therefore run the risk of causing harm to some in the population. A greater appreciation of the complexity of the diet–disease relationship is therefore of high importance.

30-fold risk that is associated with obesity (Joost *et al.*, 2007). It should also be borne in mind that other genetically determined factors may modulate the influence of the SNP. In the case of the C677T polymorphism of MTHFR, the influence on disease risk varies between ethnic groups (Klerk *et al.*, 2002). Some SNPs may increase risk of one chronic disease yet protect against another. Cardiovascular disease-prone TT MTHFR variant-carrying individuals appear to have some protection against cancers of the large intestine (Joost *et al.*, 2007). Research Highlight 1.2 describes how SNPs in MTHFR interact with diet to determine risk of breast cancer.

Understanding all these processes is important. Throughout this book, you will encounter examples of uncertainty and variation in the effectiveness of nutritional interventions to prevent or manage disease. This is because the impact of diet upon physiological and metabolic processes will vary due to the genetic variation in the population and because even straightforward nutrient–gene interactions may generate opposing responses to nutrient signals under different circumstances. Some polymorphisms related to disease risk sometimes appear to have influences that are specific to sex, menopausal status or race. It is also the case that the expressed phenotype may be life-stage specific. The Bsm1 SNP in the vitamin D receptor is strongly predictive of bone health and the response to calcium in children but has no association with bone health in adults (Ferrari *et al.*, 1998). It is therefore clear that the genotype can be an important determinant of disease risk. However, the instances of where it is the sole or major driver of risk are rare and, in most cases, genetic inheritance is just one of the many components that determine the overall risk profile for chronic disease.

1.4 Personalized nutrition

Personalized nutrition is a concept describing the use of information about individuals to produce targeted nutrition advice or interventions to improve health (Ordovas *et al.*, 2018). Personalized nutrition advice or interventions might be based on biological information about individuals (their genotype or phenotype) or information about their behaviours (dietary preferences, personal motivations and objectives). Genotype information includes data about common polymorphisms, as described in Section 1.3.2, but can also consider how those polymorphisms interact with each other or are regulated by the epigenome. Phenotype describes the observable characteristics of the individual. In terms of nutrition and health, these measures of phenotype might include age, sex, metabolic state, stage of life, body fatness, microbiome composition or disease state. Table 1.7 defines some of the terms associated with personalized nutrition.

In developing personalized nutrition, obtaining robust information, whether biological or behavioural, is the key first step to formulating targeted advice or interventions. With this information personalized nutrition may be applied in different ways. At the whole population level, it provides a way to target interventions at people with specific characteristics. The traditional one size fits all approach, for example fortifying water supplies with fluoride to prevent dental caries, may benefit a

Table 1.7 Personalized nutrition and the 'omics.

Term	Definition
Stratified nutrition	Tailoring dietary advice or interventions to groups of people based upon their shared characteristics, such as age, body mass index or sex.
Personalized nutrition	Tailoring dietary advice or interventions to individual people based upon information about their genotype, phenotype or behaviours.
Precision nutrition	The tailoring of dietary advice based on quantitative data about the specific genotype of the individual, for example single nucleotide polymorphisms.
Nutrigenetics	An approach to personalized nutrition which focuses on the response to food or nutrients, based upon variation in genotype.
Nutrigenomics	The study of all genetic factors which determine the individual response to foods or nutrients.
Metabolomics	The study and analysis of the metabolites produced by tissues. This is an approach to characterizing the phenotype response to diet and other factors.
Microbiomics	The study of the microbiome in the human gut or other tissues. The composition of the microbiome can determine the individual response to foods or nutrients.
Epigenomics	The expression of genes can be regulated by modifications to DNA, termed epigenetic regulation. In personalized nutrition, epigenomics is the study of epigenetic changes that determine the individual response to foods or nutrients.

minority of the population and cause harm to some. A more targeted personalized nutrition approach could ensure that only those who may benefit receive an intervention (Figure 1.8). The Food4Me study evaluated the efficacy of a personalized nutrition approach to behaviour change in more than 1600 people living in Europe (Celis-Morales *et al.*, 2017) It showed that a personalized nutrition approach was significantly more motivating for recipients to make lifestyle changes and was more effective in improving healthy food behaviours than generic one size fits all advice. Similarly, Doets *et al.* (2019) compared the effects of generic lifestyle modification advice and personalized nutrition in older Dutch adults. The personalized nutrition approach was more effective that generic advice in several areas, including reducing body fatness.

Personalized nutrition may also be useful in managing the diets of individuals who have specific disease states, such as type 2 diabetes or very individualized demands for nutrition, for example elite sportspeople. Providing advice which specifically integrates the metabolic, physiological and psychosocial requirements of the recipient will improve adherence and efficacy.

Early ideas about personalized nutrition were heavily focused on the potential for genotypic information to be used to predict diet–disease relationships and individual risk (Kaput and Rodriguez, 2004). Many commercial enterprises were established to exploit these ideas, for example providing dietary advice based upon MTHFR genotype (see Research Highlight 1.2). We would now describe this approach to personalized nutrition as precision nutrition (Table 1.7), which is considered by many to be impractical (Betts and Gonzalez, 2016). The effects of genetics on most (though not all) disease states are modest, are the product of multiple interacting gene variants and are insufficient to use as the basis for dietary advice or nutritional management. For example, genetic variation contributes approximately 10% of the overall risk of type 2 diabetes (Morris *et al.*, 2012), while obesity contributes far more. It makes little sense to base advice to patients with diabetes or individuals who are prediabetic on the basis of genotype rather than dealing with the excess weight.

Personalized nutrition strategies are increasingly moving away from the precision measures towards other types of information which can be simply used to identify people or groups of people for

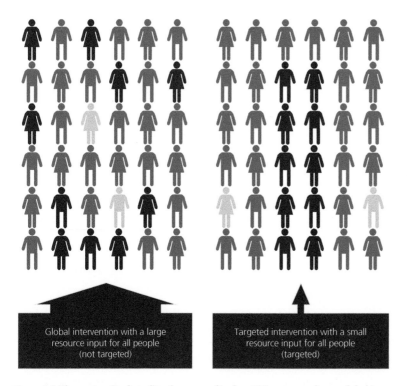

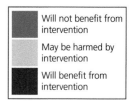

Figure 1.8 The contrasting benefits of a personalized nutrition approach to a global intervention. A global intervention will impact upon all people in a population with benefits only for a minority and the possibility of causing harm to some. A more targeted approach based on specific characteristics requires fewer resources to implement and reduces the possibility of harmful outcomes.

advice on nutrition (Adams *et al.*, 2019). Indeed, in the Food4Me study (Celis-Morales *et al.*, 2017), using simple information was more successful in driving behaviour change that more complex genotypic information. For personalized nutrition to be useful and established it will be necessary to have useful tools to enable groups in the population to base dietary decisions on their phenotypic, genotypic and behavioural characteristics. There are a number of digital tools and platforms being developed and made commercially available for the purpose of integrating this individual information with dietary advice, and these are starting to appear in clinical settings (Abrahams and Matushieski, 2020).

Personalized nutrition is still at an early stage in its development. There is clearly potential for its use in public health as it is well documented that individual variation in the response to food and nutrient exists. However, the evidence base for precision nutrition approaches is currently too weak, so this remains an impractical option. In the meantime, a stratified nutrition approach may offer greater potential for personalized nutrition in shaping public health nutrition interventions.

1.5 Assessment of nutritional status

The assessment of nutritional status is necessary in a variety of different settings. Working with individuals in a clinical setting, it may be necessary to assess dietary adequacy to plan the management of disease states or to make clinical diagnoses. Public health nutritionists require data on dietary adequacy at a group level to make assessments of the contribution of nutritional factors to disease risk in the population and to develop public health policies or intervention strategies. Nutritional assessment is also a critical research tool used in determining the relationships between diet and disease. These situations, which rely on considerations of the likelihood of nutritional deficit or excess at the individual or population level, use tools that aim either to measure intakes of nutrients or the physiological manifestations of nutrient deficit or excess within the body. Tools for nutritional assessment include anthropometric measures, dietary assessments, determination of biomarkers and clinical examination.

1.5.1 Anthropometric measures

Anthropometric methods make indirect measurements of the nutritional status of individuals and groups of individuals, as they are designed to estimate the composition of the body. Table 1.8 provides a summary of the commonly used anthropometric techniques. Many of these techniques have been designed to estimate the lean or fat mass which are present within the body. Information about relative fatness or leanness can be a useful indicator of nutritional status since excess fat will highlight storage of energy consumed in excess, while declining fat stores and loss of muscle mass are indicative of malnutrition. Extremes within anthropometric measures (e.g. the emaciation of cachexia or morbid obesity) are

Table 1.8 Anthropometric measures used to estimate body composition and nutritional status.

Technique	Component of body composition estimated	Limitations
Body mass index (weight/height^2)	Weight relative to height	Does not distinguish between lean and fat mass. Does not measure the composition of the body.
Skinfold thicknesses	Fat mass	Requires skill in measurement. Makes assumptions about the even distribution of fat in the subcutaneous layer.
Waist circumference or waist/hip ratio	Fat distribution	A good indicator of abdominal fat deposition. Requires set protocols for measurement.
Mid-upper arm circumference	Muscle mass	Prone to measurement error. Unsuitable for some groups (e.g. adolescents) with rapidly changing fat and muscle patterns. Good indicator of acute malnutrition.
Bioimpedance	Fat mass	Influenced by hydration status of subjects.
Underwater weighing	Body density, fat and lean mass	Requires subjects to undergo training for an unpleasant procedure. Underestimates fat mass in muscular individuals.
Isotope dilution	Body water	Influenced by fluid intake of subject. Analytically difficult and expensive.
Scanning techniques (NMR, CT, DXA)	Proportions and distribution of lean and fat mass	Expensive, restricted access to scanners. Use ionizing radiation so unsuitable for children and pregnant women.

CT, computed tomography; DXA, dual-energy X-ray absorptiometry; NMR, nuclear magnetic resonance.

useful indicators of disease risk or progression in a clinical setting. In children, serial measures of height and weight can provide sensitive measures of growth and development that can be used to highlight and monitor nutritional problems. The most robust anthropometric measures are challenging as they require specialist equipment. As a result, most surveys and research projects that examine large groups of people use simply determined measures such as BMI (weight in kg divided by height in m²). As shown in Figure 1.9, BMI is widely used as a measure of body fatness and to classify overweight and obesity, but it is a non-specific measure that can be misinterpreted (see Sections 6.4 and 8.4.1).

1.5.2 Estimating dietary intakes
Estimation of dietary intakes, either to determine intakes of specific macro- or micronutrients or to assess intakes of particular foods, is a mainstay of human nutrition research. A range of different methods are applied, depending on the level of detail required. All approaches are highly prone to measurement error.

1.5.2.1 Indirect measures
The least accurate measures of intake are those that make indirect estimates of the quantities of foodstuffs consumed by populations. These techniques are used to follow trends in consumption between national populations or within a national population over a period.

Food balance sheets are widely used by the United Nations Food and Agriculture Organization (FAO) to monitor the availability of foods, and hence nutrients, within most nations of the world and are published on an annual basis. They allow temporal trends to be monitored easily and apply a standardized methodology on a global scale. A food balance sheet is essentially compiled from government records of the total production, imports and exports of specific foodstuffs. This allows the quantity of that foodstuff available to the population to be calculated (available food = production + imports − exports). Dividing that figure by the total number of people in the population allows the daily availability per capita to be estimated. Figure 1.10 shows data abstracted from the FAO food balance sheets, indicating how daily availability of protein varies with different regions of the world.

Food balance sheets are subject to considerable error due to assumptions that are made in their compilation. It will be incorrectly assumed that the nutrient composition of a food will be the same regardless of where it is produced. For example, the selenium content of cereals from North America is considerably greater than in the same cereals from Europe, as European soils are relatively impoverished in this mineral. The balance sheets also assume that all available food will be completely consumed by humans and do not allow for wastage or feeding to animals. It is also fallacious to assume that available food will be equally distributed to all people in

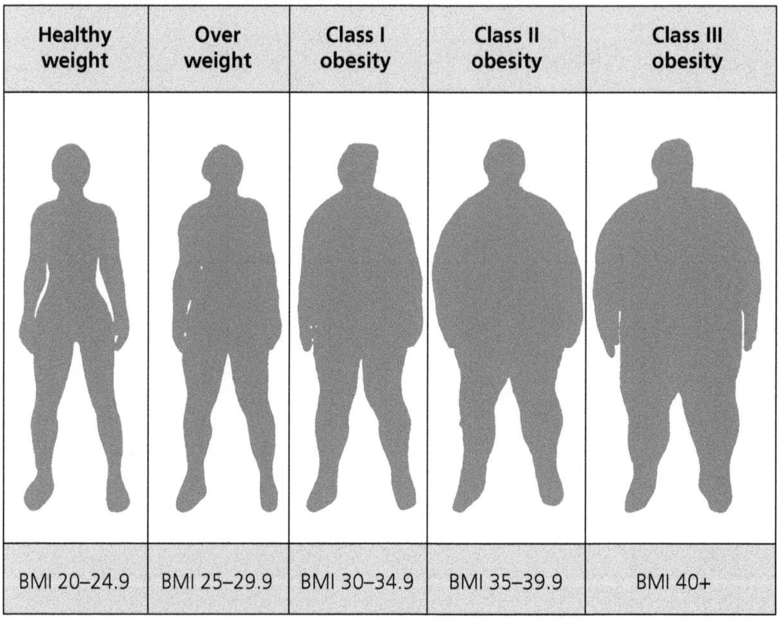

Healthy weight	Over weight	Class I obesity	Class II obesity	Class III obesity
BMI 20–24.9	BMI 25–29.9	BMI 30–34.9	BMI 35–39.9	BMI 40+

Figure 1.9 Body mass index (BMI) is commonly used to define and classify overweight and obesity (calculated as kg/m²).

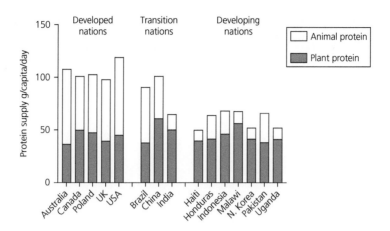

Figure 1.10 Availability protein in selected countries. Per capita availability of protein from United Nations Food and Agriculture Organization global food balance sheets, 2017. Note the disparities in the availability of higher-quality animal protein.

a population and the sheets make no distinction between food available to men and women, to adults and children or to rich and poor.

Food accounts are a similar approach to estimating food availability but, instead of collecting data on a national scale, they are used to measure the food available to a household or an institution (e.g. a nursing home). By compiling an inventory of food stored at the start of a survey, monitoring food entering the setting (often measured by looking at invoices and receipts from food shopping) and taking into account any food grown in the setting, it is possible to calculate the food available per person over the period of the survey. As with the food balance sheet, this method does not allow accurate estimation of individual food intakes and does not allow for food wastage, but the food account can provide data on dietary patterns of families or similar groups at low cost and over an extended period.

1.5.2.2 Direct measures

Direct measures of nutrient intake collect data from individuals or groups of individuals and, in addition to their obvious application to clinical circumstances, are well suited to research in human nutrition and epidemiology. Although more robust than the indirect estimates described earlier, all direct measures of intake are prone to bias and error and results must always be interpreted with caution. These methods may be particularly useful for studying individuals or populations in different settings and study types (Table 1.9).

1.5.2.2.1 Dietary recall methods

The dietary recall method is not only one of the best methods for examining nutrient intakes in a clinical setting, but it may also be used in research. One of

the major disadvantages of the method is the need for a trained interviewer to spend time with the patient or research subject to elicit detailed information on all food and drink consumed over a recent period (Table 1.9). An interview will explore all food and beverages consumed during that period and ask for descriptions of cooking methods, portion sizes, use of condiments and eating between meals. Protocols such as the US Department of Agriculture five-pass method take the subjects through the recall period several times using different techniques to ensure that a full record is obtained (Conway *et al.*, 2004). Most dietary recalls will be based on intakes over the preceding 24 hours but in some cases may look at 48- or 72-hour periods. Information obtained in this way can then be coded for detailed analysis of energy and nutrient intakes using appropriate nutritional analysis software or food tables. Dietary recall methods can generate detailed information on the types of food consumed and portion sizes. The use of photographic food atlases showing portion sizes for commonly consumed foods can enhance the quality of this quantitative information. Spending time interviewing a subject also makes it relatively easy to obtain recipes used in cooking and information about cooking techniques (e.g. use of oils in frying). Like all methods of estimating nutrient intake, the dietary recall is prone to inaccuracy due to under- and over-reporting of food intake by certain groups of people. It is also dependent upon the memory of the subject and so loses accuracy when attempting to estimate habitual intakes.

1.5.2.2.2 Food record methods

Food records or diaries, administered to subjects for completion in their own time, are widely regarded

Table 1.9 Advantages and disadvantages of dietary assessment methods.

Method	Advantages	Disadvantages
Dietary recall	Inexpensive; can be detailed; useful in clinical settings; can be repeated in the same individual; does not influence food intake.	One recall seldom representative; relies on memory; intensive data entry; prone to under- and over-reporting; requires trained interviewer.
Food frequency questionnaire	Can be self-administered; can use automated data entry; inexpensive for large population studies; represents usual intake over long periods.	May not capture portion sizes; not useful for estimating absolute nutrient intake; subject must be literate; multiple foods may be covered by a single listed item; depends on memory.
Food record	Does not depend on memory; data can be detailed and precise; captures intake over several days; can estimate nutrient intakes with good precision.	Act of recording may alter diet; subject must be literate; intensive data entry; high burden on subject can lower response rates; prone to under- and overreporting.

as the most powerful tool for estimation of nutrient intakes. Subjects keep records for extended periods of time (usually three to seven days) and note down all foods and beverages consumed at the time they are consumed. Portion sizes can be recorded in a number of different ways, with the subject most frequently either noting an estimated intake in simple household measures (e.g. two tablespoons of rice, one cup of sugar) or an intake estimated through comparison to a pictorial atlas of portion sizes. Inaccuracies in estimates of portion sizes are a major problem associated with food record methods, particularly with some subgroups in the population, and methods should be chosen that best serve the purpose of the dietary survey. To improve the quality of the data, intake can be accurately determined by weighing the food on standardized scales, taking into account any wastage (a weighed food record). Surveys of small groups of well-motivated people in a metabolic unit lend themselves well to weighed record methods, while in large surveys of free-living individuals, these are rarely practical. Participants require calibrated scales for the weighing and need some degree of skill and knowledge to make an accurate record. The act of weighing is inconvenient and may also shape eating behaviour. Over a period of days, it may deter food consumption. In some settings, it is possible for a researcher to do the weighing, thereby reducing influences upon the subject consuming the food.

Pictorial food atlases have long been in use and have been validated and made available for specific populations, for example the Young Person's Food Atlas (Foster et al., 2017). Generally, records made by subjects using atlas images to indicate portion size give good agreement with weighed food records (Frobisher and Maxwell, 2003). A systematic review of methods used to estimate portion sizes found that the photo-image based approaches were more accurate than other methods (Amoutzopoulos et al., 2020). With the advent of digital cameras on mobile phones, these devices are increasingly being incorporated into food records as a means of determining portion size. Zakrewski-Fruer et al. (2017) took the approach of supplying participants in a randomized controlled trial (RCT) with digital cameras to photograph all food and beverage consumption. The participants were asked to use the images to help them recall intake when completing food diaries, and the researchers used the images to verify what had been recorded. Olafsdottir et al. (2016) compared weighed records of food servings and wastage in school canteen settings with digital images. The images were then cross-referenced to photographic atlases to estimate portion sizes. The method gave good agreement with weight data. Kong et al. (2017) considered the validity of using smartphone images with a social media application and found very strong agreement between image data and weighed records for energy, fat, protein and carbohydrate estimation. It is likely that subjects completing an image-based record of food and beverage consumption will become a standard protocol for food records in future.

Food records have a number of strengths compared with other methods of estimating intake. Complex data on meal patterns and eating habits can be obtained through study of food diaries, and this information can supplement estimates of nutrient intake. By obtaining records for periods of five to seven days, the intakes of most micronutrients can be estimated with some degree of confidence (Table 1.9), in addition to energy and macronutrients. For some nutrients, it is suggested that records of 14 or more days may be required (Block, 1989). The major disadvantage of the food record approach is the reliance on the subject to complete the record fully and accurately. Maintaining a food record is burdensome, and it is often noted that the degree of detail and hence accuracy will be greater in the first two to three days of a seven-day record compared with later days. The act of recording intake, especially if a weighed record is used, can change the eating behaviour of subjects and hence lead to an underestimate of habitual intakes.

Like other direct methods, the food record is prone to under- and over-reporting of energy and nutrient intakes among certain subgroups in the population, due to the tendency of individuals to report intakes that will reflect them in the best possible light to the researcher. Women who are obese and overweight are frequently found to under-report intakes in dietary surveys. Murakami and Livingstone (2015) carried out an analysis of the US National Health and Nutrition Examination Survey 2003–2012 data in children and adolescents and found that under-reporting was more prevalent among obese and overweight and older children. Over-reporting was more associated with normal weight, younger children and children from poorer families. A comparison of actual measures of energy intake in 327 adults, compared with self-report or interviewer-led assessment (Brassard *et al.*, 2018) found that up to 52% of adults under-reported when self-reporting intake, and that one third still under-reported when interviewed by a researcher.

1.5.2.2.3 Food frequency questionnaire methods

Food frequency questionnaire methods involve the administration of food checklists to individuals, or groups of individuals, as a means of estimating their habitual intake of foods or groups of foods. Subjects work through the checklist and, for each foodstuff, indicate their level of consumption (i.e. number of portions) on a daily, weekly or monthly basis (Figure 1.11). Semiquantitative food frequency questionnaires also collect information on typical portion size.

Food frequency questionnaires can vary in their complexity and length. Often, a questionnaire will consist of 100–150 food items and will therefore allow for a comprehensive coverage of the dietary patterns of a subject. Some questionnaires are much shorter and may be focused upon a particular food group or the main sources of a specific type of nutrient. For example, Block *et al.* (1989) developed a questionnaire with just 13 items to identify individuals who had high intakes of fat. This was used as a preliminary screening tool to select subjects for a more detailed investigation.

Food frequency questionnaires have many desirable attributes for researchers wishing to estimate intakes in large populations (Table 1.9). They are self-administered by the subject, are generally not

	Once per week	2–4 per week	5–6 per week	Daily	Once per month	Once per 3 months	Never
White bread	◯	◯	◯	●	◯	◯	◯
Brown bread	◯	◯	◯	◯	●	◯	◯
Wholemeal bread	◯	●	◯	◯	◯	◯	◯
Burger bun	●	◯	◯	◯	◯	◯	◯
Bagel	◯	●	◯	◯	◯	◯	◯
Pitta	◯	◯	◯	◯	◯	●	◯
Tortilla	●	◯	◯	◯	◯	◯	◯
Chapatti	◯	◯	◯	◯	◯	◯	●
Brioche	◯	◯	◯	◯	◯	◯	●

Figure 1.11 A food frequency questionnaire is used to estimate the habitual consumption of foodstuffs within the diet of an individual.

time consuming and are unlikely to influence eating behaviours. Data entry can sometimes be automated, reducing the analytical burden for the researcher. Moreover, the food frequency questionnaire provides an estimate of habitual intake over a period of months or even years, as opposed to the snapshot obtained by looking at a food record representing just a few days. However, the food frequency questionnaire can be a weak tool when considering portion sizes and is therefore less effective for estimating micronutrient intakes than a food record. Food frequency questionnaires must also be valid for the population to be studied, as the range of foods consumed will vary with age and various other social and demographic factors. For example, if attempting to survey nutrient intakes in a population with a wide ethnic diversity, the foods and food groups included on the questionnaire need to reflect that level of diversity. A questionnaire that fails to include staple foods consumed by particular ethnic groups will inevitably underestimate their intake. For this reason, new food frequency questionnaires undergo extensive validation that includes comparing food frequency data with parallel analysis of dietary recalls and/or weighed food records in the same individuals.

1.5.3 Biomarkers of nutritional status

Biomarkers of nutritional status are measures of either the biological function of a nutrient or the nutrient itself in an individual or in samples taken from individuals. These measures can often provide the earliest indicator of a nutrient deficit, as they register subnormal values ahead of any clinical symptoms. Biomarkers are therefore useful in monitoring the prevalence of nutrient deficiency, measuring the effectiveness of the treatment of deficiency and assessing preventive strategies. Given the huge difficulties of making accurate assessments of dietary intakes, as described earlier, biomarkers provide a useful means of validating dietary data and are often measured as adjuncts to dietary surveys. The UK National Diet and Nutrition Survey Rolling Programme 2008–2017 used a comprehensive array of blood biomarkers to assess nutritional status, including ferritin and haemoglobin for iron, red cell and serum folate, red cell glutathione reductase for riboflavin and serum vitamin B12 (Bates *et al.*, 2019). The doubly labelled water method (Koebnick *et al.*, 2005) can be used to validate energy intakes estimated using dietary records or other means (Figure 1.12).

Biomarkers of nutritional status are often regarded as being more objective than other indices.

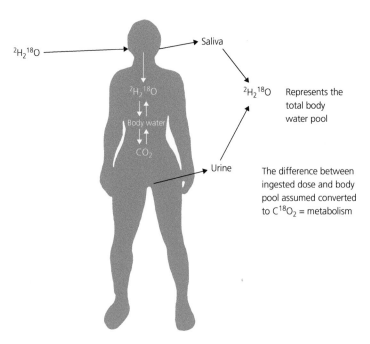

Figure 1.12 The doubly labelled water method is a technique used to assess energy expenditure. Subjects consume water containing stable isotopes of hydrogen and oxygen. This water reaches equilibrium with the body water. Measures of the doubly labelled water in saliva and urine enable estimation of the loss of $^{18}O_2$ from body water. That loss can only occur through production of labelled carbon dioxide. Carbon dioxide production is a measure of metabolism. *Source:* based on Koebnick *et al.* (2005).

They include functional tests and measurements of nutrient concentration in easily obtained body fluids or other materials. The latter type of measurement can be a static test, which is performed on one occasion, or it may be repeated at intervals to monitor change over time. The relative merits of these approaches are discussed later in this section.

Functional tests measure biological processes that are dependent upon a specific nutrient. If that nutrient is present at suboptimal concentrations in the body, it would be expected that the specific function would decline. The dark adaptation test is classic example of a functional test to determine vitamin A status. The dark adaptation test measures visual acuity in dim light after exposure to a bright light that desensitizes the eye. The reformation of rhodopsin within the retina is dependent upon the generation of cis-retinol, and thus, the visual adaptation in the dark will be related to vitamin A status. Measurement of the excretion of xanthurenic acid is a functional test for vitamin B6 (pyridoxine) status. Xanthurenic acid is a breakdown product of tryptophan and kynurenine and is formed via pyridoxine-dependent reactions.

Non-functional measures of biomarkers typically involve direct measures of specific nutrients in simply obtained samples from individuals. These are most commonly samples of blood (plasma, serum or red cells) or urine but could include faeces, hair or, more rarely, biopsy material from the adipose tissue or muscle. Static tests provide a snapshot of the nutrient concentration in the sample at a given point in time and could be misleading as they often provide an indicator of immediate intake rather than habitual intake. For example, plasma zinc concentrations will vary hugely from day to day, reflecting continuing metabolic fluxes, and fall by up to 20% following a meal (King, 1990). Wherever possible, repeated tests should be taken to increase confidence in the measured biomarker, or tests should be performed in a sample that provides a stronger indicator of habitual intake. In the case of zinc, plasma measurements are of limited value, as most zinc is held in functional forms within tissues and less than 1% of the total pool is in circulation. Red or white blood cell zinc concentrations could be used as a more robust biomarker, as could white cell metallothionein concentrations (metallothionein is a key zinc-binding protein). Hair can be used to assess zinc status, together with manganese, copper and cadmium, as there are no functional biomarkers for these metals (Pico *et al.*, 2019). Fat biopsies can be used to estimate long-term fat-soluble vitamin intake. Martinaitye *et al.* (2017) reported that long-term supplementation with vitamin D was strongly reflected in increases in the vitamin D content of adipose tissue samples. Similarly, the EURAMIC study (Kardinaal *et al.*, 1993) used measures of α-tocopherol and β-carotene in biopsies of adipose tissue to assess intakes of these vitamins. As fat-soluble vitamins are stored in adipose tissue, this gave an indicator of habitual intake over several weeks.

The levels of a measured biomarker are only useful in estimating nutritional status if there is a linear relationship between the measurement and the intake. In addition to this and the need to make measurements in a relevant sample, it is important to appreciate the non-dietary influences on the biomarker that could skew the interpretation of any measurement. Some measurements could be perturbed by the presence of disease or the use of medications to treat disease. For example, serum albumin concentration can be used as a marker of dietary protein intake but the test is poor and non-specific. Serum albumin declines with low protein intakes and, in clinical settings, can provide a predictor of morbidity and mortality associated with protein–energy malnutrition. However, as described earlier in this chapter, serum albumin concentrations also fall with infection and inflammation and, in seriously ill patients, albumin could be administered as an element of any intravenous fluid infusion. Either situation would render albumin useless as a marker of nutritional status. Like any measure of nutritional status, biochemical indices can lack specificity and should ideally be used as part of a battery of tests based upon dietary assessments, biochemical measures, anthropometry and, if appropriate, clinical assessment.

1.5.4 Clinical examination

Performing a thorough physical examination and obtaining a detailed patient history are an effective method of determining symptoms associated with malnutrition in individuals. This approach can be most useful when dealing with children, where the paucity of nutrient stores can mean that clinical symptoms develop very quickly, as opposed to in adults, where the symptoms are generally a sign of chronic malnutrition. Obtaining a patient history can highlight key points that are missed when assessing dietary intake or using anthropometric measures. Reported loss of appetite, loss of blood, occurrence of diarrhoea, steatorrhoea or nausea and vomiting may all be indicators or potential causes of malnutrition and should trigger further investigation. Physical examination can assess the degree of emaciation of a potentially malnourished individual. Careful assessment of the hair, skin, nails, eyes, lips, tongue and mouth can also highlight specific nutrient deficiencies. Bleaching of the hair is indicative of protein malnutrition, while cracking of the lips can suggest deficiency of B vitamins such as riboflavin. Pallor of the skin and spooning of the nails are clinical signs of iron deficiency. Evidence of rough spots on the conjunctiva of the eye will accompany early stages of vitamin A deficiency.

1.6 Nutritional epidemiology: understanding diet–disease relationships

1.6.1 The importance of the evidence base

Nutrition is a subject where everyone has an opinion, sometimes based on beliefs, sometimes on experience and often on information obtained from unreliable media. It is natural that we should all take an interest, as we all eat food, and contemporary populations have a good understanding that the quality of the diet is related to health.

The provisional nature of nutritional science, where the evidence base often shifts and comprises conflicting data, means that the population can be confused by apparently contradictory messages. For example, a media report may highlight that drinking coffee is protective against cancer one day, and the very next highlight that coffee increases the risk of dementia. Media coverage is too superficial to put across a measured account which looks at the strength of the evidence in a single research report, to consider the quality of how research has been performed, or to provide a synthesis of all that is known about a particular area of study. For the general public, the natural response is to either engage in regular and ill-thought-through changes to diet, or to conclude that scientists don't know what they are talking about and to reject all advice.

This creates the perfect environment for individuals with no background in science to influence behaviour and exploit health concerns for monetary gain. Fad diets, unnecessary supplements and complementary therapies with no efficacy are big business opportunities. The dietary supplement industry is worth US$195 billion globally, for example, while diet books regularly dominate the bestseller lists. These products are authored or endorsed by celebrity chefs, TV or film stars, maverick doctors and other unqualified individuals, and the market seems boundless.

While this market has existed for some time, there is a growing and insidious side to the messaging on which it relies. In the past, the trade was largely in quick fixes for weight loss, but the modern trend, projected through social media, is to imply that nutritional scientists are in a sinister cabal with the food industry to promote an unhealthy agenda. It has even been asserted that the dietary guidance pursued in westernized countries for the past 30 years is a kind of genocide (Carlson, 2008). If such a conspiracy exists, this author has not been invited to take part. Although totally fatuous and unable to explain, for example, why deaths from heart disease in the UK have declined by 75% since the 1960s, this kind of view has become part of the zeitgeist in western countries and has spawned a huge interest in low carbohydrate, high fat diets, and diet patterns which were developed to manage specific disease states, for example gluten-free and lactose-free diets. For the majority of people, these apparently 'healthy' diet trends will bring no benefit, but will also do no harm beyond being more expensive to achieve and limiting food choices. For some though, adopting a restrictive dietary pattern at the wrong stage of life, or against a background of chronic disease, could be dangerous to health and wellbeing.

Dietary advice should only be given by those who are qualified to do so. In the UK, for example, 'dietitian' is a protected title that can only be used by registered health professionals. Dietitians use their expertise to change behaviour and devise eating plans for patients who have underlying illness. 'Nutritionist' is not, as yet, a protected title, meaning that anyone can self-title themselves and trade commercially. The role of a trained nutritionist lies in providing the scientific evidence base for the field, shaping public health (disease prevention) initiatives, working with non-governmental organizations, sports people and the food industry. The boundaries between the nutritionist and dietitian roles are clear and, professionally, these workers must recognize the limits of their own expertise and practice and must refer individuals or populations to other practitioners where appropriate.

No one can work professionally in the nutrition field without a thorough understanding of the critical and central role of scientific evidence to the discipline. The following sections explain how the nutrition evidence base is generated, why it can be complex and sometimes conflicting, and why views may change as our knowledge and methodologies increase and improve.

1.6.2 Nutritional epidemiology

Epidemiology is the branch of medical science that studies the causes of health and disease in populations rather than in individuals. At the simplest level, epidemiology can be used to examine geographical and temporal trends in disease to determine initial clues to the causes of disease and then use more sophisticated techniques to examine those possible causes. Nutritional epidemiology focuses on nutrition and nutrition-related factors as both causal and preventive factors in disease. Understanding nutritional epidemiology is important, as the findings from such work are used as the main evidence base to develop public health strategies, health education advice and government policy on nutrition. For example, international policies to combat iodine deficiency through universal salt iodization would not be possible without robust epidemiology to show that the strategy would be both effective and safe.

Nutritional epidemiology studies focus on two key measurements: the exposure and the outcome. Exposure refers to a nutrition-related factor that may be related to disease. This could be a marker of body composition (e.g. BMI), a specific nutrient (e.g. folic acid), a dietary pattern (e.g. vegetarianism) or a food-related behaviour (e.g. alcohol consumption). The outcome is the disease of interest, which can be measured as confirmed diagnosis of ill health (morbidity), as risk factors for disease (e.g. raised blood pressure as a risk factor for heart disease) or as death from a disease (mortality).

1.6.3 Cause and effect

Establishing which foods and nutrients may be causally related to disease processes is a critical aim for nutritional epidemiology. Without knowledge of how nutrients and nutrition-related factors influence disease processes, it is impossible to design effective interventions that prevent disease or nutrition-based treatments for established disease. It can be relatively simple to identify associations or correlations between factors but less easy to determine which are biologically or clinically meaningful. It is always important to appreciate that correlation does not indicate causal relationship. For example, we might look for evidence that the amount of meat in the diet is related to the risk of developing oesophageal cancer and, in a simple sense, could correlate the meat intakes of different populations with the occurrence of oesophageal cancer in those populations. One approach might be to find populations with low rates of cancer and populations with high rates of cancer and compare their meat intakes. The correlation we observe may be genuine or may be spurious, and much more information needs to be considered in designing a robust study to evaluate the relationship (e.g. the size of the sample needed, the method used to collect data on meat intake and the duration of the study) and interpreting the data obtained (considering alternative reasons for the correlation such as obesity or smoking habits).

1.6.4 Bias and confounding

Figure 1.13 shows the complexity of establishing a robust study for investigating a diet–disease relationship. Components of that figure, such as sample size and who to sample, duration of study and consideration of the accuracy of measurement, are all representatives of a phenomenon called bias, which can limit the usefulness of epidemiological studies. Studies which fail to control different types of bias, either at the point where the study is designed and initiated or during the analysis of the data, may draw spurious conclusions and may be of no value in identifying diet–disease relationships.

Different types of bias may be present within a study. Bias is generally classified as 'selection bias', 'measurement bias' or 'confounding bias'. Selection bias refers to factors that relate to how the people involved in the study were recruited. It is rarely possible to assess diet and disease in a whole population, so inevitably a smaller sample has to be assessed. We may, for example, be interested in the links between cancer and meat intake across the whole of the UK but cannot possibly examine all 66 million people in the population. Instead, a study is likely to consider a few thousand individuals to represent that whole population. Selection bias occurs when there is a difference in the relationship between the exposure (diet) and outcome (disease) between the people who took part in the study and those who did not. For example, there may be no relationship between meat and oesophageal cancer in young adults, but a strong relationship could be present in older adults. To avoid such bias, a wide age range should be sampled.

Measurement bias (also called information bias) occurs when there are errors in the measurement of exposure or outcome that lead to misclassification of individuals. For example, if the method for measuring meat intake is inaccurate, individuals could be classed as high consumers when really they are not. Measurement bias is a major problem for nutrition–disease studies as the methods for considering food intake are prone to misreporting by study participants (either deliberate or due to poor memory, specifically termed recall bias) or differences in the measurement between interviewers. In the case of the meat–oesophageal cancer relationship (Figure 1.13), for example, considering oesophageal cancer as a single outcome as opposed to two different diseases would also lead to measurement bias. Adenocarcinoma may have a different relationship to meat intake than squamous cell carcinoma.

Confounding bias describes the situation where a third factor explains the relationship between exposure and outcome. To be truly considered as a confounding factor, the additional factor must be

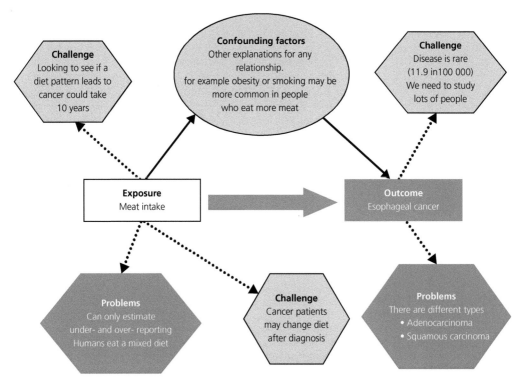

Figure 1.13 Measuring the relationship between a nutritional exposure and a disease outcome is complex, necessitating careful epidemiological designs. These designs must consider appropriate sampling in terms of size of population, length of study, measurement of diet and measurement of disease outcome. *Source:* based on Scientific Advisory Committee on Nutrition (2015).

related to both exposure and outcome but must not lie on the causal pathway between the two. The classic example of confounding is shown in Figure 1.14, where the relationship between alcohol and cancer may be explained by the fact that tobacco smoking causes cancer and people who consume high amounts of alcohol are also more likely to be heavy smokers. Some epidemiological studies are able to limit confounding bias at the design stage (see the following text), but usually confounding is adjusted for when analysing data.

1.6.5 Quantifying the relationship between diet and disease

As outlined in the following text, there is a variety of approaches used in nutritional epidemiology to explore the relationships between diet and disease. Each of these approaches yields information which quantifies the impact of specific nutrition-related factors (dietary patterns, specific nutrient intakes, obesity) upon disease outcomes (disease diagnosis, death) or risk factors for disease (blood pressure, elevated circulating biomarkers). Understanding the nature of these measured outcomes is critical for interpretation of the findings of epidemiological studies.

Some studies will yield relatively simple measures of outcome. For example, a study which measures blood pressure or elevated cholesterol concentrations in a group of people exposed to a factor and a group who are not will make a straightforward measure of whether the markers differ in the two groups of people. Considering differences in diagnosis or death, however, involves measures of 'risk' which are less familiar to those new to the subject.

One approach to quantifying risk is to provide data on prevalence or incidence rates (Table 1.10). These are essentially measures of the likelihood that individuals in a population will develop a disease (morbidity) or die from a disease (mortality), and an epidemiological study might, for example, compare the prevalence of cancer in meat eaters compared with non-meat eaters. Prevalence and incidence have different meanings. Prevalence is the measure of how likely an individual is to have a particular disease and is calculated as the number of cases in a population divided by the number of people in the population. Thus, if in the UK there are 9600 cases of oesophageal cancer, the prevalence is 9600 divided by 66 000 000, or 0.000145. This would be

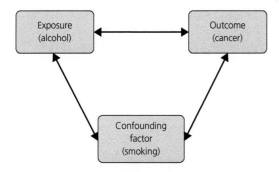

Figure 1.14 A confounding factor is an additional factor that may explain the relationship between an exposure and an outcome. The confounding factor is related to both outcome and exposure but does not lie on the causal pathway between the two.

simplified to 14.5 per 100 000 population. Incidence describes the probability of a person being diagnosed with a disease during a given period or, in effect, the number of newly diagnosed cases. For example, if over the course of one year there are 2500 new cases of oesophageal cancer diagnosed in the UK, the incidence would be 2500 divided by 66 000 000, or 0.000038. This simplifies to 3.8 new cases per 100 000 people per year.

A more commonly used approach to express the degree of risk associated with a nutrition-related factor is represented by odds ratios, relative risk (RR) and hazard ratios (Table 1.10). These are all variations on the same theme, whereby risk is expressed as the likelihood in one group (e.g. meat eaters) relative to a reference group (e.g. non-meat eaters). This is generally easy to understand as an odds ratio of 10, indicating that people exposed to a particular factor are 10 times more likely to experi-

ence a disease event. An odds ratio of 0.2 means that people exposed to a particular factor are 80% $(1 - 0.2 = 0.8 \times 100 = 80\%)$ less likely to experience a disease event. However, all calculated ratios are estimates and must be interpreted with reference to the confidence intervals (CI) that are calculated (Figure 1.15). These intervals give a measure of how reliable those estimates are. There are important differences between odds ratios, hazard ratios and relative risk ratios, and they are all calculated in different ways (Table 1.10). As a result, they are not interchangeable terms, and they are often used with specific study types. Odds ratios are calculated in most case–control studies, while relative risk is more often used in much larger cohort studies or with RCTs.

1.6.6 Study designs in nutritional epidemiology

There are a number of different approaches that can be taken to explore diet–disease relationships in human populations, and these vary in their capacity to determine causality of relationships (Table 1.11). Figure 1.16 shows a hierarchy of research designs that has the study designs with the lowest methodological quality (animal studies and in vitro studies, ecological studies) at the bottom and the highest methodological quality (RCTs and meta-analyses) at the top. Data from all studies need to be interpreted with this hierarchy in mind. Work performed in animals must always be viewed through the lens of species differences between animals and humans. Studies of large populations of free-living individuals (cohort studies) will inevitably be subject to unaccounted-for confounding factors and other bias, which can only be eliminated though an RCT.

Table 1.10 Definitions of key terms in epidemiology.

Term	Definition
Relative risk	An indicator of the risk of an event (e.g. disease) occurring in one group compared with another. It is the ratio of the probability* of an event occurring in an exposed group and the probability of an event occurring in a control group.
Odds ratio	An indicator of the risk of an event (e.g. disease) occurring in one group compared with another. It is the ratio of the odds† of an event occurring in an exposed group and the odds of an event occurring in a control group
Hazard ratio	An indicator of the risk of an event (e.g. death) occurring in one group compared to another. It is calculated from the rates at which events occur over a period of time in the two groups
Incidence rate	Incidence measures the risk of developing a disease within a given measure of time (e.g. the number of new cases of cancer per year)
Prevalence rate	Prevalence measures the proportion of people within a population who have a particular disease. It is usually expressed as the number of affected people for a given population size (e.g. the number of cancer cases per 100 000 population)

* Probability is a measure of how likely an event is and is calculated as number of adverse outcome/total number of outcomes. It is usually expressed as a value from 0 to 1.
† Odds are also measures of how likely an event is but are calculated as probability of an event/1 minus the probability.

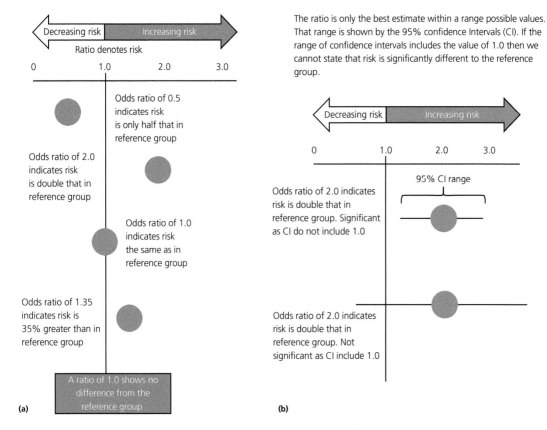

Figure 1.15 Understanding the odds ratio (OR). a) Odds ratio is a descriptor of the risk of event compared with a reference group. For the reference point or group, the OR is set at 1.0. If the OR is less than 1.0, that indicates decreased risk. If it is more than 1.0, it indicates increased risk. b) OR is an estimate of risk; the quality of that estimate will depend upon methodological factors and biological variation. The range of possible values for the OR is represented by 95% confidence intervals. These intervals are used to distinguish between OR estimates that show a significant relationship between exposure and risk and those which do not. *Source:* adapted from Institute of Medicine (2011).

Table 1.11 Factors to consider when designing a study to examine diet–disease relationships.

Study type	Typical complexity*	Typical duration†	Typical cost‡	Use
Animal/in vitro study	Moderate	Short	Low	Early test of hypotheses (equivalent to randomized controlled trial). Mechanistic study.
Meta-analysis	Low	Short	Low	Synthesis greater body of evidence to develop robust view of strength of diet–disease relationship.
Ecological	Low	Short	Low	Development of hypothesis.
Cross-sectional	Low	Short	Low	Test for existence of simple association between diet and disease.
Case–control	Moderate	Short	Low	Determine strength of a diet–disease relationship.
Cohort	High	Long	High	Examine contribution of dietary factors to future disease risk.
Randomized controlled trial	Moderate	Moderate	High	Establish causal nature of any diet–disease relationship.

* Complexity of studies may depend on means of collecting data (data extraction through to laboratory measures), need to manage study population (no population for reviews or ecological designs, through to following cohort for decades) and size of research team required (possibly one person for in vitro study, through to dozens of staff for complex prospective cohort).
† Short: 1–6 months; Moderate: 6–12 months; High: > 12 months.
‡ Low: £5–50k; Moderate: £50–250k; High: > £250k.

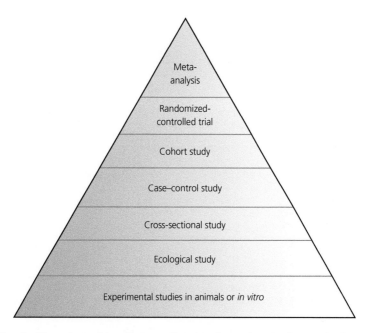

Figure 1.16 Hierarchy of evidence in nutrition–disease studies. Experiments in animals or in vitro have the lowest methodological quality, while randomized controlled trials and meta-analyses are of highest quality.

While considering the hierarchy of evidence is important when judging the validity of a diet–disease relationship, it is also important to avoid slavish faith in this hierarchy. Studies in each category could be excellent in their design or hopelessly flawed. A perfectly thought through and executed case–control study, which accounts for its limitations, can be of great value to the research field. In contrast, an RCT with a poor design (for example an inadequate randomization protocol or poor participant compliance) is of no value at all. Systematic reviews can be poorly executed and can fail to spot bias.

Knowing that there are clear differences in the value of different approaches to studying diet and disease (Figure 1.16), it is natural to wonder why not all studies follow the gold standard of an RCT. The choice of study type is invariably a pragmatic one, in which the researchers have to weigh up the relative difficulty (an ecological study is considerably less challenging than a case–control design); practical time-span (a cohort may require decades, but a cross-sectional study gives a rapid result); cost (ecological studies are resource light, but a decades long cohort can require many millions in funding to complete successfully) and may be a burden on the participants (RCTs require an intervention and adherence to protocol, while other designs are less burdensome). Table 1.12 shows the circumstances in which a particular research design may be most appropriate. When studies require invasive sampling for determining the contribution of nutritional

factors to disease mechanisms, an animal or cell culture-based approach is generally superior.

1.6.6.1 Ecological studies

An ecological study is an observational study which seeks to compare the general characteristics of whole populations to determine the factors that explain variation in disease risk between those populations (Table 1.12). For example, there may be gross differences in coronary heart disease death among the countries of Europe, and we may wish to determine whether those differences arise due to variation in diet. Alternatively, we may wish to determine why rates of coronary heart disease death in one location in 2012 are much lower than in 1992. To approach these questions, data about outcome will generally be extracted from government or international databases, and data about exposure will be collected from national diet and nutrition surveys or international sources such as the FAO food balance sheets. Importantly, these are summary data about large groups of people rather than data that have been collected on individuals (Figure 1.17). These data are then used to examine simple correlations between exposures and outcomes.

Ecological studies are ideal for examining new ideas and developing hypotheses that can be explored using approaches with greater methodological quality and capacity for determining causality. They have many weaknesses, however, not least the fact that the findings generated from group data are not necessarily applicable to individuals in a

Table 1.12 Study designs in nutritional epidemiology.

Study design	Approach taken
Ecological study	Nutritional exposures and disease outcomes are considered in populations that are grouped by geographical area or time period. Only population averages and not individual data are analysed.
Cross-sectional study	A descriptive study which measures nutritional exposure and disease outcome in a single population at a specific point in time.
Case–control study	A study which compares nutritional exposures in a population with a specific disease to a similar reference population without disease.
Cohort study	An observational study which follows a population over time. This allows nutritional exposure measured at the beginning (baseline) to be related to disease that develops over the course of the study. Follow-up from baseline may be over many years.
Randomized controlled trial	An experimental study in which a randomly selected group of people are administered nutrients, foodstuffs or other interventions focused on nutrition and are compared with a matched control group over a period of follow-up.

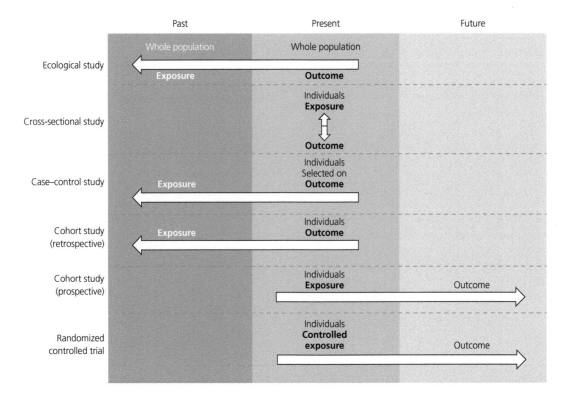

Figure 1.17 Research designs in epidemiology.

population (this is termed the ecological fallacy). The way in which data are collected leads to numerous problems; for example, the data on dietary exposure may have been collected in different ways in different countries (heterogeneity of exposure) and may not be truly comparable. The exposure and outcome may not have even been determined in exactly the same populations (e.g. data on diet in 1992 was collected in England, Wales and Scotland, but data on heart disease was collected in the whole UK – England, Wales, Northern Ireland and Scotland). Ecological studies are also highly prone to uncontrollable confounding factors.

1.6.6.2 Cross-sectional studies
A cross-sectional study is an observational study in which the exposure and outcome are measured simultaneously in a group of individuals (Figure 1.17).

The cross-sectional study will then attempt to relate disease outcomes to current dietary factors (Table 1.12). This can be a quick and inexpensive approach to examine simple diet–disease relationships. For example, it could very quickly show a relationship between BMI and energy intake. However, it is not possible to state with any certainty whether a relationship is causal. Is high energy intake a cause of high BMI or do people with a high BMI consume more energy to meet a greater demand? Another problem of the cross-sectional study is that the individuals who have a disease may change their behaviour because of the disease and hence mask the relationship. Subjects with high blood pressure, for example, may be advised by their doctors to reduce salt intake, thereby hiding a simple relationship between salt and blood pressure.

1.6.6.3 Case–control studies

Case–control studies are observational studies which deliberately sample a group of people who are confirmed to have a disease of interest (cases) for comparison with a group of people without the disease (controls; Table 1.12). The exposure of the two groups to dietary factors in the past will then be compared to see whether risk of disease can be related to those factors (Figure 1.17). For example, a group of people with high blood pressure can be compared with a group with normal blood pressure by considering salt intakes over the preceding 10 years. This approach could address the question of whether long-term, habitual salt intake is a causal factor in the development of high blood pressure.

The case–control study is a quick and inexpensive approach to epidemiology as a relatively small number of subjects is required. This is because the selection of people with the disease ensures a good representation of the diseased population which may not be possible with a cohort study (see the following text). When the disease of interest is rare, the case–control design becomes especially powerful, as it draws together a population that is unlikely to be sampled in a cohort study. The case–control study can also consider more than one exposure variable in the diet. There are significant problems with case–control designs, however, of which the most important is the fact that while outcome is usually well defined, the exposure must be established retrospectively. As described earlier, assessment of diet in individuals is problematic, and this becomes even more prone to recall bias when looking back over many years. The other major problem is the recruitment of a suitable control group. Matching closely to the cases (e.g. similar ages, same sex) is important for reducing confounding bias.

The control group should also come from the same geographical area as the cases so that it represents the same population as the cases were recruited from. Often, they are patients with other conditions who are recruited from the same clinics and hospitals as the cases. Good studies will carefully examine the health of the controls to ensure that they do not have the disease of interest (undiagnosed cases). Poor selection of controls can greatly undermine the quality of a case–control study.

1.6.6.4 Cohort studies

Cohort studies are also referred to as longitudinal studies, as they seek to study a large group of people over a set period (Figure 1.17). They identify exposures in a population and then by following the cohort over time identify outcomes as they occur and compare the incidence of disease in exposed individuals with unexposed individuals (Table 1.12). The Framingham Heart Study, for example, recruited 5209 men and women aged 30–62 years in the town of Framingham, Massachusetts, in 1948. These subjects have been examined every two years since the inception of the study, allowing determination of the major cardiovascular risk factors that predict heart disease morbidity and mortality (blood pressure, blood cholesterol, obesity, diabetes, physical inactivity).

Cohort studies may report findings from prospective cohorts or retrospective cohorts. A prospective cohort is generally recruited for a specific purpose and collects baseline data and conducts follow-up measurements at intervals over several years before reporting final outcomes. A retrospective cohort will generally involve collecting disease outcome data in a large group of people and then tracing back events by collecting historical records that provide the exposure data. For example, a prospective cohort to examine the relationship between diet and cancer would recruit a population, characterize their diet and follow for a period to see if occurrence of cancer was related to diet many years before. A retrospective cohort would look at a population of people, including people with and without cancer, and look back to see if the diets of subjects from 10 to 20 years earlier differed among cancer sufferers and those without cancer. Retrospective cohorts are generally smaller and less expensive to study than prospective cohorts but are more prone to confounding bias due to the passing of time and incomplete historical record-keeping.

1.6.6.5 Randomized controlled trials

RCTs are generally regarded as the gold-standard method for an epidemiological study (Table 1.12).

RCTs are essentially clinical experiments in which individuals are randomly assigned to be a control (no treatment) or to receive some form of intervention as a controlled exposure (Figure 1.17). In nutritional epidemiology, that intervention will generally be the administration of a supplemental nutrient (e.g. antioxidant, essential fatty acid) or a behavioural intervention related to food intake or weight control (e.g. increased physical activity, adoption of a meat-free diet).

The nature of the RCT design means that it can provide strong evidence of cause and effect. If control and intervention groups are carefully matched for key characteristics, there will generally be no issue of confounding and as the experimenters have control over the exposure, there are few issues of bias in the measurement of that exposure. Problems can arise due to non-compliance with the protocol. Participants may, for example, not take supplements as directed. RCTs in nutrition are, however, often less effective than similar studies where the treatments are drugs (clinical trials). This is because the diet–disease relationships can often be quite weak and can take years to develop. It is generally not feasible to carry out a supplementation trial over many years due to expense, because the subjects may become disaffected or disturbed by minor adverse effects and may drop out, and because the nature of the intervention may become apparent to the control group, prompting them to change their diet and behaviour in a way that detracts from the analysis (e.g. although not allocated to receive a folate supplement, the controls may consume more natural sources in the belief that it will be healthier). While drug trials can be easily blinded so that the participants and researchers are not aware of allocation to control or test groups, this is sometimes not possible within a nutrition trial (e.g. an exercise intervention cannot be disguised as something else). Thus, the intervention can introduce behavioural changes among participants, which can distort study findings.

1.6.6.6 Systematic review and meta-analysis

Systematic review is an approach to research that makes use of existing evidence to address a specific research question. In the same way as a laboratory experiment, clinical trial or single epidemiological study, the systematic review will use rigorous methodology to ensure that the quality of the finished review is reliable and robust. Systematic reviews synthesize the findings of all available research on a particular topic in an unbiased manner and produce an impartial summary of the findings, which fully considers flaws and gaps in the evidence base. This is an extremely powerful tool for evaluating the balance of evidence, particularly in areas where there is apparent controversy and uncertainty. The use of explicit, systematic methods in reviews limits bias (systematic errors) and reduces chance effects. This provides more reliable results upon which to draw conclusions, as these can be based on the totality of the available evidence rather than the elements that suit the bias of a narrative review. Systematic reviews use modern electronic database searches to access all published works related to a research question. These works and any material obtained from other sources (e.g. direct communication with experts in the field to obtain unpublished material) comprise the data that are subsequently analysed.

Systematic reviews are often combined with the analytical technique called meta-analysis. Meta-analysis enables researchers to exploit greater statistical power by effectively combining the results of several studies to generate a larger and robust sample. This enables inconsistency between studies to be both quantified and overcome and more precise measures of risk to be calculated. An example of the power of meta-analysis to resolve contentious issues is shown in Research Highlight 1.3. Other chapters of this book make frequent reference to meta-analysis.

The 2007 World Cancer Research Fund Expert Report detailed a systematic review of the evidence on salt and stomach cancer, which included data from 3 cohort studies, 21 case–control studies and 12 ecological studies. This systematic review was able to generate a meta-analysis that included data from two of the cohorts and nine of the case–control studies (World Cancer Research Fund, 2007). Using the combined data sets, the expert group found that there was a small but significant relationship apparent in the cohort studies (RR 1.08, 95% CI 1.00–1.17) and a close to significant relationship apparent in the case–control studies (RR 1.01, 95% CI 0.99–1.04). On this basis, the reviewers were able to conclude that there is a probable causal relationship between high salt intake and stomach cancer. Without a robust, unbiased review process and well-conducted meta-analysis, this conclusion would have been impossible to reach.

1.6.6.7 Scoping reviews

Scoping reviews are another form of research synthesis in which the researcher pulls together all the research in a particular area, using similar methodology to a systematic review. The aim of a scoping review is different though, and the purpose is to consider the amount of research that has been performed in an area, what type of research has been done and where the gaps in knowledge are. The outcome of a

Research Highlight 1.3   The power of meta-analysis.

A role for magnesium in the development of cardiovascular disease has long been suspected, with reports from the animal literature suggesting that low intakes increase the progression of atherosclerosis in susceptible mouse strains and some cross-sectional studies of humans indicating an inverse relationship between magnesium intake and blood pressure. A number of studies have suggested that people who have low concentrations of magnesium in their habitual source of drinking water are at greater risk of cardiovascular death (Chakraborti *et al.*, 2002).

Studies that have specifically addressed the question of whether low magnesium intake is a risk factor for cardiovascular disease have found conflicting results. Abbott *et al.* (2003), for example, reported that among men aged 45–68 at baseline, risk of cardiovascular disease over the next 30 years was increased by 50–80% in those in the lowest quintile of magnesium intake. Similarly, Chiuve *et al.* (2011) found that in the Nurses' Health Study, which followed 88 375 women for 26 years, the risk of cardiovascular disease was 37% lower in the women in the highest quartile of magnesium intake compared with those in the lowest. In contrast, Kaluza *et al.* (2010) found no association between intake and disease in a follow-up of 23 366 middle-aged men. Song *et al.*, (2005) followed women for 10 years and similarly reported no association between magnesium and cardiovascular outcomes.

Qu *et al.* (2013) completed a meta-analysis of 19 studies which considered the relationship between cardiovascular disease and either magnesium intake or serum magnesium concentrations. This review encompassed 532 979 participants and over 19 000 cardiovascular events. The meta-analysis found that if magnesium intake increased from 100 to 400 mg/day, then the risk of cardiovascular events decreased significantly (OR 0.85, 95% CI 0.78–0.92). This example illustrates the power of meta-analysis to generate a clearer picture of a diet–disease relationship and to quantify the strength of that relationship. Often, this is the only realistic way to resolve conflicting indications from a diverse evidence base, often generated using variable methodologies, classifications and time spans and markedly different populations.

scoping review will usually be to recommend further investigations to researchers and policy makers. While similar methodologies are used, scoping reviews are not set up to answer specific research questions and use broader inclusion criteria than a systematic review.

1.7 Dietary reference values

Dietary reference values (DRVs) are standards that are set by the health departments of governments in a number of countries around the world. DRVs are guidelines that can be used to define the composition of diets that will maintain good health. There are many complex systems of DRVs used in different countries. These vary according to national health priorities and policies: predominant health status, socioeconomic status, body mass and rates of growth; and local factors, for example, the composition of foods or other lifestyle influences, which determine the absorption and hence bioavailability of nutrients (Pavlovic *et al.*, 2007).

DRVs are used in a variety of different ways. While some systems, such as those developed for the UK, are generally intended to be used only with populations or subgroups within populations, others (e.g. the US dietary reference intakes) are widely used in providing dietary guidance for individuals. On a population level, the DRVs are useful yardsticks with which to assess the adequacy of the diet of a population and hence protect individuals within

that population against the adverse consequences of either deficiency or excess. By using DRVs as standard measures against which dietary survey data can be compared, it is possible to estimate the prevalence of risk of deficiency for specific nutrients within a population.

In some countries, there are regular surveys of national dietary patterns among age- and sex-specific groups; for example, the UK national diet and nutrition surveys (Bates *et al.*, 2019), the French INCA surveys (ANSES, 2017) or the US National Health and Nutrition Examination Surveys (Ahluwalia *et al.*, 2016). The majority of European countries run such surveys, focusing on mixed populations of children and adults (Rippin *et al.*, 2018). Findings from such surveys are compared with the DRVs to highlight potential nutrient deficiencies. In other countries, food supply data at the national level, such as the food balance sheets collected by the FAO, can be used to crudely estimate the average per capita availability of energy and the macronutrients and compared with international standards. Although such data are prone to error, as described earlier, they can be used for tracking trends in the food supply and determining availability of micronutrient-rich foods. By comparison of such data with DRVs, it is possible to uncover evidence of gross inadequacies in the quality of the diet across whole populations (but not subgroups such as children or older adults). Standards for nutrient provision based upon DRVs can also be used in the planning of food supplies to regions (e.g. in humanitarian aid) or in menu planning for caterers in hospitals, schools or other institutional settings. Many of the food labelling schemes used in supermarkets are based upon published DRVs for specific nutrients.

1.7.1 The UK dietary reference values system

In 1979, the UK set a series of DRVs termed the recommended daily amounts (RDAs). In 1991, a new series of DRVs were published to replace these RDA values, as they were considered to be prone to misunderstanding and misuse. The term 'recommended' wrongly suggests a level of intake that an individual must consume on a daily basis to avoid adverse consequences. The new system of DRVs produced by the Committee on Medical Aspects of Food Policy (COMA; Department of Health, 1991) therefore dropped the word recommended and the system was developed to indicate different levels of intake that would be suitable for healthy populations, according to age and sex.

In setting the DRVs, COMA reviewed research for each macro- and micronutrient to determine the levels of intake that are necessary to maintain normal health and physiological function. In considering the available evidence, the key issues to be explored for each nutrient were: (1) What level of intake is necessary to maintain circulating or tissue concentrations within normal ranges? (2) What level of intake is necessary to avoid clinical deficiency in individuals or in populations? (3) What level of intake has been established as being effec-

tive in treating clinical deficiency? (4) What level of intake has been shown to maintain normality in a biomarker of adequacy?

As shown in Figure 1.18, the relationship between nutrient intake and disease risk is not linear. At low levels of intake, the probability of adverse consequences (deficiency disease, loss of physiological function) is elevated. With rising intakes, the probability of such consequences declines to zero as intakes provide the requirements of most of the individuals in a population. At higher intakes, the probability of adverse consequences associated with overnutrition begins to rise. In developing a set of DRVs appropriate for a population like the UK, in which the economic wealth of the population makes overnutrition more likely than undernutrition, this continuum between risk and intake must be recognized.

In common with the United States and other countries (see the following text), the UK DRVs were developed to map to the expected distribution of nutrient requirements in a population. As shown in Figure 1.19, this would usually be expected to follow a normal distribution, which actually relates to the left-hand side of the distribution of risk plotted against intake. In this context, the mean value (midpoint) in a normal distribution would represent a level of nutrient intake at which the requirements of 50% of the people in a population would be met. Within the UK DRV system, this point is termed the estimated average requirement (EAR). When a population is consuming a nutrient at a level close to

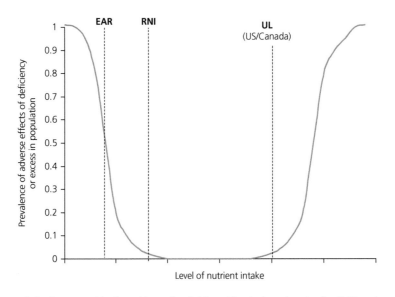

Figure 1.18 The association between risk of nutrition-related risk and level of nutrient intake. EAR, estimated average requirement; RNI, reference nutrient intake; UL, tolerable upper limit.

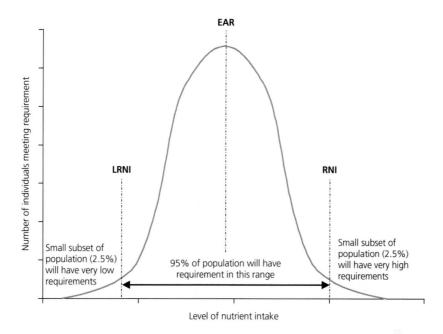

Figure 1.19 The normal distribution as a basis for dietary reference values (DRVs). UK DRVs are based upon an assumed normal distribution of individuals' nutrient requirements and level of nutrient intake. The estimated average requirement (EAR) is set at the centre (mean) of the distribution. The lower reference nutrient intake (LRNI) and reference nutrient intake (RNI) values are placed two standard deviations below and above the mean, respectively. The nutrient requirements of all but 5% of the population should therefore be met by levels of intake between these two values.

the EAR, it can be assumed that for 50% of people this will be sufficient, but that for up to 50% nutritional status would be compromised.

The other DRVs are set at points that are two standard deviations either side of the mean. The reference nutrient intake (RNI) is the upper value and within the normal distribution would represent a level of intake that should meet the requirements of 97.5% of the population. When a population is consuming a nutrient at a level close to the RNI, it can be assumed that for most individuals, this intake will be sufficient or will exceed true requirements, but that for the 2.5% of individuals with extremely high requirements, nutritional status would be compromised. The lower RNI (LRNI) lies at the lower end of the normal distribution and represents a level of intake that would meet the requirements of just 2.5% of the population. If a population was consuming a nutrient at a level close to the LRNI, it could be assumed that for most individuals, this would be insufficient and that deficiency disease would be rife.

For some nutrients (e.g. pantothenic acid, biotin and molybdenum), COMA had insufficient data to be able to derive estimates of requirements but recognized the biological importance of these compounds in the diet. In the absence of extensive information, the safe intake was set. This is an upper limit of intake set at a point likely to prevent deficiency and avoid toxicity. Safe intakes are of greatest importance to vulnerable groups in the population such as infants and children (Department of Health, 1991).

The DRVs are published as a comprehensive series of tables (Department of Health, 1999), which, for most nutrients, provide reference values for males and females separately and for different age groups (typically 0–12 months, 1–3 years, 4–6 years, 7–10 years, 11–14 years, 15–18 years, 19–50 years and 50+ years). To reflect increased demands for nutrients during pregnancy and lactation, some tables show additional increments of intake for pregnant and breastfeeding women. For micronutrients and trace elements, published values include all three terms (LRNI, EAR and RNI). With respect to protein, only EAR and RNI values were determined. Given that excess energy consumption is a driver of obesity and related disorders, it is undesirable to set reference values at an upper point such as the RNI, as a population that consumed energy at that level would be expected to have a high prevalence of related adverse effects such as obesity. DRV tables for energy therefore include only the EAR value and include modifiers to allow for levels of physical activity.

Humans have a requirement for essential fatty acids, and children can develop clinical deficiency of linoleic acid. There are DRVs that indicate minimum intakes of essential fatty acids, but as low intakes of the majority of lipids are not associated with adverse health effects, the three main DRV terms are not applied to fats and carbohydrates. Instead, COMA sets population average guidelines for consumption of saturated, monounsaturated and polyunsaturated fats based on percentage of dietary energy provided by those sources. These guidelines represent maximum intakes in the light of the established risk of cardiovascular disease with high-fat intakes (see Section 8.3). This element of the UK DRV system differs from other components, as it firmly indicates guidelines for individuals to follow rather than appropriate ranges for healthy populations (Whitehead, 1992). In the same way, COMA set guidance values for sugars and complex carbohydrates based on percentages of dietary energy intake. Population averages are designed to encourage lower intakes of free sugars (mono- and disaccharides added to food, sugars in unsweetened fruit juices, honey and syrups) and fats, while increasing intakes of starch and fibre. In 2015, the Scientific Advisory Committee on Nutrition revised the population averages for carbohydrates. Overall, the guideline for 50% of daily energy to be derived from carbohydrate was unchanged but, as shown in Table 1.13, the guideline for free sugars was reduced from 10% to 5% of daily energy. The same report recommended a major increase in the population average intake for dietary fibre from 18 g/day for adults to 30 g/day (Table 1.13).

In the UK, the DRVs are not intended to be guidelines for individuals. It is generally considered a fruitless activity to make estimates of nutrient intakes for individuals, given the problems with obtaining accurate data on food intake and because it is impossible to estimate what the true requirements for any individual are likely to be. In making assessments of dietary intakes of groups within a population, the RNI is considered to be the most important benchmark for comparison. The nearer the average intake of a group within a survey is to the RNI, the less likely it is that any individual within that group will have an inadequate intake. However, the LRNI value provides a better indicator of the likely risk of widespread deficiency, whether clinical or subclinical. The nearer the average intake of the group is to the LRNI, the greater is the probability that some individuals within that group are not consuming that nutrient at a level adequate to meet their requirements.

Many studies provide examples of the DRVs in use for highlighting nutritional shortfalls or excess in populations. Mendonca et al. (2016) used a multiple pass recall approach (two 24-hour recalls) to assess the diets of 793 men and women aged 75 years. They found that 95% consumed vitamin D below the RNI; 52.8% consumed selenium below the LRNI, and the LRNI was not met by 20% for magnesium and potassium, and by 10% for zinc, vitamin A and vitamin B12. All these nutrients play key roles in maintaining bone and cardiovascular health and musculoskeletal function, so the study was able to raise the need for this group in the population to consume a more nutrient dense diet. Pot et al., 2012 analysed data on fat intake from the first year of the UK National Diet and Nutrition Survey rolling programme and compared it with previous UK surveys and the DRVs. They found that, with the exception of men aged 19–64 years and girls aged 11–18 years, total fat consumption was close to the DRV. In contrast, intakes of saturated fat exceeded the DRV and intakes of monounsaturated fatty acids were below the DRV for all population groups. In this way, the analysis was able to demonstrate that while the UK diet was improving over time, there was still excessive intake of fatty acids associated with poor cardiovascular health. Similarly, Derbyshire (2017) carried out analysis of national diet and nutrition survey data, focusing on intakes of red meat and micronutrients in females aged 11–64 years. Among those consuming less than 40 g meat per day, a high proportion consumed micronutrients below the LRNI (iron 37.7%, zinc 18.9%, selenium 51.3%, potassium 31.2%, vitamin B2 17.9%). The study was therefore able to conclude that as national guidelines encourage the population to eat less meat, there may consequently be a developing issue with shortfalls in important micronutrients.

Table 1.13 UK average population intakes for free sugars and fibre.

Age (y)	Intake (g/d)
Free sugars	No more than 5% of dietary energy
4–5	<19
5–11	<24
>11	<30
Dietary fibre	
2–5	15
5–11	20
11–16	25
>16	30

Source: Scientific Advisory Committee on Nutrition (2015).

Although not intended for use with individuals, the DRVs could still be used in a clinical setting. When working with healthy individuals, assessments of dietary intakes that indicate intakes below or close to the LRNI could indicate a dietary problem and might be a stimulus for a more in-depth assessment of biochemical or clinical indicators of nutritional status. In planning a diet for an individual, the delivery of nutrients at the level of the RNI would be a basic priority to ensure optimal health.

1.7.2 Dietary reference values in other countries

The UK system described earlier is just one example of DRVs defined with the purpose of guiding the provision of healthy nutrition on a population-wide scale. Many other countries use similar systems that have also been derived to map against the normal distribution of nutrient intakes against provision of nutrient demands. This approach is generally applicable for westernized countries where the nutrition-related health concerns are usually focused on the consequences of nutrient excess rather than nutrient deficiency. Table 1.13 summarizes the dietary reference terms used in North America, Europe, Australia and New Zealand.

Among the countries of the European Union, there is considerable variation in the terminology used to describe DRVs and in the precise nature of recommendations made for particular population groups, most particularly children. The European Food Safety Authority undertook a 10-year process to completely review DRVs for European Union countries and to implement a unified system of terminology and values for nutrients. A series of publications released between 2010 and 2017 (available collectively in the *EFSA Journal*; European Food Safety Authority, 2017) set out references for macro- and micronutrients. The terminology adopted for these references is summarized in Table 1.14.

As in the UK, the countries of North America reviewed their existing reference values, originally set in 1941, and replaced them with a new comprehensive format in the early 1990s (Kennedy and Meyers, 2005). In Canada and the United States, the EAR and RDA terms are exact equivalents of the UK EAR and RNI terms but are used in a different manner to that seen in the UK. North American references, termed 'dietary reference intakes' are intended to be used as tools for assessing and planning diets or as the basis for food-based dietary guidelines. EAR is a term that would be used to estimate the prevalence of inadequate intakes in a population, but RDA is a term specifically intended for use with individuals. A habitual intake below this level would be associated with increased risk of dietary inadequacy. In population surveys, however, comparing mean intakes to the RDA would tend to overestimate the likely prevalence of deficiency, as it is a figure set at a level where the requirements of 97.5% of the population are being met. This means that a significant proportion of the population is likely to be exceeding requirement (Kennedy and Meyers, 2005). For example, if the RDA for iron intake in children is 11.2 mg/day and the mean intake for a population is found to be

Table 1.14 Definitions of dietary reference value terms used in the UK, North America, Europe and Oceania.

Region	Dietary reference term	Definition
UK	LRNI	Lower reference nutrient intake
	RNI	Reference nutrient intake
	EAR	Estimated average requirement
	Safe intake	
United States/Canada	EAR	Estimated average requirement
	RDA	Recommended daily allowance
	AI	Adequate intake
	UL	Tolerable upper limit
Australia/New Zealand	EAR	Estimated average requirement
	RDI	Recommended daily intake
	AI	Adequate intake
	EER	Estimated energy requirement
	UL	Upper level of intake
European Union	PRI	Population reference intake
	AR	Average requirement
	LTI	Lower threshold intake
	AI	Adequate intake
	RI	Reference intakes for macronutrients

8.4 mg/day, it should not be assumed that deficiency will have a high prevalence. The majority of children in the population may be consuming well below the RDA value and still be achieving requirement. The tolerable upper limit is defined as the highest average daily nutrient intake level that is unlikely to result in adverse health effects for almost all individuals in a population. Effectively, individuals could use this as a guide to limit their intake, and at the population level, it provides a benchmark against which estimates can be made of the likelihood of problems related to overnutrition. The term 'adequate intakes' is similar to the UK safe intake in that it is used only where there is insufficient data to determine the EAR for a particular nutrient. The North American equivalent of the UK population average intake is the acceptable macronutrient distribution range (AMDR), which is used to indicate the range of intakes for macronutrients which is associated with reduced risk of chronic disease. Table 1.15 shows the AMDR values for fats, protein and carbohydrates.

In Australia and New Zealand, the system of DRVs is broadly similar to that used in North America, except that a fifth term, estimated energy requirement, is defined for energy. This comprises two separate terms. The estimated energy requirement for maintenance (EERM) is the energy intake that is estimated to maintain balance in healthy individuals or populations at a given level of physical activity and body size. The desirable estimated energy requirement (DEER) is the level of energy intake that should maintain energy balance in healthy individuals or populations of a defined sex, age, weight, height and level of physical activity, consistent with optimal health. Although complex, this is an important distinction, as the EERM represents an actual energy requirement of an individual or group of individuals, while the DEER allows calculation of energy references that can be used to guide weight loss in a clinical situation (National Health and Medical Research Council of Australia, 2019). The Australian and New Zealand NRIs also include suggested dietary targets and AMDRs for the macronutrients.

All the DRV systems discussed above are not static and expert panels regularly revisit the evidence and, where necessary, issue updated values. An example of this is the UK update of the population average intakes for carbohydrates (Scientific Advisory Committee on Nutrition, 2015). Similarly, Australia and New Zealand released new reference values for fluorine and sodium in 2017.

In less affluent countries where there is a high burden of malnutrition-related disease, the priorities of governments are different, and DRVs are set at levels that are more appropriate for a setting where maintaining and monitoring food security are the main applications of the figures. Often, the values used in these situations are obtained from the FAO and focus heavily on setting levels of intake that will provide the basic requirements of most of the population and therefore avoid widespread clinical nutrient deficiency.

Table 1.15 North American acceptable macronutrient distribution ranges.

	Dietary energy (%)		
Age (y)	1–3	4–18	Adult
Fat	30–40	25–35	20–35
n-6 fatty acids	5–10	5–10	5–10
n-3 fatty acids	0.6–1.2	0.6–1.2	0.6–1.2
Protein	5–20	10–30	10–35
Carbohydrate	45–65	45–65	45–65

Source: adapted from Institute of Medicine (2011).

SUMMARY

- Nutritional balance depends upon the supply of nutrients being able to meet the physiological and metabolic demand for nutrients to be used as structural components or as substrates and cofactors for metabolism. Undernutrition or overnutrition arises through disturbance of this balance.
- Undernutrition can result from either a decrease in intake or an increase in the demand for nutrients. Increased demands are often a consequence of physiological insult or stressors, including trauma, pregnancy and lactation.
- Prolonged undernutrition can lead to micronutrient deficiency or malnutrition, which are common among infants and women in developing countries and among older adults and poor in developed nations.
- The way in which the body responds to food and nutrients is strongly influenced by genetic factors. SNPs result in common gene variants that can influence diet–disease relationships. This means that more individualized approaches to dietary guidelines may be more effective than general population guidelines.
- Stage of life is one of the most important determinants of nutritional status, as the nature of demands for nutrients and the way in which those demands are met undergo profound changes over the human lifespan.
- Personalized or stratified nutrition interventions are more targeted approaches to public health nutrition interventions, which are more effective than a 'one size fits all' strategy.

- Nutritional status can be assessed by using anthropometric methods, by using different methods of measuring intake, through clinical examination or by measuring specific biomarkers. All methods are limited in their scope and are prone to inaccuracy.
- Exploring relationships between diet and disease relies on well-designed epidemiological studies. Simple ecological and cross-sectional studies can provide clues to diet–disease associations, but more robust cohort studies and randomized controlled trials are necessary to confirm causal relationships.
- DRVs are standards for nutrient intake, which are set by governments. These standards are widely used as the basis of nutrition-related advice and interventions. They can be used as research tools, as guidance for meal planners and caterers and for the monitoring of food security at a national level.

References

Abrahams, M. and Matusheski, N.V. (2020). Personalised nutrition technologies: a new paradigm for dietetic practice and training in a digital transformation era. *Journal of Human Nutrition and Dietetics* **33**, : 295–298.

Abbott, R.D., Ando, F., Masaki, K.H. *et al.* (2003). Dietary magnesium intake and the future risk of coronary heart disease (the Honolulu Heart Program). *American Journal of Cardiology*, **92**: 665–669.

Ackermans, M.M., Zhou, H., Carels, C.E. *et al.* (2011). Vitamin A and clefting: putative biological mechanisms. *Nutrition Reviews* **69**: 613–624.

Adams, S.H., Anthony, J.C., Carvajal, R. *et al.* (2019). Perspective: guiding principles for the implementation of personalized nutrition approaches that benefit health and function. *Advances in Nutrition* **11**: 25–34.

Ahluwalia, N., Dwyer, J., Terry, A. *et al.* (2016). Update on NHANES dietary data: focus on collection, release, analytical considerations, and uses to inform public policy. *Advances in Nutrition* **7**: 121–134.

Alfthan, G., Eurola, M., Ekholm, P. *et al.* (2015). Effects of nationwide addition of selenium to fertilizers on foods, and animal and human health in Finland: from deficiency to optimal selenium status of the population. *Journal of Trace Elements in Medicine and Biology* **31**: 142–147.

Amoutzopoulos, B., Page, P., Roberts, C. *et al.* (2020). Portion size estimation in dietary assessment: a systematic review of existing tools, their strengths and limitations. *Nutrition Reviews* **78**: 885–900.

ANSES (2017). INCA studies: for a better understanding of French eating habits and consumption patterns. https://www.anses.fr/en/content/inca-studies. (accessed 30 March 2021).

Bates, B., Collins, D., Cox, L. *et al.* (2019). *National Diet and Nutrition Survey: Years 1 to 9 of the Rolling Programme (2008/2009 – 2016/2017): Time trend and income analyses.* London: Public Health England.

Betts, J.A. and Gonzalez, J.T. (2016). Personalised nutrition: what makes you so special? *Nutrition Bulletin* **41**: 353–359.

Black, R.E., Allen, L.H., Bhutta, Z.A. *et al.* (2008). Maternal and child undernutrition: global and regional exposures and health consequences. *Lancet* **371**: 243–260.

Black, R.E., Victora, C.G., Walker, S.P. *et al.* (2013). Maternal and child undernutrition and overweight in low-income and middle-income countries. *Lancet*, **382**: 427–451.

Block, G. (1989). Human dietary assessment: methods and issues. *Preventive Medicine* **18**: 653–660.

Block, G., Clifford, C., Naughtton, M.D. *et al.* (1989). A brief dietary screen for high fat intake. *Journal of Nutrition Education* **21**: 199–207.

Brassard, D., Lemieux, S., Charest, A. *et al.* (2018). Comparing interviewer-administered and web-based food frequency questionnaires to predict energy requirements in adults. *Nutrients* **10**: pii: E1292.

Carlson, J.E. (2008). *Genocide: How Your Doctor's Dietary Ignorance Will Kill You!!!!* Booksurge Publishing.

Celis-Morales, C., Marsaux, C.F., Livingstone, K.M. *et al.* (2017). Can genetic-based advice help you lose weight? Findings from the Food4Me European randomized controlled trial. *American Journal of Clinical Nutrition* **105**: 1204–1213.

Chakraborti, S., Chakraborti, T., Mandal, M. *et al.* (2002). Protective role of magnesium in cardiovascular diseases: a review. *Molecular and Cell Biochemistry* **238**: 163–179.

Chiuve, S.E., Korngold, E.C., Januzzi, J.L. Jr *et al.* (2011). Plasma and dietary magnesium and risk of sudden cardiac death in women. *American Journal of Clinical Nutrition* **93**: 253–260.

Chowdhury, R., Sinha, B., Sankar, M.J. *et al.* (2015). Breastfeeding and maternal health outcomes: a systematic review and meta-analysis. *Acta Paediatrica* **104**: 96–113.

Conti, G., Chirico, V., Lacquaniti, A. *et al.* (2014). Vitamin D intoxication in two brothers: be careful with dietary supplements. *Journal of Pediatric Endocrinology and Metabolism* **27**: 763–767.

Conway, J.M., Ingwersen, L.A. and Moshfegh, A.J. (2004). Accuracy of dietary recall using the USDA five-step multiple-pass method in men: an observational validation study. *Journal of the American Dietetic Association* **104**: 595–603.

Derbyshire E. (2017). Associations between red meat intakes and the micronutrient intake and status of uk females: a secondary analysis of the uk national diet and nutrition survey. *Nutrients* **18**: 768.

Department of Health. (1991). *Dietary Reference Values for Energy and Nutrients for the United Kingdom.* London: Stationery Office.

Department of Health. (1999) *Dietary Reference Values for Energy and Nutrients for the United Kingdom*, London: Stationery Office.

Doets, E.L., de Hoogh, I.M., Holthuysen, N. *et al.* (2019). Beneficial effect of personalized lifestyle advice compared to generic advice on wellbeing among Dutch seniors: an explorative study. *Physiology and Behaviour* **210**: 112642.

European Food Safety Authority. (2017). Dietary reference values. *EFSA Journal* Virtual issues https://efsa.onlinelibrary.wiley.com/doi/toc/10.1002/(ISSN)1831-4732.021217 (accessed 30 March 2021).

El-Bastawissi, A.Y., Peters, R., Sasseen, K. *et al.* (2007). Effect of the Washington Special Supplemental Nutrition

Program for Women, Infants and Children (WIC) on pregnancy outcomes. *Maternal and Child Health Journal* **11**: 611–621.

Ericson, U., Sonestedt, E., Ivarsson, M.I. *et al.* (2009). Folate intake, methylenetetrahydrofolate reductase polymorphisms, and breast cancer risk in women from the Malmö diet and cancer cohort. *Cancer Epidemiology Biomarkers and Prevention* **18**: 1101–1110.

Faber, M., Phungula, M.A., Venter, S.L. *et al.* (2002). Home gardens focusing on the production of yellow and dark-green leafy vegetables increase the serum retinol concentrations of 2–5-y-old children in South Africa. *American Journal of Clinical Nutrition* **76**: 1048–1054.

Ferrari, S.L., Rizzoli, R., Slosman, D.O. *et al.* (1998). Do dietary calcium and age explain the controversy surrounding the relationship between bone mineral density and vitamin D receptor gene polymorphisms? *Journal of Bone and Mineral Research* **13**: 363–370.

Folta, S.C., Seguin, R.A., Chui, K.K. *et al.* (2015). National dissemination of strong women-healthy hearts: a community-based program to reduce risk of cardiovascular disease among midlife and older women. *American Journal of Public Health* **105**: 2578–2585.

Foster, E., Hawkins, A., Barton, K.L. *et al.* (2017). Development of food photographs for use with children aged 18 months to 16 years: Comparison against weighed food diaries: the young person's food atlas (UK). *PLoS One* **12**: e0169084.

Frobisher, C. and Maxwell, S.M. (2003). The estimation of food portion sizes: a comparison between using descriptions of portion sizes and a photographic food atlas by children and adults. *Journal of Human Nutrition and Dietetics* **16**: 181–188.

Godfrey, K., Robinson, S., Barker, D.J. *et al.* (1996). Maternal nutrition in early and late pregnancy in relation to placental and fetal growth. *British Medical Journal* **312**: 410–414.

Grimble, R.F. (2001). Stress proteins in disease: metabolism on a knife edge. *Clinical Nutrition* **20**: 469–476.

Hambidge, K.M., Huffer, J.W., Raboy, V. *et al.* (2004). Zinc absorption from low-phytate hybrids of maize and their wild-type isohybrids. *American Journal of Clinical Nutrition* **79**: 1053–1059.

Hassan, M.A. and Killick, S.R. (2004). Negative lifestyle is associated with a significant reduction in fecundity. *Fertility and Sterility* **81**: 384–392.

Hefferon, K.L. (2015). Nutritionally enhanced food crops; progress and perspectives. *International Journal of Molecular Science* **16**: 3895–3914.

Hurst, R., Siyame, E.W., Young, S.D. *et al.* (2013). Soil-type influences human selenium status and underlies widespread selenium deficiency risks in Malawi. *Scientific Reports* **3**: 1425.

Institute of Medicine. (2011). *Dietary Reference Intakes (DRIs): Acceptable macronutrient distribution ranges*. Washington DC: National Academy of Sciences.

Joost, H.G., Gibney, M.J., Cashman, K.D. *et al.* (2007) Personalised nutrition: status and perspectives. *British Journal of Nutrition* **98**: 26–31.

Joy, E.J., Broadley, M.R., Young, S.D. *et al.* (2015). Soil type influences crop mineral composition in Malawi. *Science of the Total Environment* **505**: 587–595.

Joy, E.J.M., Kalimbira, A.A., Gashu, D. *et al.* (2019). Can selenium deficiency in Malawi be alleviated through consumption of agro-biofortified maize flour? Study protocol for a randomised, double-blind, controlled trial. *Trials*, **20**,795.

Kakkoura, M.G., Demetriou, C.A., Loizidou, M.A. *et al.* (2015). Single-nucleotide polymorphisms in one-carbon metabolism genes, Mediterranean diet and breast cancer risk: a case–control study in the Greek-Cypriot female population. *Genes and Nutrition* **10**: 453.

Kaluza, J., Orsini, N., Levitan, E.B. *et al.* (2010). Dietary calcium and magnesium intake and mortality: a prospective study of men. *American Journal of Epidemiology* **171**: 801–807.

Kapil, U., Sharma, T.D. and Singh, P. (2007). Iodine status and goiter prevalence after 40 years of salt iodisation in the Kangra District, India. *Indian Journal of Pediatrics* **74**: 135–137.

Kaput, J. and Rodriguez, R.L. (2004). Nutritional genomics: the next frontier in the postgenomic era. *Physiology and Genomics* **16**: 166–177.

Kardinaal, A.F., Kok, F.J., Ringstad, J. *et al.* (1993). Antioxidants in adipose tissue and risk of myocardial infarction: the EURAMIC study. *Lancet* **342**: 1379–1384.

Kennedy, E. and Meyers, L. (2005). Dietary reference intakes: development and uses for assessment of micronutrient status of women: a global perspective. *American Journal of Clinical Nutrition* **81**: 1194S–1197S.

King, J.C. (1990). Assessment of zinc status. *Journal of Nutrition* **120**(Suppl. 11): 1474–1479.

Klerk, M., Verhoef, P., Clarke, R. *et al.* (2002). MTHFR 677C→T polymorphism and risk of coronary heart disease: a meta-analysis. *Journal of the American Medical Association* **288**: 2023–2031.

Koebnick, C., Wagner, K., Thielecke, F. *et al.* (2005). An easy-to-use semi-quantitative food record validated for energy intake by using doubly labelled water technique. *European Journal of Clinical Nutrition* **59**: 989–995.

Kong, K., Zhang, L., Huang, L. *et al.* (2017). Validity and practicability of smartphone-based photographic food records for estimating energy and nutrient intake. *Asia Pacific Journal of Clinical Nutrition* **26**: 396–401.

Kumar, S., Palve, A., Joshi, C. *et al.* (2019). Crop biofortification for iron (Fe), zinc (Zn) and vitamin A with transgenic approaches. *Heliyon* **5**: e01914.

Langley-Evans, S.C. (2015). Nutrition in early life and the programming of adult disease: a review. *Journal of Human Nutrition and Dietetics* **28**(Suppl. 1): 1–14.

Lenz, A., Franklin, G.A. and Cheadle, W.G. (2007). Systemic inflammation after trauma. *Injury* **38**: 1336–1345.

Lonn, E., Yusuf, S., Arnold, M.J. *et al.* (2006) Homocysteine lowering with folic acid and B vitamins in vascular disease. *New England Journal of Medicine* **354**: 1567–1577.

Lowe, N., Gupta, S. and Brazier, A. (2020). Zinc deficiency in low and middle income countries: prevalence and approaches for mitigation. *Journal of Human Nutrition and Dietetics* **33**: 624–643.

Ma, E., Iwasaki, M., Junko, I. *et al.* (2009). Dietary intake of folate, vitamin B6, and vitamin B12, genetic polymorphism of related enzymes, and risk of breast cancer: a case-control study in Brazilian women. *BMC Cancer* **9**: 122.

Martinaityte, I., Kamycheva, E., Didriksen, A. *et al.* (2017). Vitamin D stored in fat tissue during a 5-year intervention affects serum 25-hydroxyvitamin d levels the following year. *Journal of Clinical Endocrinology and Metabolism* **102**: 3731–3738.

Mayer, J.E. (2007). Delivering golden rice to developing countries. *Journal of AOAC International* **90**: 1445–1449.

Mendonça, N., Hill, T.R., Granic, A. *et al.* (2016). Micronutrient intake and food sources in the very old: analysis of the Newcastle 85+ Study. *British Journal of Nutrition* **116**: 751–761.

Millward, D.J., Fereday, A., Gibson, N. *et al.* (1997). Aging, protein requirements, and protein turnover. *American Journal of Clinical Nutrition* **66**: 774–786.

Morris, A.P., Voight, B.F., Teslovich, T.M. *et al.* (2012). Large-scale association analysis provides insights into the genetic architecture and pathophysiology of type 2 diabetes. *Nature Genetics* **44**: 981–990.

MRC Vitamin Study Group. (1991). Prevention of neural tube defects: results of the Medical Research Council Vitamin Study. MRC Vitamin Study Research Group. *Lancet* **338**: 131–137.

Muñoz, N., Plummer, M., Vivas, J. *et al.* (2001) A case–control study of gastric cancer in Venezuela. *International Journal of Cancer* **93**: 417–423.

Murakami, K. and Livingstone, M.B. (2015). Prevalence and characteristics of misreporting of energy intake in US children and adolescents: National Health and Nutrition Examination Survey (NHANES) 2003–2012. *British Journal of Nutrition* **115**: 294–304.

National Health and Medical Research Council of Australia. (2019). Nutrient Reference Values for Australia and New Zealand. Dietary energy. https://www.nrv.gov.au/dietary-energy (accessed 30 March 2921).

Ohly, H., Broadley, M.R., Joy, E.J.M. *et al.* (2019). The BiZiFED project: biofortified zinc flour to eliminate deficiency in Pakistan. *Nutrition Bulletin* **44**: 60–64.

Olafsdottir, A.S., Hörnell, A., Hedelin, M. *et al.* (2016). Development and validation of a photographic method to use for dietary assessment in school settings. *PLoS One* **11**: e0163970.

Ordovas, J.M., Ferguson, L.R., Tai, E.S. *et al.* (2018). Personalised nutrition and health. *BMJ* **361**: bmj.k2173.

Pandav, C.S., Yadav, K., Salve, H.R. *et al.* (2018). High national and sub-national coverage of iodised salt in India: evidence from the first National Iodine and Salt Intake Survey (NISI) 2014–2015. *Public Health Nutrition* **21**: 3027–3036.

Patro-Gołąb, B., Zalewski, B.M., Kołodziej, M. *et al.* (2016). Nutritional interventions or exposures in infants and children aged up to 3 years and their effects on subsequent risk of overweight, obesity and body fat: a systematic review of systematic reviews. *Obesity Reviews* **17**: 1245–1257.

Pavlovic, M., Prentice, A., Thorsdottir, I. *et al.* (2007). Challenges in harmonizing energy and nutrient recommendations in Europe. *Annals of Nutrition and Metabolism* **51**: 108–114.

Pearce, J., Langley-Evans, S.C. (2013). The types of food introduced during complementary feeding and risk of childhood obesity: a systematic review. *International Journal of Obesity* **37**: 477–485.

Picó, C., Serra, F., Rodríguez, A.M. *et al.* (2019). Biomarkers of nutrition and health: new tools for new approaches. *Nutrients* **11**: 1092.

Pot, G.K., Prynne, C.J., Roberts, C. *et al.* (2012). National Diet and Nutrition Survey: fat and fatty acid intake from the first year of the rolling programme and comparison with previous surveys. *British Journal of Nutrition* **107**: 405–415.

Qu, X., Jin, F., Hao, Y. *et al.* (2013). Magnesium and the risk of cardiovascular events: a meta-analysis of prospective cohort studies. *PLoS One* **8**: e57720.

Richardson, R.A. and Davidson, H.I. (2003). Nutritional demands in acute and chronic illness. *Proceedings of the Nutrition Society* **62**: 777–781.

Rippin, H.L., Hutchinson, J., Evans, C.E.L. *et al.* (2018). National nutrition surveys in Europe: a review on the current status in the 53 countries of the WHO European region. *Food and Nutrition Research* **62**: doi: 10.29219/fnr.v62.1362.

Romijn, J.A. (2000). Substrate metabolism in the metabolic response to injury. *Proceedings of the Nutrition Society* **59**: 447–449.

Scientific Advisory Committee on Nutrition. (2015). *Carbohydrates and Health*. London: Stationery Office.

Sebotsa, M.L., Dannhauser, A., Jooste, P.L. *et al.* (2005). Iodine status as determined by urinary iodine excretion in Lesotho two years after introducing legislation on universal salt iodization. *Nutrition* **21**: 20–24.

Seshadri, S. (2001). Prevalence of micronutrient deficiency particularly of iron, zinc and folic acid in pregnant women in South East Asia. *British Journal of Nutrition* **85** (Suppl. 2): S87–S92.

Song, Y., Manson, J.E., Cook, N.R., *et al.* (2005). Dietary magnesium intake and risk of cardiovascular disease among women. *American Journal of Cardiology* **96**: 1135–1141.

Tsugane, S., Sasazuki, S., Kobayashi, M. *et al.* (2004). Salt and salted food intake and subsequent risk of gastric cancer among middle-aged Japanese men and women. *British Journal of Cancer* **90**: 128–234.

UNICEF. (2019). Malnutrition. https://data.unicef.org/topic/nutrition/malnutrition (accessed 30 March 2021).

West, K.P. (2003). Vitamin A deficiency disorders in children and women. *Food and Nutrition Bulletin* **24**(Suppl. 4): S78–S90.

Whitehead, R.G. (1992). Dietary reference values. *Proceedings of the Nutrition Society* **51**: 29–34.

Wild, T., Rahbarnia, A., Kellner, M. *et al.* (2010). Basics in nutrition and wound healing. *Nutrition*, **26**, 862–866.

World Cancer Research Fund. (2007). *Food, Nutrition, Physical Activity, and the Prevention of Cancer: A Global Perspective*, Washington, DC: WCRF/AICR.

World Health Organization. (2017). World Life Expectancy, Malnutrition death rates. https://www.worldlifeexpectancy.com/cause-of-death/malnutrition/by-country (accessed 30 March 2021).

Zagré, N.M., Delpeuch, F., Traissac, P. *et al.* (2003). Red palm oil as a source of vitamin A for mothers and children: impact of a pilot project in Burkina Faso. *Public Health Nutrition* **6**: 733–742.

Zakrzewski-Fruer, J.K., Plekhanova, T., Mandila, D. *et al.* (2017). Effect of breakfast omission and consumption on energy intake and physical activity in adolescent girls: a randomised controlled trial. *British Journal of Nutrition*, **118**, : 392–400.

Additional reading

If you would like to find out more about the material discussed in this chapter, the following sources may be of interest.

Department of Health. (1991). *Dietary Reference Values of Food Energy and Nutrients for the United Kingdom: Report of the Panel on Dietary Reference Values of the Committee on Medical Aspects of Food.* London: Stationery Office.

Galakis, C. (2019). *Trends in Personalized Nutrition.* London: Academic Press.

Goldacre, B. (2009). *Bad Science.* London: Fourth Estate.

Institute of Medicine. (2001). *Dietary Reference Intakes: Applications in Dietary Assessment.* Washington, DC: National Academies Press.

Lee, R.D. and Nieman, D.C. (2012). *Nutritional Assessment.* New York, NY: McGraw-Hill.

Margetts, B.M. and Nelson, M. (2009). *Design Concepts in Nutritional Epidemiology.* Oxford: Oxford Medical Publications.

Warner, A. (2017). *The Angry Chef: Bad Science and the Truth about Healthy Eating.* London: Oneworld Publications.

CHAPTER 2

Before life begins

LEARNING OBJECTIVES

This chapter will enable the reader to:
- Describe how trends in modern healthcare have made it both possible and desirable to change diet and lifestyle in preparation for pregnancy
- Show an understanding of the endocrine control of both female and male reproductive functions
- Discuss the contribution of body fatness to initiation and maintenance of normal reproductive cycling in women
- Critically review the evidence that commonly consumed agents such as alcohol and caffeine may have an adverse effect on female fertility
- Discuss the possible contribution of antioxidant nutrients to optimal fertility in both men and women
- Show an understanding of dietary factors and non-nutrient components of food that may have an adverse impact on male fertility
- Describe the importance of reducing intake of vitamin A for reducing risk of embryonic malformation in the earliest stages of pregnancy
- Discuss the key evidence that informs debates surrounding policies designed to reduce the prevalence of neural tube defects through increasing population intakes of folate

2.1 Introduction

The twentieth century saw a profound change in the manner in which human reproductive health and function is managed. Medicalization of the process of childbirth and the management of pregnancy transformed human reproduction. In the early part of the century, death rates among newborn infants in the UK were as high as 150–200 per 1000 births, and pregnancy-related complications were the major cause of death among young women, with death rates of 5–6 per 1000 births (Office for National Statistics, 1997). Improved medical care, hygiene, diet and housing conditions have brought death rates among infants down to 4–6 per 1000 births, and maternal deaths are now very rare events (<0.1 per 1000 births). Maternal and neonatal deaths are falling, but remain high in developing countries (Figure 2.1).

These changes have also transformed the priorities for researchers and health professionals working in the field of human reproduction. With less emphasis on the avoidance of catastrophic pregnancy outcomes, it is now of prime importance to promote good health in pregnant women and to ensure achievement of the optimal maternal environment for the development of the baby. In terms of nutrition, it is becoming clear that many of the important changes that women should consider making to their diets need to be implemented before conception. In most western countries, the majority (60%) of pregnancies are planned and this allows scope for optimizing nutrition. Attaining optimal body weights, avoiding potentially harmful substances and increasing intakes of nutrients that are of greatest importance to fetal development are all most effective when achieved while planning a pregnancy.

Nutrition may also be of major importance in achieving conception for many couples. Nutritional status, and in particular female body fatness, plays a role in determining fertility. This chapter sets out the key nutrition-related issues that impact upon the ability of men and women to conceive a child. Estimates of infertility rates vary considerably between developed and developing countries but, globally, 15% of women seeking to conceive cannot do so within 12 months, with higher prevalence in Central and Eastern Europe, Central and South Asia and North Africa (Agarwal *et al.*, 2015; Mascarenhas *et al.*, 2012). Some 12% of US women of childbearing age report having undergone fertility treatment and 1% of all US

Nutrition, Health and Disease: A Lifespan Approach, Third Edition. Simon Langley-Evans.
© 2021 John Wiley & Sons Ltd. Published 2021 by John Wiley & Sons Ltd.
Companion website: www.wiley.com/go/langleyevans/lifespan3e

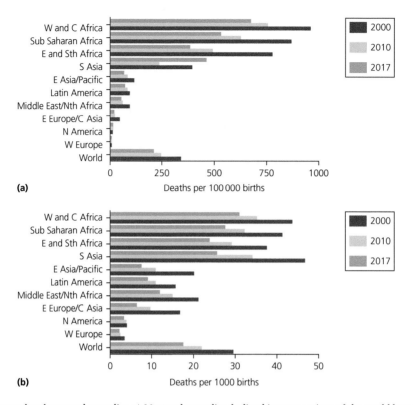

(a)

(b)

Figure 2.1 Maternal and neonatal mortality. a) Maternal mortality declined in most regions of the world between 2000 and 2017, but remains markedly higher in the developing countries. b) There is considerable global variation in neonatal mortality, with highest mortality in the African nations. *Source:* data from Unicef (2019a; 2019b).

babies are born following assisted reproductive treatments. In parts of Europe, this figure is as high as 3%. Primary infertility, the term used to describe cases in which couples are unable to conceive within one year of unprotected sex, is considerably less prevalent than secondary infertility (85% of all cases), in which fertility issues impact upon women who have previously had a child. Table 2.1 shows the main causes of infertility in men and women.

Table 2.1 Causes of infertility.

Female causes	Male causes
Anovulation	Abnormal sperm production
Menstrual irregularities	Problems with delivery of sperm
Infections	Infections
Damage related to cancer treatment	Damage related to cancer treatment
Endometriosis	
Polycystic ovary syndrome	
Primary ovary insufficiency	
Embryo implantation failure	

50% of infertility is explained by solely female factors and 20–30% by solely male factors. The remainder of infertility cases result from both male and female factors.

Consistent with the changing priorities in relation to how reproduction is managed in developed countries, the chapter also considers the dietary changes that women should consider ahead of conception to optimize their nutrient reserves for pregnancy and minimize the likelihood of embryonic exposure to harmful agents in the first few weeks of life.

2.2 Nutrition and female fertility

2.2.1 Determinants of fertility and infertility

Female fertility is primarily determined by factors that are seemingly unrelated to nutritional status. Whereas men generally retain some degree of fertility throughout their adult lives, women have a fixed reproductive span that runs from menarche (the onset of reproductive cycling) to menopause (when reproductive cycling ends). Infertility or subfertility in women can arise due to problems with the endocrine regulation of reproductive system function or due to other medical conditions that impair reproductive capacity. These medical conditions include infections of the reproductive tract, ovarian disease, trauma to the reproductive organs, endometriosis and polycystic ovary syndrome (PCOS). Although these reproductive events appear to be primarily determined by age and ill health, it is becoming clear that nutritional status can have some impact on the timing of menarche, and hence duration of reproductive span, and upon the maintenance of normal reproductive cycling.

2.2.1.1 The endocrine control of female reproduction

The endocrine regulation of female reproductive function is extremely complex, and this text attempts to give only a simple overview. Within the ovaries, women have primary follicles containing immature oocytes that are present from the time of birth. The hormones involved in the regulation of the menstrual cycle function to facilitate the maturation of a small number of these oocytes, the release of a single mature ovum in each cycle and the preparation of the uterine lining for the implantation of a fertilized egg. The menstrual cycle comprises two distinct phases, with follicle and egg maturation occurring in the follicular phase. After

ovulation, the cycle enters the luteal phase, in which the corpus luteum (remnants of the follicle which released the mature ovum at ovulation) acts as the main controller of the uterine environment. It can either promote the maintenance of a suitable environment for implantation or pregnancy, or in the absence of fertilization, it can degenerate and promote the sloughing of the uterine lining and hence menstrual bleeding.

The endocrine factors that regulate the menstrual cycle are shown in Figure 2.2. The hypothalamus is the central integrator of the cycle, acting through production of gonadotrophin-releasing hormone (GnRH). This stimulates the production of two hormones from the anterior pituitary. Follicle-stimulating hormone (FSH) acts on the ovaries to stimulate the maturation of the follicles and to drive the production of oestrogens. Oestrogens also stimulate follicular development and act upon the uterus to build up the endometrial lining. During the follicular phase, oestrogen concentrations tend to be low, but this is still sufficient to lower the production of FSH from the anterior pituitary and

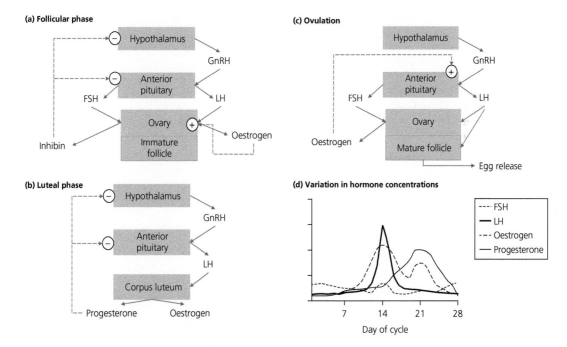

Figure 2.2 The endocrine control of female reproductive function. The menstrual cycle lasts for an average of 28 days. This can be divided into a) the follicular phase (days 1–13), during which oestrogen, luteinizing hormone (LH) and follicle-stimulating hormone (FSH) stimulate follicular development; b) ovulation, driven by high concentrations of LH and oestrogen, occurs on day 14; and c) the luteal phase (days 15–28), which is driven by hormone production from the corpus luteum and produces high concentrations of progesterone and oestrogen to prepare the uterine lining for implantation of a fertilized embryo. In the absence of fertilization, feedback inhibition of progesterone promotes the degeneration of the corpus luteum and menstrual bleeding. d) The shifting concentrations of key hormones through the cycle. GnRH, gonadotrophin-releasing hormone.

GnRH from the hypothalamus, through a negative feedback mechanism. The other anterior pituitary hormone produced in response to GnRH secretion is luteinizing hormone (LH). The ovaries are a target for LH where, like FSH, it stimulates follicular development. The ovaries also produce the hormone inhibin in response to LH, and this selectively inhibits the secretion of FSH (Figure 2.2). This, together with the effects of oestrogen, means that LH concentrations tend to rise towards the midpoint in the cycle, while FSH concentrations tend to fall.

While effects of oestrogen upon the hypothalamus and anterior pituitary involve negative feedback, oestrogens exert positive feedback effects on the ovaries to generate more oestrogen (Figure 2.2). This means that by the midpoint in the menstrual cycle, oestrogen concentrations spike dramatically. Rising levels of oestrogens have a paradoxical effect upon the hypothalamus and anterior pituitary and now start to stimulate secretion of LH and to a lesser extent FSH. The resultant surge in LH is the trigger for ovulation. The mature follicle ruptures and releases the ovum. At the same time, the corpus luteum is formed and the cycle now enters the luteal phase.

During the luteal phase, the key anterior pituitary factor is LH, which stimulates the corpus luteum to produce initially low levels of oestrogens and progesterone. The concentrations of these sex steroids rise gradually and progesterone, in particular, reaches a very high concentration. This inhibits the further production of GnRH and hence LH and FSH, and thereby prevents the maturation of further follicles should a pregnancy occur (Figure 2.2). If there is no pregnancy, the corpus luteum degenerates as LH is no longer produced to maintain it and hence production of progesterone and oestrogen ends.

2.2.1.2 Disordered reproductive cycling

Disordered menstrual cycling can arise for a number of reasons. Stress, excessive or intense exercise, smoking, ovarian or uterine disease, use of certain medications and treatments such as chemotherapy, drug abuse, illness and emotional traumas have all been shown to impact upon hypothalamic and ovarian production of hormones. Any problems with secretion of LH, FSH or oestrogens will impact upon the normal reproductive cycle, with several possible outcomes. In some women, menstrual cycles cease entirely (amenorrhoea), or the cycle may become excessively long, perhaps lasting for 45–90 days instead of the usual 28 (oligorrhoea). If there is insufficient production of LH or oestrogen, there may be an absence of ovulation (anovulation). As will become clear in later sections, poor nutritional status is a major cause of menstrual cycle disorders and hence is an important factor in unexplained (idiopathic) infertility in women.

2.2.1.3 Polycystic ovary syndrome

PCOS is one of the more common medical causes of female subfertility and infertility. Women with PCOS develop clusters of immature follicles within the ovaries, all of which fail to develop and eventually form fluid-filled cysts. Generally, women with PCOS will either be anovulatory or will have infrequent periods and oligorrhoea. One of the features of the syndrome is the production of high concentrations of male sex hormones (androgens), which can often manifest physically as excess facial or chest hair growth (hirsutism), loss of head hair and acne (Table 2.2). In addition to producing abnormally high levels of testosterone, women with PCOS generally overproduce LH.

Obesity, and therefore nutritional status, is a major determinant of risk of PCOS, although it has also been related to a family history of the condition. There is a high prevalence of obesity among women with PCOS (Pasquali *et al.*, 2006), and abdominal fat deposition appears to confer particularly high risk. Women with central obesity of this nature tend to develop insulin resistance, which is characterized by excessively high levels of circulat-

Table 2.2 Characteristics of polycystic ovary syndrome.

Physiological and metabolic symptoms	Reproductive impact (increased risk)	Associated disease states (increased risk)
Enlarged ovaries with fluid-filled cysts	Oligomenorrhea or amenorrhea	Type-2 diabetes
Weight gain	Anovulation	Cardiovascular disease
Hypercholesterolaemia	High androgen secretion	Endometrial cancer
Hirsutism- face, chest, back and buttocks	Subfecundity	Depression
Alopecia: head	Miscarriage	
Oily skin and acne	Gestational diabetes	
	Caesarean section	

Polycystic ovary syndrome is a heterogenous condition and most women will suffer some, but not all symptoms.

ing insulin. Insulin inhibits synthesis of sex hormone binding globulin in the liver. This protein plays a key role in controlling the access of sex hormones to their target tissues and, in the absence of sex hormone binding globulin, concentrations of free androgens rise. Obesity also favours increased synthesis of androgens and other mechanisms operating in adipose tissue serve to drive hyperandrogenaemia.

Weight loss in women with PCOS is effective in restoring normal endocrine functions and reproductive cycling (Figure 2.3). Pasquali *et al.* (2006)

reported that a 12-month period of dieting to promote significant weight loss in women with PCOS significantly improved symptoms (partial restoration of menstrual cycles, reduction in hirsutism) and that these changes were associated with markedly lower circulating insulin concentrations, improved insulin sensitivity and lower testosterone concentrations. As described in Research Highlight 2.1, many studies have examined the optimal weight loss strategy for treatment of PCOS. Although there is some evidence that varying the macronutrient composition of the diet may influence some features of PCOS, weight

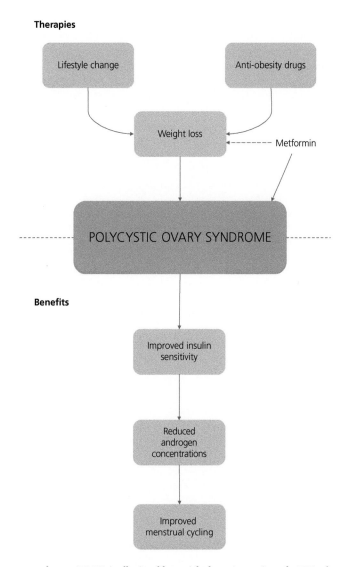

Figure 2.3 Polycystic ovary syndrome (PCOS) is alleviated by weight loss. Approximately 50% of women with PCOS are overweight and obese. PCOS symptoms can be reduced by weight loss, achieved through increased physical activity and dietary change or by treatment with metformin. Metformin is an anti-diabetic drug, which acts by suppressing hepatic gluconeogenesis.

loss through caloric restriction remains the most important approach to managing PCOS, regardless of the overall dietary composition (Moran *et al.*, 2012).

As insulin resistance has a central role in PCOS, there are good pharmaceutical options to supplement weight loss interventions as a means of improving fertility. Drugs which improve insulin sensitivity can also alleviate features of PCOS. Metformin is the most commonly used of these drugs. It improves insulin sensitivity by inhibiting hepatic gluconeogenesis. Studies show that metformin can restore menstrual cycles in 50% of women with PCOS (Fruzzetti *et al.*, 2017) and can significantly improve pregnancy and live birth rates (Sharpe *et al.*, 2019). Other insulin-sensitizing drugs, such as myo-inositol and pioglitazone may be equally effective and suitable for use in women who cannot tolerate the gastrointestinal adverse effects of metformin treatment (Fruzzetti *et al.*, 2017; Xu *et al.*, 2017).

2.2.2 Importance of body fat

Body fatness is a major factor determining the span of reproductive life in women and as illustrated by the example of PCOS, determines some of the risk of developing menstrual cycle disturbances. It was noted several decades ago that young women who partake in high-intensity sport or dance activities tend to exhibit delayed menarche and will later be at greater risk of amenorrhoea or anovulation. Amenorrhoea is also observed in women who are excessively thin, or who undergo extreme weight loss, either as a result of eating disorders (e.g. anorexia nervosa) or through other restrictive dietary practices. Weight loss equivalent to around 10–15% of normal weight for height in women is associated with menstrual cycle abnormalities. Obesity is also

associated with amenorrhoea. Together, these observations suggest that both too much and too little body fat can have an adverse impact on female fertility (Frisch, 1987).

Young women at the present time are significantly taller and heavier than their counterparts in earlier centuries, and with this change in growth, they are attaining greater proportions of body fat at earlier ages. This secular trend is associated with a trend for menarche to occur at an earlier age. In the nineteenth century, the average age for first menses was between 17 and 18 years. By the 1920s, this had declined to 14 years and by the 1990s was between 12 and 13 years. In developed countries, a steady decline in age at menarche was observed across the twentieth century with girls initiating menstruation approximately 15 months earlier in the 1990s than in the 1920s (Figure 2.4). The proportion of girls entering puberty before age 10, which was extremely rare in the 1940s, was approximately 2% in 1990. In populations that have undergone a rapid economic transformation, the boost in nutrition that follows has been accompanied by a rapid decrease in age at menarche (see China and South Africa, Figure 2.4). The main contributor to the decline in age at menarche is believed to be increased body fatness in the population. Chang-Mo *et al.* (2012) reported that in a Korean population, menarche before 12 years of age was up to sevenfold more likely in girls who were taller, heavier and of greater body mass index (BMI) at ages 8 and 9. Girls who matured early were approximately 5 kg heavier than girls who reached menarche after 12 years and had a greater percentage body fat at age 13.

The growth spurt during adolescence is obviously associated with a significant increase in both height and weight but is also a time when body

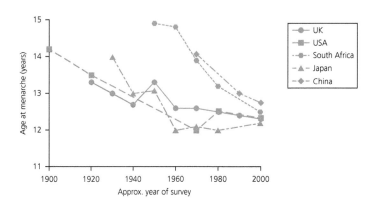

Figure 2.4 Secular trends in menarche 1900–2000 in selected countries. *Sources:* data from Whincup *et al.* (2001); Hosokawa *et al.* (2012); Bodicoat *et al.* (2014); Jones *et al.* (2009).

Research Highlight 2.1 Polycystic ovary syndrome, weight loss diets and reproductive function.

Overweight and obesity are strongly associated with risk of polycystic ovary syndrome (PCOS). While the syndrome is heterogenous, with different causes and symptom patterns, 40–60% of women with PCOS are overweight or obese and, in those who are lean, PCOS often manifests due to greater visceral adiposity (Motta, 2012). Weight loss remains the most effective means of improving symptoms and reproductive outcomes. A weight loss of as little as 5% of initial body weight can bring about positive changes. Panidis *et al.* (2008) reported that a 24-week energy-restricted diet combined with orlistat treatment improved insulin sensitivity and lowered testosterone concentrations.

While the benefits of weight loss in PCOS are well established, there has been a considerable amount of research into whether any particular diet is more effective than others. Low carbohydrate, high protein and modified fatty acid diet patterns have all been investigated. Kasim-Karakas *et al.* (2004) reported that a three-month period following a polyunsaturated fatty acid-enriched diet had no impact upon insulin sensitivity or reproductive outcomes. While Paoli *et al.* (2020) found that a ketogenic diet (high fat, high protein, low carbohydrate) promoted weight loss, improved insulin sensitivity and raised secretion of oestrogen and progesterone, their study design was weak; it lacked a control group, had too few subjects and too short an intervention.

A number of studies have suggested that low carbohydrate diets are a beneficial means of promoting weight loss and improving reproductive status in women with PCOS. However, the systematic review of Frary *et al.* (2016) concluded that, although such diets could promote greater weight loss than standard energy-restricted diets, they did not influence parameters of fertility. Similarly, Moran *et al.* (2003) compared the effects of diets of low- or high-protein content against a 6 MJ per day energy-restricted diet for 16 weeks, followed by 4 weeks of a weight-maintenance diet. While energy restriction improved menstrual function, varying the protein content of the diet carried no additional benefit. Marsh and Brand-Miller (2005) reported that high-protein diets worsened insulin resistance and did not enhance reproductive function any more than a high-carbohydrate weight-loss diet. A meta-analysis of studies which have considered variation in diet composition in management of PCOS, concluded that while different diets produce subtle differences in features of the syndrome, such as depression, dietary composition does not influence weight loss or menstrual function (Moran *et al.*, 2012). Current advice is therefore to reduce energy density of the diet, increase aerobic exercise and consider the use of weight loss drugs or metformin to enhance insulin sensitivity.

composition undergoes major changes. In girls, there is a relative increase in the proportion of body fat, which increases from around 5 kg in total to 11 kg. Lean body mass increases to a much lesser extent. Frisch *et al.* (1973) studied adolescent girls and found that on attainment of stable reproductive cycling, all had approximately 22% body fat, regardless of their absolute height or weight. These studies identified this proportion of body fat as being the minimum required to maintain stable menstrual cycling, and hence women restricting diet to promote weight loss and women engaged in intense physical activity develop amenorrhoea and other cycle problems as they fall below this fat threshold. There is a difference between menarche and attainment of stable and regular cycles, and the minimum threshold of body fat required to trigger menarche is lower, at 17% of body weight (Frisch, 1987).

There are therefore minimal levels of body fat required to support reproductive function in women. It is easy to see how such a system has evolved in humans. Body fat is essentially a store of metabolizable energy and provides a metabolic indicator of the nutritional environment and fitness of a woman to support a pregnancy and later breastfeed an infant. Mechanisms that prevent conception during times of famine would have been a considerable survival advantage to early humans. Allal *et al.* (2004) showed that in developing countries such as

the Gambia, delayed reproductive maturity and hence a later first pregnancy allow women to grow to a greater height. Greater maternal stature is associated with reduced infant death.

2.2.3 Role of leptin

There is a simple hormonal signal that links the body fatness of women to the hypothalamic–pituitary–ovarian axis that ultimately governs their fertility. Leptin is one of a group of peptide hormones, termed adipokines, produced from adipose tissue. Other adipokines, including resistin and adiponectin, have been suggested to play a role in controlling fertility. Adiponectin, for example, appears to play a role in follicle maturation and preparation of the uterus for implantation. While the role of leptin in regulating menstrual cycle function is well established, effects of other adipose tissue-derived hormones upon human reproductive function have not been clearly demonstrated (Mitchell *et al.*, 2005). Leptin is the product of the *ob* gene, which is only expressed in adipose tissue. As a result, plasma concentrations of leptin are closely correlated with the overall level of body fat. Leptin is a satiety hormone, which acts at the hypothalamus to suppress appetite and increase energy expenditure through thermogenesis. Satiety effects are mediated indirectly as leptin, within the arcuate nucleus of the hypothalamus, stimulates release of further satiety-inducing peptides, including neuropeptide Y and agouti-related peptide.

The first clues for a role of leptin in controlling fertility came from studies of a range of genetically obese rodents. The *ob/ob* mouse produces a defective leptin that is unable to bind the leptin receptors, while the *db/db* mouse and *fa/fa* rat have defective receptors which do not fully mediate the effects of leptin on binding. All these rodent strains exhibit problems with fertility. The female *ob/ob* mouse is totally infertile as it never achieves puberty and cannot produce mature follicles. These mice have abnormal levels of FSH and GnRH in circulation. Similarly, the female *fa/fa* rat is rarely fertile, having a suppressed LH surge and lower FSH secretion, preventing normal ovulation.

In humans, changes in leptin concentrations occur around the time of puberty, but only in girls. As a result, women have higher leptin concentrations (normal range 5–20 ng/ml) than are seen in men, at all ages. This reflects their higher proportions of body fat at any given weight or height. As adipose tissue is the only site of leptin synthesis, circulating concentrations of the hormone are always directly proportional to fat mass. However, it is clear that leptin has a function in controlling fertility, as studies show that irrespective of fat mass, concentrations vary across the menstrual cycle. Leptin secretion is greater in the luteal phase than in the follicular phase (Asimakopoulos *et al.*, 2009). Leptin concentrations are also strongly associated with menarche. Gavela-Perez *et al.* (2016) studied a cohort of Spanish girls and found that even after correction for BMI, prepubertal leptin concentrations predicted timing of menarche. Girls who achieved menarche before

the age of 12 had markedly high leptin than those who did not have their first period until after the age of 13. Generally, menarche is associated with an increase in body fat mass and this drives a further increase in leptin, which serves to maintain regular cycles. Bandini *et al.* (2008) reported that among a group of US girls, before menarche fat contributed 24.6% of body weight and mean leptin concentration was 8.4 ng/ml. After menarche, these values increased to 27% and 12 ng/ml, respectively.

Figure 2.5 shows how leptin influences the hypothalamic–pituitary–ovarian axis. Leptin receptors are present in key nuclei of the hypothalamus and in the anterior pituitary, and it therefore directly influences the secretion of GnRH, LH and FSH. In the absence of leptin, the normal pulsatile secretion of all these factors is lost (Goumenou *et al.*, 2003). The *ob/ob* mouse, lacking leptin, is analogous to the excessively thin woman, and both will have fertility problems for the same reasons.

Given the stimulatory role of leptin upon the reproductive axis, the negative effects of excess body fat appear to be paradoxical. Obese individuals typically exhibit very high concentrations of leptin. The explanation for the negative effect on fertility is provided by the concept of leptin resistance. The effects of leptin within the brain are mediated through its binding to two different forms of the leptin receptor. The short-form receptor Ob-Ra has a transport role and carries leptin across the blood–brain barrier, thereby providing access to the hypothalamic tissues. The long-form Ob-Rb receptor is membrane bound and mediates the physiological effects of leptin via several signal transduction mechanisms (Figure 2.6). One of these mechanisms

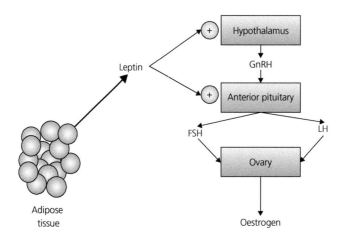

Figure 2.5 Adipose tissue-derived leptin and the hypothalamic–pituitary–ovarian axis. Leptin from adipose tissue promotes production of gonadotrophin-releasing hormone, follicle-stimulating hormone and luteinizing hormone and therefore has a stimulatory effect on the hypothalamic–pituitary–ovarian axis.

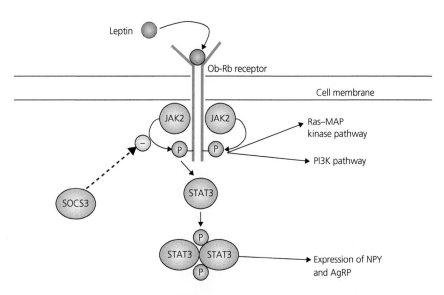

Leptin

Ob-Rb receptor

Cell membrane

JAK2   JAK2

− → P   P

Ras–MAP kinase pathway

PI3K pathway

SOCS3

STAT3

P

STAT3   STAT3

P

Expression of NPY and AgRP

Figure 2.6 Leptin receptor signalling cascade. Binding of leptin to the membrane-bound Ob-Rb receptor activates multiple signalling pathways, including the phosphoinositol-3 kinase (PI3K) pathway and the Ras–mitogen-activated protein (Ras–MAP) kinase pathway. Binding of leptin activates Janus kinase-2 (JAK2), which phosphorylates signal transducer and activator of transcription-3 (STAT3). Formation of phosphorylated STAT3 complexes drives activation of transcription of target genes including neuropeptide Y (NPY) and agouti-related peptide (AgRP). Leptin resistance develops through leptin up-regulation of the expression of suppressor of the cytokine signalling-3, which inhibits the JAK2–STAT3 pathway. SOCS3, suppressor of the cytokine signalling-3. P, phosphate.

is the Janus kinase (JAK)–signal transducer and activator of transcription-3 (STAT3) pathway. Binding of leptin stimulates phosphorylation of STAT3 and hence gene transcription to mediate cellular responses. Leptin resistance involves impairment of both Ob-Ra and Ob-Rb functions (El-Haschimi *et al.*, 2000). Impaired Ob-Ra function is poorly understood but clearly reduces the amount of leptin reaching target sites. Leptin up-regulates expression of suppressor of the cytokine signalling-3 (SOCS3), which is an inhibitor of the JAK– STAT3 pathway. Thus, the very high concentrations of leptin associated with obesity will suppress leptin action in the hypothalamus and remove the stimulatory effect of the hormone on the hypothalamic–pituitary–ovarian axis, leading to disordered reproductive cycling. The *fa/fa* rat, which has leptin receptor defects, provides an analogy to the obese woman, and their reproductive cycle defects are similar.

2.2.4 Antioxidant nutrients

A free radical is any molecule that has unpaired electrons, and as such, these molecules are highly reactive and short lived. Free radicals and associated oxidants formed from oxygen within biological systems are termed reactive oxygen species (ROS). These include the superoxide (O_2^{-}) and hydroxyl (OH·) radicals, hydrogen peroxide, nitric oxide (NO)

and lipid hydroperoxides (Halliwell, 1999). As will be seen in later chapters, the reactive nature of ROS gives them the capacity to cause widespread cellular and tissue damage that is associated with the development and progression of many disease states.

Exposure to ROS is an unavoidable feature of life in oxygen, as they are mainly formed as a by-product of mitochondrial respiration. Other important sources of ROS in biological systems are shown in Table 2.3. ROS have the capacity to damage all components of cells, as they will react with all types of macromolecules (Figure 2.7). Thus, they damage proteins (e.g. protein–protein cross-linking), nucleic acids (e.g. DNA strand scission) and phospholipids in membranes (lipid peroxidation).

Life in oxygen is only possible due to the presence of antioxidant species that have the capacity to neutralize ROS (Table 2.3). Most aspects of antioxidant protection are to some extent influenced by the diet and nutritional status. The antioxidant enzymes generally have metal ions at their active sites (e.g. CuZn superoxide dismutase), and scavenging antioxidants such as ascorbate, ß-carotene and vitamin E are all obtained directly through the diet. These scavenging species must be constantly replenished, as interaction with ROS leads to their destruction.

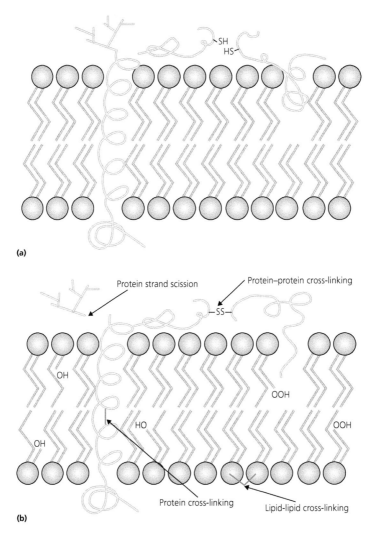

Figure 2.7 Reactive oxygen species are damaging within biological systems. a) A section of membrane in a mammalian cell comprises the phospholipid bilayer with a transmembrane protein and cell surface proteins. b) After interaction with a reactive oxygen species, the section of membrane is heavily damaged due to the chain reactions established by the oxidation of macromolecules. Oxidative damage to the lipid bilayer (lipid peroxidation) will impact upon membrane properties such as permeability. Damage to proteins will alter conformation and impact upon receptor, signalling, transport and enzyme functions.

Table 2.3 Reactive oxygen species.

Reactive oxygen species		Antioxidants		
Free radicals	**Non-radicals**	**Enzymes**	**Scavengers**	**Ion binding proteins**
Superoxide (O_2^-)	Hydrogen peroxide (H_2O_2)	Superoxide dismutase	Ascorbate	Albumin
Hydroxyl radical (OH)	Ozone (O_3)	Catalase	Polyphenols	Ferritin
Peroxyl radical (RO_2)	Hypochlorous acid (HOCl)	Glutathione peroxidase	α-Tocopherol	Transferrin
Alkoxyl radical (RO)	Hypobromous acid (HOBr)		β-Carotene	Caeruloplasmin
Nitric oxide (NO)			Lutein	

Reactive oxygen species are either generated endogenously through processes such as respiration and the respiratory burst of immune cells or can be derived from exogenous sources (pollutants, drugs, food contaminants). Enzymatic antioxidants are present in most cells and some forms occur in circulation. Scavenging antioxidants are generally derived from the diet and are found in body fluids and the cytosol of most cells. Ion binding proteins are transport proteins that provide antioxidant protection by removing free iron and copper ions, which can generate free radical species when they react with oxygen.

Oxidative stress, the situation where ROS activity is not fully buffered by the presence of antioxidants, is a known feature of normal reproductive function in women. ROS play a key role in several aspects of the menstrual cycle, including follicle maturation, ovulation, development of the endometrium for implantation and synthesis of progesterone by the corpus luteum (Ruder *et al.*, 2009). While ovulation will not occur without ROS, excess production or inadequate antioxidant status is associated with poor fertility. Endometriosis is a condition in which the tissue that lines the uterus grows in the fallopian tubes and areas outside the reproductive tract, causing pain, irregular bleeding and subfertility. Observational studies suggest that the condition is associated with increased oxidative stress (Scutiero *et al.*, 2017), although this is not necessarily a causal relationship. Most studies conclude that even in mild endometriosis, there is greater evidence of oxidative damage during the follicular phase of the menstrual cycle (Ferreira *et al.*, 2019). Amreen *et al.* (2019) showed that as the severity of endometriosis increased, the presence of oxidative damage markers in blood and follicular fluid also increased, while activities of key antioxidant enzymes were decreased.

To ensure that antioxidant stress is controlled, the reproductive system is rich in antioxidants. Follicular fluid is rich in scavenging antioxidants and the endometrium expresses superoxide dismutase as part of the normal response to progesterone (Ebisch *et al.*, 2007). Follicular fluid may be especially important (Ruder *et al.*, 2009), with reports that successful oocyte retrieval and embryo transfer in assisted reproduction are related to the total antioxidant capacity of follicular fluid. Melatonin is a derivative of tryptophan that is synthesized by all cells. It has antioxidant activity and is found at high concentrations in the ovary and follicular fluid. Melatonin supplementation for women who are about to undergo assisted reproductive therapies has been shown to increase the numbers of oocytes harvested, improve fertilization rates and increase the numbers of high quality embryos available for implantation (Tamura *et al.*, 2020). Animal studies suggest that adding melatonin to culture medium used for in vitro fertilization also improves outcomes.

Subfertility is generally the product of inadequate gamete production or quality, or a hostile environment for fertilization or implantation. A role for antioxidants in optimizing these aspects of female reproductive health has been suggested by virtue of the importance of controlled oxidative processes in menstrual cycle function. Investigations that have considered whether dietary antioxidants can improve outcomes for women who are subfertile have been limited by quality issues. Many fail to include a placebo group in the experimental design or recruit very small sample sizes. A number of these studies report no effect of antioxidant supplementation (Bentov *et al.*, 2014), but a few report positive outcomes (Nasr, 2010). A meta-analysis of over 50 antioxidant supplementation trials concluded that, despite low-quality evidence, antioxidants did increase clinical pregnancy rates compared with placebo or no treatment (odds ratio, OR, 1.52, 95% confidence interval, CI, 1.31–1.76). However, this is a relatively small effect size, which would improve pregnancy rates in women with subfertility from 22% (placebo) in a given reproductive cycle to between 27 and 33% (Showell *et al.*, 2017). The benefit of antioxidant supplementation was found to be greatest in women with PCOS and the strongest effects were seen with L-carnitine, coenzyme Q and mixed antioxidant supplements. The mode of action is likely to be through increasing the quality of eggs released at ovulation or by creating a better environment for fertilization. Sperm are vulnerable to oxidative damage and so antioxidant concentrations in the fallopian fluid may influence their ability to reach and fertilize an egg (Agarwal *et al.*, 2005).

2.2.5 Caffeine and alcohol

In many parts of the world, it is part of the normal culture to consume alcohol and/or caffeine in the form of beverages. These widely consumed agents are known to be highly active substances that are capable of exerting toxic effects at high levels and major metabolic and physiological responses at low to moderate levels of consumption. Both alcohol and caffeine consumption have been linked to problems with female fertility and indeed may interact with each other in lowering the chances of conception.

Caffeine is pharmacologically active, acting as a central nervous system stimulant. It is consumed in a variety of forms, principally tea and coffee, but also as an additive to soft drinks and in some over-the-counter medicines. Several animal studies have shown that caffeine can have adverse reproductive effects and that it is potentially hazardous to the early embryo. However, in humans, it is more difficult to interpret the findings of studies that relate caffeine intake to reproductive function and to develop a credible explanation of how it could reduce fertility. Certainly, caffeine can deplete the body of certain micronutrients through either inhibition of absorption (e.g. iron and zinc) or through increasing losses (e.g. calcium and thiamine), but these nutrients have no clear role in determining female fertility. Research Highlight 2.2

Table 2.4 Impact of alcohol on fertility in women and men.

Units* consumed	Classification	Impact on female fertility	Impact on male fertility
Women, up to 1/day; men, up to 2/day	Moderate consumer	Increased risk of miscarriage	No effect
Women, 4 in 2 hours; men, 5 in 2 hours	Binge drinker	Increased risk of miscarriage Lower chance of conception[†]	Lower sperm count Fewer sperm with normal morphology
5 or more binge episodes per month	Heavy consumer	Increased risk of miscarriage Lower chance of conception[†]	Lower semen volume Lower sperm count Fewer sperm with normal morphology

* One unit of alcohol corresponds to 12.5g of ethanol; one unit would be a 25-ml measure of spirits, 237 ml of beer; A 125-ml serving of wine contains 1.5 units.
[†] Chance of conception within 12 months of ceasing contraception.

discusses the possible association between caffeine and fertility in women.

A range of cohort and case–control studies have evaluated the impact of alcohol consumption on fertility in both men and women. The general findings are summarized in Table 2.4. Studies which have considered the impact of alcohol in women have produced conflicting results. Grodstein *et al.* (1997), for example, reported that 4–7 units of alcohol per week was associated with ovulatory problems (OR 1.3, 95% CI 1.1–1.7) and endometriosis (OR 1.6, 95% CI 1.1–2.3). Taylor *et al.* (2011) reported a large effect of alcohol, which was dependent upon the phenotype for the detoxification enzyme N-acetyl-transferase. In women who were 'fast' acetylators, alcohol had no detrimental effect on fertility but in 'slow' acetylators, consuming more than one alcoholic drink per day reduced fecundability by 82%. In contrast, Mikkelsen *et al.* (2016) showed that in a large cohort of Danish women, there was no effect of up to three drinks per day on ability to conceive. Other studies also concluded that there was no effect of alcohol consumption on fertility in women with no reported fertility problems. Lyngso *et al.* (2019b) also found that consuming low to moderate amounts of alcohol had no effect on the success of fertility treatments. A systematic review and meta-analysis of studies considering alcohol and female fertility found a dose-dependent effect. Each unit of alcohol consumed per day reduced fecundability by 2% (Fan *et al.*, 2017). Comparing women who were drinkers with those who were not showed a 13% reduction in fecundability. The effect was greater (23%) in women who were moderate to heavy drinkers.

Some studies have attempted to evaluate whether the form in which alcohol is consumed determines the impact on fertility. Wine, and to some extent beer, delivers polyphenols which have an antioxidant activity, which would be lacking when spirits are consumed. Juhl *et al.* (2003)

reported that spirits increased time to conception in women who were attempting to become pregnant (OR of delayed conception 2.4, 95% CI 1.0–5.73). In contrast, wine drinkers were less likely than non-drinkers to have delayed conception. However, this study did not adequately adjust for the confounding influence of socioeconomic status, which is a major determinant of behaviour in relation to alcohol. The meta-analysis of Fan *et al.* (2017) could not find any association between types of alcoholic beverage and fertility in women.

Although the evidence surrounding alcohol and caffeine in relation to female fertility is inconclusive, current advice is that women who wish to become pregnant should reduce intake of both alcohol and caffeine, with six cups of tea per day, three cups of coffee per day and one to two units of alcohol per week suggested as sensible limits.

2.3 Nutrition and male fertility

2.3.1 Determinants of fertility and infertility

While the origins of infertility in women are often complex and difficult to define, male fertility is readily assessed through simple measures of sperm production and quality. In general terms, the fertility of men depends on the quantity of sperm produced (defined either as sperm concentration per millilitre of ejaculate or as total numbers of sperm produced per ejaculation) or the characteristics of the sperm produced (Table 2.5). The latter can be measured in terms of sperm motility (the capacity of the sperm to swim) and sperm morphology (assessments of the proportion of sperm cells with a normal healthy structure).

The process of sperm production is termed spermatogenesis, which takes place in the seminiferous tubules within the male reproductive tract. These

Research Highlight 2.2   Caffeine and female fertility

There has been a long-standing concern that high consumption of caffeine through coffee, tea, energy drinks and medication, may have a detrimental impact upon female fertility. The first indication of a possible problem came from the study of Olsen (1991), which suggested that eight or more cups of coffee per day was associated with greater odds of subfecundity (OR 1.35, 95% CI 1.02–1.45). Other studies appeared consistent with this observation. For example, Hassan and Killick (2004) reported a 70% greater risk of subfecundity with seven or more cups of coffee per day, after correction for confounding factors. Such research was problematic as the definition of a 'cup' of coffee and how much caffeine it delivers, varies between studies, but Bolúmar et al. (1997) used estimates of actual caffeine intake in 3187 European women to demonstrate a significant 45% reduction in fecundability when comparing intakes in excess of 500 mg per day, with 100 mg per day or less. In all these studies, the effect of caffeine appeared to be either increased by or dependent upon tobacco smoking as a further detrimental exposure. More recent analyses have used more robust methodologies and often larger cohorts to investigate the issue. Soylu et al. (2018) followed 7574 women over a period of 17–19 years and found no risk of infertility associated with tea or coffee consumption. Similarly, Hatch et al. (2012) and Wesselink et al. (2016) found that women's consumption of caffeine was unrelated to their ability to conceive. Some of the most important studies to address this issue have focused on the effects of caffeine in women undergoing assisted reproductive therapies such as in vitro fertilization or intrauterine insemination. Ricci et al. (2018) found that the caffeine intakes of 339 couples did not influence their ability to conceive or carry a live birth. The much larger study of Lyngsø et al. (2019a) actually found a benefit associated with caffeine for women undergoing assisted reproductive therapy. Women consuming five or more cups of coffee per day were more likely to become pregnant (RR 1.49 95% CI 1.05–2.11) and carry a live birth (RR 1.53, 95% CI 1.06–2.21) than women who consumed no coffee.

The balance of evidence therefore suggests that caffeine does not have a significant adverse effect on female fertility. However, as some studies have shown an association of caffeine with spontaneous abortion in early pregnancy (Cnattingius et al., 2000), a reduction in consumption during the pre-conception period may be a worthwhile precaution for women to consider.

Table 2.5 Normal parameters for fertile sperm.

Sperm parameter	Description	Reference range (WHO)
Semen volume	Volume of ejaculate	1.5–7.6 ml
Total sperm count	Total sperm present in an ejaculation	39–928 million
Sperm concentration	Number of sperm per millilitre of semen	15–259 million/ml
Total motility	Proportion of sperm cells showing forward motion	40–81%
Progressive motility	Proportion of sperm cells swimming forward in a straight line	32–75%
Morphology	Proportion of sperm with normal undamaged appearance	4–48%

WHO, World Health Organization.

tubules contain two specific cell types that drive the process. Germ cells are the cells that have the capacity to develop into sperm cells. These cells are supported by Sertoli cells, which surround the germ cells, providing a protective barrier, and secrete nutrients and hormones. Spermatogenesis begins with the most primitive stage of germ cells which are termed spermatogonia. These cells go through rounds of mitotic and meiotic divisions before undergoing differentiation to produce mature sperm cells with specialized tail, mid-and head sections that can perform the required swimming and fertilization functions (Figure 2.8).

Spermatogenesis begins in males at around the time of puberty and will then continue throughout the adult lifespan. The process is regulated by a variety of hormonal factors which are produced by the hypothalamic–pituitary–gonadal axis (Figure 2.9).

The hypothalamus produces GnRH in a pulsatile manner, with concentrations peaking every 90 minutes. Thus, a new batch of sperm cells can be produced every hour and a half throughout adult life. GnRH acts on the anterior pituitary to stimulate production of LH and FSH, each of which has different functions. LH acts directly on the Leydig cells of the testis to stimulate production of the main androgenic steroid, testosterone. In this context, testosterone is responsible for the stimulation of spermatogenesis, but this hormone is critical to male reproduction in other ways, as it initiates puberty, stimulates the male sex drive and promotes the development of the male secondary sexual characteristics. Testosterone stimulates spermatogenesis through action on the Sertoli cells. These cells are also a target for FSH which has the same function. This endocrine axis is subject to negative

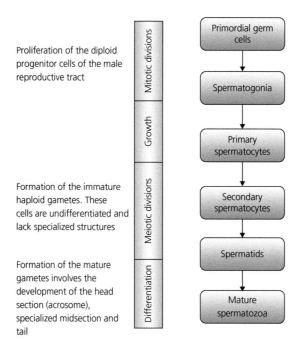

Proliferation of the diploid progenitor cells of the male reproductive tract

Formation of the immature haploid gametes. These cells are undifferentiated and lack specialized structures

Formation of the mature gametes involves the development of the head section (acrosome), specialized midsection and tail

Figure 2.8 Endocrine control of male reproductive function. In males, pulsatile hypothalamic production of gonadotrophin-releasing hormone stimulates the release of follicle-stimulating hormone and luteinizing hormone, which stimulate the production of testosterone and the development of mature sperm in the testes. Testis-derived inhibin-B and testosterone have negative feedback effects in the anterior pituitary and hypothalamus and thereby regulate the hypothalamic–pituitary–testicular axis.

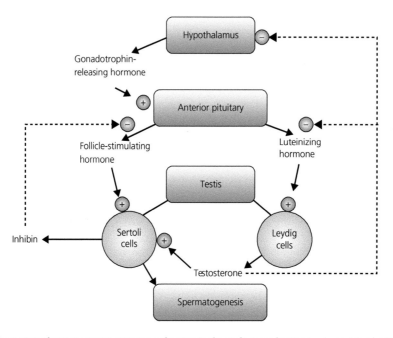

Figure 2.9 The formation of mature sperm. Sperm production in the male reproductive tract consists of mitotic and meiotic divisions followed by a differentiation phase in which sperm acquire their specialized structures.

feedback regulation at two key points. Testosterone negatively feedbacks on production of both GnRH and LH, while FSH secretion is directly controlled by the production of inhibin-B from the Sertoli cells. As Sertoli cells require both FSH and testosterone stimulation to maintain spermatogenesis, inhibin-B effectively limits sperm production by reducing FSH production.

The male reproductive system may be particularly vulnerable to adverse effects of poor nutrition or environmental exposures by virtue of the way in which it develops and functions. The repeated production of new sperm over rapid intervals throughout adult life means that short-term influences on spermatogenesis may become important in determining fertility. Fetal life and early infancy may, however, represent more important points in life when food-borne influences may have the greatest impact on later fertility. Initially, both male and female embryos develop a common ductal system, termed the Müllerian duct, that will ultimately go on to form the reproductive system. In males, early formation of Sertoli cells results in the production of anti-Müllerian hormone, causing the Wolffian duct to develop. This eventually forms the male reproductive organs. Masculinization of the reproductive tissues also depends on production of testosterone and its binding to the androgen receptor. There are many defects of this process that have been identified, which in the most extreme cases will lead to ambiguous genitalia, intersex and infertility (Sharpe, 1999). Development of male fertility therefore depends heavily on Sertoli cell numbers and function, which peak at around one year of age.

Earlier in the chapter, it was stated that a high proportion of female subfertility and infertility can be attributed to specific medical conditions. There are also conditions which affect the male reproductive tract that can impact upon fertility, of which the most important are hypospadias and cryptorchidism. These appear to be the product of adverse influences on early life development (Sharpe, 1999). Hypospadias is a defect in which the opening of the urethra is misplaced and may be at any point along the shaft of the penis. This is one of the most common birth defects of the male genitalia, occurring in as many as 1 in 125 boys. Like hypospadias, cryptorchidism is a defect associated with early development of the reproductive tract. Cryptorchidism refers to a failure of the testes to descend from the abdomen into the scrotum. This occurs in approximately 3% of babies but will resolve in the majority, leaving around 1% of mature adults with the condition. Both of these conditions can reduce male fertility (e.g. around 10% of men with cryptorchidism

will be subfertile) and there is some evidence that the incidence of these conditions and other defects of the reproductive tract (e.g. testicular cancers) is on the increase (Sharpe, 1999). While cases of cryptorchidism doubled between 1960 and 2002, this increase appears to have abated. However, there is considerable evidence that the increasing prevalence of male fertility problems continues to rise. Nassar *et al.* (2007) reported that the prevalence of hypospadias in Australian boys increased from 20 per 10 000 population in the 1980s to 36 per 10 000 in the 2000s. In Denmark, hypospadias prevalence rose from 3 per 10 000 to 17 per 10 000 between 1986 and 2009 (Nissen *et al.*, 2015). An international assessment that took data from 27 populations found that the global prevalence of hypospadias increased 1.6-fold between 1980 and 2010 (Yu *et al.*, 2019).

It is estimated that problems with male fertility explain around 20–30% of subfecundity in couples attempting to conceive a child. Initial reports from the United States of a steady decline in sperm counts in the second half of the twentieth century raised concerns that male fertility may be declining in developed countries. Other reports suggested that the European average sperm count in the 1940s and 1950s was around 170 million cells/ml, but this had declined to 60 million cells/ml by 1990 (Sharpe and Irvine, 2004). The assertion that male fertility is falling has been disputed by many researchers, as surveys conducted across five decades may have failed to use equivalent methodologies and populations. However, methodological differences do not fully explain the observations as more recent surveys, using robust methodologies in a number of developed and developing countries indicate small but significant declines in sperm counts over the past two to three decades (Figure 2.10). A meta-analysis found that average sperm counts in men from Europe, North America, Australia and New Zealand declined by 0.7 million sperm/ml per year between 1973 and 2011, constituting an overall decline of 50–60% (Levine *et al.*, 2017).

These trends clearly raise the question of why this has occurred and, here, attention must shift to the environmental changes that have occurred in western populations over the same period. While there are a number of environmental factors that may be of importance, one of the main changes from the 1950s to the end of the twentieth century was the industrialization of food production and the profound change to the type of diet consumed by the population. As developing countries go through improvements in their economies and alongside this adopt a more westernized diet, sperm counts appear to fall accordingly.

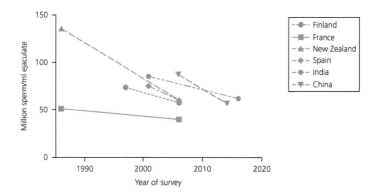

Figure 2.10 Contemporary trends in sperm counts. The assertion that sperm counts fell sharply between the 1940s and 1990s has been widely disputed. However, data from recent surveys using robust methodologies often indicate a progressive decline over a more recent period. *Sources:* data from Shine *et al.* (2008); Jørgensen *et al.* (2011); Geoffroy-Siraudin *et al.* (2012); Mendiola *et al.* (2013); Wang *et al.* (2017); Mishra *et al.* (2018).

2.3.2 Obesity

Obesity is a major problem for all western countries, and the rising trends in overweight and obesity largely mirror the time period over which male fertility has been in decline. Rates of overweight and obesity have roughly doubled every 10 years over the past few decades in developed countries. It is currently estimated that 43% of men aged 20 years and over are obese (BMI >30 kg/m²) in the United States (Hales *et al.*, 2020) and, in England, 27% of men are obese, with 40% being overweight (BMI 25–29.99 kg/m²; NHS Digital, 2019).

BMI appears to be strongly associated with indices of sperm quantity and quality. Men who are underweight have low circulating testosterone concentrations and consequently fail to maintain normal spermatogenesis. Several studies similarly show that being overweight lowers sperm counts. A study of normal fertile men showed that BMI greater than 30 kg/m² was associated with significant detriment to most semen parameters, including a 38% lower total sperm count, relative to men of normal weight (BMI 20–24.99 kg/m²; Ramaraju *et al.*, 2018). Effects of lower magnitude have been reported by other studies, including Ma *et al.* (2019), who reported that sperm counts were 3.9% lower in men who were overweight compared with those of normal weight. The meta-analysis of Guo *et al.* (2017) found that there was a dose-dependent relationship between sperm parameters and BMI. For every 5 kg/m² increase in BMI, total sperm count declined by 2.4%. Evidence suggests that abdominal obesity may be a particular risk factor for infertility, with waist–hip ratio correlating strongly with sperm count and progressive motility (Keszthelyi *et al.*, 2020). Together, these data suggest that to some extent the reported decline in male fertility

between the 1980s and 2010s can be attributed to the accompanying steep increase in the prevalence of overweight and obesity. Sperm samples from men who are overweight and obese have also been reported to show more evidence of oxidative damage. Table 2.6 summarizes the effects of obesity on sperm quality in humans.

Obesity has important effects on the endocrine control of spermatogenesis. Men with excess body fat have lower circulating testosterone concentrations and produce lower quantities of sex hormone binding proteins, which play a key role in the transport of testosterone to the gonads. The lowering of testosterone appears to be driven by a reduced secretion of LH in response to GnRH pulses. There is a cyclical relationship between obesity and sex hormone production in men (Figure 2.11) as, while excess body fat lowers testosterone production, the lower androgen stimulation of the adipose tissue reduces lipolysis and hence promotes further fat deposition. Obesity in men is also associated with a

Table 2.6 Impact of obesity on sperm parameters.

Sperm parameter	Change in men with BMI >30 kg/m² compared to BMI 20–24.9 kg/m²
Semen volume	↓
Total sperm count	↓
Sperm concentration	↓
Total motility	↓
Progressive motility	↓
DNA fragmentation	↑
Abnormal morphology	–

–, no difference; ↑, increased with obesity; ↓, decreased with obesity.

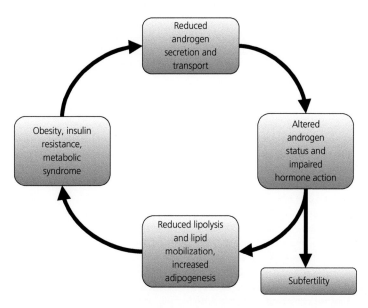

Figure 2.11 The relationship between male obesity and subfertility. Obesity and insulin resistance are a cause of infertility as they interfere with the normal secretion and transport of androgens. As androgens are activators of lipolysis, further adiposity is stimulated by impaired action of the androgens.

lower production of inhibin-B. While this might initially be thought to promote spermatogenesis by reducing negative feedback on FSH production (Figure 2.9), lower inhibin-B production is likely to be indicative of lower Sertoli cell numbers and hence reduced capacity for spermatogenesis.

2.3.3 Alcohol

Excess consumption of alcohol has been linked to subfertility in males, in studies of both humans and animals. Studies that compare men who are fertile and those who are subfertile indicate that alcohol consumption is generally higher in the subfertile population, but there is little evidence that moderate alcohol consumption has a direct effect upon sperm production. As shown in Table 2.4, alcohol has negative effects, but generally only in those who are heavy or binge drinkers. Binge drinking is associated with lower total sperm counts and a reduction in the proportion of sperm with normal morphology. In heavy drinkers, there is evidence of lower semen volume and sperm count, and a greater proportion of damaged sperm cells. The full mechanism responsible for the association between alcohol and male infertility is not well established in humans, but studies of animals indicate that chronically high alcohol intakes lower testosterone production and that ethanol may be directly toxic to testicular tissues. Certainly, the increased numbers of sperm with abnormal morphology associated with excess alcohol may be suggestive of a spermatotoxic effect.

2.3.4 Zinc

Zinc is an essential micronutrient required for the production of a wide range of enzymes, receptors and structural proteins. Zinc is an active site component of over 200 different metalloenzymes and is chiefly involved in stabilization of protein structures, synthesis of DNA and RNA, formation of chromatin, protein synthesis, digestive processes (notably the pancreatic enzymes), antioxidant defences (cofactor for superoxide dismutase) and oxygen transport.

Zinc is postulated to play a role in several components of male reproductive function, and zinc deficiency in some parts of the Middle East has been classically linked to delayed sexual maturation in adolescent boys. The testes have a very high zinc content compared with other organs and tissues, and zinc concentrations are particularly high in the seminal fluid produced by the prostate gland. Data on the role of zinc in maintaining fertility in human males is sparse. There are reports, however, that men with low sperm counts (<20 million cells/ml) have reduced seminal zinc concentrations compared with individuals who are normospermic (Fuse *et al.*, 1999) and seminal zinc concentration is positively correlated with sperm quality. It has been suggested that a small proportion of idiopathic infertility in men may be explained by poor zinc status.

Intervention studies that have considered the impact of zinc supplementation on fertility suggest some improvements in sperm counts, motility and morphology, and increased testosterone concentrations. In the study of Wong *et al.* (2002), administration of 66 mg/day zinc sulphate over six months had no impact on indices of sperm quality or quantity in fertile men but in subfertile men, supplementation increased numbers of sperm with normal motility and morphology by 74%. Despite this major increase, the mean sperm counts in these subfertile men remained below the 20 million cells/ml that the World Health Organization (WHO) uses as the cut-off to define subfertility.

Zinc is increasingly used as a component of commercially available antioxidant supplements to support male fertility. These supplements are discussed in the following section. Zinc is incorporated by virtue of being a cofactor for antioxidant enzymes such as superoxide dismutase. However, the data on zinc is equivocal. Balanced against the study of Wong *et al.* (2002), described above, are reports that suggest limited efficacy. A six-month trial of 30 mg zinc with 5 mg folate per day compared with placebo found no beneficial effect on semen parameters or live births when the supplement was given to male partners in couples undergoing fertility treatment. There was evidence of greater sperm DNA fragmentation in the supplemented group (Schisterman *et al.*, 2020).

2.3.5 Antioxidant nutrients

Free radicals and other ROS were discussed in the context of female fertility earlier in this chapter. While ROS are generally perceived as having negative, tissue-damaging effects in biological systems, it is important to realize that endogenously generated ROS also play a number of important physiological roles. The manufacture of sperm is one such role, and ROS produced within immature sperm cells are important in the production of the tail sheath that encloses the mitochondria of the midsection, which will ultimately generate adenosine triphosphate and provide the motile function of the sperm cells. ROS are also important in the functions of spermatozoa during fertilization and are generated to promote attachment to oocytes and to generate the acrosome reaction, which allows the sperm to penetrate the zona pellucida layer of the oocyte.

As ROS are critical for normal sperm functions, mature sperm cells are less protected with antioxidants than most other cell types, although the immature cells are rich in the antioxidant enzymes superoxide dismutase, glutathione peroxidase (GPx) and catalase. Mature cells are therefore vulnerable to damage by ROS, which will principally cause fragmentation of DNA, the primary morphological abnormality noted in subfertile men.

Immature sperm cells are vulnerable as they are producing ROS for differentiation and are present in a membrane-rich tissue. Biological membranes are rich in polyunsaturated fatty acids, which are a major target for ROS-mediated damage. There is clearly a delicate balance between oxidative and antioxidant processes in sperm cells and their associated support tissues.

It is biologically plausible to suggest that antioxidant nutrients may have a beneficial effect on male fertility, but unfortunately there are few studies of high quality which have assessed the strength of this hypothesis (Showell *et al.*, 2011). A number of studies have compared subfertile men with healthy, normospermic donors and reported that subfertile men have higher concentrations of ROS and lower concentrations of antioxidant nutrients in semen samples (Moustafa *et al.*, 2004). Other studies have shown that the addition of antioxidants, for example, glutathione or α-tocopherol to culture media used in artificial reproductive technologies, boosts conception rates by increasing the motility of spermatozoa (Ozawa *et al.*, 2006). Studies which have investigated antioxidant potential of semen itself have demonstrated that antioxidants may improve quality. Among subfertile men, greater sperm concentration was accompanied by higher semen antioxidant capacity (Silberstein *et al.*, 2016). A study of 55 men grouped according to seminal plasma antioxidant potential showed that sperm motility was greater in those with high potential, but other sperm parameters were not different to those of men with low seminal antioxidant potential.

There are few studies that have considered the impact of antioxidant intakes within a normal diet upon indices of male fertility. Salas-Huetos *et al.* (2017) reviewed observational studies that have explored this impact and concluded that dietary patterns which are rich in antioxidant nutrients (fish, shellfish, vegetables, fruit, poultry, cereals) are associated with better male fertility. However, this analysis lacked the depth to demonstrate an antioxidant effect, as opposed to a healthy diet that maintains a healthy weight. Other studies have sought to investigate the association between specific nutrient intakes and sperm quality, and have suggested that higher intakes of vitamin C, α-tocopherol and β-carotene are associated with greater sperm counts and measures of sperm motility (Eskenazi *et al.*, 2005).

Many studies have evaluated the effects of antioxidant supplementation on male fertility. Unfortunately, many of these studies suffer from poor experimental design (a lack of placebo control), low sample size and the use of doses that are super-physiological. Steiner *et al.* (2020) targeted infertile men who had normally ovulatory partners, using a mixed supplement containing vitamin C, vitamin E, folate, zinc, carnitine, selenium and lycopene. After three months of supplementation there were no improvements in sperm parameters or in the success of fertility treatments. In contrast, three months of administration of a complex supplement containing vitamin C, beta-carotene, vitamin E, folate, vitamin K, vitamin B6, vitamin B12, riboflavin, niacin, thiamine, biotin, lycopene, N-acetylcysteine, carnitine, coenzyme Q, zinc, iodine, selenium, molybdenum, manganese, copper and chromium improved sperm concentrations, motility and morphology, and reduced oxidative damage in sperm (Arafa *et al.*, 2020). Despite these improvements, the average values for sperm quality remained below the WHO cut-offs for fertility. A triple-blind randomized controlled trial of 600 mg/day alpha-lipoic acid in men with infertility, improved seminal antioxidant capacity and most parameters of sperm quality over a 12-week period (Haghighian *et al.*, 2015).

A meta-analysis of all randomized controlled trials of antioxidant supplementation concluded that although the quality of evidence was very low, supplements may improve the chances of conception and live birth (Smits *et al.*, 2019). Antioxidant supplements increased the odds of live birth (OR 1.79, 95% CI 1.20–2.50). In effect, antioxidant supplements increase the chances of successful pregnancy in any given cycle from 12% in placebo groups to 14–26% in supplemented groups. This area of research is therefore suggestive of benefits associated with increased antioxidant consumption, but more high-quality research is needed to firm up the potential benefits and the nature of the key nutrients or foodstuffs.

2.3.6 Selenium

It is well established from animal studies that selenium is a key nutrient for the maintenance of male fertility. Selenium deficiency in animals, or the knockout of key genes in mice that lead to production of selenoproteins, leads to lower sperm production and poor sperm motility. Selenium appears to be particularly important in the formation of the tailpiece in mammalian sperm. As described above, this is a process that involves the generation of ROS and a balance between oxidative and antioxidative processes is critical in normal differentiation of the spermatids. Selenium is a cofactor for the antioxidant enzyme GPx and, in sperm, the GPX4 isoform appears particularly important in tail formation (Beckett and Arthur, 2005). Although there is clear evidence that many men with subfertility who have sperm defects have abnormalities of GPX4 in their sperm, it is unlikely that in most cases this is due to limiting intakes of selenium in the diet.

In populations where habitual selenium intakes are low (e.g. Scotland), there is no strong evidence of lower fertility. A detailed study of men whose selenium status was controlled for a period of 120 days while living on a metabolic unit (Hawkes and Turek, 2001) suggested that while a high-selenium diet produced large increases in seminal selenium concentrations, sperm motility actually decreased. This suggests that the common recommendation to consume rich sources of selenium (e.g. Brazil nuts) for men preparing for fatherhood may be ineffective.

2.3.7 Phytoestrogens and environmental oestrogens

In developed countries, populations are constantly exposed to a range of chemical agents that have endocrine-disrupting properties. Endocrine disruptors are agents that interfere with normal hormonal functions within the body, either by having a direct hormonal effect or by opposing the actions of endogenous hormones (anti-hormones). Human exposure to endocrine disruptors comes from a wide range of different sources (Table 2.7), most of which are unavoidable due to their presence in the food chain, atmosphere and water supply.

Table 2.7 Environmental sources of human exposure to endocrine-disrupting chemicals.

Source	Examples	Putative effects
Atmosphere (inhalation), cosmetics	Polyaromatic hydrocarbons, parabens (in shampoos, perfumes, deodorants)	Suppress oestrogen metabolism, oestrogen mimics
	Phthalates	Suppress testosterone synthesis
	Nitromusks	Inhibit hypothalamic–gonadotrophic axis
Food chain	Plasticizers (phthalates)	Suppress testosterone synthesis
	Polyaromatic hydrocarbons, pesticides and fungicides	Suppress oestrogen metabolism, oestrogenic and anti-androgenic effects
Water supply	Atrazine (herbicide) 17β-oestradiol	Oestrogen mimic, oestrogenic effect

Endocrine disruptors are known from studies of the impact of human activity on wildlife to be particularly potent within the reproductive organs. For example, tributyltin, an antifouling agent used on ships, was found to be an anti-hormone blocking production of oestrogen and masculinizing shellfish. The excretion of oestrogen metabolites in urine from women using certain oral contraceptives has been blamed for the feminization of male fish found around sewage outlets. Clear examples of effects of endocrine disruptors on human male fertility are more difficult to demonstrate, but there are a number of agents that have been proposed as potentially harmful. These agents are described in the following sections.

2.3.7.1 Phthalates

Phthalates are a class of chemicals used to make plastics. They are widely used in the production of cosmetics, toys and all manner of goods that require flexible plastics. Phthalates are known to adversely affect the male reproductive system in animals, inducing both hypospadias and cryptorchidism and leading to reduced testosterone production and sperm counts (Sharpe and Irvine, 2004). Exposure to phthalates during human fetal development has been linked to feminization of baby boys, and this has led to widespread concern at the potential for these agents to enter formula milk consumed by infants during the critical phase of reproductive development. However, levels of phthalates in formula milks have been shown to be low and are now monitored. Studies show that phthalates also appear in breast milk, as they are excreted following maternal exposure.

There is also some evidence of associations between phthalate exposure and fertility in mature men. The mode of phthalate action is simply to inhibit testosterone production. Measurements of phthalate metabolites have proved to be inversely proportional to sperm quality. Thurston *et al.* (2016) reported that adult exposure to mono-isobutyl phthalate was associated with reduced sperm motility, but the effect was small and no other phthalate species appeared to be harmful. Other studies have shown urinary phthalates and the use of plastic food storage containers to be negatively associated with semen volume and sperm concentration (Caporossi *et al.*, 2020).

2.3.7.2 Phytoestrogens

Phytoestrogens are plant-derived compounds that have a weak oestrogenic activity by virtue of a similar molecular structure to oestrogens (Figure 2.12). Within the human diet, they are ingested either in

the form of lignans, which are present in vegetable matter, or as soya-derived isoflavones, which include genistein, daidzein and naringenin. Intakes of isoflavones within the diet vary immensely both within and between different populations. Average intakes for omnivores in the UK are around 1 mg per day, while vegetarians have much higher intakes at around 7–8 mg per day. In Japan and Southeast Asia, soya is consumed as a staple food, for example, as tempeh or tofu, and intakes are around 25–100 mg per day.

The oestrogenic effects of phytoestrogens have a number of positive effects upon health in women, which are dealt with elsewhere in this book. There have been concerns over their impact upon male reproductive health, particularly as within a western diet soya is becoming very widely used as an ingredient in processed foods and as a meat or dairy substitute. These concerns arise primarily from studies of animals suggesting that phytoestrogens may have effects on young, developing males but not on mature individuals. Several studies have shown in rats and mice that comparing the offspring of pregnant animals fed diets containing soya to those fed a soya-free diet reveals differences in testicular weight, circulating FSH and capacity to successfully mate with females. Atanassova *et al.* (2000) found that adverse effects of genistein on indices of fertility in male rats were at their greatest when it was administered during puberty. In contrast, Tan *et al.* (2006) studied the impact of feeding soy formula milk to baby marmosets and found no gross effects upon their reproductive organs in later life. While many studies on animals suggest that exposure to phytoestrogens in early life delays puberty and impacts detrimentally on reproductive performance and fertility, many such experiments have used doses that are very high compared with the range of human consumption. In contrast, Fielden *et al.* (2003) fed male mice genistein at levels equivalent to human consumption and found no adverse effects on their fertility.

In humans, dietary phytoestrogens appear to have pronounced effects on endocrine markers in women but not in men. There is no evidence in Asian countries, where intakes are high, that fertility is impaired. This may in part be due to the low prevalence of obesity in such populations. Evidence relating to phytoestrogens and male fertility in humans is somewhat mixed in terms of outcome. A study of the male partners in subfertile couples showed that, after adjustment for confounding factors, men who consumed more soy-based foods had markedly lower sperm counts but normal sperm morphology and motility (Chavarro *et al.*, 2008). A study of more than

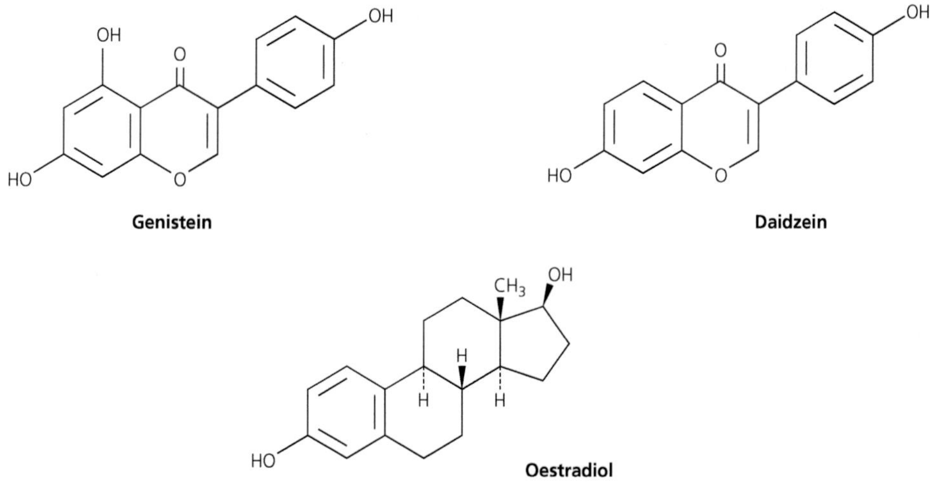

Figure 2.12 The structures of oestrogen and phytoestrogens. Phytoestrogens such as genistein and daidzein (the principal soya isoflavones) have a similar chemical structure to oestrogens, allowing binding to the oestrogen receptors.

1000 Chinese men found that high urinary excretion of phytoestrogens was a feature of those men with idiopathic infertility, with lower total sperm counts, sperm concentrations and motility observed in the highest quintile of daidzein excretion (Xia *et al.*, 2013). Similarly, semen phytoestrogen concentrations were inversely associated with semen quality in another study of Chinese men (Yuan *et al.*, 2019). High semen genistein or naringin concentrations were associated with low sperm concentrations, total sperm counts and motility. In contrast, controlled trials in which soy isoflavones were administered to men with normal fertility found little impact. Mitchell *et al.* fed men 40 mg of soy isoflavones for two months and showed no change in testicular volume, sex hormone concentrations or sperm quality. Similarly, administration of high concentrations of soy isolates for eight weeks, sufficient to increase urinary isoflavone concentrations, had no impact on any indices of sperm quality or total sperm count (Beaton *et al.*, 2010).

While data on exposure of older men to phytoestrogens do not consistently support the evidence of risk inferred from animal studies, an impact of phytoestrogen exposure during infancy cannot be excluded. Early life exposure to isoflavones through sources other than soy milk formula in infancy is difficult to evaluate, but there are some data suggesting an association with reproductive abnormalities. A study of the Avon Longitudinal Study of Parents and Children cohort, a large study of pregnancy and childhood in the Bristol area of the UK, suggested that vegetarian mothers were almost five times more likely to have baby boys with hypospadias than omnivorous mothers (North and Golding, 2000). This finding may be attributed either to the high phytoestrogen content of the maternal diet or to greater ingestion of pesticides and other contaminants on fruit and vegetable matter. There are no data available on fertility rates or markers of semen quality from individuals exposed to high levels of phytoestrogen in fetal life or infancy.

It is widely assumed that a western dietary pattern is harmful to male fertility, particularly given the association between BMI and sperm parameters. There is therefore some interest in evaluating whether a vegetarian or vegan diet may be beneficial. However, there is little research available. A study of 474 men living in the Loma Linda Blue Zone (an area in California with a high density of largely vegetarian Seventh Day Adventists), considered sperm parameters in omnivores compared with lacto-ovo vegetarians and a very small number (five) of vegans (Orzylowska *et al.*, 2016). The vegetarians had lower total sperm counts than the omnivores and their samples showed lower sperm motility (omnivores 52.2%, vegetarians 33.2%). The vegans in this sample had lower total sperm counts than the lacto-ovo vegetarians. The reasons for this apparently detrimental impact of a vegetarian diet are unclear, but could relate to greater intakes of phytoestrogens, or greater prevalence of underweight. Lower BMI has been associated with lower sperm counts.

2.3.7.3 Pesticides

A huge range of organic pesticides are present within the environment, and many of these are known to have endocrine-disrupting properties. Of greatest concern are those which have the potential to enter the food chain as contaminants. Vinclozolin is an example of a pesticide that has been linked to male fertility problems in animals (Gray *et al.*, 1999). Vinclozolin is a fungicide used in the production of oil seed rape, peas, and fruits such as grapes. Studies of this agent in rats and other species show that, at doses that may be consumed by humans, it can feminize males and damage their reproductive capacity. As with phthalates, the early stages of fetal development appear to be a sensitive period for exposure. Although there is no clear evidence of harmful effects in humans, approvals for use of this agent on strawberries, tomatoes, lettuce and raspberries were withdrawn by the UK and European Commission in the 1990s.

The potential for pesticides in food to be of detriment to male fertility is one reason why some in the population advocate consumption of only organic produce. A series of studies which have compared farmers, who have the greatest exposure to pesticides, with other occupations have suggested that pesticide workers may have impaired fertility with lower sperm counts and motility (Hossain *et al.*, 2010). However, direct comparison of organic and non-organic farmers has suggested that such findings are artefacts of poor experimental design (Larsen *et al.*, 1999). There is no robust evidence to indicate that pesticide contamination of items in the human food chain is a contributor to the observed decline in population level male fertility.

2.4 Preparation for pregnancy

2.4.1 Why prepare for pregnancy?

With modern healthcare and an increasing emphasis on maintaining and promoting health, rather than treating disease, provision of advice and care during the preconceptual period is becoming more commonplace in developed countries. The main aim of any work in this area will be to maximize the health of both prospective parents, and this will maximize their fertility (as described previously) and minimize the potential for the early embryo to be exposed to potentially harmful agents. To achieve this aim, it is necessary to address the controllable risk factors for adverse pregnancy outcomes while parents are still planning a pregnancy (Table 2.8). Clearly, not all such factors are directly related to nutrition, but social, environmental and behavioural elements are all interlinked and impact upon individuals' attitudes, choices and opportunities in relation to lifestyle and diet.

In addition to maximizing fertility, it is important to eliminate the potential for an early embryo to be exposed to factors that could exert harmful effects should a conception occur. To this end, the preparatory phase before conception should ideally involve lifestyle changes for both men and women. Although women are preparing and providing the environment in which the fetus will develop, their chances of success in making lifestyle changes will be considerably greater if they do so in partnership. Men are therefore responsible for much more than maximizing their own fertility and should cooperate with women in maintaining a healthy body weight, in ensuring that immunizations against infections that might harm the fetus (e.g. rubella) are up to date and in reducing exposures to alcohol and tobacco smoke. From a dietary point of view, there are two important changes that should be made to minimize risk of birth defects. These are increasing intakes of folic acid and reducing exposure to high doses of vitamin A, both of which are described in more detail in the following sections.

2.4.2 Maternal weight management

In addition to adverse effects upon female fertility, maternal overweight and excessive weight gain in pregnancy is a major risk factor for poor pregnancy outcomes, as will be described in Chapter 3. Weight during pregnancy and the rate of weight gain during pregnancy are closely linked to weight prior to pregnancy, and prepregnancy weight is strongly associated with risk of gestational diabetes and hypertensive complications in pregnancy (Li *et al.*, 2013) and may also predict the health of children in later life (Hinkle *et al.*, 2013). The recommendations on pregnancy weight gain made by the US Institute of Medicine (2009) are stratified by prepregnancy BMI (see Section 3.4.2.1), reflecting the important contribution of weight prior to conception upon pregnancy outcomes.

Although lower weight gain in pregnancy is advised for women who are overweight or obese, weight loss is not advised during pregnancy, as this may limit provision of nutrients to the developing fetus. Weight loss advice is instead targeted at women prior to conception. In 2010, the National Institute for Health and Care Excellence issued a guideline that health professionals should identify women with BMI over 30 kg/m^2 prior to pregnancy and advise a 5–10% weight loss prior to conception (National Institute for Health and Care Excellence, 2010). This guidance aims to improve conception rates and reduce pregnancy complications.

2.4.3 Vitamin A and liver

Vitamin A is one of the essential nutrients in the diet, but intake should be restricted during pregnancy because of a well-established association with

Table 2.8 Factors that impact on parental health during the periconceptual period.

Factors	Examples
Controllable:	
Environmental: the influence of home and workplace	Hygiene, sanitation, occupational chemical exposure
Lifestyle: the health choices and behaviours of the parents	Smoking, alcohol, diet, exercise
Uncontrollable:	
Social: the circumstances in which the parents live	Family income, access to healthcare, education
Physiological: the underlying health circumstances of the parents	Genetic disorders, age, obstetric disorders, infection

birth defects. In the diet, vitamin A is available in two forms, the first being animal-derived retinol and the second plant-derived carotenoids. Due to this diversity of sources, vitamin A intakes are generally described in terms of retinol activity equivalents (RAE) with one RAE being equivalent to 1 μg retinol or 6 μg β-carotene. Generally, intakes of vitamin A are measured as milligramme retinol equivalents or international units (iu, with one RAE equivalent to 3.3 iu). Once within the body, vitamin A undergoes extensive metabolism (Figure 2.13). In addition to mediating some of the classically defined functions, such as formation of rhodopsin within the retina, it is an important regulator of gene expression through the retinoic acid and retinoid X receptors.

Vitamin A first was shown to be a teratogen in studies of animals. The administration of high doses of retinol and all-trans retinoic acid during pregnancy induced abnormalities in almost all tissues of fetal mice, rats, hamsters, rabbits and non-human primates (Soprano and Soprano, 1995). The demonstration that the same effects occur in humans has generally relied on the observation of the adverse effects of certain pharmacological agents. Retinoid derivatives are widely used in the treatment of skin conditions such as severe acne. Pregnant women who used products containing 12-*cis*retinoic acid had babies with craniofacial abnormalities such as cleft lip, with heart defects and with abnormalities of the central nervous system. Such products are therefore contraindicated in women who are pregnant or considering having a child.

There are very few recorded cases in which overconsumption of dietary vitamin A can be firmly

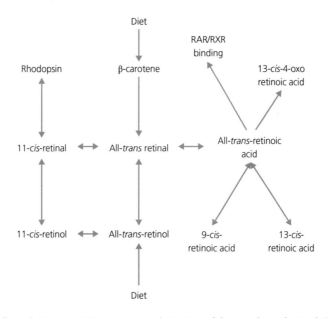

Figure 2.13 The metabolism of vitamin A. Dietary sources of vitamin A deliver preformed retinol (from animal sources) or β-carotene. Retinol from the diet or formed within the liver is used to generate rhodopsin in the retina and is converted to retinoic acid which modulates gene expression via the RAR/RXR receptors. Retinoic acid can be metabolized to a number of intermediates that are known to have teratogenic properties in animals and humans.

attributed as the cause of birth defects in humans. However, where this is the case (Soprano and Soprano, 1995), the defects generated tend to be highly variable and to occur across multiple organ systems, including the heart. Martinez-Frias and Salvador (1990) compared Spanish women who had given birth to babies with congenital malformations (cases) with women whose babies were normally developed (controls). The overwhelming majority of cases were unrelated to vitamin A teratogenicity, but among women who had taken megadose supplements of vitamin A, there were significant associations between consumption and malformations. At doses below 40 000 iu, there was no increased risk, but over 40 000, the odds of malformation were increased 2.7-fold (Figure 2.14). The greatest risk was associated with consumption of vitamin A alone, at doses of over 60 000 iu. Further studies indicate that the danger to fetal development lies with consumption of preformed retinol during the phases of embryonic development when the organs initially form (organogenesis). Retinol, intake in excess of 10 000 iu was found to increase risk of major cardiac defects by 9.2-fold (95% CI 4.0–21.2) but the risk was all from supplement use (Botto *et al.*, 2001). Rothman *et al.* (1995) noted that greater risk of cranial–neural crest defects began to appear at doses as low as 5000 iu and concluded that, at this dose, 1 in 57 pregnant women using supplements would give birth to a child with a malformation. The threshold intake for safe consumption is difficult to pinpoint but may lie between 8000 and 10 000 iu (Mills *et al.*, 1997). Some studies indicate that risk is negligible within extended ranges of intake, with no evidence of increased risk

of orofacial clefts reported in the highest 5% of consumers (Johansen *et al.*, 2008). In the light of these observations, it is strongly advised that pregnant women, or those planning a pregnancy, should avoid vitamin A containing supplements. Typical multivitamins available over the counter contain approximately 8000–9000 iu. Although the Martinez-Frias and Salvador (1990) study and similar works suffer from the generic problems associated with case–control studies (choice of control group can be problematic, study cannot firmly demonstrate causal relationships, exposure to nutrient has to be done retrospectively and may be inaccurate), together with the data from animal and pharmacological studies, it appears that excessive levels of vitamin A consumption do play a causal role in development of fetal abnormalities.

Liver is a major source of preformed retinol within the diet, and a 100-g portion of beef liver may deliver 32 000 iu vitamin A in a single meal. The vitamin A content of liver has increased since the 1980s because of intensive farming, and so the associated risk in modern times is likely to be greater than in the past, when pregnant women were actively encouraged to eat liver as a source of iron. In particular, liver appears to increase circulating concentrations of two of the most teratogenic isomers of retinoic acid, namely, 13-*cis*-retinoic acid and 13-*cis*-4-oxoretinoic acid. Arnhold *et al.* (1996) showed that feeding male volunteers fried turkey liver significantly elevated concentrations of all metabolites of retinol within a short period of time. Similarly, Hartmann *et al.* (2005) found that feeding non-pregnant women 120 000 iu vitamin A in a liver meal greatly increased plasma 13-*cis*-retinoic

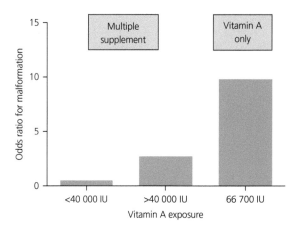

Figure 2.14 Vitamin A supplementation and fetal malformations. The relationship between vitamin A supplementation and fetal malformations was explored in a population of Spanish women. The data show odds of malformations associated with vitamin A in a multivitamin supplement, higher levels of vitamin A in a multivitamin supplement and megadose supplements of vitamin A alone. *Source:* data from Martinez-Frias and Salvador (1990).

acid and 13-*cis*-4-oxo-retinoic acid concentrations. Clearly, with these observations, alongside the studies of Martinez-Frias and Salvador (1990), caution is appropriate, and liver should be avoided by women planning a pregnancy. An important consideration is that consumption of liver appears to increase circulating retinoic acid metabolites in women, to a much greater extent than consumption of a vitamin A supplement of equivalent dosage (van Vliet *et al.*, 2001).

The association between vitamin A and birth defects is particularly challenging for populations in regions where vitamin A deficiency is prevalent. Vitamin A deficiency results in night blindness for many pregnant women in developing countries and contributes to poor pregnancy outcomes and greater risk of infectious disease for their infants. Vitamin deficiency also increases risk of preterm birth and anaemia (Radika *et al.*, 2002). To ameliorate these problems, the WHO has developed a protocol for safe vitamin A supplementation (Table 2.9).

2.4.4 Folic acid and neural tube defects

Neural tube defects (NTDs) are among the most common fetal abnormalities observed in western populations. These conditions, of which the most significant are spina bifida and anencephaly, currently affect 0.3 births in every 1000 in the UK, representing around 150–200 cases every year. However, the true number of NTDs is considerably higher (around 4 cases per 1000 births) and most affected fetuses are terminated after diagnosis with antenatal ultrasound scans.

Spina bifida and anencephaly are different manifestations of the same developmental problem. During normal development, the embryonic neural tube, which will go on to become the brain and the spinal cord, undergoes a process of folding and closing to form an enclosed neural canal. This closure of the neural tube will normally occur in the fourth

Table 2.9 World Health Organization protocol for vitamin A supplementation.

Target group	Dose (iu)	Frequency
Infants		Once
6–11 months	100 000	
12–59 months	200 000	Every 4–6 months
Pregnant women*	Up to 10 000	Daily[†]
	Up to 25 000	Weekly[†]

Oral supplements are provided as oily drops of retinyl palmitate.
* Only to be used in communities where vitamin A deficiency is a significant problem.
[†] Only for the last three months of pregnancy.

week of gestation, a time which is generally too early for the mother to be aware of her pregnancy. Failure of the neural tube to close results in permanent disability, the severity of which depends on the location of the tube lesion. A lesion high up along the neural tube will result in anencephaly, a condition in which the cerebral arches of the brain will be absent (Figure 2.15). Babies with anencephaly will inevitably die, either during gestation or within a few hours of birth. Lesions lower down the neural tube will result in spina bifida. As the spinal cord is not fully encased in bone, it is vulnerable to injury and damaged spinal nerves and cord are associated with paralysis, incontinence and, in some cases, delayed cognitive development and learning disabilities.

As discussed in Research Highlight 2.3, low maternal intake of folic acid is one of several risk factors for NTDs. The demands of the fetus for folate around the time of the closure of the neural tube are high as folates are important cofactors for the synthesis of purine nucleotides and thymidylate which are required for cell division. If folate is a limiting nucleotide at this time, then neural tube closure may be irreversibly compromised. The link between folic acid and NTDs was firmly established through intervention trials using varying doses of folic acid in combination with other micronutrients (Laurence *et al.*, 1981; Czeizel and Dudas, 1992). The MRC Vitamin Study Group (1991) performed a randomized, double-blind trial of 1817 women in 33 centres, across 7 countries. All women had a previous history of a pregnancy with NTD and were randomized to either a placebo group; a group given a supplement of folic acid alone (4 mg/day); a group provided with a supplement containing vitamins A, D, B1, B2, B6 and C and nicotinamide or a fourth group provided with the same multivitamin supplement plus folate. Supplementation to 12 weeks of gestation produced the greatest beneficial effect when folate was given alone (72% reduction in NTD risk). Folate as an element of a multivitamin supplement was effective, but less so than as a single nutrient.

On the basis of the MRC study and the work of Czeizel and Dudas (1992), it is clear that increasing dietary supply of folic acid will reduce the risk of a pregnancy being affected by an NTD. Accordingly, the reference nutrient intake for folic acid increases during pregnancy from 200 to 600 mg per day. However, as neural tube closure is an early event in embryonic development, any increase in maternal supply has to occur prior to conception to ensure risk is minimal. To this end, there are two strategies that can be used to protect the population: supplementation and fortification.

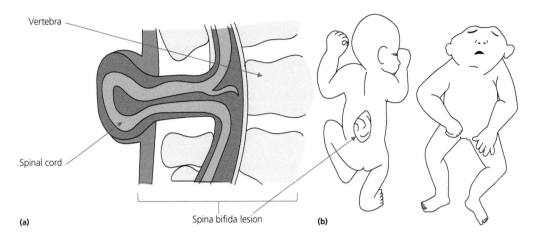

Vertebra

Spinal cord

(a)

Spina bifida lesion

(b)

Figure 2.15 The main neural tube defects, spina bifida (a) and anencephaly (b) are caused by the failure of the neural tube to close during embryonic development. In spina bifida this occurs at the level of the spinal cord, resulting in lesions where the cord is not encased in bone. In anencephaly the defect results in the cerebral arches being absent and the condition is invariably fatal.

Research Highlight 2.3 Risk factors for neural tube defects.

The risk of a neural tube defect (NTD)-affected pregnancy is multifactorial (Agopian *et al.*, 2013), with greater risk associated with a family history of such defects, particular ethnic backgrounds, obesity, poorly controlled diabetes before pregnancy, gestational diabetes, low intakes of folate, use of anticonvulsant drugs for epilepsy, opioid abuse and maternal hyperthermia (e.g. use of saunas). The role of genetics is considerable, and women who have previously had an NTD-affected pregnancy are at 100-fold greater risk in subsequent pregnancies. A number of genetic susceptibilities have been identified which include some of the enzymes involved in folic acid metabolism, genes associated with glucose homeostasis and insulin resistance (Lupo *et al.*, 2012). The genetic risk predictors are complex as multiple genotypes may interact within the mother and between mother and fetus to determine how the neural tube develops. A study of Chinese women showed that single nucleotide polymorphisms in genes which regulate glucose metabolism are associated with NTDs. For example, the AA variant of the GCKRrs780094 (glucokinase regulator) was associated with 1.83-fold greater risk of spina bifida (95% CI 1.16–2.28; Fu *et al.*, 2015).

The major avoidable risk factors are obesity and folate intake. The impact of obesity is considerable and may be linked to the metabolic impact of excess body fatness upon glucose homeostasis. Gao *et al.* (2013) reported an OR of 2.45 for NTD associated with overweight. According to Donnan *et al.* (2017), risk of spina bifida was increased with obesity prior to pregnancy (OR 2.24 95% CI 1.86–2.74) and a huge study of all 1.33 million pregnancies in Florida between 2005 and 2009 demonstrated a 1.36-fold greater risk of spina bifida with prepregnancy obesity (Block *et al.*, 2013). A systematic review of 39 articles by Stothard *et al.* (2009) found that risk of all NTD was increased by 1.87-fold (95% CI 1.62–2.15) in obese women (OR for spina bifida 2.24, 95% CI 0.86–2.69). Risk was shown to be considerably higher in women with two features of the metabolic syndrome (Ray *et al.*, 2007) or in women with excessive sugar intakes prior to conception. Parnell *et al.* (2017) suggested that the risk of NTD was only elevated with obesity if the pregnancy was also complicated by gestational diabetes.

Obesity may also modify risk of NTD through changes in folate metabolism, transport and storage. Benefits of folate supplementation are only seen in women of normal weight and are absent in overweight or obese groups (Wang *et al.*, 2013). Tinker *et al.* (2012) reported that in women with higher BMI, serum folate concentrations were lower than in women of ideal BMI, while red cell folate concentrations were elevated. Lower serum folate has been noted in maternal obesity, with a negative correlation between BMI and folate concentrations, irrespective of maternal intake from diet, or supplements (O'Malley *et al.*, 2018). These findings suggest that obesity may impact upon the distribution and availability of folate to the developing embryo and some studies indicate that it may also impact upon the effects of folate in the epigenetic regulation of gene expression (Park *et al.*, 2017). Given such findings, recommendations for folic acid supplementation might need to be different for women with a higher BMI. However, there is also evidence that the relationship between obesity and NTD risk is independent of any influence of folate. By comparing the prevalence of NTD in obese women in the United States prior to and after the introduction of mandatory fortification of grains with folic acid, Ray *et al.* (2005) showed that the risk associated with obesity increased after the folate status of the population had improved. This would indicate that folate-independent mechanisms increase NTD risk in overweight women.

2.4.4.1 Supplementation with folic acid

Supplementation with folic acid prior to conception and in the early stages of pregnancy is the approach to NTD prevention in most European countries. In 1992, the UK Chief Medical Officer first announced a firm recommendation that women who are considering pregnancy should take a 400 μg per day supplement of folic acid for 3 months prior to conception and for the first 12 weeks of pregnancy to reduce risk of NTD. This strategy was devised with the intention that it would cover the period of neural tube closure (often occurring before a woman knows she is pregnant) and reduce risk by approximately half. Supplementation was considered necessary as achieving 400 μg per day extra intake through diet alone would require impossible increases in consumption of fruit and vegetables. Women with a prior history of NTD were advised to take a 4-mg per day supplement, the dose noted to be effective in the MRC Vitamin Study Group (1991) trial.

The impact of folic acid supplementation in the UK on NTD prevalence was modest, with a decline that was barely distinguishable from a general downward trend associated with improved antenatal screening and other factors (Figure 2.16). This limited success highlights the main difficulty with supplementation on a population-wide scale, which is providing the necessary health education and awareness campaigns to ensure a high level of compliance. Younger women, women of lower educational achievement and women who smoke are the population groups that are least likely to use folate supplements (Langley-Evans and Langley-Evans, 2001). Moreover, with 40% of pregnancies reported to be unplanned, the impact of periconceptual supplementation is inevitably reduced.

2.4.4.2 Fortification with folic acid

As described previously, the major problem with a prevention strategy based on supplementation is that full coverage of all the at-risk population can never be achieved. In the UK, it was found that even after many years to allow for training of health professionals and promotion of supplementation through health education, the policy did not achieve the expected reduction in risk. The alternative to supplementation, which depends upon individuals making an active decision to change dietary behaviour, is fortification of staple foods that are widely consumed by the target population.

Fortification of wheat flours has been adopted worldwide as a public health nutrition strategy in 81 countries including Canada (1998, addition of 150 μg folate per 100 g grain), Chile (1998, 220 μg folate per 100 g grain), Costa Rica (180 μg folate per 100 g grain) and South Africa (2003, 150 μg folate per 100 g grain). The level of fortification varies between countries to reflect national trends in consumption of wheat products. Fortification with folate became mandatory in the United States in 1998 (140 μg folate per 100 g grain) and proved highly effective in reducing the prevalence of NTDs (Figure 2.16). Pfeiffer *et al.* (2005) examined the impact of this

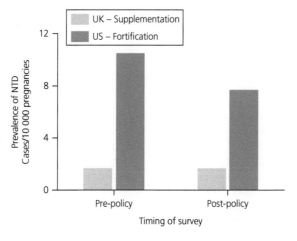

Figure 2.16 US fortification with folic acid has been more effective than supplementation in the UK in the prevention of neural tube defects (NTD). In 1992, the UK introduced guidelines recommending supplementation with folic acid in preparation for pregnancy to reduce the risk of neural tube defects. The United States introduced mandatory fortification of grains with folic acid in 1998. UK data correspond to 1990 (pre-policy) and 1999 (post-policy) and show a decline of 2%. US data correspond to 1995–1996 (pre-policy) and 1999–2000 (post-policy) and show a decline of 27%. *Sources:* data from Centers for Disease Control and Prevention (2004); Morris and Wald (1999).

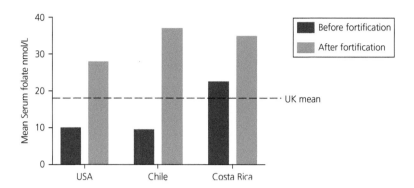

Figure 2.17 Change in folate status in women of reproductive age in countries implementing mandatory fortification of grains with folic acid. UK mean shown for reference. *Sources:* data from Hertrampf *et al.* (2003), Centers for Disease Control and Prevention (2004); Chen and Rivera (2004).

policy on folate status in the US population and found that fortification reduced the prevalence of low serum folate concentrations dramatically, with benefits observed in all ethnic groups, in both sexes and in people of all ages. Figure 2.17 shows mean serum folate concentrations in three countries where mandatory folate fortification has been introduced. Marked increases from pre-fortification levels are observed in all studies. In countries such as the UK, where no fortification occurs, the mean folate concentration is significantly lower. Alongside increases in population folate status, fortification achieves the intended goal of reducing NTD prevalence. Between 1995, when a period of optional fortification began, and 2002, intakes of folate in the US population doubled. The prevalence of spina bifida declined by 36% among Hispanic women (the highest-risk group in the United States) and 34% among the white population (Williams *et al.*, 2005). Dramatic declines in NTD prevalence have been reported for Canada (46%), Chile (50%) and Costa Rica (35%). In contrast, among 19 countries of the European Union, which have not adopted mandatory fortification, the prevalence of NTDs has remained stable at 9.1 cases per 10 000 births, based on data collected between 1991 and 2011 (Khoshnood *et al.*, 2015).

Fortification through wheat flours may not reach all women of childbearing age, so other fortified products are required to achieve full coverage in the population. In the United States, although NTD levels declined sharply among Hispanic women, this group remained at higher risk than other ethnic groups. The staple for this population is corn masa flour, which is not included in mandatory fortification. In 2016, a voluntary fortification scheme was introduced to target corn masa products and tortillas, but uptake by manufacturers has been very

poor (Redpath *et al.*, 2018) so Hispanic women who follow a traditional diet and are considering pregnancy should consume supplements at a rate of 400 µg per day for three months prior to conception and throughout the first trimester of pregnancy (Kancherla *et al.*, 2019).

Where fortification of staple foods with folate has been introduced, there are reports of benefits to the wider adult population in terms of cardiovascular health and cancer risk (See Section 8.4.4.3.4). This shows a reach for this policy that extends beyond the intended target group. To date 81 countries have adopted mandatory folate fortification policies to reduce the prevalence of NTDs and all of these have done so without major objections from their populations or evidence of significant detriment to health. The UK and countries in the European Union have not adopted this approach, although a UK government consultation launched in 2019 appears to pave the way for a policy change. There are two key concerns about the adverse consequences of folate overconsumption that have led to caution on the part of European governments.

First, there have been reports that following introduction of fortification in North America, or with supplementation of folic acid at 400 µg per day, there was an increase in risk of colorectal and breast cancer (Charles *et al.*, 2004; Mason *et al.*, 2007). This may be because some tumours remain in a premalignant state for long periods in individuals with poor folate status, becoming malignant only when intake increases and availability of nucleotide precursors meets demand for tumour cell division. The other concern is that improving folate status in older adults may mask the haematological symptoms of vitamin B12 deficiency, increasing the risk of pernicious anaemia.

The experience from the United States, however, is that folate fortification had no impact on the prevalence of low B12 status in the elderly population. Intakes of folic acid up to 1 mg per day are not associated with delayed diagnosis of vitamin B12 deficiency (Scientific Advisory Committee on Nutrition, 2006). Consumption in countries with fortification tends to be well below that level (e.g. median intake in post-fortification United States is around 450 μg per day). Less than 5% of US adults over 65 years consume more than 1 mg/day, and this is achieved only through supplementation. Wald *et al.* (2018) argue that the 1 mg per day tolerable upper limit that is observed by the European governments is just an arbitrary value with no underpinning evidence of risk above that level of consumption. It is argued that with mandatory fortification only a small proportion of the population could exceed this level of intake. With overwhelming evidence that poor folate status is the main driver of birth defects and associated neonatal deaths and calls for establishment of fortification programmes in developing countries, it is unlikely that the European governments will resist this public health intervention for very much longer.

- Zinc and selenium are key nutrients associated with male fertility. Suggested relationships of indices of fertility with increased intakes of antioxidant nutrients are of interest but are as yet inconclusive.
- Vitamin A is a teratogen associated with central nervous system and heart defects in the human embryo. Women considering pregnancy should avoid rich sources of vitamin A, such as liver, and vitamin A supplements.
- Optimizing maternal weight prior to conception is regarded as a means of reducing the risk of adverse outcomes for mothers and children during pregnancy, as well as enhancing fertility.
- Folic acid protects the embryo from NTDs during the first few weeks of development. In many parts of the world, public health strategy has been based on prevention of these defects through supplementation of women who are planning a pregnancy. Fortification is a more effective strategy, but in some countries has not been adopted due to concerns about detriment to some groups in the population.

SUMMARY

- Reduced risk of infant and maternal deaths during pregnancy has shifted priorities of medical care towards optimizing parental health to maximize fertility and reduce risk of fetal abnormalities.
- In women, the key determinant of fertility is a healthy body weight. Low levels of body fat or excessive adiposity disrupt the actions of leptin upon the hypothalamic–pituitary–ovarian axis and prevent normal reproductive cycling.
- Consumption of substances such as caffeine and alcohol in moderate amounts has little impact upon female fertility, but heavy alcohol use may be detrimental to chances of conception. Heavy alcohol consumption and binge drinking reduces sperm quality in men.
- Antioxidant nutrients are important in assisted reproduction. A low-quality evidence base suggests that higher intakes, including supplements, may improve fertility in both women and men.
- Male fertility appears to be decreasing and the prevalence of abnormalities of the male reproductive tract is increasing. This may be associated with increased exposure to endocrine disruptors in the food chain and environment. Obesity reduces male fertility through reductions in androgen synthesis and transport.

References

Agarwal, A., Gupta, S. and Sharma, R.K. (2005). Role of oxidative stress in female reproduction. *Reproductive Biology and Endocrinology* **3**: 28–48.

Agarwal, A., Mulgund, A., Hamada, A. and Chyatte, M.R. (2015). A unique view on male infertility around the globe. *Reproductive Biology and Endocrinology* **13**: 37.

Agopian, A.J., Tinker, S.C., Lupo, P.J. *et al.* (2013). Proportion of neural tube defects attributable to known risk factors. *Birth Defects Research A: Clinical and Molecular Teratology* **97**: 42–46.

Allal, N., Sear, R., Prentice, A.M. and Mace, R. (2004). An evolutionary model of stature, age at first birth and reproductive success in Gambian women. *Proceedings Biological Sciences* **271**: 465–470.

Amreen, S., Kumar, P., Gupta, P. *et al.* (2019). Evaluation of oxidative stress and severity of endometriosis. *Journal of Human Reproduction Science* **12**: 40–46.

Arafa, M., Agarwal, A., Majzoub, A. *et al.* (2020). Efficacy of antioxidant supplementation on conventional and advanced sperm function tests in patients with idiopathic male infertility. *Antioxidants* **9**: E219.

Arnhold, T., Tzimas, G., Wittfoht, W. *et al.* (1996). Identification of 9-cis-retinoic acid, 9,13-di-cis-retinoic acid, and 14- hydroxy-4,14-retro-retinol in human plasma after liver consumption. *Life Science* **59**: PL169–PL177.

Asimakopoulos, B., Milousis, A., Gioka, T. *et al.* (2009). Serum pattern of circulating adipokines throughout the physiological menstrual cycle. *Endocrine Journal* **56**: 425–433.

Atanassova, N., McKinnell, C., Turner, K.J. *et al.* (2000). Comparative effects of neonatal exposure of male rats to potent and weak (environmental) estrogens on spermatogenesis at puberty and the relationship to adult testis size and fertility: evidence for stimulatory effects of low estrogen levels. *Endocrinology* **141**: 3898–3907.

Bandini, L.G., Must, A., Naumova, E.N. *et al.* (2008). Change in leptin, body composition and other hormones around menarche: a visual representation. *Acta Paediatrica* **97**: 1454–1459.

Beaton, L.K., McVeigh, B.L., Dillingham, B.L. *et al.* (2010). Soy protein isolates of varying isoflavone content do not adversely affect semen quality in healthy young men. *Fertility and Sterility* **94**:1717–1722.

Beckett, G.J. and Arthur, J.R. (2005). Selenium and endocrine systems. *Journal of Endocrinology* **184**: 455–465.

Bentov, Y., Hannam, T., Jurisicova, A. *et al.* (2014). Coenzyme Q10 supplementation and oocyte aneuploidy in women undergoing IVF-ICSI treatment. *Clinical and Medical Insights in Reproductive Health* **8**: 31–36.

Block, S.R., Watkins, S.M., Salemi, J.L. *et al.* (2013). Maternal pre-pregnancy body mass index and risk of selected birth defects: evidence of a dose-response relationship. *Paediatric Perinatology and Epidemiology* **27**: 521–531.

Bodicoat, D.H., Schoemaker, M.J., Jones, M.E. *et al.* (2014). Timing of pubertal stages and breast cancer risk: the Breakthrough Generations Study. *Breast Cancer Research* **16**: R18.

Bolúmar, F., Olsen, J., Rebagliato, M. *et al.* (1997). Caffeine intake and delayed conception: a European multicentre study on infertility and subfecundity. European Study Group on Infertility Subfecundity. *American Journal of Epidemiology* **145**: 324–334.

Botto, L.D., Loffredo, C., Scanlon, K.S. *et al.* (2001). Vitamin A and cardiac outflow tract defects. *Epidemiology* **12**: 491–496.

Caporossi, L., Alteri, A., Campo, G. *et al.* (2020). Cross-sectional study on exposure to BPA and phthalates and semen parameters in men attending a fertility center. *International Journal of Environmental Research and Public Health* 2020; **17**: 489.

Centers for Disease Control and Prevention. (2004). Spina bifida and anencephaly before and after folic acid mandate: United States, 1995–1996 and 1999–2000. *MMWR Morbidity and Mortality Weekly Report* 53(17): 362–365.

Chang-Mo, O., In-Hwan, O., Kyung-Sik, C. *et al.* (2012). Relationship between body mass index and early menarche of adolescent girls in Seoul. *Journal of Preventive Medicine and Public Health* **45**: 227–234.

Charles, D., Ness, A.R., Campbell, D. *et al.* (2004). Taking folate in pregnancy and risk of maternal breast cancer. *British Medical Journal* **329**: 1375–1376.

Chavarro, J.E., Toth, T.L., Sadio, S.M. *et al.* (2008). Soy food and isoflavone intake in relation to semen quality parameters among men from an infertility clinic. *Human Reproduction* **23**: 2584–2590.

Chen, L.T. and Rivera, M.A. (2004). The Costa Rican experience: reduction of neural tube defects following food fortification programs. *Nutrition Reviews* **62**: S40–S43.

Cnattingius, S., Signorello, L.B., Annerén, G. *et al.* (2000). Caffeine intake and the risk of first-trimester spontaneous abortion. *New England Journal of Medicine* **343**: 1839–1845.

Czeizel, A.E. and Dudas, I. (1992). Prevention of the first occurrence of neural-tube defects by periconceptional vitamin supplementation. *New England Journal of Medicine* **327**: 1832–1835.

Donnan, J., Walsh, S., Sikora, L. *et al.* (2017). A systematic review of the risk factors associated with the onset and natural progression of spina bifida. *Neurotoxicology* **61**: 20–31.

Ebisch, I.M., Thomas, C.M., Peters, W.H. *et al.* (2007). The importance of folate, zinc and antioxidants in the pathogenesis and prevention of subfertility. *Human Reproduction Update* **13**: 163–174.

El-Haschimi, K., Pierroz, D.D., Hileman, S.M. *et al.* (2000). Two defects contribute to hypothalamic leptin resistance in mice with diet-induced obesity. *Journal of Clinical Investigation* **105**: 1827–1832.

Eskenazi, B., Kidd, S.A., Marks, A.R. *et al.* (2005). Antioxidant intake is associated with semen quality in healthy men. *Human Reproduction* **20**: 1006–1012.

Fan, D., Liu, L., Xia, Q., *et al.* (2017). Female alcohol consumption and fecundability: a systematic review and dose-response meta-analysis. *Scientific Reports* **7**: 13815.

Ferreira, E.M., Giorgi, V.S.I., Rodrigues, J.K. *et al.* (2019). Systemic oxidative stress as a possible mechanism underlying the pathogenesis of mild endometriosis-related infertility. *Reproductive Biomedicine Online* **39**: 785–794.

Fielden, M.R., Samy, S.M., Chou, K.C. *et al.* (2003). Effect of human dietary exposure levels of genistein during gestation and lactation on long-term reproductive development and sperm quality in mice. *Food Chemistry and Toxicology* **41**: 447–454.

Frary, J.M., Bjerre, K.P., Glintborg, D. *et al.* (2016). The effect of dietary carbohydrates in women with polycystic ovary syndrome: a systematic review. *Minerva Endocrinology* **41**: 57–69.

Frisch, R.E. (1987). Body fat, menarche, fitness and fertility. *Human Reproduction* **2**: 521–533.

Frisch, R.E., Revelle, R. and Cook, S. (1973). Components of weight at menarche and the initiation of the adolescent growth spurt in girls: estimated total water, lean body weight and fat. *Human Biology* **45**: 469–483.

Fruzzetti, F., Perini, D., Russo, M. *et al.* (2017). Comparison of two insulin sensitizers, metformin and myo-inositol, in women with polycystic ovary syndrome (PCOS). *Gynecology and Endocrinology* **33**: 39–42.

Fu, Y., Wang, L.L., Yi, D. *et al.* (2015). Association between maternal single nucleotide polymorphisms in genes regulating glucose metabolism and risk for neural tube defects in offspring. *Birth Defects Research A: Clinical and Molecular Teratology* **103**: 471–478.

Fuse, H., Kazama, T., Ohta, S. *et al.* (1999). Relationship between zinc concentrations in seminal plasma and various sperm parameters. *International Urology and Nephrology* **31**: 401–408.

Gao, L.J., Wang, Z.P., Lu, Q.B. *et al.* (2013). Maternal overweight and obesity and the risk of neural tube defects: a case-control study in China. *Birth Defects Research A: Clinical and Molecular Teratology* **97**: 161–165.

Gavela-Pérez, T., Navarro, P., Soriano-Guillén, L. *et al.* (2016). High prepubertal leptin levels are associated with earlier menarcheal age. *Journal of Adolescent Health* **59**: 177–181.

Geoffroy-Siraudin, C., Loundou, A.D., Romain, F. *et al.* (2012). Decline of semen quality among 10 932 males consulting for couple infertility over a 20-year period in Marseille, France. *Asian Journal of Andrology* **14**: 584–590.

Goumenou, A.G., Matalliotakis, I.M., Koumantakis, G.E. *et al.* (2003). The role of leptin in fertility. *European Journal of Obstetrics Gynecology and Reproductive Biology* **106**: 118–124.

Gray, L.E., Ostby, J., Monosson, E. *et al.* (1999). Environmental antiandrogens: low doses of the fungicide vinclozolin alter sexual differentiation of the male rat. *Toxicology and Industrial Health* **15**: 48–64.

Grodstein, F., Goldman, M.B. and Cramer, D.W. (1994). Infertility in women and moderate alcohol use. *American Journal of Public Health* **84**: 1429–1432.

Guo, D., Wu, W., Tang, Q. *et al.* (2017). The impact of BMI on sperm parameters and the metabolite changes of seminal plasma concomitantly. *Oncotarget* **8**: 48619–48634.

Haghighian, H.K., Haidari, F., Mohammadi-Asl, J. *et al.* (2015). Randomized, triple-blind, placebo-controlled clinical trial examining the effects of alpha-lipoic acid supplement on the spermatogram and seminal oxidative stress in infertile men. *Fertility and Sterility* **104**: 318–324.

Hales, C.M, Carroll M.D., Fryar, C.D. *et al.* (2020). *Prevalence of Obesity and Severe Obesity Among Adults: United States, 2017–2018*. NCHS Data Brief 360. Hyattsville, MD: National Center for Health Statistics.

Halliwell, B. (1999). Antioxidant defence mechanisms: from the beginning to the end (of the beginning). *Free Radical Research* **31**: 261–272.

Hartmann, S., Brors, O., Bock, J. *et al.* (2005). Exposure to retinoic acids in non-pregnant women following high vitamin A intake with a liver meal. *International Journal of Vitamin and Nutrition Research* **75**: 187–194.

Hassan, M.A. and Killick, S.R. (2004). Negative lifestyle is associated with a significant reduction in fecundity. *Fertility and Sterility* **81**: 384–392.

Hatch, E.E., Wise, L.A., Mikkelsen, E.M. *et al.* (2012). Caffeinated beverage and soda consumption and time to pregnancy. *Epidemiology* **23**: 393–401.

Hawkes, W.C. and Turek, P.J. (2001). Effects of dietary selenium on sperm motility in healthy men. *Journal of Andrology* **22**: 764–772.

Hertrampf, E., Cortés, F., Erickson, J.D. *et al.* (2003). Consumption of folic acid-fortified bread improves folate status in women of reproductive age in Chile. *Journal of Nutrition* **133**: 3166–3169.

Hinkle, S.N., Sharma, A.J., Kim, S.Y. *et al.* (2013). Maternal prepregnancy weight status and associations with children's development and disabilities at kindergarten. *International Journal of Obesity* **37**: 1344–1351.

Hosokawa, M., Imazeki, S., Mizunuma, H. *et al.* (2012). Secular trends in age at menarche and time to establish regular menstrual cycling in Japanese women born between 1930 and 1985. *BMC Womens Health* **12**: 19.

Hossain, F., Ali, O., D'Souza, U.J. *et al.* (2010). Effects of pesticide use on semen quality among farmers in rural areas of Sabah, Malaysia. *Journal of Occupational Health* **52**: 353–360.

Institute of Medicine (2009). *Weight Gain During Pregnancy: Reexamining the Guidelines*, Washington, DC: National Academies Press.

Johansen, A.M., Lie, R.T., Wilcox, A.J. *et al.* (2008). Maternal dietary intake of vitamin A and risk of orofacial clefts: a population-based case-control study in Norway. *American Journal of Epidemiology* **167**: 1164–1170.

Jones, L.L., Griffiths, P.L., Norris, S.A. *et al.* (2009). Age at menarche and the evidence for a positive secular trend in urban South Africa. *American Journal of Human Biology* **21**: 130–132.

Jørgensen, N., Vierula, M., Jacobsen, R. *et al.* (2011). Recent adverse trends in semen quality and testis cancer incidence among Finnish men. *International Journal of Andrology* **34**: e37–e48.

Juhl, M., Olsen, J., Andersen, A.M. *et al.* (2003). Intake of wine, beer and spirits and waiting time to pregnancy. *Human Reproduction* **18**: 1967–1971.

Kancherla, V., Averbach, H., Oakley, G.P. (2019). Nationwide failure of voluntary folic acid fortification of corn masa flour and tortillas with folic acid. *Birth Defects Research* **111**: 672–675.

Kasim-Karakas, S.E., Almario, R.U. *et al.* (2004). Metabolic and endocrine effects of a polyunsaturated fatty acid-rich diet in polycystic ovary syndrome. *Journal of Clinical Endocrinology and Metabolism* **89**: 615–620.

Keszthelyi, M., Gyarmathy, V.A., Kaposi, A. *et al.* (2020). The potential role of central obesity in male infertility: body mass index versus waist to hip ratio as they relate to selected semen parameters. *BMC Public Health* **20**: 307.

Khoshnood, B., Loane, M., de Walle, H. *et al.* (2015). Long term trends in prevalence of neural tube defects in Europe: population based study. *BMJ* **351**: h5949.

Langley-Evans, S.C. and Langley-Evans, A.J. (2001). Use of folic acid supplements in the first trimester of pregnancy. *Journal of the Royal Society for the Promotion of Health* **122**: 181–186.

Larsen, S.B., Spano, M., Giwercman, A. *et al.* (1999). Semen quality and sex hormones among organic and traditional Danish farmers. ASCLEPIOS Study Group. *Occupational and Environmental Medicine* **56**: 139–144.

Laurence, K.M., James, N., Miller, M.H. *et al.* (1981). Double-blind randomised controlled trial of folate treatment before conception to prevent recurrence of neural-tube defects. *British Medical Journal* **282**: 1509–1511.

Levine, H., Jørgensen, N., Martino-Andrade, A. *et al.* (2017). Temporal trends in sperm count: a systematic review and meta-regression analysis. *Human Reproduction Update* **23**: 646–659.

Li, N., Liu, E., Guo, J. *et al.* (2013). Maternal prepregnancy body mass index and gestational weight gain on pregnancy outcomes. *PLoS One* **8**: e82310.

Lupo, P.J., Canfield, M.A., Chapa, C. *et al.* (2012). Diabetes and obesity-related genes and the risk of neural tube defects in the national birth defects prevention study. *American Journal of Epidemiology* **176**: 1101–1109.

Lyngsø, J., Kesmodel, U.S., Bay, B. *et al.* (2019a). Impact of female daily coffee consumption on successful fertility treatment: a Danish cohort study. *Fertility and Sterility* **112**: 120–129.

Lyngsø, J., Ramlau-Hansen, C.H., Bay, B. *et al.* (2019). Low-to-moderate alcohol consumption and success in fertility treatment: a Danish cohort study. *Human Reproduction* **34**: 1334–1344.

Ma, J., Wu, L., Zhou, Y. *et al.* (2019). Association between BMI and semen quality: an observational study of 3966 sperm donors. *Human Reproduction* **34**: 155–162.

Marsh, K. and Brand-Miller, J. (2005). The optimal diet for women with polycystic ovary syndrome? *British Journal of Nutrition* **94**: 154–165.

Martinez-Frias, M.L. and Salvador, J. (1990). Epidemiological aspects of prenatal exposure to high doses of vitamin A in Spain. *European Journal of Epidemiology* **6**: 118–123.

Mascarenhas, M.N., Flaxman, S.R., Boerma, T. *et al.* (2012). National, regional, and global trends in infertility prevalence since 1990: a systematic analysis of 277 health surveys. *PLoS Medicine* **9**: e1001356.

Mason, J.B., Dickstein, A., Jacques, P.F. *et al.* (2007). A temporal association between folic acid fortification and an increase in colorectal cancer rates may be illuminating important biological principles: a hypothesis. *Cancer Epidemiology Biomarkers and Prevention* **16**: 1325–1329.

Mendiola, J., Jørgensen, N., Mínguez-Alarcón, L. *et al.* (2013). Sperm counts may have declined in young university students in Southern Spain. *Andrology* **1**: 408–413.

Mikkelsen, E.M., Riis, A.H., Wise, L.A. *et al.* (2016). Alcohol consumption and fecundability: prospective Danish cohort study. *BMJ* **354**: i4262.

Mills, J.L., Simpson, J.L., Cunningham, G.C. *et al.* (1997). Vitamin A and birth defects. *American Journal of Obstetrics and Gynecology* **177**: 31–36.

Mishra, P., Negi, M.P.S., Srivastava, M. *et al.* (2018). Decline in seminal quality in Indian men over the last 37 years. *Reproductive Biology and Endocrinology* **16**: 103.

Mitchell, M., Armstrong, D.T., Robker, R.L. *et al.* (2005). Adipokines: implications for female fertility and obesity. *Reproduction* **130**: 583–597.

Moran, L.J., Noakes, M., Clifton, P.M. *et al.* (2003). Dietary composition in restoring reproductive and metabolic physiology in overweight women with polycystic ovary syndrome. *Journal of Clinical Endocrinology and Metabolism* **88**: 812–819.

Moran, L.J., Ko, H., Misso, M. *et al.* (2012). Dietary composition in the treatment of polycystic ovary syndrome: a systematic review to inform evidence-based guidelines. *Journal of the Academy of Nutrition and Dietetics* **113**: 520–545.

Morris, J.K. and Wald, N.J. (1999). Quantifying the decline in the birth prevalence of neural tube defects in England and Wales. *Journal of Medical Screening* **6**: 182–185.

Motta, A.B. (2012). The role of obesity in the development of polycystic ovary syndrome. *Current Pharmaceutical Design* **18**: 2482–2491.

Moustafa, M.H., Sharma, R.K., Thornton, J. *et al.* (2004). Relationship between ROS production, apoptosis and DNA denaturation in spermatozoa from patients examined for infertility. *Human Reproduction* **19**: 129–138.

MRC Vitamin Study Group. (1991). Prevention of neural tube defects: results of the Medical Research Council Vitamin Study. *Lancet* **338**: 131–137.

Nasr, A. (2010). Effect of N-acetyl-cysteine after ovarian drilling in clomiphene citrate-resistant PCOS women: a pilot study. *Reproductive Biomedicine Online* **20**: 403–409.

Nassar, N., Bower, C., Barker, A. (2007). Increasing prevalence of hypospadias in Western Australia, 1980–2000. *Archives of Diseases in Childhood* **92**: 580–584.

NHS Digital (2019). Statistics on obesity, physical activity and diet, England, 2019. Part 3: Adult overweight and obesity. https://digital.nhs.uk/data-and-information/publications/statistical/statistics-on-obesity-physical-activity-and-diet/statistics-on-obesity-physical-activity-and-diet-england-2019/part-3-adult-obesity (accessed 1 April 2021).

National Institute of Health and Care Excellence. (2010). *Weight Management Before, During and After Pregnancy*. Public Health Guideline PH27. London: NICE.

Nissen, K.B., Udesen, A., Garne, E. (2015). Hypospadias: prevalence, birthweight and associated major congenital anomalies. *Congenital Anomalies* **55**: 37–41.

North, K. and Golding, J. (2000). A maternal vegetarian diet in pregnancy is associated with hypospadias. The ALSPAC Study Team. Avon Longitudinal Study of Pregnancy and Childhood. *BJU International* **85**: 107–113.

Office for National Statistics. (1997). *Health of Adult Britain, 1841–1994*, London: Stationery Office.

Olsen, J. (1991). Cigarette smoking, tea and coffee drinking, and subfecundity. *American Journal of Epidemiology* **133**: 734–739.

O'Malley, E.G., Reynolds, C.M.E., Cawley, S. *et al.* (2018). Folate and vitamin B12 levels in early pregnancy and maternal obesity. *European Journal of Obstetrics Gynecology and Reproductive Biology* **231**: 80–84.

Orzylowska, E.M., Jacobson, J.D., Bareh, G.M. *et al.* (2016). Food intake diet and sperm characteristics in a blue zone: a Loma Linda Study. *European Journal of Obstetrics Gynecology and Reproductive Biology* **203**: 112–115.

Ozawa, M., Nagai, T., Fahrudin, M. *et al.* (2006). Addition of glutathione or thioredoxin to culture medium reduces intracellular redox status of porcine IVM/IVF embryos, resulting in improved development to the blastocyst stage. *Molecular Reproduction and Development* **73**: 998–1007.

Panidis, D., Farmakiotis, D., Rousso, D. *et al.* (2008). Obesity, weight loss, and the polycystic ovary syndrome: effect of treatment with diet and orlistat for 24 weeks on insulin resistance and androgen levels. *Fertility and Sterility* **89**: 899–906.

Paoli, A., Mancin, L., Giacona, M.C. *et al.* (2020). Effects of a ketogenic diet in overweight women with polycystic ovary syndrome. *Journal of Translational Medicine* **18**: 104.

Park, H.J., Bailey, L.B., Shade, D.C. *et al.* (2017). Distinctions in gene-specific changes in DNA methylation in response to folic acid supplementation between women with normal weight and obesity. *Obesity Research in Clinical Practice* **11**: 665–676.

Parnell, A.S., Correa, A., Reece, E.A. (2017). Pre-pregnancy obesity as a modifier of gestational diabetes and birth defects associations: a systematic review. *Maternal and Child Health Journal* **21**: 1105–1120.

Pasquali, R., Gambineri, A. and Pagotto, U. (2006). The impact of obesity on reproduction in women with polycystic ovary syndrome. *BJOG* **113**: 1148–1159.

Pfeiffer, C.M., Caudill, S.P., Gunter, E.W. *et al.* (2005). Biochemical indicators of B vitamin status in the US population after folic acid fortification: results from the National Health and Nutrition Examination Survey 1999–2000. *American Journal of Clinical Nutrition* **82**: 442–450.

Ramaraju, G.A., Teppala, S., Prathigudupu, K. *et al.* (2018). Association between obesity and sperm quality. *Andrologia* **50**: doi: 10.1111/and.12888.

Ray, J.G., Wyatt, P.R., Vermeulen, M.J. *et al.* (2005). Greater maternal weight and the ongoing risk of neural tube defects after folic acid flour fortification. *Obstetrics and Gynecology* **105**: 261–265.

Ray, J.G., Thompson, M.D., Vermeulen, M.J. *et al.* (2007). Metabolic syndrome features and risk of neural tube defects. *BMC Pregnancy and Childbirth* **19**: 21.

Redpath, B., Kancherla, V., Oakley, G.P. (2018). Availability of corn masa flour and tortillas fortified with folic acid in Atlanta after national regulations allowing voluntary fortification. *JAMA* **320**: 1600–1601.

Radhika, M.S., Bhaskaram, P., Balakrishna, N. *et al.* (2002). Effects of vitamin A deficiency during pregnancy on maternal and child health. *BJOG* **109**: 689–693.

Ricci, E., Noli, S., Cipriani, S. *et al.* (2018). Maternal and paternal caffeine intake and ART outcomes in couples referring to an Italian fertility clinic: a prospective cohort. *Nutrients* **10**: pii:E1116.

Rothman, K.J., Moore, L.L., Singer, M.R. *et al.* (1995). Teratogenicity of high vitamin A intake. *New England Journal of Medicine* **333**: 1369–1373.

Ruder, E.H., Hartman, T.J. and Goldman, M.B. (2009). Impact of oxidative stress on female fertility. *Current Opinion in Obstetrics and Gynecology* **21**: 219–222.

Schisterman, E.F., Sjaarda, L.A. and Clemons, T. (2020). Effect of folic acid and zinc supplementation in men on semen quality and live birth among couples undergoing infertility treatment: a randomized clinical trial. *Journal of the American Medical Association* **323**: 35–48.

Scientific Advisory Committee on Nutrition. (2006). *Folate and Disease Prevention*. London: Stationery Office.

Scutiero, G., Iannone, P., Bernardi, G. *et al.* (2017). Oxidative stress and endometriosis: a systematic review of the literature. *Oxidative Medicine and Cellular Longevity* **2017**: 7265238.

Sharpe, R.M. (1999). Fetal and neonatal hormones and reproductive function of the male in adulthood. In *Fetal Programming, Influences on Development and Disease in Later Life* (ed. P.M.S. O'Brien, T. Wheeler and D.J.P. Barker), 187–194. London: RCOG Press.

Sharpe, R.M. and Irvine, D.S. (2004). How strong is the evidence of a link between environmental chemicals and adverse effects on human reproductive health? *BMJ* **328**: 447–451.

Sharpe, A., Morley, L.C., Tang, T. *et al.* (2019). Metformin for ovulation induction (excluding gonadotrophins) in women with polycystic ovary syndrome. *Cochrane Database of Systematic Reviews* (12): CD013505

Shine, R., Peek, J. and Birdsall, M. (2008). Declining sperm quality in New Zealand over 20 years. *New Zealand Medical Journal* **121**: 50–56.

Showell, M.G., Brown, J., Yazdani, A. *et al.* (2011). Antioxidants for male subfertility. *Cochrane Database of Systematic Reviews* (1): CD007411.

Showell, M.G., Mackenzie-Proctor, R., Jordan, V. *et al.* (2017). Antioxidants for female subfertility. *Cochrane Database of Systematic Reviews* (7): CD007807.

Silberstein, T., Har-Vardi, I., Harlev, A. *et al.* (2016). Antioxidants and polyphenols: concentrations and relation to male infertility and treatment success. *Oxidative Medicine and Cellular Longevity* **2016**: 9140925.

Smits, R.M., Mackenzie-Proctor, R., Yazdani, A. *et al.* (2019). Antioxidants for male subfertility. *Cochrane Database of Systematic Reviews* (3): CD007411.

Salas-Huetos, A., Bulló, M., Salas-Salvadó, J. (2017). Dietary patterns, foods and nutrients in male fertility parameters and fecundability: a systematic review of observational studies. *Human Reproduction Update* **23**: 371–389.

Soprano, D.R. and Soprano, K.J. (1995). Retinoids as teratogens. *Annual Review of Nutrition* **15**: 111–132.

Soylu, L., Jensen, A., Juul, K.E. *et al.* (2018). Coffee, tea and caffeine consumption and risk of primary infertility in women: a Danish cohort study. *Acta Obstetrica Gynecologica Scandinavia* **97**: 570–576.

Steiner, A.Z., Hansen, K.R., Barnhart, K.T. *et al.* (2020). The effect of antioxidants on male factor infertility: the Males, Antioxidants, and Infertility (MOXI) randomized clinical trial. *Fertility and Sterility* **113**: 552–560.

Stothard, K.J., Tennant, P.W., Bell, R. *et al.* (2009). Maternal overweight and obesity and the risk of congenital anomalies: a systematic review and meta-analysis. *JAMA* **301**: 636–650.

Tamura, H., Jozaki, M., Tanabe, M. *et al.* (2020). Importance of melatonin in assisted reproductive technology and ovarian ageing. *International Journal of Molecular Science* **21**: E1135.

Tan, K.A., Walker, M., Morris, K. *et al.* (2006). Infant feeding with soy formula milk: effects on puberty progression, reproductive function and testicular cell numbers in marmoset monkeys in adulthood. *Human Reproduction* **21**: 896–904.

Taylor, K.C., Small, C.M., Dominguez, C.E. *et al.* (2011). Alcohol, smoking, and caffeine in relation to fecundability, with effect modification by NAT2. *Annals of Epidemiology*, **21**: 864–872.

Thurston, S.W., Mendiola, J., Bellamy, A.R. *et al.* (2016). Phthalate exposure and semen quality in fertile US men. *Andrology* **4**: 632–638.

Tinker, S.C., Hamner, H.C., Berry, R.J. *et al.* (2012). Does obesity modify the association of supplemental folic acid with folate status among nonpregnant women of childbearing age in the United States? *Birth Defects Research A: Clinical and Molecular Teratology* **94**: 749–755.

UNICEF (2019a). Maternal mortality September 2019. https://data.unicef.org/topic/maternal-health/maternal-mortality (accessed 1 April 2021).

UNICEF (2019b). Neonatal mortality September 2020. https://data.unicef.org/topic/child-survival/neonatal-mortality (accessed 1 April 2021).

van Vliet, T., Boelsma, E., de Vries, A.J. *et al.* (2001). Retinoic acid metabolites in plasma are higher after intake of liver paste compared with a vitamin A supplement in women. *Journal of Nutrition* **131**: 3197–3203.

Wald, N.J., Morris, J.K., Blakemore, C. (2018). Public health failure in the prevention of neural tube defects: time to abandon the tolerable upper intake level of folate. *Public Health Reviews* **39**: 2.

Wang, M., Wang, Z.P., Gao, L.J. *et al.* (2013). Maternal body mass index and the association between folic acid supplements and neural tube defects. *Acta Paediatrica* **102**: 908–913.

Wang, L., Zhang, L., Song, X.H. *et al.* (2017). Decline of semen quality among Chinese sperm bank donors within 7 years (2008–2014). *Asian Journal of Andrology* **19**: 521–525.

Wesselink, A.K., Wise, L.A., Rothman, K.J. *et al.* (2016). Caffeine and caffeinated beverage consumption and fecundability in a preconception cohort. *Reproductive Toxicology* **62**: 39–45.

Williams, L.J., Rasmussen, S.A., Flores, A. *et al.* (2005). Decline in the prevalence of spina bifida and anencephaly by race/ethnicity: 1995–2002. *Pediatrics* **116**: 580–586.

Wong, W.Y., Merkus, H.M., Thomas, C.M. *et al.* (2002). Effects of folic acid and zinc sulfate on male factor subfertility: a double-blind, randomized, placebo-controlled trial. *Fertility and Sterility* **77**: 491–498.

Xia, Y., Chen, M., Zhu, P. *et al.* (2013). Urinary phytoestrogen levels related to idiopathic male infertility in Chinese men. *Environment International* **59**: 161–167.

Xu, Y., Wu, Y., Huang, Q. (2017). Comparison of the effect between pioglitazone and metformin in treating patients with PCOS: a meta-analysis. *Archives of Gynecology and Obstetrics* **296**: 661–677.

Yu, X., Nassar, N., Mastroiacovo, P. *et al.* (2019). Hypospadias prevalence and trends in international birth defect surveillance systems, 1980–2010. *European Urology* **76**: 482–490

Yuan, G., Liu, Y., Liu, G. *et al.* (2019). Associations between semen phytoestrogens concentrations and semen quality in Chinese men. *Environment International* **129**: 136–144.

Additional reading

If you would like to find out more about the material discussed in this chapter, the following sources may be of interest.

Du Plessis, S.S., Agarwal, A., Sabanegh, E.S. (eds) (2014). *Male Infertility: A Complete Guide to Lifestyle and Environmental Factors*. New York, NY: Springer.

Hollins-Martin, C.J., Van Den Akker, O.B.A., Martin, C.R. *et al.* (eds) (2014). *Handbook of Diet and Nutrition in the Menstrual Cycle, Periconception and Fertility*, Wageningen: Wageningen Academic Publishers.

Thompson, L.U. and Ward, W.E. (eds) (2007). *Optimising Women's Health Through Nutrition*. Boca Raton, FL: CRC Press.

CHAPTER 3

Pregnancy

LEARNING OBJECTIVES

This chapter will enable the reader to:
- Describe the physiological adaptations that occur during pregnancy and their role in maintaining the placenta and fetus.
- Show an appreciation of the increased maternal demand for energy, protein and micronutrients during pregnancy.
- Discuss the adaptations to maternal physiology and behaviour that enable nutrient demands to be met even in relatively undernourished women.
- Demonstrate an understanding of the importance of iron for the maintenance of normal pregnancy.
- Describe the nutrition-related factors that determine the risk of miscarriage and stillbirth.
- Show an understanding of the risk to the infant associated with preterm delivery and describe the role of nutrition in determining this risk.
- Describe the hypertensive disorders of pregnancy and discuss the physiological and metabolic processes that lead to pre-eclampsia.
- Discuss the potential for nutritional intervention for the prevention of pre-eclampsia.
- Discuss the high incidence of nausea and vomiting and pregnancy, describing the possible hormonal causes and impact of these symptoms and associated eating behaviours upon pregnancy outcomes.
- Demonstrate an awareness of the fetal disorders that are related to excessive maternal consumption of alcohol.
- Highlight the hazards associated with obesity in pregnant women.

3.1 Introduction

Human pregnancy is a period of remarkable adaptations which impact physiology and metabolism in a manner that is unlike any other scenario at any stage of life. Pregnancy not only involves the development of a new individual from the single-celled zygote formed by gamete fusion at the moment of conception but is also a period of profound alterations within the maternal system, as considerable changes to the endocrine milieu dictate adaptations that maintain and support the pregnancy, prevent immunological rejection of the fetus and ensure that maternal homeostasis is maintained. Human gestation lasts for 40 weeks, timed from the last menstrual period of the mother. Birth in fact occurs 38 weeks following conception. The 40 weeks of gestation are divided into three trimesters, which correspond to the main phases of embryonic and fetal development. The first trimester (conception to 12 weeks) is the period of maximum vulnerability for the embryo as, at this stage, it has to implant into the uterine lining, establish the supporting placenta and undergo development from a cluster of cells to an individual of approximate human morphology with a vascular system and a number of functional organs. The first trimester is the stage where the formation of all organ systems is initiated (organogenesis).

During the first trimester of pregnancy, women acquire an additional organ. The placenta is a major organ system, which may weigh as much as 1.5 kg by the time of birth. It is formed from a pooling of fetal and maternal tissue and provides the interface across which nutrients, gases, immune signals and hormones can be transferred in both directions. During implantation, the chorionic layer of the embryo projects villi into the lining of the uterus, a process that is aided by the release of cytokines that enable the embryo, firstly to adhere to the uterus, and secondly to invade the tissue (Figure 3.1). Within the chorionic villi, the embryo establishes a network of arterioles and venules that will eventually form the umbilical artery and umbilical vein,

Nutrition, Health and Disease: A Lifespan Approach, Third Edition. Simon Langley-Evans.
© 2021 John Wiley & Sons Ltd. Published 2021 by John Wiley & Sons Ltd.
Companion website: www.wiley.com/go/langleyevans/lifespan3e

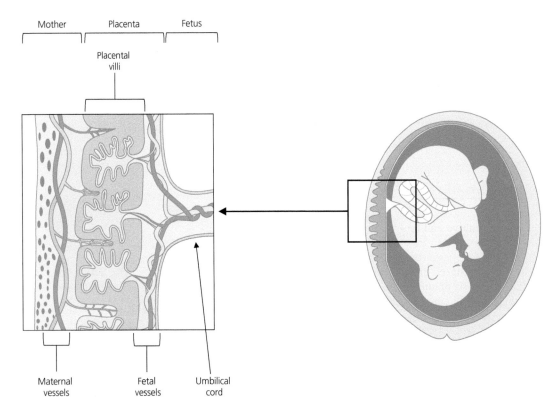

Figure 3.1 The placenta provides the interface between mother and fetus. Villous structures in the placental tissue enable diffusion and active transport of oxygen, waste products and nutrients between maternal and fetal circulation.

within the cord that links fetus to placenta. On the maternal side of the developing placenta, uterine tissue is modified so that uterine arteries feed a series of blood sinuses that form around the chorionic villi. These sinuses fill with maternal blood, which is then drained via the uterine veins. The chorionic villi enclosing the embryonic and fetal vessels are thus in close proximity to maternal blood, allowing exchange of materials. Gases such as oxygen and carbon dioxide and most nutrients in maternal circulation can passively diffuse across the two barriers formed within the placenta (the chorionic membrane and the epithelial cells of the fetal blood vessels). Some nutrients, particularly the minerals, cross the placenta by active transport. The placenta is therefore responsible for supplying the developing fetus with the nutrients and oxygen it requires and also removes the waste products of fetal metabolism.

The placenta has other functions. It effectively acts as a barrier to the passage of many potentially harmful agents. Water-soluble material requiring active transport will be effectively barred from the fetal circulation, so only fat-soluble toxins and teratogens (e.g. alcohol) are likely to cross from mother to fetus. The placenta is also a key endocrine organ, synthesizing many of the hormones that shape maternal physiology during pregnancy.

The second trimester (13–27 weeks of gestation) is the period where most of the emphasis of fetal development is on growth, with the average fetus increasing in mass approximately from 25 to 875 g. By the end of this period, the fetus is considered viable; that is, it has a reasonable chance of survival if born prematurely, despite the fact that many organ systems are immature. During the third trimester (28–40 weeks), growth remains rapid and the fetus will quadruple in weight. Some of this increase in weight is due to increased body size (i.e. truncal growth), but there is also deposition of stores of fat and other nutrients during this period. The third trimester sees the maturation of all organ systems in preparation for birth (Table 3.1).

The maternal hormonal environment is transformed during pregnancy. Initially, the remnants of the corpus luteum and the chorionic layer of the embryo are the main sources of progesterone, oestrogen and human chorionic gonadotrophin (hCG). These hormones act upon the uterine lining and prepare the maternal environment for implanta-

Table 3.1 Development of the human organs during gestation.

Organ	Organogenesis begins (weeks)	Formation complete (weeks)
Brain	3	28
Heart	3	6
Lungs	5	24–28
Liver	3–4	12
Gastrointestinal tract	3	24
Kidneys	4–5	12
Limbs	4–5	8
Eyes	3	20–24
Genitals	5	7
Spinal cord	3–4	20

tion of the embryo and formation of the placenta. Most of the events in the first trimester are controlled by hormones of ovarian origin. These hormones are produced in response to embryonic chorion synthesis of luteinizing hormone to maintain the corpus luteum. Beyond the first trimester, pregnancy is dominated by progesterone produced by the placenta. Oestrogen concentrations also rise to more than the peak level seen at ovulation. The maternal adrenals undergo change and increase the production of cortisol and aldosterone, which has important consequences for metabolism, transport and processing of nutrients. The placenta itself releases hormones, such as placental growth hormone, that have important metabolic functions. In addition to these agents, there is a wide range of hormonal products that have important effects upon the maternal brain and which modify homeostatic processes. These include corticotrophin-releasing hormone, galanin, renin, cholecystokinin, leptin, thyroid-stimulating hormone, serotonin and growth hormone.

This chapter describes the physiological and metabolic changes that occur during pregnancy and how they alter maternal requirements for nutrients. Discussion also focuses on the importance of maternal nutrition in maintaining a healthy pregnancy and the relationships between nutrition-related factors and adverse pregnancy outcomes.

3.2 Physiological demands of pregnancy

Pregnancy is a period of intense physiological adaptations and involves constant responses to the need for oxygen and nutrients, and to the changing hormonal environment. Overall, pregnancy is an anabolic state and hormones produced by the placenta ensure that nutrients are metabolized in a manner that allows maintenance of maternal homeostasis,

provide support for the growth of the placenta and fetus and prepare the maternal system for later lactation (Most *et al.*, 2019). Many of the adaptations that are necessary to maintain a successful pregnancy occur at a very early stage of gestation. Although growth of the fetus is limited in the first trimester, as described earlier, this is the period where implantation occurs and the placenta becomes established. The maternal cardiovascular, renal and respiratory systems undergo major change early in pregnancy, to be able to support placental perfusion and delivery of oxygen and nutrients that will drive the later growth of the fetus.

3.2.1 Maternal weight gain and body composition changes

Weight gain in pregnancy can be highly variable, but typically will be of the order of 12.5 kg. Most of this weight gain occurs during the second half of gestation. Only one third of the weight gain is due to the growth of the fetus and most of the increase is attributable to maternal changes (Figure 3.2). Some of the changes to maternal weight are explained by altered cardiovascular and renal functions, which serve to increase the blood volume and drive retention of water in the interstitial compartment. There are also major increases in the size of the uterus as the pregnancy proceeds, and the breasts can increase in weight by up to 0.5 kg. This latter change appears to be an adaptation to ensure that the breasts are ready for lactation after the birth of the baby. Women also deposit large reserves of fat, typically in the abdomen, thighs and back. These reserves start to be mobilized in later stages of pregnancy to drive fetal growth; they also act as an energy source for later lactation.

As described later in this chapter, maternal weight gain is an important predictor of pregnancy outcome. Insufficient or excessive weight gains are associated with poor outcomes for both mother and fetus. Desirable weight gains are therefore in a

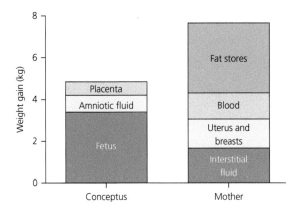

Figure 3.2 Components of maternal weight gain during pregnancy. *Source:* Institute of Medicine (2009).

Table 3.2 Optimal weight gain for women in pregnancy is dependent upon their pre-pregnancy BMI.

BMI at conception (kg/m2)	Optimal maternal weight gain (kg)*
<18.5	13–18
18.5–24.9	11–16
25–29.9	7–11
>30	5–9

Data source: Institute of Medicine (2009). Reproduced with permission of The National Academies Press.
* Optimal weight gain ranges are those associated with favourable pregnancy outcomes for mother and fetus and which lead to birth weight of 3.1–3.6 kg.

range that optimizes maternal survival, reduces complications in pregnancy and labour and gives the greatest fetal growth and protection from morbidity and mortality (Goldstein *et al.*, 2017; Santos *et al.*, 2019). It is suggested that the optimal range for maternal weight gain is dependent upon maternal body mass index (BMI) prior to pregnancy. Women who are underweight prior to pregnancy should aim for a greater degree of weight gain, while the overweight may need to control weight gain to some degree (Table 3.2).

3.2.2 Blood volume expansion and cardiovascular changes

During pregnancy, there is a need for the maternal cardiovascular system to adapt to supply enlarged organs and maintain the perfusion of the placenta. This ensures an adequate exchange of materials with the fetal compartment. Placentation necessitates an increase in the overall volume of blood within the maternal system, which is achieved through a repartitioning of water between the intracellular and extracellular compartments. Overall,

body water increases by 1.5 litres (pre-pregnant body water volume is 2.6 litres) within the first 20 weeks of pregnancy and continues to rise throughout gestation. The volume of water held in cells (intracellular fluid) is unchanged, and the increased fluid volume is partitioned between the interstitial spaces and the blood plasma.

Increased blood plasma volume has a number of important consequences. First, the fluid expansion enables the delivery of the increased workload required of the heart during pregnancy. The heart needs to deliver more oxygen to tissues than before pregnancy and the increased vascularization of the uterus and placenta require a greater cardiac output. The heart increases in volume by approximately 20% during pregnancy and this enables a greater stroke volume (the amount of blood pumped from the ventricles with each contraction). The pulse rate increases, typically rising from 70 beats per minute in the non-pregnant state to 85 beats per minute by late pregnancy. The combination of raised heart rate and stroke volume increases cardiac output by 40%. Cardiac output is an important contributor to blood pressure, but the latter remains largely unchanged, as the peripheral resistance to blood flow is reduced.

The other main consequence of increased plasma volume is a change in the composition of the blood. Overall, the plasma volume increases by 40–50% over the course of pregnancy, which results in a reduction in the concentrations of many plasma proteins, most notably albumin. To meet the increased demand for oxygen transport, there is greater production of red blood cells and, as a result, the total amount of haemoglobin in circulation increases (Figure 3.3). However, as the 20% increase in red-cell volume achieved by full-term gestation is considerably less than the increase in blood volume,

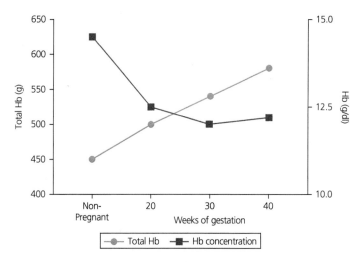

Figure 3.3 Changes in iron status during pregnancy. The total amount of haemoglobin (Hb) in circulation increases, but due to rising plasma volume, the haemoglobin concentration decreases.

the number of red cells per millilitre blood and overall haemoglobin concentration fall as gestation advances. This makes diagnosis of iron deficiency anaemia more challenging in pregnancy, as the stage of gestation has to be considered. For example, a haemoglobin concentration of 10.5 g/dl would be indicative of anaemia in a non-pregnant woman and in a woman at 20 weeks of gestation, but would be considered within normal ranges at 30 weeks of pregnancy.

3.2.3 Renal changes
Modifications in the function of the kidneys are among the earliest physiological responses to pregnancy. The purpose of these adaptations is to support the cardiovascular changes, modify maternal fluid balance and increase capacity for excretion of metabolic waste. Tubular reabsorption of water and electrolytes is increased during pregnancy and although pregnant women experience more frequent micturition due to the pressure of the uterus upon the bladder, the actual daily volume of urine produced is only 80% of that seen in non-pregnant women. Chapman *et al.* (1998) observed that blood flow through the maternal kidneys, and hence the glomerular filtration rate, was significantly increased by 6 weeks of gestation and that renal function reached the maximum for pregnancy by as early as 8–12 weeks. Increased renal blood flow and reduced arterial resistance in the kidneys are important mechanisms through which maternal cardiac output can be increased without producing dangerous increases in blood pressure. The kidneys show distinct functional changes as pregnancy progresses.

Hyperfiltration in the third trimester results from several mechanisms working together (Odutayo and Hladunewich, 2012).

3.2.4 Respiratory changes
A number of changes take place to improve maternal gaseous exchange. These adaptations ensure that the maternal blood is enriched with oxygen and is effectively cleared of carbon dioxide. This maximizes concentration gradients across the placental membranes and aids delivery of oxygen and removal of carbon dioxide from the fetal system. The maternal diaphragm takes on a greater range of movement and the ribs flare outwards. This means that during early to mid-pregnancy there is a greater tidal movement of air during each breath and effectively more fresh air is inhaled and more used air exhaled with each breath. As pregnancy proceeds, the mass of the uterus and fetus presses upon the diaphragm and limit this tidal movement, but respiratory efficiency is maintained by a slightly more rapid rate of breathing.

The efficient removal of carbon dioxide from the maternal blood is of importance for the nutrition of the fetus as well as for gaseous exchange across the placenta. Carbon dioxide is transported in the blood as bicarbonate ions (HCO_3^-). With less of this anion in circulation, there is a reduced requirement for appropriate cations (Na^+, K^+ and Ca^{2+}) to be in circulation and these cations are therefore available for transfer to the fetus for growth and skeletal mineralization. Maternal blood concentrations of cations therefore fall from around 155 m.equiv/l before pregnancy to 147 m.equiv/l mid-gestation.

3.2.5 Gastrointestinal changes

The maternal gastrointestinal tract is influenced by the high prevailing concentrations of progesterone and oestrogen. These produce adaptations that increase the capacity of the gut to absorb nutrients and hence increase availability for incorporation into maternal or fetal structures and stores. In the stomach, the secretion of gastric juices is reduced, but gastric emptying is slowed. This means that ingested food is churned within the stomach for a longer period and is more effectively pulped. This improves digestion lower down the tract. The motility of both the small and large intestines is reduced, and this exposes food materials to digestive enzymes for longer time and increases the duration of time during which nutrients can be absorbed and water recovered.

3.2.6 Metabolic adaptations

Demands for energy and protein are increased during pregnancy and these increased demands are partly met through adaptations in the metabolism of macronutrients. There is an accretion of approximately 0.5 kg of protein during pregnancy, around half of which is deposited in the conceptus (fetus and placenta). As described in the preceding section, pregnancy is associated with decreased gastrointestinal motility and this improves the absorption of amino acids from ingested food. Absorbed amino acids are transported to the liver, where normally they would be used in protein synthesis, or deaminated so that any excess is excreted via the urine in the form of urea. During pregnancy, the enzymes responsible for deamination are inhibited first by hCG and later by placental growth hormone. This means that more amino acids enter the maternal circulation, which can be used for expansion of maternal tissues and the placenta or exported to the fetal compartment.

The hormonal changes that accompany pregnancy serve to create a state of insulin resistance. By the second and third trimesters, pregnant women secrete 2–2.5-fold more insulin than in the non-pregnant state (Barbour, 2003). Despite this, the disposal of glucose in the skeletal muscle and liver is suppressed and, as a result, the circulating glucose concentration remains high, ensuring the supply to the fetal tissues. The mechanisms through which the insulin resistance of pregnancy develops are not fully understood. Normal glucose uptake by tissues such as skeletal muscle is dependent upon the translocation of glucose transporter 4 (GLUT4) to the cell membrane following insulin binding to the insulin receptor (Figure 3.4). The insulin signal to GLUT4 depends on the binding of phosphorylated insulin receptor substrate-1 (IRS1) to phosphoinositol 3 kinase (PI3K). Formation of the IRS1–PI3K complex is the key event that activates GLUT4 translocation. In pregnancy, it is apparent that the formation of this complex is inhibited, which essentially limits glucose uptake by maternal tissues, establishing preferential uptake for the fetal organs (Barbour, 2003).

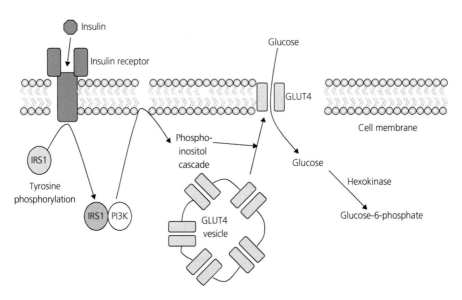

Figure 3.4 The role of glucose transporter 4 (GLUT4) in glucose transport. GLUT4 translocation is a key step in the movement of glucose across cell membranes. In pregnancy, the formation of insulin receptor substrate-1 (IRS1)–phosphoinositol-3 kinase (PI3K) complexes is inhibited, leading to insulin resistance.

In addition to these metabolic adaptations that promote maximum availability of energy substrates to support the pregnancy, there are behavioural adaptations that similarly make more energy available to the developing fetus. It is generally reported that pregnant women alter their profile of food choices and consume smaller portions of food on a more frequent basis. while this is driven by physical constraint as the fetus fills the abdominal space, smaller more frequent meals help to maintain raised blood glucose throughout the day. Furthermore, as pregnancy advances, most women reduce the levels of physical activity, even if they were previously highly active (Borodulin et al., 2008). A study of over 10 000 pregnant women across the United States found that by 22–30 weeks of gestation, only 6.7% of the women were achieving guidelines for moderate exercise (150 minutes per week; Catov et al., 2018). Declining physical activity reduces overall energy expenditure.

3.3 Nutrient requirements in pregnancy

It should be clear from the preceding sections that pregnancy is a time of major remodelling of maternal tissues, deposition of new tissue in the uterus and in the form of the placenta, and of considerable metabolic change. As a result, maternal demands for all nutrients would be expected to increase markedly. It is, however, becoming clear that in normal pregnancy, the same suite of adaptations that leads to increased nutrient demand also optimizes bioavailability and use of nutrients. As a result, major changes to maternal intake are generally unwarranted.

3.3.1 Energy, protein and lipids

Pregnancy considerably increases the maternal demand for energy to drive the growth of the fetus and placenta, the deposition of fat reserves for lactation and the expansion of maternal tissues. The increase in maternal body size in itself will increase the basal metabolic rate and will increase the amount of energy required for physical activity. Estimates of the total energy cost of pregnancy vary greatly but, in general, most studies support the early work of Hytten and Leitch (1971) who estimated that the increase in basal metabolism (30 000 kcal, 126 MJ) and the extra requirement associated with increasing body size (40 000 kcal, 167 MJ) totalled 70 000 kcal (293 MJ) over the whole gestation period. This equates to an extra requirement of 250 kcal per day (1.04 MJ per day).

Studies of pregnant women in developed countries show that this energy demand is not met by increased intakes of energy. Durnin (1991) reported that women typically did not increase intake at all until the third trimester, and even then, increases were only of the order of 100 kcal per day (0.42 MJ per day). Despite an apparent shortfall of energy intake, the women had normal pregnancy outcomes. Similarly, Stråvik et al. (2019) and Langley-Evans and Langley-Evans (2003) reported that pregnant women consumed between 1780 and 2010 kcal per day (7.4 and 8.4 MJ per day), which compares to an estimated average requirement of 1940 kcal per day (8.1 MJ per day) for non-pregnant women. The fact that many women successfully carry pregnancy safely without attaining reference intakes for energy strongly suggests that pregnancy is associated with adaptive responses to conserve energy.

Conservation of energy may involve reductions of either basal metabolism or physical activity (King, 2000). Prentice and Goldberg (2000) suggested that there is wide variation in the metabolic response to pregnancy. While most women increase basal metabolic rate as would be expected with increasing tissue mass, some women actually exhibit a decrease during early gestation. This form of energy-conserving response is most common among women who are undernourished with limited fat stores and high demands for physical activity to ensure survival (e.g. women depending on subsistence agriculture in developing countries). In developed countries where the food supply is secure, it seems that most energy conservation is likely to occur through reduction in overall levels of physical activity or improved efficiency of movement. The analysis of Most et al. (2019) found that decreases in physical activity are relatively modest, at around 5%. Across pregnancy, women become less likely to engage in sports activity and activities such as swimming. Yoga and antenatal exercise classes are the activities most commonly reported (Catov et al., 2018), but a high proportion are inactive by the end of the second trimester (Swift et al., 2017). Where weight-bearing activity does take place, pregnant women do more respiratory work and the metabolic impact is greater (Davenport et al., 2009), but it is generally observed that in habitual activity pregnant women move more efficiently, altering their gait so that stride length is shorter and speed is reduced (Forczek and Staszkiewicz, 2012). The response to pregnancy is highly variable but, overall, adaptations serve to ensure that the metabolic demands of pregnancy are met without increasing intake.

It is clear that the control of energy balance in pregnancy is subject to a diverse range of influences and there is a high level of inter-individual variation. This is explained by the fact that energy requirements and processes that match intake to expenditure are influenced by rates of maternal weight gain, fetal growth rates, maternal lifestyle and activity levels, maternal body composition and genetic factors (King, 2000). In the UK, the Committee on Medical Aspects of Food Policy suggested an additional increment of 200 kcal per day (0.84 MJ per day) to be added to the estimated average requirement (Department of Health, 1999). This assumed an average pregnancy weight gain of 12.5 kg and a fetus of average weight at birth. Women who are underweight prior to pregnancy and those who are unable to reduce physical activity may require greater increases in energy intake. In the United States, the recommended daily amount (RDA) for pregnancy includes an increment of 300 kcal per day, targeted at the second and third trimesters.

There are undoubtedly major requirements for protein during pregnancy. Growth of the fetus, placenta, and maternal tissues all require protein deposition. However, there are no recommendations for major changes to maternal intakes in developed countries. In the UK, the reference nutrient intake increment for pregnancy is a mere 6 g per day, while in the United States, an RDA increment of 10 g per day is advised (Millward, 1999). With intakes of protein in developed countries ranging from 60 to 110 g per day, there seems no need for dietary change to meet the demands for protein. However, women in developing countries and women from poor backgrounds may struggle to obtain dietary protein requirements. As described in Chapter 4, this may be associated with long-term disease risk in their offspring.

The dietary supply of essential fatty acids may become important during pregnancy. These lipids give rise to the n-6 and n-3 series of fatty acids, which have major biological functions (Figure 3.5). The long-chain polyunsaturated fatty acids (LCPUFAs) from these series give rise to the pro- and anti-inflammatory eicosanoids and hence modulate cell-signalling pathways. LCPUFAs are also involved in the regulation of gene expression through their interaction with transcription factors (Wainwright, 2002). In humans, LCPUFAs are

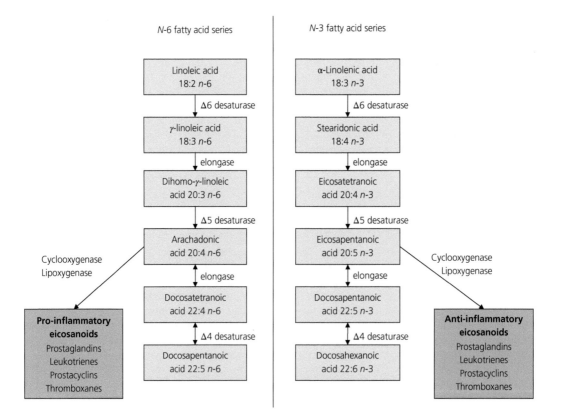

Figure 3.5 Biosynthesis of long-chain polyunsaturated fatty acids from essential fatty acids.

heavily concentrated in the brain and retina, where they account for approximately 35% of the total fatty acid profile. The fetal and neonatal brain has particularly high demand for arachidonic acid (n-6 series) and docosahexaenoic acid (DHA; n-3) series. While these can be synthesized de novo from the essential dietary fatty acids (Figure 3.5), in the fetal brain the activity of these pathways is low. There is consequently a dependence upon their transfer across the placenta from the maternal circulation. The accrual of DHA, in particular, in the fetal brain and retina occurs largely during the third trimester. DHA is incorporated into phosphatidylethanolamine and phosphatidylserine in these tissues (Innis, 2005).

Transfer of LCPUFAs from mother to fetus appears to occur at a rate that is closely correlated with maternal intake. Maternal concentrations are predictive of arachidonic acid and DHA concentrations in umbilical cord plasma and red cells at birth (Connor et al., 1996). The best sources of LCPUFAs in the diet are oily fish, eggs, meat and certain seed oils. Maintaining an adequate supply to the fetus appears to be critical to neurodevelopment as maternal intakes are predictive of brain fatty acid composition and size in the fetus (Wainwright, 2002). Depletion of DHA has been associated with reduced visual function and learning defects in children. A number of studies suggest that maternal n-3 LCPUFA supplementation in pregnancy may have benefits for fetal neurodevelopment. However, the evidence is far from conclusive and findings are inconsistent (Chmielewska et al., 2019).

While an extensive literature focuses on the effects of LCPUFA on infant development, there is also a body of evidence linking consumption of n-3 LCPUFA with improved pregnancy outcomes. Vinding et al. (2019) carried out a randomized controlled trial of LCPUFA 2.4 g per day compared with an olive oil placebo, and noted that gestation length was increased on average by two days and birth weight increased by 97 g. In contrast, van Wijngaarden et al. (2014) reported no association between weight at birth and maternal whole blood LCPUFA concentrations at 28 weeks of gestation. There are positive associations between maternal DHA intake and measures of adiposity in newborns (Perreira da Silva et al., 2015), which suggests that LCPUFA may play a role in determining fetal growth patterns. Maternal circulating DHA concentrations in the first trimester of pregnancy are positively associated with birth weight. Women giving birth to low-birth-weight infants have lower n-3 LCPUFA and greater n-6 PUFA concentrations (Meher et al., 2016). Many randomized controlled trials

Table 3.3 Additional vitamin requirements for pregnancy

Micronutrient	UK RNI	Pregnancy increment
Thiamin (mg/d)	0.8	0.1
Riboflavin (mg/d)	1.1	0.3
Niacin (mg/d)	13	–
Vitamin B6 (mg/d)	1.2	–
Vitamin B12 (µg/d)	1.5	–
Folate (µg/d)	200	100
Vitamin C (mg/d)	40	10
Vitamin A (µg/d)	600	100
Vitamin D (µg/d)	10	10

RNI, reference nutrient intake.

have investigated the impact of n-3 LCPUFA on other pregnancy outcomes. Carlson et al. (2013) found that DHA 600 mg per day over the second half of pregnancy increased the length of gestation and markedly reduced the risk of preterm delivery. A systematic review of 70 randomized controlled trials considering LCPUFA intake from food or supplements confirmed a protective effect of n-3 LCPUFA against preterm birth and low birth weight (<2500 g) deliveries (Middleton et al., 2018).

3.3.2 Micronutrients

Pregnancy increases demand for micronutrients to support maternal body composition changes, metabolic demands and the requirements for fetal growth and development. Additional requirements for vitamins are well established and are reflected in additional increments in dietary reference values (Table 3.3). Mineral requirements are also increased but for well-nourished women, mineral nutrition is unlikely to be solely dependent on current dietary intake. Some stores of most minerals are held in bone and can be released to meet the demands of pregnancy.

3.3.2.1 Iron

Maternal requirements for iron during pregnancy are high, with the fetus taking up as much as 400 mg over its full gestation, and up to 175 mg accumulating in the placenta (Whittaker et al., 1991). With further allowances for maternal production of red blood cells and blood losses during delivery, an extra 430–1000 mg is required in a normal pregnancy. To some extent, these requirements are delivered through savings associated with the cessation of menstrual cycling, but women still require an extra 1 mg per day in the first trimester, rising to 6 mg per day in late gestation (Figure 3.6). Little adjustment to the diet is generally required, as absorption of iron across the gut increases markedly from 7.6% of

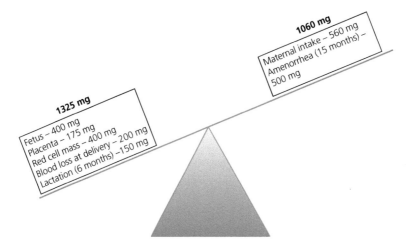

Figure 3.6 Contributors to maternal iron status during pregnancy. Replenishment of iron stores will be less in women who do recommence menstruation sooner (not breastfeeding) but may be aided by improved absorption of dietary iron in the third trimester of pregnancy.

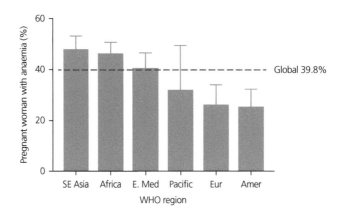

Figure 3.7 Prevalence of iron deficiency anaemia globally and by World Health Organization region (E Med, Eastern Mediterranean; Eur, Europe; Amer, Americas).

ingested iron in the first trimester to 37.4% by 36 weeks of gestation.

Poor maternal iron status is a recognized risk factor for preterm delivery, low birth weight and neonatal death, particularly in the developing countries. The global prevalence of iron deficiency anaemia in pregnancy is close to 40%, and in some parts of the world more than half of pregnant women will be affected (Figure 3.7). The timing of onset of iron deficiency anaemia is important in predicting outcome. This reflects the fact that deficiency exerts its effects through changes in maternal plasma volume expansion, which is at a critical phase in the second trimester. Smith *et al.* (2019) examined a cohort of 515 270 pregnancies, of which 12.8% were complicated by mild, moderate or severe anaemia. At all levels of severity, anaemia was associated with greater risk of complications such as pre-eclampsia, preterm birth, small-for-gestational age birth, caesarean section, neonatal and perinatal death. Preterm birth is a commonly reported outcome associated with iron deficiency anaemia. A comparison of the lowest and highest quartiles of serum ferritin in a cohort of pregnant women in South Africa found that the risk of preterm delivery was markedly higher in the women with poor iron status (odds ratio, OR, 3.57, 95% confidence interval, CI, 1.24–10.34; Symington *et al.*, 2019).

The relationship between iron status and adverse pregnancy outcome appears to be U-shaped, as high markers of iron status, such as elevated haemoglobin concentrations, are associated with preterm birth, low birth weight and stillbirth (Dewey and Oaks, 2017). Again, this may reflect issues with the normal physiological response of plasma volume to pregnancy. Elevated haemoglobin is not likely to be an indicator or iron overload, but in this scenario it is evidence of insufficient haemodilution. Lower plasma volume would result in inadequate perfusion of the placenta and hence limit fetal uptake of oxygen and nutrients.

Including iron supplementation as an element of antenatal care is a practice that varies between low–middle income (developing) countries and developed nations. In the latter, the practice has largely been abandoned as routine. Most women are well nourished so supplements are not required. Iron supplementation has undesirable adverse effects, such as constipation, and is expensive to administer at a population level. Normal practice is to target supplementation at women with a clear need, with confirmed iron deficiency or carrying twin pregnancies. While supplements are effective in improving iron status, there is limited evidence of their efficacy in preventing adverse pregnancy outcomes, largely because anaemia is detected after plasma volume expansion is complete. There is considerable evidence that many pregnant women take supplements regardless of iron status. Spary-Kainz et al. (2019) found that 67% of women in an Austrian cohort took supplements, although only 11% had anaemia. Many had been advised to do so by a medical professional, despite there being no need.

In developing countries, the use of antenatal iron supplements can save the lives of babies and their mothers. Anaemia is a risk factor for postpartum haemorrhage, which is the most common cause of maternal death. Numerous studies show the efficacy of supplementation. For example, Chikakuda et al. (2018) reported that the risk of low birth weight was reduced in women who consumed iron supplements daily in Malawi. The World Health Organization (WHO) recommends that iron supplementation is combined with folic acid in any region where malaria is endemic. This is effective in preventing anaemia and adverse pregnancy outcomes (Bourassa et al., 2019). In malarial areas, there are risks associated with iron supplementation, however, as it is reported that being iron replete can increase the risk of infection (Fowkes et al. 2019) and the risk of preterm delivery (Brabin et al., 2019). It is vital that pregnant women at risk of malaria are supported through other means to prevent infection, such as bed nets to exclude the mosquito vector, as an adjunct to iron supplementation.

3.3.2.2 Calcium and other minerals

The fetus accumulates large quantities of most minerals during late gestation. The fetal skeleton deposits calcium, magnesium and phosphorus in the last trimester of pregnancy, and high uptakes of zinc, copper and other trace metals are also noted. In some countries, notably the United States, these increased demands associated with pregnancy have prompted the inclusion of pregnancy increments over and above the published RDA values. In the UK, however, there are no extra allowances for pregnancy, as it is assumed that maternal adaptations are capable of providing sufficient mineral to maintain fetal demands.

Pregnancy is associated with improved absorption of most micronutrients from the digestive tract due to the increased gastrointestinal transit times. Increased absorption and the mobilization of minerals from stores in the maternal skeleton ensure the fetal supply. In the case of magnesium, for example, the fetus accumulates an average of 8 mg per day over the full gestation. To meet this demand, with an average absorption of 50% of dietary magnesium, and to meet the demand for magnesium from the placenta and other maternal structures, pregnancy increases overall demand by 26 mg per day (Department of Health, 1999). Given that average intakes are in the range 200–280 mg per day, this is a small extra demand that should be easily met by release from the skeleton, where 60% of magnesium is stored.

The same principle applies to calcium, phosphorus, copper and zinc. Demand for zinc is considerable in late gestation at 5.6–14 mg per day, which is in excess of normal ranges of intake. However, zinc supplementation studies have shown little or no benefit for pregnant women and their babies. Similarly, studies of pregnant women with mild to moderate zinc deficiency show that there are no adverse consequences. It is therefore assumed that the increased requirement is met by mobilizing stores (Department of Health, 1999).

The only circumstances in which mineral nutrition may become problematic in pregnancy are when the mother is still in her growing stage. Adolescent pregnancy is a risk factor for many adverse outcomes of pregnancy, and much of the risk is associated with competition for nutrients between the growing fetus and the maternal system. Antenatal mineral supplementation may therefore be appropriate for this age group.

Iodine is an essential nutrient for fetal development, where it is particularly important in the development of the central nervous system during the first trimester of pregnancy. Severe maternal iodine deficiency is associated with fetal death or with cretinism in the affected baby. In countries such as the UK, where iodine deficiency is assumed to be rare, the extra 25 μg per/day iodine required during pregnancy is comfortably delivered by dietary sources. However, in countries where iodine status tends to be poor, pregnancy is a time when careful intervention should be implemented. Most countries where iodine deficiency disorders are a problem have implemented fortification schemes, such as the highly successful universal salt iodization programme (see Section 1.2.3.4). This programme adds iodine to salt used in food production and for home consumption and has coverage in over 120 countries. WHO has estimated that 68% of the five billion people who live in countries where iodine deficiency disorders occur have access to iodized salt at an average cost of US$0.05 per year.

Several studies have, however, suggested that fortification programmes such as universal salt iodization either fail to reach a significant number of pregnant women, particularly in developing countries, or lack the capacity to produce sufficient increases in iodine status in pregnant women. WHO states that urinary iodine excretion of 100–199 μg/l is indicative of healthy iodine status in non-pregnant adults, and that this should increase to 150–249 μg/l in pregnant women. Routine fortification at a high level increases the risk of hyperthyroidism, particularly in older adults, so the level of iodine added to salt has to be carefully monitored and controlled at a local level to reduce adverse effects. Thus, demands for pregnancy may not be met. Where effective campaigns of salt iodization, iodine supplementation and awareness raising take place, requirements for iodine at the population level can be met. In India, fortification has been largely successful (Jaiswal *et al.*, 2015) and, similarly, a campaign in a region of Spain which had previously had a high prevalence of iodine deficiency, increased use of iodized salt and supplements to cover 98.5% of pregnant women (Ollero *et al.*, 2020).

Actions to address iodine status in pregnancy are not universally successful. Despite the introduction of iodized salt in 1997, the median urinary iodine concentration in pregnant women in Poland was reported to be only 111.6 μg/l, which is adequate for non-pregnant women but not for gestation (Trofimiuk-Muldner *et al.*, 2020). Similarly, a report showed Israeli women to be consuming only 75% of the WHO recommendation for iodine, despite having access to fortified sources (Lazarus, 2020). A lack of awareness may be a critical factor making women vulnerable to iodine insufficiency (McMullan *et al.*, 2019). Changing dietary patterns may also lead to insufficiency in surprising places. Traditionally, the diet of Iceland has been iodine-rich due to high consumption of fish and milk.

Recent shifts in dietary preferences at population level mean that these sources are no longer staple foods. Adalsteinsdottir *et al.* (2020) reported that the median urinary iodine concentration for almost 1000 pregnant women was only 89 μg/l.

3.3.2.3 Vitamin D

Pregnant women have increased requirements for vitamin D, by virtue of the increased mobilization of calcium for transfer across the placenta to drive growth of the fetal skeleton. Pregnancy is associated with changes in the metabolism of vitamin D. Concentrations of the biologically active form, 1,25-dihyroxy vitamin D3 (1,25-dihydroxycholecalciferol; Figure 3.8), increase, while circulating 25-hydroxy vitamin D3 (25-hydroxycholecalciferol) decreases. Pregnant women show a marked seasonal variation in vitamin D status in climates where sunlight is markedly lower in the winter months and, as a result, their babies are at greater risk of defects associated with calcium metabolism and dental problems associated with vitamin D deficiency (Department of Health, 1999). Babies born to women with vitamin D deficiency are generally also deficient, and the consequences of this for their development have yet to be defined (Karras *et al.*, 2020).

The prevalence of vitamin D deficiency among pregnant women in northern climates where winter sunlight exposure is poor, is high. In the UK, Javaid *et al.* (2006) reported that 31% of pregnant women were vitamin D insufficient (concentration <25–50 nmol/l) and 18% deficient (<25 nmol/l). Similarly, Emmerson *et al.* (2018) found 7% deficiency and 27% insufficiency among white-skinned women in northwest England. Surprisingly, prevalence has been shown to be high in parts of the world with rich sunlight exposure. A prevalence of 48% insufficiency was reported for pregnant women in Doha (Bener *et al.*, 2013) and in Greece at least one third of pregnant women were deficient (Karras *et al.*, 2020). In a Malaysian population sample, 43% of women were vitamin D deficient and those who had adequate status were heavily dependent upon fortified food sources and supplements to achieve this (Woon *et al.*, 2019). A very large study from Shanghai, China, found that only 1.6% of 34 417 pregnant women had adequate vitamin D status (Li *et al.*, 2020).

In common with similar recommendations in other countries, women in the UK are advised to either increase their intake of vitamin D-fortified foods or to consume a supplement of 10 μg/day. Poor vitamin D status is associated with adverse

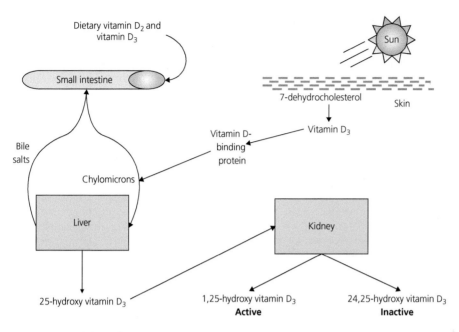

Figure 3.8 Metabolism of vitamin D.

outcomes of pregnancy, including preterm delivery, pre-eclampsia and gestational diabetes mellitus (Wei *et al.*, 2013).

3.4 Diet in relation to pregnancy outcomes

Human gestation is long and has evolved to maximize the growth of the brain and produce an infant that is well developed and relatively mature compared with many other mammalian species. The long gestation brings with it an extended period during which the developing infant is vulnerable to adverse factors that impact upon the mother. Many of these adverse factors can compromise the pregnancy by imposing physiological and metabolic stressors upon a maternal system that is already operating outside normal functional limits. Although modern medical care has drastically reduced the impact of an adverse environment upon maternal and fetal health, pregnancy remains a hazardous process. Nutrition-related factors play an important role in determining the outcomes of pregnancy.

3.4.1 Miscarriage and stillbirth
Miscarriage is defined as the natural end of pregnancy at a stage of fetal development before the fetus is capable of survival. With modern medical technology, fetuses of 23–24 weeks' gestation may

be considered viable, so miscarriage refers to loss of pregnancy prior to this stage. Later in pregnancy, the fetus may die either prior to or during delivery. The former case is termed late fetal death, while the latter is referred to as stillbirth. The death of a baby within the first 28 days after delivery is termed neonatal death.

There are a number of indicators that nutrition-related factors are predictive of miscarriage or later loss of the fetus. Miscarriages occur in approximately 15% of pregnancies and their causes are generally unexplained. The major risk factors for miscarriage in the first trimester of pregnancy are a previous history of miscarriage, assisted conception, being an older woman, alcohol consumption, and having a low BMI prior to pregnancy. For women with BMI less than 18.5 kg/m² the risk of miscarriage is significantly greater than for women with a prepregnancy BMI of 18.5–24.99 kg/m² (relative risk 1.23, 95% CI 1.09–1.38; Cohain *et al.* 2017). Being underweight was also reported to be a risk factor for stillbirth in a cohort of more than half a million Chinese women (OR 1.59, 95% CI 1.18–2.25; Pan *et al.*, 2016). It is suggested that being underweight is a risk factor for miscarriage in early pregnancy due to the lower concentrations of circulating leptin. In addition to stimulating the secretion of sex steroids, leptin plays a key role in the development of the placenta and implantation of the embryo.

Data linking maternal overweight and obesity to loss of pregnancy is equivocal. In women who are overweight, the risk of stillbirth is slightly increased. Weight gain is associated with risk, with insufficient gestational weight gain identified as a major risk for stillbirth (Pickens *et al.*, 2019). While Johansson *et al.* (2018) could find no direct association of maternal obesity with risk of stillbirth, it is clear that lower gestational weight gain is protective in obese women. This protective effect was clear in among women who were morbidly obese, where low gestational weight gain reduced the risk of stillbirth (Yao *et al.*, 2017). This observation strongly indicates that there is a U-shaped relationship between BMI going into pregnancy and risk of fetal loss.

Caffeine has been recognized as a possible risk factor for miscarriage and consequently the UK Department of Health has recommended an intake of no more than 300 mg caffeine/day (approximately three mugs of instant coffee). Such advice is consistent with the evidence base, which suggests significant risk. Bucks-Louis *et al.* (2016) found a 74% increased risk of miscarriage with consumption of more than two caffeinated beverages per day. Meta-analyses confirm the risk, with an estimated 7% risk of pregnancy loss for each additional 100 mg/day of caffeine consumed (Chen *et al.*, 2016).

Heavy consumption of alcohol is a known risk factor for both miscarriage and stillbirth, but even light consumption may be detrimental, so all alcohol should be avoided in pregnancy. An analysis of 91 427 pregnancies in the Danish national birth cohort 1996–2002 found that as little as 1.5 units of alcohol per week increased risk of pregnancy loss in the second trimester (RR 1.13, 95% CI 1.0–1.20), and consumption of four or more units per week increased risk of first-trimester pregnancy loss by almost three-fold (Feodor Nilsson *et al.*, 2014). Women who conceive through in vitro fertilization are at higher risk of pregnancy loss than those who conceive naturally. One report has shown that daily alcohol use increased that risk by more than two-fold (Dodge *et al.*, 2017).

Some degree of protection against miscarriage may be obtained through appropriate dietary advice and change at the start of pregnancy. A systematic review of the literature to explore the influence of nutritional advice to pregnant women, and of supplemental energy and protein during pregnancy on pregnancy outcomes reported no significant effects of advice or supplements on risk of miscarriage but found that nutritional advice and balanced supplements of energy and protein reduced the occurrence of both stillbirth and neonatal death (Ota *et al.*, 2015).

There is a conflicting literature on the effects of vitamin supplementation or increasing micronutrient intake from food, upon risk of miscarriage. Women who consumed fresh fruit and vegetables on a daily basis were half as likely to suffer a miscarriage as women who did not consume these foods daily. In contrast, Nohr *et al.* (2014) found that women who consumed multivitamin supplements in the periconceptual period were at greater risk of losing their pregnancy (OR 1.29, 95% CI 1.12–1.48). This risk was not seen with supplements of folic acid, which in the US Nurses' Health Study (Gaskins *et al.*, 2014) decreased risk of miscarriage by 20%. In contrast to Nohr *et al.* (2014), Keats *et al.* (2019) found that mixed micronutrient supplementation did not impact on risk of early miscarriage and slightly reduced the risk of stillbirth (RR 0.95, 95% CI 0.86–1.04). The meta-analysis of Balogun *et al.* (2016), which included 40 studies of vitamin supplementation during pregnancy, found no significant risk or benefits with respect to miscarriage but women receiving multivitamins plus iron and folic acid had a reduced risk of stillbirth.

3.4.2 Premature labour

Babies who are born before 37 weeks of gestation are termed premature or preterm. Preterm delivery is the main cause of perinatal death and neonatal morbidity in developed countries. It is also associated with significant levels of disability among children. As such, premature birth is associated with a major human cost and has a significant economic impact upon health services, due to the expense of neonatal intensive care.

Intrauterine growth restriction leading to a baby who is small for gestational age is commonly associated with preterm delivery. There are many other known risk factors for premature labour, including maternal infection, psychological trauma of the mother and maternal smoking (Table 3.4), but around one third of cases have no known cause. Lifestyle factors, including nutrition-related factors and excessive physical activity, are believed to contribute to some of these cases.

3.4.2.1 Prepregnancy body mass index and pregnancy weight gain

Maternal BMI is a major indicator of risk for a number of adverse outcomes of pregnancy, including preterm birth. Being overweight or obese is of greatest concern (Figure 3.9; Figure 3.10), with clear relationships between complications of pregnancy and poor pregnancy outcomes. Being underweight is also a risk factor for poor outcomes. It is estimated that globally there are close to 39 million pregnancies

Table 3.4 Risk factors for preterm delivery.

Risk factors	Explanation of risks
Multiple births	Twins and other multiple pregnancies are often delivered early for medical management
Premature rupture of membranes	Delivery necessary to avoid infection
Obstetric emergencies	Maternal bleeding, placental abruption or other placental problems require delivery of baby
Cervical incompetence	The weight of the uterus in late pregnancy may not be supported by the cervix, leading to delivery
Pre-eclampsia	Delivery is the only option to prevent maternal and foetal death
Maternal age	Mothers under the age of 15 or older than 35 are at greater risk of preterm delivery
Stress	Only extremely traumatic psychological stressors will cause premature labour

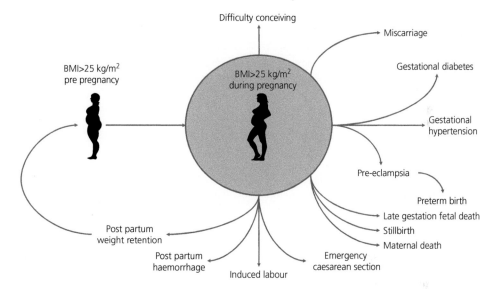

Figure 3.9 Obesity in pregnancy is a risk factor for adverse outcomes (BMI, body mass index).

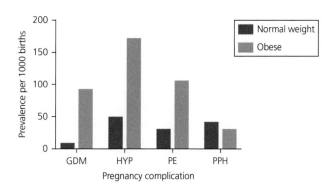

Figure 3.10 Prevalence of pregnancy and labour complications in obese women (body mass index, BMI, >30 kg/m²) and women of normal weight (BMI 20–24.99 kg/m²). GDM, gestational diabetes; HYP, gestational hypertension; PE, pre-eclampsia; PPH, post-partum haemorrhage.

per year that are complicated by maternal obesity (Chen *et al.*, 2018b). In some countries, the estimated prevalence of overweight and obesity in pregnancy is over 60% (e.g. South Africa 64%, Mexico 65%). Estimates of overweight and obesity for the United States vary between 55% and 62.9% (Chen *et al.*, 2018b; Deputy *et al.*, 2018). In Australia, it is estimated that 20.6% of pregnant women are obese (Australian Institute of Health and Welfare, 2020). Among English women prevalence of overweight and obesity increases from 35% among women aged 16–24 years to 61% among those aged 35–44 years, highlighting the high risk among women of reproductive age (East Midlands Maternity Network, 2020). It is widely recognized that, among pregnant women who are severely obese, interventions to control weight gain may be important in preventing major complications of pregnancy and improving pregnancy outcomes (see Research Highlight 3.1).

Studies of the relationship between prepregnancy BMI and weight gain in pregnancy suggest that the risk of preterm delivery may be increased at either extreme of the ranges. Obesity and overweight are widely regarded as risk factors for preterm delivery. The association with risk of preterm delivery in these cases appears to be a result of the increased prevalence of complications of pregnancy that stems from the greater blood pressures and relative insulin resistance that accompany obesity. These are more likely to necessitate medical intervention and premature induction of labour. While smaller studies have indicated that there is limited association between maternal obesity and preterm birth, larger cohorts show strong evidence of detriment. A study of the large Danish national birth cohort (100 000 women, studied between 1996 and 2002) showed that a prepregnancy BMI in the obese range (over 30 kg/m^2) significantly increased the risk of both induced and spontaneous preterm birth by approximately 50% (Nohr *et al.*, 2007). Analysis of data from more than half a million pregnancies in Ontario, Canada, indicated that maternal obesity had a significant impact on risk of preterm delivery (RR 1.14, 95% CI 1.10–1.17; Berger *et al.*, 2020). Similarly, a study of Chinese women, with overweight and obesity defined using Asian cut-offs, showed greater risk of preterm birth. For those who were overweight (BMI 23–27.5 kg/m^2), the relative risk was 1.22 (95%CI 1.08–1.37) and for obesity (BMI >27.5 kg/m^2) 1.30 (95% CI 1.01–1.60; Su *et al.*, 2020).

Maternal underweight has been shown in some studies to increase the risk of preterm birth to the same extent as obesity. The study of Nohr *et al.* (2007) showed a 40% increase in risk comparing women with a prepregnancy BMI of less than 18.5 kg/m^2 with those with a BMI between 18.5 and 24.9 kg/m^2. Lower weight gain in pregnancy was also associated with greater risk. Other studies are consistent with this finding but often report a lower degree of risk (Sebire *et al.*, 2001). The risk associated with underweight and poor maternal weight gain is almost certainly attributable to maternal undernutrition and a lack of sufficient reserve of energy and other nutrients to meet demands for fetal growth. Merlino *et al.* (2006) demonstrated, in a small cohort of women, that underweight women were at greater risk of preterm delivery when in their second pregnancy rather than their first pregnancy. This risk was greatly increased if weight loss corresponding to five BMI units (kg/m^2) had occurred between first and second pregnancies. Although this is indicative of a role for undernutrition in promoting preterm birth, studies that have considered iron deficiency anaemia (Scholl and Reilly, 2000) or the impact of protein and energy status (Kramer and Kakuma, 2003) have not identified a clear and unequivocal role for specific nutrients.

3.4.2.2 Alcohol and caffeine consumption

Caffeine is a widely consumed stimulant, which may be consumed by pregnant women in the form of beverages (e.g. coffee, tea and soft drinks) or in over-the-counter medications. Caffeine is widely reported as being hazardous in pregnancy, if consumed in large quantities. In the UK, women are advised to restrict intake to 300 mg per day or less from all sources, to avoid risk of miscarriage in early pregnancy or preterm delivery later in gestation. Other countries, such as Australia, have adopted lower recommended limits (Peacock *et al.*, 2018). As described in Section 3.4.1, associations between caffeine and miscarriage risk are well established, but the relationship with preterm birth and other adverse pregnancy outcome is controversial.

The idea that caffeine may be a risk factor for preterm labour and adverse effects on the fetus is plausible, since caffeine is known to cross the placental barrier to act in fetal tissues, increases maternal catecholamine production and diminishes placental blood flow. Moreover, in pregnancy, the metabolism of caffeine is inhibited, producing a more protracted response to any given dose. Coffee is the main source of caffeine in the diet, although this varies between cultures. Although most women become averse to coffee and tea and reduce intake during their pregnancy, it is still consumed to some extent by 70–80% of pregnant women.

Research Highlight 3.1 The management of weight in pregnancy.

Maternal obesity during pregnancy increases the risk of adverse pregnancy outcomes, including miscarriage, gestational diabetes and hypertensive disorders (Yu *et al.*, 2006; Sommer *et al.*, 2014; Berger *et al.*, 2020) and is a significant risk factor for maternal and fetal death (Yao *et al.*, 2019). Where they exist, guidelines for maternal weight gain are generally based on the US Institute of Medicine (2009) recommended ranges, with mothers with obesity advised to limit weight gain to 5–9 kg across pregnancy, compared with the 12.5–16 kg recommendation for women of healthy weight, or they emphasize the importance of managing weight before conception or after delivery (National Institute of Health and Care Excellence, 2010). Weight loss is not advised during pregnancy as this may pose a risk to fetal nutrition and development.

The antenatal period puts women into greater contact with health professionals and is therefore an ideal time for health education. Mothers are generally open and more readily motivated to make lifestyle changes that could benefit the health of themselves and their baby (Ritchie *et al.*, 2010; Wilkinson and McIntyre, 2012; May *et al.*, 2014; Wilkinson *et al.*, 2015). Although the need to manage weight among pregnant women who are overweight and obese is recognized, opportunities to engage with women may be missed. Swift *et al.* (2017) found that pregnant women with obesity were happy to receive advice about excessive weight gain, but that receiving such advice was rare. Although they were more likely to discuss weight with a health professional than women who were overweight, only 30% had done so in their first or second trimester.

Some studies have evaluated the impact of antenatal diet, exercise or weight management programmes upon pregnancy outcomes, but generally yield inconsistent results. Generally, such interventions succeed in the objective of reducing gestational weight gain through dietary change, increasing physical activity or providing counselling. McGowan *et al.* (2013) allocated women to low glycaemic index diets, while Ferrara *et al.* (2020) provided telehealth sessions. These interventions reduced weight gain but had no impact on perinatal complications. In contrast, Assaf-Balut *et al.* (2020) allocated women to low-fat dairy substitutes, which had no impact on either weight gain or pregnancy outcomes. The meta-analysis of the International Weight Management in Pregnancy Collaborative Group (2017) considered 36 randomized controlled trials including 12 526 women and found that while interventions limited gestational weight gain and risk of caesarean delivery, there were no significant effects on the risk of developing gestational diabetes, hypertension or pre-eclampsia.

Two large randomized controlled trials have evaluated the impact of comprehensive dietary, physical activity and lifestyle advice on pregnancy outcomes in women with obesity. The Australian LIMIT trial randomized 2212 women to standard care or an intervention led by a research dietitian. This approach failed to limit gestational weight gain and had no significant impact on pregnancy or delivery complications (Dodd *et al.*, 2011). In the UK, 1158 women were recruited to the UPBEAT trial, which promoted a lower glycaemic index diet and achieved long-term improvements in diet quality and activity levels (Mills *et al.*, 2019). However, like LIMIT, UPBEAT did not result in any reduction in risk of gestational diabetes, large-for-gestational age births or any other pregnancy complications (Poston *et al.*, 2015). In contrast, the UK Bumps and Beyond intervention (McGiveron *et al.*, 2015) showed that an intensive midwife and health educator-led programme greatly reduced pregnancy weight gain in women who were morbidly obese and achieved a 90–95% decrease in hypertensive disorders of pregnancy. This programme led to antenatal weight loss in some women, but this was not associated with any adverse outcomes for mothers and babies. However, when the same intervention was introduced to a of population of women that was more ethnically diverse, using a team of health professionals to drive the intervention as opposed to specialist behaviour practitioners, no benefits were observed. This suggests that successful interventions with pregnant women with obesity may depend on building strong relationships and on one-to-one sessions. This sort of pragmatic, more personalized intervention may be more successful than protocols that are more regimented to meet the requirements of a randomized controlled trial. Enrolment in any intervention tends to be low and pregnant women with obesity are especially intimidated and put off by dietitian-led programmes, as they prefer pregnancy to be a normal, non-medical life event.

Early studies which suggested that caffeine may impair fetal growth and increase risk of preterm birth were largely discounted, as they were poorly adjusted for confounding factors and relied on retrospective recall of consumption. More recent prospective studies have proven more suggestive of risk. The very large Norwegian Mother and Child Cohort Study (67 569 mother–infant pairs) found that intakes of caffeine over 200 mg/day were associated with greater need for medical intervention at birth and babies who were small for gestational age (Modzelewska *et al.*, 2019). A large Irish cohort study (Chen *et al.*, 2018a) also reported a higher risk of low birth weight (OR 1.47, 95% CI 1.14–1.90) and preterm birth (OR 1.36, 95% CI 1.07–1.74) with caffeine consumption, when comparing highest with lowest categories of intake. The latter observation was similar to the findings of a Japanese study, which showed that risk of preterm delivery increased by 28% with every 100 mg per day increment in caffeine consumption (Okubo *et al.*, 2015). Caffeine consumption tends to be greater in women who smoke tobacco, and smoking is itself an important risk factor for both low birth weight and preterm delivery. However, the study of Chen *et al.* (2018a) importantly found that associations between caffeine intake, low birth weight and preterm birth held firm even among women who had never smoked. A meta-analysis of eight cohort and four case–control studies found a significant association between caffeine and low birth weight, with every 100 mg per day increase in consumption increasing risk by 3% (Rhee *et al.*, 2015). The balance of evidence suggests that caffeine may carry risks beyond those associated with early miscarriage, and advice to limit intake seems sensible for the whole of pregnancy.

Alcohol consumption during pregnancy has a number of adverse impacts, of which the most important are the fetal alcohol syndrome (see Section 3.8.3) and alcohol-related birth defects. As discussed in Research Highlight 3.2, there are concerns that consumption of alcohol below the threshold for induction of fetal alcohol syndrome may have harmful effects in pregnancy.

3.4.2.3 Oral health

The risk of preterm delivery increases in all situations where an inflammatory response is mounted within the maternal system. The pro-inflammatory cytokines and prostaglandins that are released in response to infection promote the premature rupture of the amniotic and chorionic membranes. This may lead to the spontaneous initiation of premature labour or prompt the need for a medically induced preterm delivery.

Periodontitis is an oral health problem that represents one of the most common chronic disease states on a global scale. Milder forms of periodontitis are noted in 50% of the population at some stage of life, and more advanced destructive periodontitis is noted in 5–10% of people. Periodontitis is essentially an inflammation of the gums, which in mild cases manifests as gingivitis. In the more advanced form, the disease results in destruction of gum tissue and underlying bone, leading to tooth loss. Periodontitis is the result of infection of the gum tissues by anaerobic bacterial species such as *Porphyromonas gingivalis*. This infection results in activation and recruitment of neutrophils to the gums. The subsequent release of reactive oxygen species causes local host tissue injury, and the associated inflammatory response has systemic effects (Sculley and Langley-Evans, 2003). Periodontitis-related inflammation has been linked to development of other conditions, including coronary heart disease (Beck *et al.*, 1996).

Systemic activation of the immune system and elevated concentrations of inflammatory agents may be a trigger for preterm delivery in pregnant

Research Highlight 3.2   The relationship between alcohol consumption and poor pregnancy outcomes.

The consumption of excessive amounts of alcohol in pregnancy, whether as part of a habitual daily activity or in the form of regular binge-drinking episodes, has clear adverse effects. These include preterm birth, birth defects, stillbirth and fetal alcohol syndrome (Foltran *et al.*, 2011). The impact of lower-level alcohol use is less well understood, and the detrimental effects may be hidden until after delivery. While some studies indicate that relatively low intakes of alcohol are associated with lower weight at birth, particularly weights lower than 2 kg (Umer *et al.*, 2020), there is no clear consensus that this is the case. Similarly, while Umer *et al.* (2020) reported that low-level alcohol consumption increased the odds of preterm birth by almost two-fold (OR 1.88, 95% CI 1.23–2.89), other studies find no risk associated with either continuous low alcohol use or occasional binge drinking (Weile *et al.*, 2020). The meta-analysis of Patra *et al.*, (2011) found no evidence that intakes of up to 10 g alcohol per day (one drink) were related to low birth weight, or that intakes of up to 18 g/day were associated with preterm birth. Beyond those cut-offs, however, the risks were dose dependent and significant.

The longer-term effects of low-level alcohol exposure may be hidden during pregnancy and at birth, but may be profound in later life. While Parviainen *et al.* (2020) reported a relationship between maternal alcohol consumption and risk of long-bone fracture in childhood, most effects of exposure appear to manifest in neural development and future cognition and behaviour. Shuffrey *et al.* (2020) showed that the brain activity of newborns (up to 48 hours of age) differed in those whose mothers had been regular low consumers of alcohol. Developmental delay and communication problems are commonly reported in exposed infants (Netelenbos *et al.*, 2020) and offspring of mothers who consumed any alcohol in the first 18 weeks of gestation were shown to be at greater risk of depressive illness between the ages of 18 and 24 years (Easey *et al.*, 2020).

The current advice to women who are planning a pregnancy or who are pregnant is to abstain from alcohol completely. The risks are not fully defined and the critical time frame in which adverse effects may be mediated may lie in the period of embryonic development, before pregnancy is confirmed.

women. Unravelling the true contribution of periodontitis to risk is problematic, as the condition is far more common in cigarette smokers than non-smokers. Smoking is in itself a risk factor for preterm delivery and other complications of pregnancy. Pitiphat *et al.* (2008) reported that, after robust adjustment for smoking, women with periodontal disease were more likely to have a baby that was born prematurely or at full term but small for gestational age (OR 2.26, 95% CI 1.05–4.85). Periodontitis has also been identified as a risk factor for pre-eclampsia. The meta-analysis of Sgolastra *et al.* (2013) suggested a more than doubled risk of pre-eclampsia in women with periodontitis, but low methodological quality of the papers reviewed weakened the strength of the observation. Periodontitis may also be associated with intrauterine growth restriction and low birth weight (Kumar *et al.*, 2013), but these observations are not seen in all studies (Abati *et al.*, 2013) and appear to be population specific. Further evidence favouring a contribution of periodontitis to risk comes from some small intervention studies which have shown that effective treatment of periodontal disease during pregnancy can reduce the risk of preterm delivery and the delivery of infants who are small for gestational age (López *et al.*, 2002; Jeffcoat *et al.*, 2003).

The mechanisms to explain the associations between periodontal disease and pregnancy complications are not well understood. There are two favoured possibilities, which involve either direct interaction between the oral pathogens or their products with the fetal–placental unit, or effects of pro-inflammatory cytokines upon the fetal–placental unit (Sanz and Kornman, 2013). Individuals with periodontal disease have high circulating concentrations of tumour necrosis factor alpha and prostaglandin E2, which could promote placental dysfunction.

3.4.3 Hypertensive disorders of pregnancy

Rising blood pressure is a common feature of pregnancy and reflects the changing renal function requirement to maintain placental perfusion and alterations in fluid balance. In some women, the increased blood pressure crosses the threshold of systolic pressure over 140 mmHg and diastolic pressure over 90 mmHg at which hypertension is clinically diagnosed. When hypertension has onset in the latter part of pregnancy, this is termed gestational hypertension (Table 3.5). If hypertension has an onset in the first six weeks of pregnancy and persists throughout gestation, it is termed chronic hypertension of pregnancy. Neither of these conditions is of major significance in terms of maternal or fetal health.

In contrast, pre-eclampsia is an extremely dangerous condition that threatens the lives of both mother and fetus. Pre-eclampsia occurs in 2–7% of pregnancies (Poston, 2006) and is characterized by the development of hypertension after 20 weeks of gestation and urinary excretion in excess of 300 mg protein in 24 hours. In some cases, blood pressure may not rise above the 140/90 mmHg threshold for hypertension diagnosis but will rise sharply (more than 30 mmHg) over a few weeks. Although not used as diagnostic criteria for pre-eclampsia, affected women will also develop severe oedema and metabolic disturbances.

Pre-eclampsia is a progressive condition that cannot be reversed or controlled. Without intervention, women are at risk of developing eclampsia. Eclampsia is the end stage of the pre-eclampsia disorder and is characterized by maternal seizures and coma due to oedema of the brain. Eclampsia can result in multiple organ failure, renal collapse, abruption of the placenta and death of both mother and baby. In the medical management of

Table 3.5 Hypertensive conditions during pregnancy.

Condition	Gestational age at appearance (weeks)	Blood pressure (mmHg)*	Proteinuria†	Maternal seizures
Chronic hypertension	<20 and prior to pregnancy	>140/90	None	Not present
Gestational hypertension	>20	>140/90	None	Not present
Mild pre-eclampsia	>20	>140/90	<5g/24 hours	Not present
Severe pre-eclampsia	>20	>160/110	>5g/24 hours	Present
Eclampsia	>20	>160/110	>5g/24 hours	Present

* Blood pressure values are shown as systolic/diastolic; normal adult blood pressure should be below 140/90 mmHg.
† Normal urine should contain negligible protein.

pre-eclampsia in developed countries, the usual protocol is to monitor progress closely and deliver the baby preterm. This is the only way to bring the maternal disease to an end. As a result, pre-eclampsia is the major cause of preterm birth (accounting for around 25% of cases).

3.4.3.1 The aetiology of pre-eclampsia

The primary cause of pre-eclampsia is defective placentation (Poston, 2006). Histological examination of placental tissue from affected pregnancies suggests that there is a partial failure of the invasion of the uterine lining during the early stages of placental formation and, as a result, the formation of the maternal spiral arteries is incomplete. Blood flow through the placenta is reduced and the capacity to maintain normal perfusion of the organ is impaired. Pre-eclampsia is generally regarded as being a two-stage process (Figure 3.11) and this placental defect represents the first stage (Roberts and Gammill, 2005).

The second stage in the development of pre-eclampsia is the appearance of the maternal disorders. The impaired perfusion of the placenta is believed to result in the release of factors that impact upon vascular endothelial cell function throughout the maternal system. It is argued that one of the key drivers of this dysfunction could be oxidative injury in the placental tissue (Poston, 2006). With reduced placental perfusion, the placental tissue is likely to undergo periods of hypoxia followed by improved blood flow and renewed delivery of oxygen. This

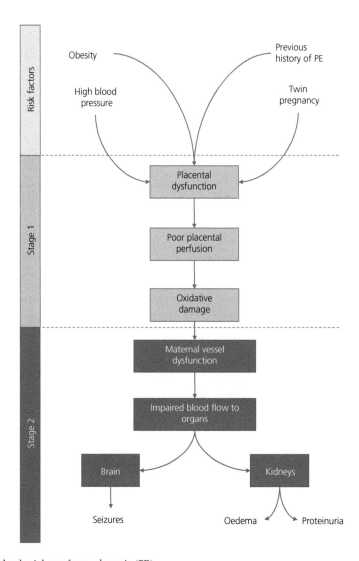

Figure 3.11 The pathophysiology of pre-eclampsia (PE).

hypoxia–reperfusion process will result in the release of free radicals and other reactive oxygen species, causing placental injury. In response to this injury, the placenta will release pro-inflammatory cytokines and activate cells of the immune system. In effect, a systemic inflammatory response is initiated.

The inflammatory response is the main driver of the maternal disorders associated with pre-eclampsia. Primarily, it generates maternal vascular endothelial dysfunction and the main consequences of this are hypertension and a reduction of the blood flow to major organs, including the brain, kidney and liver (Figure 3.11). In the liver, the inflammatory response is responsible for metabolic changes that are remarkably similar to those that are known to occur in cardiovascular disease (Roberts and Gammill, 2005). Indeed, pre-eclampsia is often compared with a speeded-up form of atherosclerosis, specifically impacting upon the placenta. Pro-inflammatory cytokines are antagonists of insulin action and, as a result, pre-eclampsia is associated with insulin resistance. Maternal circulating free fatty acid and triglyceride concentrations rise, as does low-density lipoprotein cholesterol, while high-density lipoprotein concentrations decrease. Uric acid concentrations in maternal circulation are also reported to increase dramatically with pre-eclampsia and this may be related to declining renal function (Pereira *et al.*, 2014). Hyperuricaemia was shown by Zhou *et al.* (2012) to be a strong predictor of pre-eclampsia (OR 1.99, 95% CI 1.16–3.40) but as it also is predictive of gestational diabetes, it may not be seen as a specific biomarker of risk. However, when detected in women with gestational hypertension, it is a strong predictor of progression to pre-eclampsia (Wu *et al.*, 2012). It has been suggested that hyperuricaemia may play a causal role in the development of pre-eclampsia as it occurs in pre-eclampsia before the onset of renal dysfunction and could promote oxidative stress, inflammation and endothelial cell dysfunction (Roberts *et al.*, 2005).

The true determinants of the risk that a woman may develop pre-eclampsia are unknown. It is clear that not all women with placental dysfunction go on to develop pre-eclampsia, which suggests that the presence of other factors is necessary to move from stage 1 to stage 2. Some of the risks may be genetically determined and, certainly, women with a previous history of pre-eclampsia are at increased risk. The heritability of pre-eclampsia is estimated from twin studies to be 55% (Williams and Broughton Pipkin, 2011), but no universally accepted susceptibility genes have been identified.

Polymorphisms in a number of genes in placenta have been associated with pre-eclampsia, including pentraxin 3 (an inflammatory protein; Xu and Zhang, 2020) and Cyp11B2 (an enzyme which synthesizes the steroid hormone, aldosterone; Azimi-Nezhad *et al.*, 2020). The broader significance of such findings for prevention or treatment has yet to be determined, so lifestyle factors including diet have been the major focus in research aimed at the prevention of pre-eclampsia.

3.4.3.2 Nutrition-related factors and pre-eclampsia

While it is suspected that dietary factors may be important in determining the risk of pre-eclampsia, there is no convincing research that implicates any one specific nutrient (Roberts *et al.*, 2003). Historically, it has been believed that variation in macronutrient intake was an important factor, but contributions of low-protein diets, high intakes of n-6 fatty acids or low intakes of n-3 fatty acids have largely been excluded.

Observations that women whose pregnancies are complicated by pre-eclampsia show evidence of poor micronutrient status, have prompted an interest in potential causal relationships. Low serum zinc, calcium, iron and magnesium have all been associated with pre-eclampsia, but these observations may be a consequence rather than a cause of the condition. In the case of iron, reduced concentrations of ferritin and transferrin, which are markers of poor iron status, are also indicators of inflammation, which is a feature of pre-eclampsia. However, reports continue to associate low iron with pre-eclampsia risk. Lewandowska *et al.* (2020) reported that women who developed hypertensive disorders of pregnancy had lower serum iron at 10–14 weeks of gestation than women whose pregnancies were normal. For every 100 µg/l greater iron concentration, the risk of pre-eclampsia declined significantly (OR 0.73, 95% CI 0.57–0.92). However, elevated biomarkers of iron status are also associated with greater risk of pre-eclampsia (Scholl, 2005). This may represent a failure of plasma volume expansion, limiting placental perfusion, or alternatively could be due to iron overload causing oxidative damage at the maternal-placental interface (Ng *et al.*, 2019).

Associations between magnesium and pre-eclampsia are well established, but only as a treatment. In women who develop pre-eclampsia, magnesium sulfate is administered to prevent the progression to eclampsia and is demonstrably effective (Yifu *et al.*, 2020). The role of magnesium in the development of pre-eclampsia has not been robustly established. While women with pre-eclampsia have lower circulating magnesium, the administration of magnesium supplements is not protective (de Araújo et al., 2020).

There is a stronger case for calcium playing a causal role in pre-eclampsia. It is noted that women with pre-eclampsia excrete less calcium in their urine than is normal for pregnancy, and supplementation trials have shown that using very high doses of calcium (1.5–2.0 g/day) reduces the prevalence of hypertension in pregnant women by as much as 50% but appears to reduce the risk of pre-eclampsia only in the small subset of women with very poor calcium status going into pregnancy. A systematic review and meta-analysis by Hofmeyr et al. (2018) was able to evaluate the effects of calcium supplements in women in different categories of pre-eclampsia risk and at different levels of habitual intake. Calcium supplementation appeared to be beneficial for women at high risk of gestational hypertension and in communities with low dietary calcium intake. In the light of evidence that increasing calcium intake may be of benefit in reducing risk of pre-eclampsia, WHO issued guidance in 2011, updated in 2018. The guidance stated that women who live in areas where calcium intake is habitually low (for example due to non-consumption or availability of dairy produce), should take a daily supplement of 1.5–2 g elemental calcium to prevent pre-eclampsia. However, a lack of evidence meant that it was not possible to state at what point in pregnancy the supplementation should begin (World Health Organization, 2018). High-dose calcium supplements run the risk of impairing the absorption of iron and may have a negative impact on bone mineral after delivery (von Dadelszen et al., 2012). It is therefore preferable that women increase their intakes of calcium-rich food sources and avoid agents such as caffeine and salt (sodium chloride) which promote calcium excretion. A review of the evidence regarding lower dose (<1 g/day) calcium supplementation demonstrated that this would also significantly reduce the risk of pre-eclampsia (RR 0.38 95% CI 0.28–0.52; Hofmeyr et al., 2014).

Vitamin D has also been considered as a protective nutrient in the development of pre-eclampsia but, overall, the evidence suggests that it is of limited significance. However, this may reflect the low quality of the research conducted to date and more robust trials are necessary. Observational studies give conflicting views. Zeng et al. (2020) reported lower 25-hydroxy vitamin D concentrations in women who developed pre-eclampsia compared with normal pregnancies, but the prevalence of vitamin D deficiency was high in this study. Cristoph et al. (2020) also considered a population with a high prevalence of deficiency, but found no association with risk of pre-eclampsia. Aguilar-Cordero et al. (2020) considered seven observational studies in a systematic review and found no significant association between pre-eclampsia risk and either vitamin D insufficiency or deficiency. Low quality supplementation trials also deliver variable outcomes. One trial of 50 000 iu vitamin D given every two weeks from recruitment to 36 weeks of gestation in women at high risk of pre-eclampsia prevented recurrence (Behjat Sasan et al., 2017). In contrast, a trial where the vitamin D dose was dependent on baseline 25-hydroxy vitamin D concentration, and doses as high as 120 000 iu administered at 20, 24, 28 and 32 weeks of gestation found no significant benefits (Sablok et al., 2015). Meta-analysis of the data from eight trials showed a trend towards a protective effect of supplementation, but this was not statistically significant and was based on low-quality evidence (OR 0.61 95% CI 0.36–1.04; Aguilar-Cordero et al., 2020).

Oxidative processes appear to play a key role in the development of pre-eclampsia. Pre-eclampsia arises due to defective placentation, and reactive oxygen species drive its development by promoting inflammation, activating apoptosis and generating anti-angiogenic factors that inhibit the formation of new blood vessels and the formation of maternal spiral arteries within the placenta (Poston et al., 2011). Comparison of placentas from pregnancies impacted by pre-eclampsia with normal pregnancies shows greater activity of antioxidant enzymes with pre-eclampsia. This is a common feature of tissues when oxidative injury has occurred and represents a compensatory response (Ferreira et al., 2020). While isolated studies have shown that women with low antioxidant status are at greater risk of pre-eclampsia, the evidence to suggest that antioxidant nutrients may be protective tends to be of low quality. A systematic review of 58 observational studies concluded that vitamin C and vitamin E concentrations are lower in women with pre-eclampsia, but that this is probably explained by publication bias (Cohen et al., 2015). A large-scale, multicentred, randomized placebo-controlled trial involving women at high risk of pre-eclampsia assigned participants to receive placebo or vitamin C 1000 mg per day and vitamin E 400 iu per day. However, with this trial there was no reduction in the incidence of pre-eclampsia and, alarmingly, the antioxidant supplement increased the risk of low birth weight by 15% (Poston et al., 2006). Most other studies show that supplements of vitamins C and E similarly fail to impact the risk of pre-eclampsia (Villar et al., 2009; Bastani et al., 2011; Weissgerber et al., 2013).

The lack of effect of supplementation with the antioxidant vitamins has been explained on the basis of inappropriate supplementation strategy (Poston et al., 2011), including dose and timing. However, the observation that supplements of vitamins C and E did not alter the concentrations of these vitamins in cord blood and in placenta and did not alter the overall antioxidant capacity of the placenta (Johnston et al., 2016) may be a more important indication that the nutrients do not reach the target tissue. Overall, there would appear to be no evidence to suggest that antioxidant nutrients can prevent pre-eclampsia in women at high risk. A meta-analysis of 16 randomized controlled trials using vitamin C either alone or in combination with other micronutrients found no significant benefits with respect to pre-eclampsia (Rumbold et al., 2015).

Prepregnancy BMI is the main nutrition-related predictor of risk of pre-eclampsia. Studies suggest that women who are underweight going into pregnancy are at lower risk while, in general, women who are obese have substantially elevated risk (Sebire et al., 2001). Jensen et al. (2003) reported that women with a BMI over 30 kg/m² were at 3.8-fold greater risk than those with a prepregnancy BMI of 18.5–24.9 kg/m². Weight gain in pregnancy is also critical. An intervention which targeted women with BMI over 35 kg/m² showed that limiting weight gain below 5 kg reduced the risk of pre-eclampsia by 95% (McGiveron et al., 2015). Studies that have assessed the impact of pre-eclampsia in one pregnancy on risk in subsequent pregnancies suggest that gaining weight between confinements adds to risk. An increase in BMI of 3 kg/m² doubles the risk of pre-eclampsia, even in women of normal weight. Weight loss between pregnancies decreases risk (Walsh, 2007).

The association between pre-eclampsia and obesity is most likely explained by the fact that obesity creates a pro-inflammatory state, with adipose tissue expressing a number of cytokines. Obesity is also associated with insulin resistance and endothelial dysfunction, independently of pregnancy. Thus, for women with obesity, there is a low-grade inflammatory response due to excess adiposity, superimposed upon the low-grade inflammation that occurs in normal pregnancy (Poston, 2006). This may make the progression from stage one of pre-eclampsia (placental dysfunction) to fully symptomatic pre-eclampsia, a significantly greater probability.

3.4.4 Abnormal labour

The duration of normal labour, from the first onset of contractions to delivery of the baby, can vary tremendously in length from just a few minutes to two or three days. On average, women experience labour for four to eight hours. Labour has three stages. In the first stage, contractions result in cervical dilatation, thereby opening up the birth canal for the passage of the infant. This first stage is the most protracted element of the labour. In the second stage, the baby moves through the vagina and is born. The third stage of labour is the delivery of the placenta. Risk of fetal or neonatal death is increased in protracted labour, particularly if the labour fails to progress once full cervical dilatation has occurred. In modern medical management of labour, a failure for labour to progress will result in intervention to protect the health of mother and baby. The most extreme intervention is caesarean section, but other interventions that may be used in the second stage include the use of forceps or ventouse to deliver the baby (instrumented delivery). For most women, labour begins spontaneously, but if there is no onset of labour beyond 42 weeks of gestation, it is normal for medical staff to artificially induce labour, either using hormone administration or through artificially rupturing of the amniotic membrane. This reduces the risk of adverse maternal health outcomes.

Interventions in labour are not closely related to maternal nutritional status, but it is clear that maternal BMI is a predictor of these outcomes. A survey of pregnancy outcomes in Lincoln found that women with a BMI in the obese range were significantly more likely to require caesarean delivery (Figure 3.12). There is also evidence that women with obesity are more likely to have labour-induced, ventouse or forceps deliveries and have longer hospital stays after delivery (Morgan et al., 2014). The development of complications may vary according to the stage of labour and may depend on a woman's previous reproductive history. Labour complications (induction, caesarean, epidural anaesthesia) associated with obesity in a first pregnancy may be absent in subsequent pregnancies (O'Dwyer et al., 2013). As gestational diabetes (see Section 3.8.1) is often seen in women who are obese, there is a greater prevalence of babies being large for gestational age. This size contributes to the greater need for medical intervention and also increases the prevalence of shoulder dystocia in babies born to these mothers.

In contrast, women who are underweight appear to have lower risk of labour complications than women with BMI in the ideal range. BMI less than 20 kg/m² is associated with less frequent induction

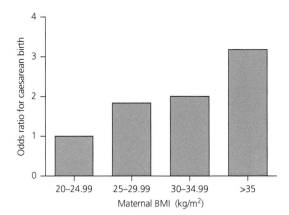

Figure 3.12 Risk of caesarean birth is greater in women who are overweight or obese. BMI, body mass index. *Source:* data from Langley-Evans and Langley-Evans (2003).

of labour, fewer instrumented deliveries and lower risk of emergency caesarean (Sebire *et al.*, 2001). Postpartum haemorrhage is one of the most serious maternal complications of labour and is the major cause of maternal mortality. Between 5% and 12% of women experiencing normal vaginal delivery will experience postpartum haemorrhage. In developed countries, medical management means that the death rate is low (less than 10 cases per million births), but in the developing world, postpartum haemorrhage accounts for around 125 000 maternal deaths every year. Postpartum haemorrhage is more common in women with obesity but being underweight reduces the risk.

3.5 Nausea and vomiting of pregnancy

3.5.1 Nausea and vomiting of pregnancy as a normal physiological process

Nausea and vomiting of pregnancy (NVP) is a commonly reported symptom associated with early pregnancy. Most studies estimate that the prevalence is somewhere between 60% and 80%, with generally higher rates of occurrence in westernized countries than in developing countries (Furneaux *et al.*, 2001). Given the high prevalence, NVP is widely regarded as a normal but unpleasant feature of pregnancy. It usually manifests somewhere between two and six weeks after conception, and for many women it is the first sign that makes them feel that they have conceived. Generally, the peak in NVP symptoms occurs between 10 and 12 weeks of gestation and for most women the condition disappears by 20 weeks. For some women, though, NVP continues throughout the pregnancy.

NVP is colloquially known as 'morning sickness', but this is a misnomer. Although most women will experience nausea or vomiting in the early morning, there are also peak times for symptoms at other points in the day, and episodes are often triggered by exposure to cooking odours or the preparation and consumption of meals. NVP is for many women a debilitating issue that can cause major interference with the pursuit of normal day-to-day activities. NVP may vary greatly in severity (Coad *et al.*, 2002). In mild cases, there may be nothing more than the sensation of nausea. Moderate cases may suffer some episodes of vomiting but in severe NVP, women may struggle to retain the meals that they have consumed. The most extreme manifestation of NVP is hyperemesis gravidarum, which is discussed in the next section. NVP is more common in some groups of women, most notably those having their first baby, women with multiple pregnancies, those of greater BMI, non-smokers and women with a family history of NVP.

The causes of NVP are not fully understood, but most evidence suggests that the symptoms arise as a consequence of the major endocrine changes that accompany the early stages of pregnancy. Oestrogen and progesterone concentrations are high at this stage and both may contribute to the development of NVP (Coad *et al.*, 2002). Progesterone is a modulator of muscle tone in the gastrointestinal tract and may promote gastric reflux by causing a reduction in the patency of the oesophageal sphincter. The mode of action of oestrogen is unclear, but it is noted that women who have a nauseous reaction to oral contraceptives based upon oestrogens are highly likely to develop NVP.

hCG is produced in early pregnancy and plays a key role in the implantation of the embryo and establishment of the placenta. Many lines of circumstantial evidence point to hCG as an important driver of NVP in the first trimester. First, there is a close temporal association between hCG secretion and NVP symptoms (Figure 3.13). The onset of NVP for most women coincides with the first appearance of hCG, and the peak in hCG concentrations in maternal circulation falls around 9–12 weeks, shortly preceding the maximum symptoms of NVP. Women with the most severe NVP are found to have elevated concentrations of hCG compared with asymptomatic women, and correlations have been shown between hCG concentrations and the severity of NVP (Furneaux *et al.*, 2001). hCG has a critical role in the establishment of pregnancy. Disturbances in the secretion of this hormone are associated with adverse pregnancy outcomes. Women who underproduce hCG are more likely to suffer spontaneous miscarriage in early pregnancy and have a greater risk of ectopic pregnancy. Extremely high hCG is also predictive of poor outcomes, including fetal death, premature birth and lower weight at birth.

As mentioned earlier, NVP symptoms are the norm rather than the exception for pregnant women in westernized countries. The very high prevalence of a condition that is so debilitating, and in rare cases lethal, to women in early pregnancy, has prompted some researchers to propose that it serves some function that increases the chances of reproductive success. One view is that NVP serves to change patterns of maternal intake and that this prompts the ingestion of foods that are optimal for the development of the placenta (Coad *et al.*, 2002). Most women with NVP quickly learn that, unlike most nausea, these symptoms are alleviated or suppressed by the regular consumption of foods that are rich in complex carbohydrates. An alternative

view expressed by Flaxman and Sherman (2000) is that NVP has evolved as a defence mechanism to protect the early embryo from maternal ingestion of food-borne pathogens or toxins. The peak period for NVP corresponds to maximum vulnerability of the fetus or embryo to abortifacients, infected foodstuffs or teratogens. NVP leads most women to avoid ingestion of caffeine-containing beverages, meats, fatty foods, burnt food or spicy food. It is argued that many of these foodstuffs would have represented a major risk for pregnant women in the early history of humankind. Whatever the mechanistic driver may be, NVP has a profound impact on the eating patterns of the women who suffer from it (Figure 3.14). Foods which trigger symptoms are avoided, while women will choose to snack frequently on the foods that alleviate their symptoms.

There is a wealth of data to support either theory of the origins of NVP, as clearly women who exhibit mild to moderate symptoms are at reduced risk of a number of poor pregnancy outcomes. Czeizel and Puhó (2004) observed that women reporting that they had suffered from NVP had longer gestation periods and had a lower prevalence of premature delivery. This finding confirms observations of a cohort of 300 British women (Figure 3.15), where an absence of NVP was associated with a 3.26-fold (95% CI 1.19–8.91) greater risk of premature delivery and slightly increased risk of caesarean delivery. Within this study, it was apparent that NVP had no major impact upon women's actual consumption of nutrients in the first trimester of pregnancy. The only significant difference was that NVP sufferers consumed less alcohol (an important teratogen) than women who were asymptomatic.

A range of studies have explored possible associations between NVP and risk of poor pregnancy outcome, particularly miscarriage before 20 weeks

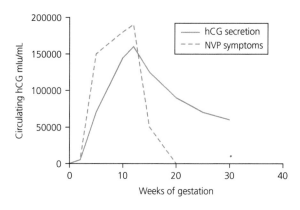

Figure 3.13 The temporal association between symptoms of nausea and vomiting in pregnancy (NVP) and concentrations of human chorionic gonadotrophin (hCG).

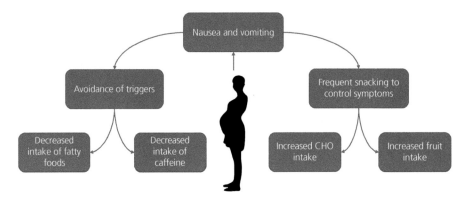

Figure 3.14 Nausea and vomiting of pregnancy brings about changes in eating behaviour. These shape nutrient intakes and ingestion of potentially harmful substances. CHO, carbohydrates.

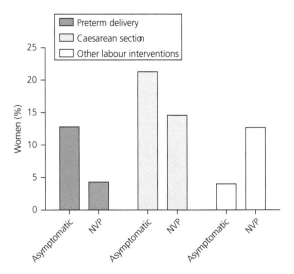

Figure 3.15 Nausea and vomiting in pregnancy (NVP) is associated with reduced risk of preterm delivery; 300 pregnant women were questioned about symptoms of NVP in the first trimester of pregnancy and the outcome of pregnancy was followed up. Women who reported no NVP symptoms were significantly more likely to give birth prior to 37 weeks of gestation. *Source:* data from Langley-Evans and Langley-Evans (2003).

of gestation. Hinkle *et al.* (2016) noted that the onset of symptoms was rapid after conception, with 17.8% of women reporting nausea in the second week of gestation. This rose to 57.3% by week eight, with about half of the effected group experiencing vomiting. In this cohort, NVP was associated with markedly reduced risk of clinical pregnancy loss (hazard ratio 0.2, 95% CI 0.09–0.44) in women who experienced vomiting compared with those who were asymptomatic. Similarly, Sapra *et al.* (2018) found that in women experiencing nausea and vomiting between weeks three and five after a positive pregnancy test, risk of miscarriage was reduced by up to 70%. Other pregnancy risks, including preterm birth, may also be lower in

women who suffer from NVP (Mitsuda *et al.*, 2018). While not all studies find NVP to have an apparently protective effect (Al-Memar *et al.*, 2019), a systematic review of 10 papers considering NVP and pregnancy outcomes found favourable effects of NVP on risk of miscarriages, congenital abnormalities and premature delivery (Koren *et al.*, 2014).

3.5.2 Hyperemesis gravidarum
The severity of NVP symptoms varies enormously between women, but only rarely does the extent of those symptoms become so great that there is a threat to the health of the pregnant woman or her child. Hyperemesis gravidarum lies at the extreme end of the NVP spectrum and may in fact have

completely different causes. It is characterized by intractable nausea and vomiting, which results in metabolic disturbances, ketosis, dehydration, reduction in maternal blood volume and loss of around 5% of the prepregnancy body weight (Figure 3.16). Like NVP, the onset of hyperemesis gravidarum is usually between 4 and 10 weeks of gestation and the condition resolves for most women by 20 weeks (Verberg *et al.*, 2005). For 10% of women with hyperemesis gravidarum, the condition will continue for the whole of their pregnancy. Hyperemesis gravidarum is relatively uncommon, occurring in 0.3–1.5% of pregnancies (Bailit, 2005; Dodds *et al.*, 2006). Women who suffer from hyperemesis gravidarum in their first pregnancy are at very high risk of developing the same degree of nausea and vomiting in subsequent pregnancies. Trogstad *et al.* (2005) found that the odds of recurrence were as high as 26-fold. The risk of hyperemesis gravidarum in a second pregnancy appeared to reduce if the second child had a different father to the first. This suggests an involvement of paternal genes in the development of hyperemesis gravidarum and may give some clues to the aetiology of the problem.

The severity of symptoms will generally result in hospitalization for appropriate treatment using vitamin supplements and intravenous infusion of fluids and electrolytes. Before the introduction of this therapy, hyperemesis gravidarum was a cause of maternal death for around 16 in every 100 000 pregnancies. Most women are successfully treated through fluid infusion, and if this does not lead to recovery, they are given antiemetic drugs. For around 2% of women, there is no response to treatment and it becomes necessary to terminate the pregnancy (Verberg *et al.*, 2005).

Although, with treatment, the impact of hyperemesis gravidarum on maternal health can be greatly reduced, there may be greater risks for the fetus in an hyperemesis gravidarum-complicated pregnancy. Tan *et al.* (2007) reported that the severity of hyperemesis gravidarum as measured by biomarkers of maternal fluid and electrolyte status was a determinant of pregnancy outcomes. More severe symptoms were associated with a greater prevalence of gestational diabetes, more intervention during labour and more emergency procedures. Bailit (2005) found that hyperemesis gravidarum was associated with shorter gestation, a greater prevalence of babies who were small for gestational age, and greater risk of fetal death. Within the same study, it was shown that babies born prematurely (24–30 weeks) were at greater risk of death if born to women with hyperemesis gravidarum. Examination of birth records from over two million pregnancies in Norway (Vandraas *et al.*, 2013) found a greater risk of perinatal death (OR 1.27) associated with hyperemesis gravidarum, together with lower birth weight (21.4 g smaller). Hyperemesis gravidarum-affected pregnancies were, however, significantly less likely to end in very preterm birth. In contrast, the much smaller Norwegian Mother and Child Cohort Study (Vikanes *et al.*, 2013) found no relationship between hyperemesis gravidarum and any birth outcomes.

Failure to gain weight and less effective perfusion of the placenta due to reduced blood volume

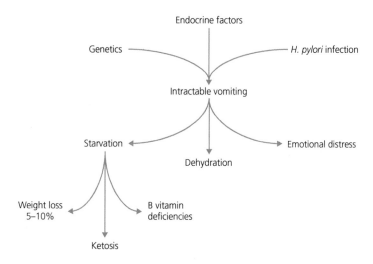

Figure 3.16 Hyperemesis gravidarum is a serious condition of unknown origin. It results in severe dehydration and reduced food intake.

expansion are the most likely routes through which risk of adverse pregnancy outcomes are associated with hyperemesis gravidarum. Certainly, there is very limited evidence that it has a major effect upon maternal nutritional status. There are reports of numerous deficiencies of vitamins and minerals. These have been attributed to raised demands of pregnancy, reduced food intakes and greater nutrient losses. However, the only consistent findings relate to thiamine and vitamin K (Verberg *et al.*, 2005).

3.6 Cravings and aversions

Just as nausea and vomiting are common symptoms experienced by pregnant women, the majority of women in the first trimester report changes in preferences for certain foodstuffs. These changes are often aversive, with women rejecting foods or beverages that might have been staples within their diet prior to pregnancy. Food cravings are strong desires to consume particular food items, which may not have been major elements of the prepregnancy diet. Surveys of the prevalence of food aversions and cravings suggest that between 50% and 60% of women will experience these changes to their eating and drinking behaviours (Furneaux *et al.*, 2001; Bayley *et al.*, 2002). Cravings appear to be universal, appearing in all cultures, but the nature of the foods involved varies by setting (Orloff and Hormes, 2014).

Aversions reported by pregnant women are most commonly to caffeine-based drinks, red and white meats, fish and eggs. Furneaux *et al.* (2001) observed that two thirds of pregnant women among a sample of 300 reported aversion to coffee, with 54% developing an aversion to tea. Other foods rejected by this sample of women included spicy foods and foods that were fatty or greasy. Cravings in early pregnancy are often for foods with a high sugar content, with sweets, chocolate and cakes being widely favoured, together with fruit and fruit juices (Hill *et al.*, 2016, Forbes *et al.*, 2018). Cravings are strongest in the first trimester of pregnancy and may change as gestation progresses, such that sweet cravings give way to cravings for salty foods in later pregnancy (Orloff and Holmes, 2014).

Some studies have suggested that women who change their diet due to cravings may be at risk of excessive gestational weight gain. Orloff *et al.* (2016) reported that up to one quarter of gestational weight gain was driven by sweet cravings, but the causality of the association may be questionable since the data were gathered through self-report via an online questionnaire. In contrast, Hill *et al.* (2016) found

that while women who craved sweet foods had higher energy intakes, their overall dietary quality was not altered and cravings were not associated with excessive weight gain or fetal outcomes. Similarly, Farland *et al.* (2015) examined eating behaviours in the Project Viva prospective cohort and found no risk associated with sweet cravings. This study found that there was a lower risk of excessive gestational weight gain in women who had cravings for salty foods.

The reasons why women develop cravings and aversions in pregnancy are not well understood. Some researchers have suggested that taste and aroma perception is altered by the hormonal changes that accompany early pregnancy and that this produces a preference for sweet foods over bitter foods and a dislike of the smell of foods high in fat (Coad *et al.*, 2002). There are also some suggestions that cravings and aversions have no biological foundation and are instead the products of cultural expectations. One proposal that has received considerable attention and popular support is that cravings and aversions are an element of the broader spectrum of NVP and contribute to fetal defence during embryonic development (Flaxman and Sherman, 2000). It is suggested that NVP symptoms lead to taste aversion learning, in which women are conditioned to avoid foods that are associated with bouts of nausea or vomiting (Bayley *et al.*, 2002). Within an evolutionary perspective, this conditioned behaviour would lead to rejection of the foods most likely to carry toxins or pathogens that might threaten fetal survival.

Support for this idea is partly provided by evidence that women suffering from NVP are more likely to report food aversions than those who do not. Bayley *et al.* (2002) noted that women whose NVP was moderate to severe were more likely to report food aversions and suffered aversions to a greater range of foods than women whose NVP was mild or absent. Importantly, the onset of food aversions appeared to coincide with the onset of NVP symptoms. In contrast, cravings were no more common in women with NVP than in those without and tended to begin much earlier in pregnancy and several weeks ahead of any NVP symptoms. These findings are not supported by all studies (Furneaux *et al.*, 2001), and in contrast to the study by Bayley *et al.* (2002), Coad *et al.* (2002) reported that women with NVP were more likely to have both food aversions and cravings than those who were asymptomatic. Weigel *et al.* (2011) found that women suffering NVP symptoms were more likely to report increased odour sensitivity and aversions to foods and were more likely to crave for fruit. The roots of cravings and aversions may be different, however, and cravings are often reported to occur in women whose NVP begins very early in pregnancy. The high-carbohydrate foods that are most commonly craved often appear to be of benefit in suppressing or controlling feelings of nausea. A study of nearly 52 000 women in the Norwegian Mother and Child Cohort (Chortatos *et al.*, 2013) found that NVP was associated with higher intakes of carbohydrates and sugary drinks. While the simplest interpretation of this is that women choose these foods to control symptoms, the authors could not discount the possibility that high consumption of these foods may be a cause of NVP.

The hypothesis that aversions, together with NVP, may protect the embryo in early pregnancy, receives support from studies of women living in rural communities in developing countries. While some foods become taboo because of the cultural belief that they may be harmful, there is clear evidence among women in rural India, that avoidance of spicy foods in early pregnancy is a genuine aversion (Placek *et al.*, 2017). Clear aversions driven by the smell or taste of food were also noted in a rural island community in Tanzania (Steinmetz *et al.*, 2012). The presence of aversive behaviour in the absence of cultural expectations is highly suggestive of a biological mechanism that has been conserved through human evolution.

3.6.1 Pica

Pica represents an extreme form of craving behaviour, which in addition to being noted in pregnancy is associated with mental illness and some micronutrient deficiencies, including iron deficiency anaemia. Pica is the ingestion of substances that have no nutritive value. Pica behaviours include the consumption of clay or soil, ice, laundry starch or other substances such as soap or chalk (Table 3.6). Pica in pregnancy appears to be a behaviour that is most commonly associated with women of low socioeconomic status, often including those from ethnic minority groups. Mikkelsen *et al.* (2006) noted that

Table 3.6 Pica behaviours.

Pica behaviours	Items that are consumed
Amylophagia	Laundry starch
Coniophagia	Dust
Geophagia*	Clay, dirt, soil
Lithophagia	Small stones, grit
Pagophagia*	Ice
Trichophagia	Hair and wool

* Most frequently reported by pregnant women.

among a large well-nourished Danish population with relatively low numbers of ethnic minorities, pica was a rare behaviour that was reported by just 0.7% of women. This was in stark contrast to figures quoted for the United States, where pica is commonplace (30–50%) in migrant women of African or African-American origin. Indeed, such is the demand for material among such women, some US stores stock clay for human consumption (Stokes, 2006). Rainville (1998) found a high prevalence of pica among deprived, mostly African-American women in Texas. Pica occurred in 77% of pregnant women, with the most common substances consumed being ice or the frost from freezers and refrigerators. Although commonplace, there was no evidence that the pica behaviours had any negative effect upon the outcome of pregnancy. However, the women with pica had lower haemoglobin concentrations at delivery than those without pica. While this US study could not with confidence identify iron deficiency as a cause or consequence of pica, due to confounding influences of maternal smoking and educational achievement, other studies show that pica and iron deficiency are closely associated. Pica was noted in around 20% of pregnant women in an Argentine study (López *et al.*, 2007), with women reported as consuming ice or dirt. As with Rainville (1998), birth weight and anthropometry among infants were not compromised by pica, but markers of iron status were greatly reduced in the women who indulged in pica behaviours. In contrast, in a study of 586 Ghanaian women, of whom 22.8% reported pica, the behaviour was associated with markedly greater risk of low birthweight babies (Abubakari and Jahn, 2016)

Associations of this nature have lent some support to the concept that pica develops as a response to nutrient deficiency. Consumption of clay, for example, could be seen as a means of ingesting the minerals present in the clay matrix. Malnutrition could thus be a trigger for pica, explaining the higher prevalence in women from deprived backgrounds. However, studies using clay slurries in artificial models of the digestive tract show that clay, for example, would tend to exacerbate malnutrition as iron, zinc and copper become bound to the clay matrix, especially under acid conditions (Stokes, 2006). Geophagia could therefore promote malnutrition rather than being a corrective behaviour. In developing countries, soil and clay are likely to carry pathogenic organisms that may cause harm to pregnant women. Young *et al.* (2007) examined infection with nematodes in an African population of pregnant women. Pica was common in these women and the main behaviours were consumption of clay (7% of women), ice (21%), uncooked rice (55%) and unripe mangoes (84%). Although there was no clear difference in risk of infection when comparing women with geophagia with those showing no pica, there was a tendency for greater levels of hookworm infection in clay eaters. Hookworm infection is an important cause of iron deficiency anaemia in African countries. In addition to infection with nematodes and parasites, consumption of soil carries a substantial risk of bacterial or fungal infection, and ingestion of contaminants including lead (Kutalek *et al.*, 2010). A study of pregnant women in New York City found that soil consumption was the most commonly exhibited pica behaviour, together with intake of brick dust, paint and plaster. This behaviour was associated with elevated blood lead levels (Thihalolipavan *et al.*, 2013).

It seems unlikely then that pica develops to replace nutrient losses or address deficiency. It is possible that these behaviours may help women deal with nausea and vomiting, but far more likely that pica is a cultural phenomenon. This could explain the very high occurrence in women of African origin (Stokes, 2006). As described above, there is no clear evidence of pica causing harm to infants. The potential for harm is clearly present though. Pica, particularly where consumption of clay or soil is involved, has the potential to introduce pathogens or toxins, such as lead, to the body. There are also reports of pica as a cause of gestational diabetes. Jackson and Martin (2000) reported two cases of pregnant women with uncontrolled diabetes in a home setting, which spontaneously reversed without treatment on admission to hospital. On investigation, it emerged that these women were consuming large quantities of laundry (corn) starch each day.

3.7 Gastrointestinal disturbances in pregnancy

As described earlier in this chapter, the gastrointestinal tract undergoes a number of functional changes during pregnancy, largely under the influence of progesterone. These changes serve to slow down transit times and hence maximize the absorption of nutrients and reabsorption of water from the tract. A combination of these effects of steroid hormones on the tract and the physical expansion of the uterus, baby and placenta as pregnancy progresses can produce a series of minor symptoms of the gastrointestinal tract. These cause discomfort to many pregnant women but only rarely impact pregnancy outcomes.

Heartburn (dyspepsia) is a symptom that afflicts many women early in gestation due to declining competency of the oesophageal sphincter. In later gestation, the pressure of the uterus upon the stomach can limit the total stomach capacity and also drive gastric reflux. The period of rapid late gestation fetal growth, where demands for nutrients and fluids are at their greatest, therefore corresponds to the time of lowest stomach capacity, so at this time women need to consume smaller but more frequent meals.

Constipation is also a common symptom of later gestation, impacting upon around one quarter of pregnancies (Bradley *et al.*, 2007). This is largely a consequence of the slow transit of faecal material through the colon and the highly efficient reabsorption of water. Dry compacted faecal material becomes harder to pass and this can also increase the risk of haemorrhoids, which are another complaint associated with pregnancy. Certain factors increase the likelihood of constipation, including low intakes of water, low fibre diets, reduced physical activity and the prescribing of iron supplements to combat iron deficiency anaemia.

3.8 High-risk pregnancies

A number of pregnancies may be considered to be at higher than normal risk and merit close monitoring and possible medical intervention to ensure a successful outcome. Women may be identified as being at high risk on the basis of pre-existing medical conditions (e.g. diabetes types 1 and 2), socioeconomic status and lifestyle factors. Maternal factors that are associated with greater risk include prepregnancy underweight or obesity, low socioeconomic status, a history of eating disorders, HIV infection, alcohol or other substance abuse.

3.8.1 Gestational diabetes

Gestational diabetes is a syndrome of insulin resistance that develops during pregnancy. In the past, it was referred to as latent diabetes, in reference to the fact that it most probably represents a state in which the metabolic stress of pregnancy causes an existing pre-diabetic state to progress to a symptomatic state. As already mentioned in this chapter, pregnancy is a state in which the mother becomes increasingly insulin resistant. This produces a metabolic scenario in which post-prandial plasma glucose concentrations are elevated and, on fasting, there is greater mobilization of triglycerides, free fatty acids and ketones (Carpenter, 2007). This ensures substrate supply to the placenta and fetus. In 2–3% of pregnancies, these metabolic changes lead to gestational diabetes. The condition is more common in women who are obese, have a family history of diabetes or have other factors that predispose to type 2 diabetes.

In most cases, gestational diabetes is a transient state that resolves with the end of pregnancy. However, women suffering from gestational diabetes are more likely to develop type 2 diabetes at a later date, and around 50% of women with gestational diabetes will also develop the condition in subsequent pregnancies (Reader, 2007). Gestational diabetes is associated with a number of adverse pregnancy outcomes and, in particular, is closely related to the hypertensive disorders of pregnancy (e.g. pre-eclampsia). These associations suggest a common aetiology that relates to inflammatory processes associated with insulin resistance and excess adiposity (Carpenter, 2007).

Gestational diabetes has a number of negative impacts on fetal and infant health. One of the most significant of these is macrosomia or 'large baby syndrome'. Babies are defined as being large for gestational age if they weigh over 4.5 kg at birth, regardless of gestational age. Babies who are large for their gestational age are more common in pregnancies associated with gestational diabetes. This makes an operative delivery more likely, as the large baby is unable to progress through the birth canal without sustaining significant injury such as shoulder dystocia, subconjunctival haemorrhage or fractures (Hadden, 2008). Gestational diabetes promotes macrosomia of the fetus through spillover of

glucose from mother to fetus across the placenta (Figure 3.17).

Infants whose mothers have gestational diabetes may also suffer a period of hypoglycaemia after birth because of the steep fall in glucose input once out of the uterus. Gestational diabetes is also associated with fetal hypocalcaemia. High prevailing insulin and insulin-like growth factor-1 concentrations in response to high glucose concentrations drive calcium into bone. The affected fetus tends to have high bone mineral mass but low circulating calcium and, in extreme cases, this can lead to convulsions after birth. In addition to these immediate hazards, there is a growing body of evidence that suggests that a fetus exposed to gestational diabetes is more likely to become obese and to develop type 2 diabetes later in life (Hussain *et al.*, 2007; see Research Highlight 3.3).

Women with gestational diabetes require careful monitoring and nutritional management to limit the risk of adverse pregnancy outcomes. Therapies aim to control blood glucose concentrations without the use of insulin injection. Management is therefore focused around control of carbohydrate intake, while maintaining appropriate rates of weight gain and intakes of other nutrients. Prospective studies from the United States and Australia have shown that such approaches are effective in limiting the need for more robust medical intervention and reducing the risk of serious perinatal complications (Reader, 2007). Physical activity is an important element of the management of gestational diabetes. There is evidence that increasing activity before

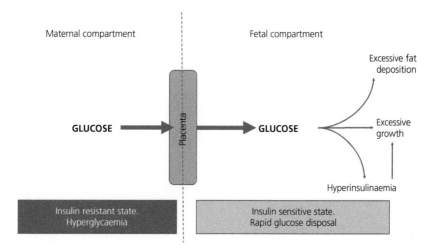

Figure 3.17 Gestational diabetes is a condition of maternal insulin resistance. Maternal insulin resistance drives glucose across the placenta to the fetal tissues. The ensuing increase in fetal insulin secretion drives excessive fetal growth and leads to a baby who is large for gestational age.

Research Highlight 3.3   Long-term impact of gestational diabetes on offspring health and wellbeing.

Gestational diabetes is a risk factor for poor maternal and fetal outcomes in pregnancy, with greater likelihood of babies who are large for gestational age, macrosomia, labour interventions and shoulder dystocia. There are also concerns that children exposed to gestational diabetes during fetal development may be at greater risk of metabolic disorders and neurobehavioural problems later in life. This area of research is challenging though, as many potential confounding factors must be considered. Most women who develop gestational diabetes are overweight or obese, so apparent long-term effects of the diabetes may be caused by maternal weight problems rather than the metabolic disorder. Similarly, obesity is a bigger problem in women of lower socioeconomic status, and this may also be a driver of problems observed in their children.

Possible long-term metabolic effects of exposure to gestational diabetes were first reported by Silverman *et al.* (1995), who noted that 10–16-year-old children of mothers with diabetes showed glucose intolerance themselves. Other studies failed to verify this finding (Landon *et al.*, 2015). The Hyperglycemia and Adverse Pregnancy Outcomes (HAPO) study reported that body composition of 11-year-olds was related to maternal gestational diabetes. The children of 672 mothers with gestational diabetes in a cohort of 4697 women showed greater adiposity by a number of measures, but this disappeared when data were adjusted for maternal prepregnancy BMI (Lowe *et al.*, 2018). Subsequent analysis of the HAPO data (Lowe *et al.*, 2018) found that children's adiposity was associated with measures of maternal glycemia in pregnancy, and that the influence of gestational diabetes was therefore independent of maternal overweight. The meta-analysis of Kawasaki *et al.* (2018), however, concluded that there was no significant association between children's BMI z-scores and maternal gestational diabetes. This area remains of interest but with no clear consensus.

Similarly, evidence that gestational diabetes exposure is a factor in neurobehavioural disorders is interesting but conflicting. Nomura *et al.* (2012) reported that among six-year-olds, gestational diabetes increased the risk of attention deficit hyperactivity disorder (ADHD) by up to 14-fold. However, this cohort was small and the relationship was only seen in the children from a poor socioeconomic background. The importance of socioeconomic status was also apparent in a study of 18–27-year-olds, which showed an adverse impact of gestational diabetes exposure on global cognitive scores (Clausen *et al.*, 2013). Despite the often low-quality evidence available from case–control studies and strong evidence of publication bias, the meta-analysis of Zhao *et al.* (2019) concluded that cohort studies had sufficient robust data to be able to conclude that gestational diabetes increased the risk of ADHD in children significantly (OR 1.64, 95%CI 1.25–5.56).

pregnancy and maintaining this during gestation can reduce risk. Care should be taken to monitor blood glucose before and after exercise, and pregnant women should avoid periods of vigorous activity in excess of 15–30 minutes.

For women with pre-existing diabetes, whether type 1 or type 2, pregnancy presents additional challenges. In terms of pregnancy outcomes, type 2 diabetes has a similar risk profile to gestational diabetes. Mothers with type 1 diabetes are at substantially greater risk of pre-eclampsia and require more interventions, such as emergency caesarean delivery (Owens *et al.*, 2015). Close monitoring and support for mothers with diabetes, beginning prior to conception, is strongly advised, and women with type 1 diabetes should avoid unplanned pregnancy. There is an increased risk of the development of diabetic retinopathy during pregnancy, and while diabetic nephropathy is unlikely to progress during gestation, impairments of renal function will contribute to development of pre-eclampsia.

To manage risk, women with diabetes need to maintain very tight control of glycaemia and will need to change their insulin regimens and other control protocols, including dietary change. They may need to be introduced to additional metformin therapy, but no other anti-diabetic drugs should be considered (Ringholm *et al.*, 2012). The nausea and vomiting of early pregnancy may make maintaining glycaemic control especially challenging. Diabetes significantly increases the risk of fetal malformations, so women with diabetes should commence taking high-dose folic acid supplements (5 mg per day) prior to conception. Putting in place robust support in the pre-conception period has been shown to improve glycaemic control and clinical outcomes (Owens *et al.*, 2012).

3.8.2 Adolescent and older mothers

Maternal age is a significant determinant of the risk of poor pregnancy outcomes and complications (Figure 3.18). Pregnant adolescents are at higher risk of giving birth to preterm babies who are small for gestational age. Some of this risk is attributable to nutrition-related factors. Adolescents who are pregnant are generally still in their own growth phase, as growth in girls continues for 4–7 years after menarche, and peaks between 11 and 13 years of age. Girls who become pregnant before the age of 14 will suffer complications resulting from their growth

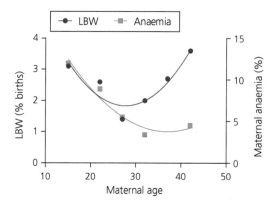

Figure 3.18 U-shaped relationship between maternal age and risk of iron deficiency anaemia and low birth weight baby (low birth weight, LBW = birth weight < 2500 g).

competing with the nutritional demands of pregnancy, particularly for energy, protein and micronutrients. Workicho *et al.* (2020) reported that around 20% of the risk of small-for-gestational age delivery was associated with lower mid–upper arm circumference, an indicator of muscle mass, in younger mothers.

Adolescent girls are at particularly high risk of poor micronutrient status, including iron deficiency anaemia, and this raises risk in pregnancy. The reasons for poor nutritional status vary by culture and setting. In developed countries, the drivers are generally the girl's push for independence, personal beliefs, social factors and the use of potentially harmful substances. In developing countries where early marriage is common, girls are often chronically undernourished before pregnancy and suffer adverse consequences of multiple pregnancies in a short space of time (Lassi *et al.*, 2017). Appropriate interventions to improve nutritional status, and hence pregnancy outcomes, include supplemental micronutrients, and protein energy supplementation.

Women of any age with a short inter-pregnancy intervals are also at risk of poor pregnancy outcomes as they cannot replenish fat and micronutrient reserves between pregnancies. recommended minimum spacing of pregnancies is 12 months in developed countries, but in impoverished populations a minimum of 24 months is more appropriate. The impact of an interval of less than 12 months was illustrated by Schummers *et al.* (2018), who observed greater risk of small for gestational age babies, preterm delivery and greater maternal mortality. There are well-established effects of short spacing upon fat reserves. Pinto *et al.* (2015) reported lower n-3 fatty acid status in women with shorter inter-pregnancy intervals.

All pregnancy-associated risks to maternal health and poor fetal outcomes increase with greater maternal age. Older mothers are more likely to develop pre-eclampsia and gestational diabetes, require intervention in labour, have higher risk of death and are more likely to suffer miscarriage or stillbirth (Kenny *et al.*, 2013; Khalil *et al.*, 2013). This risk may be driven by pre-existing maternal hypertension, obesity and insulin resistance. Obesity is a particular problem in pregnancy for women over the age of 40 years (Fredriksen *et al.*, 2018). While the nutritional influences on risk for older women are less well defined than for adolescents, the strong influence of socioeconomic status on the association between age and pregnancy outcome (Kenny *et al.*, 2013) suggests that lifestyle factors, including diet, are an important contributor.

3.8.3 Multiple pregnancies

Multiple pregnancies (twins, triplets, quadruplets or greater) are associated with significantly greater risks for a number of adverse maternal and fetal outcomes of pregnancy. Naturally occurring multiparity is relatively uncommon, with around 1 in 80 natural conceptions resulting in twin pregnancy, 1 in 80^2 (64 000) resulting in triplets and 1 in 80^3 (512 000) leading to quadruplets. However, the numbers of multiple pregnancies have increased markedly since the 1980s due to the greater use of assisted reproductive technologies (Brown and Carlson, 2000). Often, techniques such as in vitro fertilization result in the implantation of two or three fertilized embryos to maximize the chances of a successful outcome. As the majority of women undergoing assisted reproduction are older (over 35 years), the combination of multiparity and greater age has a particularly marked impact upon their risk profile.

Multiple pregnancies carry significant risk for both mother and babies (Rosello-Soberon *et al.*, 2005). There are greater risks of maternal and neonatal mortalities arising from increased risk of preterm delivery, increased prevalence of pre-eclampsia, gestational diabetes and postpartum haemorrhage (Rao *et al.*, 2004). Much of the risk of preterm delivery is related to intrauterine growth restriction, with 50% of twins and 90% of triplets being small for gestational age. The combination of being small for gestational age and prematurity is a particularly high risk for neonatal death (Brown and Carlson, 2000).

As with other outcomes of pregnancy, maternal BMI prepregnancy and weight gain during gestation are the strongest predictors of the outcome of multiple pregnancy. Weight before pregnancy is a key determinant of pregnancy weight gain and availability of maternal reserves to drive the extra fetal growth. Women with twin pregnancies who are obese are significantly less likely to have preterm birth and infants of low birth weight than those who are underweight before pregnancy (Rosello-Soberon *et al.*, 2005). Yeh and Shelton (2007) showed that in twin-bearing women with a BMI of 29 kg/m², birth weights were up to 170 g greater than in women with a BMI less than 19.8 kg/m² before conception. This study found that achieving a weight gain in excess of 25 kg across pregnancy could increase the birth weights of twins by up to 500 g and reduced the risk of the babies being born before 36 weeks of gestation and of being small for gestational age. This was emphasized by the study of Flidel-Rimon *et al.* (2005), who showed that in women expecting triplets, achieving a weight gain in excess of 16.2 kg over the first 24 weeks of gestation significantly reduced the risk of a small for gestational age baby, irrespective of the prepregnancy BMI. For triplet pregnancies, having a higher prepregnancy BMI, even if in the overweight or obese range, reduces the risk of negative pregnancy outcomes.

Final achieved birth weight in multiple pregnancies is most closely related to maternal weight gain in the first trimester, with the period 20–28 weeks of gestation also being of great importance (Luke, 2005). It is suggested that to minimize risk associated with multiparity, the early phase of pregnancy should be targeted with appropriate advice to maximize weight maternal gain. Just as with singleton pregnancies, weight gain should be greater in women of lower BMI and reduced in women who are obese. However, proposed gains are considerably greater than for singleton pregnancies. Underweight women carrying twins should aim to gain 22–28 kg over the first 28 weeks of pregnancy, at a rate of 0.5–0.8 kg per week in the first trimester (Luke, 2005). Recommended gains are 17–25, 14–23 and 11–19 kg for women in normal weight, overweight and obese BMI ranges respectively (Rasmussen *et al.*, 2009). Higher gains are desirable in multiple pregnancies, as preterm delivery is far more likely, so the period of intrauterine growth is shorter. Maximizing weight at delivery greatly reduces the risk of morbidity and mortality in preterm infants. Fox *et al.* (2010) considered the weight gain of 297 women carrying twin pregnancies and noted that those achieved a weight gain at the level recommended by the US Institute of Medicine (2009) had babies that were on average 200–250 g heavier. Preterm birth and small for gestational age births were less likely with weight gain at the recommended level. In all pregnancies, the function of the placenta declines in late gestation. In multiple pregnancies, the decline in function is more rapid. It is suggested that more rapid maternal weight gain in early pregnancy helps to establish a more robust placentation (Luke, 2005).

Women with multiple pregnancies are assumed to have significantly greater energy requirements than women with singleton pregnancies, based purely upon requirements to achieve the optimal weight gains described above. Although there are several recommendations published, there is a lack of robust evidence base available to support any nutritional guidance for multiple pregnancies (Bricker *et al.*, 2015). Brown and Carlson (2000) have suggested that, over a full pregnancy, the extra energy requirement for a twin pregnancy would be equivalent to 150 kcal per day on top of the enhanced requirement for pregnancy. Goodnight and Newman (2009) suggested a greater increment, with a recommendation of 40–45 kcal per kg body weight per day. This is the equivalent of 3150 kcal per day for a 70-kg woman and is well above the 1940 kcal per day (2140 kcal per day in the third trimester) for a singleton pregnancy. A small but rigorous study of twin pregnancies (20 women; Ghandi *et al.*, 2018) found that estimated energy requirements increased by 700 kcal per day between the first and second trimesters and then remained stable in the third trimester. These requirements were not compensated by reductions in physical activity level. The greater requirement was estimated at 2940 kcal per day. Luke (2005) suggested that energy intakes should be 3000 kcal per day for mothers with twin pregnancies who were obese and 4000 kcal per day for mothers who were underweight.

Pregnant women, in general, begin gestation with normal insulin secretion and sensitivity, but as pregnancy proceeds they develop an exaggerated insulin response to feeding. Insulin concentrations in late pregnancy can be more than three times greater in late pregnancy than in the non-pregnant state. Pregnant women are therefore insulin resistant and this metabolic adaptation helps to shunt substrates across the placenta to the fetus (Butte, 2000). This is enhanced in multiple pregnancy, and as a result, maternal glucose concentrations tend to be low and glycogen stores deplete very rapidly. Development of ketosis as metabolism switches to the use of fat, as will occur rapidly during periods of fasting in such women, is predictive of poor pregnancy outcomes (Luke, 2005). Women with multiple pregnancies are therefore advised to consume food frequently (three meals plus three snacks daily).

In keeping with the extra demand for fetal growth and deposition of maternal tissue to support that growth, micronutrient requirements for multiple pregnancy will be greater than for a singleton pregnancy. Iron status, for example, will be markedly impacted by the needs of multiple fetuses, possibly additional placentation and the greater maternal blood volume expansion. It is suggested that requirements may be 1.8-fold higher than in a singleton pregnancy (Rosello-Soberon *et al.*, 2005). The US Institute of Medicine has made recommendations relating to intakes of a number of micronutrients in women with multiple pregnancies (Table 3.7), which are over and above the standard recommendations for antenatal supplements. These recommendations are not matched by equivalent advice in other countries. The potential benefits and hazards associated with supplementation with minerals and folate have not been well defined and it may be more appropriate

for women to meet the increased need for these nutrients by consuming more nutrient-dense foods. There is a dearth of research evidence to guide the development of recommendations and associated with this there appears to be a lack of advice given to women who are bearing twins or triplets (Whitaker *et al.*, 2019). This area requires further investigation, but some reports have shown benefits of following standard antenatal advice. In a large cohort of Chinese women, consumption of 400 µg/day of supplemental folic acid was found to reduce the risk of low birth weight and small for gestational age outcomes among twins (Zhang *et al.*, 2020). There is some evidence that essential fatty acid concentrations are reduced in multiparous women, suggesting that there may be increased demands for these nutrients. Increased intakes of eggs, fatty fish and oils may therefore be appropriate (Goodnight and Newman, 2009).

Table 3.7 Recommendations for micronutrient supplementation in multiple pregnancy.

Micronutrient	Recommended supplement dose*
Iron	30 mg/day
Zinc	15 mg/day
Calcium	250 mg/day
Copper	2 mg/day
Folate	300 µg/day
Vitamin B6	2 mg/day
Vitamin C	50 mg/day
Vitamin D	5 µg/day

* To be introduced after weeks of 12 gestation.

3.8.4 Fetal alcohol spectrum disorders

This chapter has already highlighted the risks associated with alcohol consumption in pregnancy, in relation to miscarriage and preterm birth. Extremes of alcohol consumption, for example, where a pregnant woman is an alcoholic, are associated with a range of fetal abnormalities that are collectively known as the fetal alcohol spectrum (FAS) disorders. FAS disorders arise when a child has confirmed exposure to maternal alcohol consumption; the child exhibits craniofacial abnormalities, pre- and post-natal growth restriction and neurocognitive defects (Figure 3.19). The related disorders are FAS, partial FAS, alcohol-related birth defects and neurodevelopmental

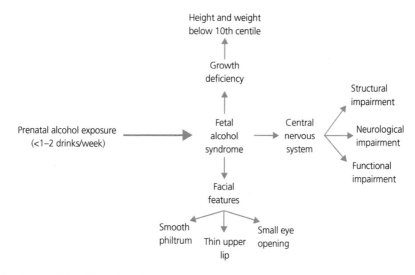

Figure 3.19 The characteristics of fetal alcohol syndrome.

disorder, in which some of the features of FAS disorders may be absent, or specific elements may be more pronounced. For example, in FAS, the confirmed exposure to maternal drinking is often absent, while in alcohol-related neurodevelopmental disorder, the neurocognitive defects are the most pronounced manifestation (Mukherjee et al., 2006).

The prevalence of these disorders is difficult to estimate as affected children can be undiagnosed until they reach school age. Estimates for prevalence varies widely, but approximately one to three births per 1000 may be affected (Hannigan and Armant, 2005). Prevalence rises to 60 per 1000 births for pregnancies where the mother is a confirmed alcoholic. For neurodevelopmental disorders and partial FAS, the prevalence is likely to be higher and is possibly as much as 30 cases per 1000 births.

Alcohol is able to freely cross the placenta by diffusion. This means that fetal tissues are effectively exposed to the same concentrations as the maternal tissues. However, the fetal system is unable to metabolize alcohol as effectively and so effects are prolonged. When alcohol exposure occurs during critical periods of organ development in the first and second trimesters of pregnancy, there can be major impacts on organ growth and morphogenesis. The central nervous system is most vulnerable to effects of alcohol and it is believed that as much as 20% of all mental restriction in developed countries could be related to FAS disorders. Affected children are born with microcephaly (small head), functional deficits (e.g. loss of hearing), and go on to have lower IQ, learning difficulties, language deficits and social and behavioural problems that often lead to disrupted schooling and alcohol and drug abuse problems (Mukherjee et al., 2006). The heart and kidneys are also major targets for alcohol-related birth defects.

The impact of FAS disorders on affected children appears to be long lasting and certainly extends into adulthood. These disorders are associated with criminal behaviour in adolescence (Momino et al., 2012), mental health problems (Easey et al., 2019) and greater risk of alcohol and drug abuse (Dodge et al., 2019). Affected individuals have impaired immunity, impaired metabolic function and increased risk of cancer in adulthood (Mead and Sarkar, 2014). In adulthood, it is clear that while some craniofacial abnormalities are resolved, stunted height and microcephaly are not and adults with FAS show a high prevalence of moderate to severe mental restriction (Spohr et al., 2007). There is emerging evidence that alcohol exposure during fetal development impacts the epigenome, changing DNA and histone marks in a heritable manner.

In this way, maternal drinking may impact more than one generation. Kvigne et al. (2008) reported that the grandchildren of women who had abused alcohol in pregnancy were at greater risk of FAS disorders. Given the potentially devastating effect of excessive alcohol consumption in pregnancy, it is alarming to note the growth of binge-drinking cultures among young women in countries such as the UK. Cessation of drinking should be a priority for women considering pregnancy, as the greatest effects of alcohol may occur during embryogenesis and may precede confirmation of conception.

SUMMARY

- Pregnancy is accompanied by major maternal adaptations that support the development of the placenta and allow fetal growth and development. These adaptations, and the growth of the fetus, greatly increase the demand for energy and nutrients.
- Changes to maternal physiology, behaviour and the mobilization of prepregnancy stores are often sufficient to meet requirements for nutrients without changes to intake.
- Optimal maternal weight gain in pregnancy is a key determinant of pregnancy outcome. Advised weight gains vary depending on prepregnancy BMI.
- Nutrition-related factors are predictive of a number of adverse pregnancy outcomes, including miscarriage and stillbirth, gestational diabetes, preterm delivery and the hypertensive disorders of pregnancy.
- Maternal obesity is a major risk factor for most of the adverse pregnancy outcomes.
- Nausea and vomiting of pregnancy is a normal feature of the early stages of most pregnancies. These symptoms may be protective and are associated with a lower risk of early miscarriage.
- Hyperemesis gravidarum is the most extreme form of nausea and vomiting in pregnancy. This condition requires robust intervention as it is associated with greater risk of both maternal and fetal death.
- Excessive alcohol consumption in pregnancy is associated with neurocognitive and other congenital disorders in the fetus.

References

Abati, S., Villa, A., Cetin, I. et al. (2013). Lack of association between maternal periodontal status and adverse pregnancy outcomes: a multicentric epidemiologic study. Journal of Maternal Fetal and Neonatal Medicine. **26**: 369–372.

Abubakari, A., Jahn, A. (2016). Maternal dietary patterns and practices and birth weight in Northern Ghana. *PLoS One* **11**: e0162285.

Adalsteinsdottir, S., Tryggvadottir, E.A., Hrolfsdottir, L. et al. (2020). Insufficient iodine status in pregnant women as a consequence of dietary changes. *Food and Nutrition Research* **64**: 10.29219.

Aguilar-Cordero, M.J., Lasserrot-Cuadrado, A., Mur-Villar, N. et al. (2020). Vitamin D, preeclampsia and prematurity: A systematic review and meta-analysis of observational and interventional studies. *Midwifery* **87**: 102707.

Australian Insitute of Health and Welfare. (2020). Australia's mothers and babies data visualisations. https://www.aihw.gov.au/reports/mothers-babies/australias-mothers-babies-data-visualisations/contents/antenatal-period/body-mass-index (accessed 3 April 2021).

Al-Memar, M., Vaulet, T., Fourie, H. et al. (2019). Early-pregnancy events and subsequent antenatal, delivery and neonatal outcomes: prospective cohort study. *Ultrasound Obstetrics and Gynecology* **54**: 530–537.

Assaf-Balut, C., Garcia de la Torre, N., Bordiu, E. et al. (2020). Consumption of fat-free dairy products is not associated with a lower risk of maternofetal adverse events. *BMJ Open Diabetes Research Care* **8**: e001145.

Azimi-Nezhad, M., Teymoori, A., Ebrahimzadeh-Vesal, R. (2020). Association of CYP11B2 gene polymorphism with preeclampsia in north east of Iran (Khorasan province). *Gene* **733**: 144358.

Bailit, J.L. (2005). Hyperemesis gravidarum: epidemiologic findings from a large cohort. *American Journal of Obstetrics and Gynecology* **193**: 811–814.

Balogun, O.O., da Silva Lopes, K., Ota, E. et al. (2016). Vitamin supplementation for preventing miscarriage. *Cochrane Database of Systematic Reviews* 2016(5): CD004073.

Barbour, L.A. (2003). New concepts in insulin resistance of pregnancy and gestational diabetes: long-term implications for mother and offspring. *Journal of Obstetrics and Gynaecology* **23**: 545–549.

Bastani, P., Hamdi, K., Abasalizadeh, F. et al. (2011). Effects of vitamin E supplementation on some pregnancy health indices: a randomized clinical trial. *International Journal of General Medicine* **4**: 461–464.

Bayley, T.M., Dye, L., Jones, S. et al. (2002). Food cravings and aversions during pregnancy: relationships with nausea and vomiting. *Appetite*, **38**: 45–51.

Beck, J., Garcia, R., Heiss, G. et al. (1996). Periodontal disease and cardiovascular disease. *Journal of Periodontitis* **67**: 1123–1137.

Behjat Sasan, S., Zandvakili, F., Soufizadeh, N. et al. (2017). The effects of vitamin D supplement on prevention of recurrence of preeclampsia in pregnant women with a history of preeclampsia. *Obstetrics and Gynecology International* **2017**: 8249264.

Bener, A., Al-Hamaq, A.O. and Saleh, N.M. (2013). Association between vitamin D insufficiency and adverse pregnancy outcome: global comparisons. *International Journal Womens Health* **5**: 523–531.

Berger, H., Melamed, N., Davis, B.M. et al. (2020). Impact of diabetes, obesity and hypertension on preterm birth: Population-based study. *PLoS One* **15**: e0228743.

Borodulin, K.M., Evenson, K.R., Wen, F. et al. (2008). Physical activity patterns during pregnancy. *Medicine and Science in Sports and Exercise* **40**: 1901–1908.

Bourassa, M.W., Osendarp, S.J.M., Adu-Afarwuah, S. et al. (2019). Review of the evidence regarding the use of antenatal multiple micronutrient supplementation in low- and middle-income countries. *Annals of the New York Academy of Science* **1444**: 6–21.

Brabin, B., Tinto, H., Roberts, S.A. (2019). Testing an infection model to explain excess risk of preterm birth with long-term iron supplementation in a malaria endemic area. *Malaria Journal* **18**: 374.

Bradley, C.S., Kennedy, C.M., Turcea, A.M. et al. (2007). Constipation in pregnancy: prevalence, symptoms, and risk factors. *Obstetrics and Gynecology* **110**: 1351–1357.

Bricker, L., Reed, K., Wood, L. et al. (2015). Nutritional advice for improving outcomes in multiple pregnancies. *Cochrane Database of Systematic Reviews.* (11): CD008867.

Brown, J.E. and Carlson, M. (2000). Nutrition and multifetal pregnancy. *Journal of the American Dietetic Association* **100**: 343–348.

Buck Louis, G.M., Sapra, K.J., Schisterman, E.F. et al. (2016). Lifestyle and pregnancy loss in a contemporary cohort of women recruited before conception: the LIFE study. *Fertility and Sterility* **106**: 180–188.

Butte, N.F. (2000). Carbohydrate and lipid metabolism in pregnancy: normal compared with gestational diabetes mellitus. *American Journal of Clinical Nutrition* **71**: 1256S–1261S.

Carlson, S.E., Colombo, J., Gajewski, B.J. et al. (2013). DHA supplementation and pregnancy outcomes. *American Journal of Clinical Nutrition* **97**: 808–815.

Carpenter, M.W. (2007). Gestational diabetes, pregnancy hypertension, and late vascular disease. *Diabetes Care* **30**(Suppl 2): S246–S250.

Catov, J.M., Parker, C.B., Gibbs, B.B. et al. (2018). Patterns of leisure-time physical activity across pregnancy and adverse pregnancy outcomes. *International Journal of Behavioural Nutrition and Physical Activity* 2018; 15(1): 68.

Chapman, A.B., Abraham, W.T., Zamudio, S. et al. (1998). Temporal relationships between hormonal and hemodynamic changes in early human pregnancy. *Kidney International* **54**: 2056–2063.

Chen, L.W., Wu, Y., Neelakantan, N. et al. (2016). Maternal caffeine intake during pregnancy and risk of pregnancy loss: a categorical and dose-response meta-analysis of prospective studies. *Public Health Nutrition* **19**: 1233–1244.

Chen, L.W., Fitzgerald, R., Murrin, C.M. et al. (2018a). Associations of maternal caffeine intake with birth outcomes: results from the Lifeways Cross Generation Cohort Study. *American Journal of Clinical Nutrition* **108**: 1301–1308.

Chen, C., Xu, X., Yan, Y. (2018). Estimated global overweight and obesity burden in pregnant women based on panel data model. *PLoS One* **13**: e0202183.

Chikakuda, A.T., Shin, D., Comstock, S.S. et al. (2018). Compliance to prenatal iron and folic acid supplement use in relation to low birth weight in Lilongwe, Malawi. *Nutrients* **10**: 1275.

Chmielewska, A., Dziechciarz, P., Gieruszczak-Białek, D. et al. (2019). Effects of prenatal and/or postnatal supplementation with iron, PUFA or folic acid on neurodevelopment: update. *British Journal of Nutrition* **122**: S10–S15.

Chortatos, A1., Haugen, M., Iversen, P.O. *et al.* (2013). Nausea and vomiting in pregnancy: associations with maternal gestational diet and lifestyle factors in the Norwegian Mother and Child Cohort Study. *BJOG* **120**: 1642–1653.

Clausen, T.D., Mortensen, E.L., Schmidt, L. *et al.* (2013). Cognitive function in adult offspring of women with gestational diabetes--the role of glucose and other factors. *PLoS One* **8**: e67107.

Coad, J., Al-Rasasi, B. and Morgan, J. (2002). Nutrient insult in early pregnancy. *Proceedings of the Nutrition Society* **61**: 51–59.

Cohain, J.S., Buxbaum, R.E., Mankuta, D. (2017). Spontaneous first trimester miscarriage rates per woman among parous women with 1 or more pregnancies of 24 weeks or more. *BMC Pregnancy and Childbirth* **17**: 437.

Cohen, J.M., Beddaoui, M., Kramer, M.S. *et al.* (2015). Maternal antioxidant levels in pregnancy and risk of preeclampsia and small for gestational age birth: a systematic review and meta-analysis. *PLoS One* **10**: e0135192.

Connor, W.E., Lowensohn, R. and Hatcher, L. (1996). Increased docosahexaenoic acid levels in human newborn infants by administration of sardines and fish oil during pregnancy. *Lipids* **31**: S183–S187.

Christoph, P., Challande, P., Raio, L. and Surbek, D. (2020). High prevalence of severe vitamin D deficiency during the first trimester in pregnant women in Switzerland and its potential contributions to adverse outcomes in the pregnancy. *Swiss Medical Weekly* **150**: w20238.

Czeizel, A.E. and Puhó, E. (2004). Association between severe nausea and vomiting in pregnancy and lower rate of preterm births. *Paediatric and Perinatal Epidemiology* **18**: 253–259.

Davenport, M.H., Steinback, C.D., Mottola, M.F. (2009). Impact of pregnancy and obesity on cardiorespiratory responses during weight-bearing exercise. *Respiratory Physiology and Neurobiology* **167**: 341–347.

de Araújo, C.A.L., Ray, J.G., Figueiroa, J.N. and Alves, J.G. (2020). BRAzil magnesium (BRAMAG) trial: a double-masked randomized clinical trial of oral magnesium supplementation in pregnancy. *BMC Pregnancy and Childbirth* **20**: 234.

Department of Health. (1999). *Dietary Reference Values for Energy and Nutrients for the United Kingdom*, London: Stationery Office.

Deputy, N.P., Dub, B., Sharma, A.J. (2018). Prevalence and trends in prepregnancy normal weight: 48 states, New York City, and District of Columbia, 2011–2015. *Morbidity and Mortality Weekly Reports* **66**: 1402–1407.

Dewey, K.G. and Oaks, B.M. (2017). U-shaped curve for risk associated with maternal hemoglobin, iron status, or iron supplementation. *American Journal of Clinical Nutrition* **106**(Suppl 6): 1694S–1702S.

Dodd, J.M., Turnbull, D.A., McPhee, A.J. *et al.* (2011). Limiting weight gain in overweight and obese women during pregnancy to improve health outcomes: the LIMIT randomised controlled trial. *BMC Pregnancy and Childbirth* **11**: 79.

Dodds, L., Fell, D.B., Joseph, K.S. *et al.* (2006). Outcomes of pregnancies complicated by hyperemesis gravidarum. *Obstetrics and Gynecology* **107**: 285–292.

Dodge, L.E., Missmer, S.A., Thornton, K.L. *et al.* (2017). Women's alcohol consumption and cumulative incidence of live birth following in vitro fertilization. *Journal of Assisted Reproduction and Genetics* **34**: 877–883.

Dodge, N.C., Jacobson, J.L. and Jacobson, S.W. (2019). Effects of fetal substance exposure on offspring substance use. *Pediatric Clinics of North America* **66**: 1149–1161.

Durnin, J.V. (1991). Energy requirements of pregnancy. *Diabetes* **40**(Suppl 2): 152–156.

Easey, K.E., Dyer, M.L., Timpson, N.J. *et al.* (2019). Prenatal alcohol exposure and offspring mental health: A systematic review. *Drug and Alcohol Dependency* **197**: 344–353.

Easey, K.E, Timpson, N.J., Munafò, M.R. (2020). Association of prenatal alcohol exposure and offspring depression: A negative control analysis of maternal and partner consumption. *Alcohol Clinical and Experimental Research* **44**: 1132–1140.

East Midlands Maternity Network. (2015). *Pregnant Women with a Raised BMI: Best practice standards of care*. Leicester: East Midlands Maternity Network.

Emmerson, A.J.B., Dockery, K.E., Mughal, M.Z. *et al.* (2018). Vitamin D status of White pregnant women and infants at birth and 4 months in North West England: A cohort study. *Maternal and Child Nutrition* **14**: e12453.

Farland, L.V., Rifas-Shiman, S.L. and Gillman, M.W. (2015). Early pregnancy cravings, dietary intake, and development of abnormal glucose tolerance. *Journal of the Academy of Nutrition and Dietetics* **115**: 1958–1964

Feodor Nilsson, S., Andersen, P.K. *et al.* (2014) Risk factors for miscarriage from a prevention perspective: a nationwide follow-up study. *BJOG* **121**: 1375–1384.

Ferrara, A., Hedderson, M.M., Brown, S.D. *et al.* (2020). A telehealth lifestyle intervention to reduce excess gestational weight gain in pregnant women with overweight or obesity (GLOW): a randomised, parallel-group, controlled trial. *Lancet Diabetes and Endocrinol.* **8**: 490–500.

Ferreira, R.C., Fragoso, M.B.T., Tenório, M.C.D.S *et al.* (2020). Biomarkers of placental redox imbalance in pregnancies with preeclampsia and consequent perinatal outcomes. *Archives of Biochemistry and Biophysics* **691**: 108464.

Flaxman, S.M. and Sherman, P.W. (2000). Morning sickness: a mechanism for protecting mother and embryo. *Quarterly Review of Biology* **75**: 113–148.

Flidel-Rimon, O., Rhea, D.J., Keith, L.G. *et al.* (2005). Early adequate maternal weight gain is associated with fewer small for gestational age triplets. *Journal of Perinatal Medicine* **33**: 379–382.

Foltran, F., Gregori, D., Franchin, L. *et al.* (2011). Effect of alcohol consumption in prenatal life, childhood, and adolescence on child development. *Nutrition Reviews* **69**: 642–659.

Forbes, L.E., Graham, J.E., Berglund, C. and Bell, R.C. (2018). Dietary change during pregnancy and women's reasons for change. *Nutrients* **10**: 1032.

Forczek, W. and Staszkiewicz, R. (2012). Changes of kinematic gait parameters due to pregnancy. *Acta Bioengineering and Biomechanics* **14**: 113–119.

Fowkes, F.J.I., Davidson, E., Agius, P.A. *et al.* (2019). Understanding the interactions between iron supplementation, infectious disease and adverse birth outcomes is essential to guide public health recommendations. *BMC Medicine* **17**: 153.

Fox, N.S., Rebarber, A., Roman, A.S., *et al.* (2010). Weight gain in twin pregnancies and adverse outcomes:

examining the 2009 Institute of Medicine guidelines. *Obstetrics and Gynecology* **116**: 100–106.

Frederiksen, L.E., Ernst, A., Brix, N. *et al.* (2018). Risk of adverse pregnancy outcomes at advanced maternal age. *Obstetrics and Gynecology* **131**: 457–463.

Furneaux, E.C., Langley-Evans, A.J. and Langley-Evans, S.C. (2001). Nausea and vomiting of pregnancy: endocrine basis and contribution to pregnancy outcome. *Obstetric and Gynecological Surveys* **56**: 775–782.

Gaskins, A.J., Rich-Edwards, J.W., Hauser, R. *et al.* (2014). Maternal prepregnancy folate intake and risk of spontaneous abortion and stillbirth. *Obstetrics and Gynecology* **124**: 23–31.

Gandhi, M., Gandhi, R., Mack, L.M. *et al.* (2018). Estimated energy requirements increase across pregnancy in healthy women with dichorionic twins. *American Journal of Clinical Nutrition* **108**: 775–783.

Goldstein, R.F., Abell, S.K., Ranasinha, S. *et al.* (2017). Association of gestational weight gain with maternal and infant outcomes: A systematic review and meta-analysis. *JAMA* **317**: 2207–2225.

Goodnight, W. and Newman, R. (2009). Optimal nutrition for improved twin pregnancy outcome. *Obstetrics and Gynecology* **114**: 1121–1134.

Hadden, D.R. (2008). Prediabetes and the big baby. *Diabetic Medicine* **25**: 1–10.

Hannigan, J.H. and Armant, D.R. (2005). Alcohol in pregnancy and neonatal outcome. *Seminars in Neonatology* **5**: 243–254.

Hill, A.J., Cairnduff, V. and McCance, D.R. (2016). Nutritional and clinical associations of food cravings in pregnancy. *Journal of Human Nutrition and Dietetics* **29**: 281–289.

Hinkle, S.N., Mumford, S.L., Grantz, K.L. *et al.* (2016). Association of nausea and vomiting during pregnancy with pregnancy loss: a secondary analysis of a randomized clinical trial. *JAMA Internal Medicine* **176**: 1621–1627.

Hofmeyr, G.J., Lawrie, T.A., Atallah, A.N. *et al.* (2018). Calcium supplementation during pregnancy for preventing hypertensive disorders and related problems. *Cochrane Database of Systematic Reviews* **2018**(10): CD001059.

Hofmeyr, G., Belizán, J. and von Dadelszen, P. (2014). Low-dose calcium supplementation for preventing preeclampsia: a systematic review and commentary. *BJOG* 8: 951–957.

Hussain, A., Claussen, B., Ramachandran, A. *et al.* (2007). Prevention of type 2 diabetes: a review. *Diabetes Research and Clinical Practice* **76**: 317–326.

Hytten, F.E. and Leitch, I. (1971). *The Physiology of Human Pregnancy*. Oxford: Blackwell.

Innis, S.M. (2005). Essential fatty acid transfer and fetal development. *Placenta* **26**(Suppl A): S70–S75.

Institute of Medicine. (2009). *Weight Gain During Pregnancy: Reexamining the Guidelines*. Washington, DC: National Academies Press.

International Weight Management in Pregnancy (i-WIP) Collaborative Group. (2017). Effect of diet and physical activity based interventions in pregnancy on gestational weight gain and pregnancy outcomes: meta-analysis of individual participant data from randomised trials *British Medical Journal* **358**: j3119.

Jackson, W.C. and Martin, J.P. (2000). Amylophagia presenting as gestational diabetes. *Archives of Family Medicine* **9**: 649–652.

Jaiswal, N., Melse-Boonstra, A., Sharma, S.K. *et al.* (2015). The iodized salt programme in Bangalore, India provides adequate iodine intakes in pregnant women and more-than-adequate iodine intakes in their children. *Public Health Nutrition* **18**: 403–413.

Javaid, M.K., Crozier, S.R., Harvey, N.C. *et al.* (2006). Maternal vitamin D status during pregnancy and childhood bone mass at age 9 years: a longitudinal study. *Lancet* **367**: 36–43.

Jeffcoat, M.K., Hauth, J.C., Geurs, N.C. *et al.* (2003). Periodontal disease and preterm birth: results of a pilot intervention study. *Journal of Periodontology* **74**: 1214–1218.

Jensen, D.M., Damm, P., Sørensen, B. *et al.* (2003). Pregnancy outcome and prepregnancy body mass index in 2459 glucose-tolerant Danish women. *American Journal of Obstetrics and Gynecology* **189**: 239–244.

Johansson, K., Hutcheon, J.A., Bodnar, L.M. *et al.* (2018). Pregnancy weight gain by gestational age and stillbirth: a population-based cohort study. *BJOG* **125**: 973–981.

Johnston, P.C., McCance, D.R., Holmes, V.A. *et al.* (2016). Placental antioxidant enzyme status and lipid peroxidation in pregnant women with type 1 diabetes: the effect of vitamin C and E supplementation. *Journal of Diabetes Complications* **30**: 109–114.

Karras, S.N., Koufakis, T., Antonopoulou, V. *et al.* (2020). Characterizing neonatal vitamin D deficiency in the modern era: A maternal-neonatal birth cohort from Southern Europe. *Journal of Steroid Biochemistry and Molecular Biology* **98**:105555.

Kawasaki, M., Arata, N., Miyazaki, C. *et al.* (2018). Obesity and abnormal glucose tolerance in offspring of diabetic mothers: a systematic review and meta-analysis. *PLoS One* **13**: e0190676.

Keats, E.C., Haider, B.A., Tam, E. *et al.* (2019). Multiple-micronutrient supplementation for women during pregnancy. *Cochrane Database of Systematic Reviews* **2019**(4): CD004905.

Kenny, L.C., Lavender, T., McNamee, R. *et al.* (2013). Advanced maternal age and adverse pregnancy outcome: evidence from a large contemporary cohort. *PLoS One* **8**: e56583.

Khalil, A., Syngelaki, A., Maiz, N. *et al.* (2013). Maternal age and adverse pregnancy outcome: a cohort study. *Ultrasound in Obstetrics and Gynecology* **42**: 634–643.

King, J.C. (2000). Physiology of pregnancy and nutrient metabolism. *American Journal of Clinical Nutrition* **71**: 1218S–1225S.

Koren, G., Madjunkova, S. and Maltepe, C. (2014). The protective effects of nausea and vomiting of pregnancy against adverse fetal outcome: a systematic review. *Reproductive Toxicology* **47C**: 77–80.

Kumar, A., Basra, M., Begum, N. *et al.* (2013). Association of maternal periodontal health with adverse pregnancy outcome. *Journal of Obstetric and Gynaecological Research* **39**: 40–45.

Kutalek, R., Wewalka, G., Gundacker, C. *et al.* (2010). Geophagy and potential health implications: geohelminths, microbes and heavy metals. *Transactions of the Royal Society of Tropical Medicine and Hygiene* **104**: 787–795.

Kvigne, V.L., Leonardson, G.R., Borzelleca, J. *et al.* (2008). Characteristics of grandmothers who have grandchildren with fetal alcohol syndrome or incomplete fetal alcohol syndrome. *Maternal and Child Health Journal* **12**: 760–765.

Landon, M.B., Rice, M.M., Varner, M.W. *et al.* (2015). Mild gestational diabetes mellitus and long-term child health. *Diabetes Care* **38**: 445–452.

Langley-Evans, A.J. and Langley-Evans, S.C. (2003). Relationship between maternal nutrient intakes in early and late pregnancy and infants weight and proportions at birth: prospective cohort study. *Journal of the Royal Society for the Promotion of Health* **123**: 210–216.

Lassi, Z.S., Mansoor, T., Salam, R.A. *et al.* (2017). Review of nutrition guidelines relevant for adolescents in low- and middle-income countries. *Annals of the New York Academy of Science* **1393**: 51–60.

Lazarus, J.H. (2020). Iodine deficiency in Israeli pregnant women: a time for action. *Israeli Journal of Health Policy Research* **9**: 20.

Lewandowska, M., Więckowska, B., Sajdak, S. *et al.* (2020). First trimester microelements and their relationships with pregnancy outcomes and complications. *Nutrients* **12**: 1108.

Li, H., Ma, J., Huang, R. *et al.* (2020). Prevalence of vitamin D deficiency in the pregnant women: an observational study in Shanghai, China. *Archives of Public Health* **78**: 31.

López, L.B., Langini, S.H. and Pita dePortela, M.L. (2007). Maternal iron status and neonatal outcomes in women with pica during pregnancy. *International Journal of Gynaecology and Obstetrics* **98**: 151–152.

López, N.J., Smith, P.C. and Gutierrez, J. (2002). Periodontal therapy may reduce the risk of preterm low birth weight in women with periodontal disease: a randomized controlled trial. *Journal of Periodontology* **73**: 911–924.

Lowe, W.L., Scholtens, D.M., Lowe, L.P. *et al.* (2018). Association of gestational diabetes with maternal disorders of glucose metabolism and childhood adiposity. *JAMA* **320**: 1005–1016.

Luke, B. (2005). Nutrition and multiple gestation. *Seminars in Perinatology* **29**: 349–354.

May, L., Suminski, R., Berry, A. *et al.* (2014). Diet and pregnancy: health-care providers and patient behaviors. *Journal of Perinatal Education* **23**: 50–56.

McGiveron, A., Foster, S., Pearce, J. *et al.* (2015) .Limiting antenatal weight gain improves maternal health outcomes in severely obese pregnant women: findings of a pragmatic evaluation of a midwife-led intervention. *Journal of Human Nutrition and Dietetics* **28**(Suppl 1): 29–37.

McGowan, C.A., Walsh, J.M., Byrne, J. *et al.* (2013). The influence of a low glycemic index dietary intervention on maternal dietary intake, glycemic index and gestational weight gain during pregnancy: a randomized controlled trial. *Nutrition Journal* **12**: 140.

McMullan, P., Hunter, A., McCance, D. *et al.* (2019). Knowledge about iodine requirements during pregnancy and breastfeeding among pregnant women living in Northern Ireland. *BMC Nutrition* **5**: 24.

Mead, E.A. and Sarkar, D.K. (2014). Fetal alcohol spectrum disorders and their transmission through genetic and epigenetic mechanisms. *Frontiers in Genetics* **5**: 154.

Meher, A., Randhir, K., Mehendale, S. *et al.* (2016). Maternal fatty acids and their association with birth outcome: a prospective study. *PloS One* **11**: e0147359.

Merlino, A., Laffineuse, L., Collin, M. *et al.* (2006). Impact of weight loss between pregnancies on recurrent preterm birth. *American Journal of Obstetrics and Gynecology* **195**: 818–821.

Mikkelsen, T.B., Andersen, A.M. and Olsen, S.F. (2006). Pica in pregnancy in a privileged population: myth or reality. *Acta Obstetrica et Gynecologica Scandinavica* **85**: 1265–1266.

Middleton, P., Gomersall, J.C., Gould, J.F. *et al.* (2018). Omega-3 fatty acid addition during pregnancy. *Cochrane Database of Systematic Reviews* (11): CD003402.

Mills, H.L., Patel, N., White, S.L. *et al.* (2019). The effect of a lifestyle intervention in obese pregnant women on gestational metabolic profiles: findings from the UK Pregnancies Better Eating and Activity Trial (UPBEAT) randomised controlled trial. *BMC Medicine* **17**: 15.

Millward, D.J. (1999). Optimal intakes of protein in the human diet. *Proceedings of the Nutrition Society* **58**: 403–413.

Mitsuda, N., Eitoku, M., Yamasaki, K. *et al.* (2018). Nausea and vomiting during pregnancy associated with lower incidence of preterm births: the Japan Environment and Children's Study (JECS). *BMC Pregnancy and Childbirth* **18**: 268.

Modzelewska, D., Bellocco, R., Elfvin, A. *et al.* (2019). Caffeine exposure during pregnancy, small for gestational age birth and neonatal outcome: results from the Norwegian Mother and Child Cohort Study. *BMC Pregnancy and Childbirth* **19**: 80.

Momino, W., Félix, T.M., Abeche, A.M. *et al.* (2012). Maternal drinking behavior and fetal alcohol spectrum disorders in adolescents with criminal behavior in southern Brazil. *Genetics and Molecular Biology* **35**(4 Suppl): 960–965.

Morgan, K.L., Rahman, M.A., Hill, R.A. *et al.* (2014). Physical activity and excess weight in pregnancy have independent and unique effects on delivery and perinatal outcomes. *PLoS One* **9**: e94532.

Most, J., Dervis, S., Haman, F. *et al.* (2019). Energy intake requirements in pregnancy. *Nutrients* **11**: 1812.

Mukherjee, R.A., Hollins, S. and Turk, J. (2006). Fetal alcohol spectrum disorder: an overview. *Journal of the Royal Society of Medicine* **99**: 298–302.

National Institute for Health and Care Excellence. (2010). *Weight Management Before, During and After Pregnancy*. Public Health Guidance PH27. London: NICE.

Netelenbos, N., Sanders, J.L., Ofori Dei, S. *et al.* (2020). A case for early screening: prenatal alcohol risk exposure predicts risk for early childhood communication delays. *Journal of Development Behavior and Pediatrics* **41**: 559–564.

Ng, S.W., Norwitz, S.G. and Norwitz, E.R. (2019). The impact of iron overload and ferroptosis on reproductive disorders in humans: Implications for preeclampsia. *International Journal of Molecular Science* **20**: 3283.

Nohr, E.A., Bech, B.H., Vaeth, M. *et al.* (2007). Obesity, gestational weight gain and preterm birth: a study within the Danish National Birth Cohort. *Paediatric and Perinatal Epidemiology* **21**: 5–14.

Nohr, E.A., Olsen, J., Bech, B.H. *et al.* (2014). Periconceptional intake of vitamins and fetal death: a cohort study on multivitamins and folate. *International Journal of Epidemiology* **43**: 174–184.

Nomura, Y., Marks, D.J., Grossman, B. *et al.* (2012). Exposure to gestational diabetes mellitus and low socio-economic status: effects on neurocognitive development and risk of attention-deficit/hyperactivity disorder in offspring. *Archives of Pediatric and Adolescent Medicine* **166**: 337–343.

Odutayo, A., Hladunewich, M. (2012). Obstetric nephrology: renal hemodynamic and metabolic physiology in normal pregnancy. *Clinical Journal of the American Society of Nephrologists* **7**: 2073–2080.

O'Dwyer, V., O'Kelly, S., Monaghan, B. *et al.* (2013). Maternal obesity and induction of labor. *Acta Obstetrica et Gynecologica Scandinavica* **92**: 1414–1418.

Okubo, H., Miyake, Y., Tanaka, K. *et al.* (2015). Maternal total caffeine intake, mainly from Japanese and Chinese tea, during pregnancy was associated with risk of preterm birth: the Osaka Maternal and Child Health Study. *Nutrition Reseach* **35**: 309–316.

Ollero, M.D., Martínez, J.P., Pineda, J. *et al.* (2020). Change over time in the iodine nutritional status of pregnant women from the Pamplona healthcare region. *Endocrinology Diabetes and Nutrition* **67**: 643–649.

Orloff, N.C. and Hormes, J.M. (2014). Pickles and ice cream! Food cravings in pregnancy: hypotheses, preliminary evidence, and directions for future research. *Frontiers in Psychology* **5**: 1076.

Orloff, N.C., Flammer, A., Hartnett, J. *et al.* (2016). Food cravings in pregnancy: preliminary evidence for a role in excess gestational weight gain. *Appetite* **105**: 259–265.

Ota, E., Hori, H., Mori, R. *et al.* (2015). Energy and protein intake in pregnancy. *Cochrane Database of Systematic Reviews* **2015**(6): CD000032.

Owens, L.A., Avalos, G., Kirwan, B. *et al.* (2012). Changing clinical practice can improve clinical outcomes for women with pre-gestational diabetes mellitus. *Irish Medical Journal* **105**(Suppl): 9–11.

Owens, L.A., Sedar, J., Carmody, L. and Dunne, F. (2015). Comparing type 1 and type 2 diabetes in pregnancy: similar conditions or is a separate approach required? *BMC Pregnancy and Childbirth* **15**: 69.

Pan, Y., Zhang ,S., Wang, Q. *et al.* (2016). Investigating the association between prepregnancy body mass index and adverse pregnancy outcomes: a large cohort study of 536 098 Chinese pregnant women in rural China. *BMJ Open* **6**: e011227.

Parviainen, R., Auvinen, J., Serlo, W. *et al.* (2020). Maternal alcohol consumption during pregnancy associates with bone fractures in early childhood: a birth-cohort study of 6718 participants *Bone* **137**: 115462.

Patra, J., Bakker, R., Irving, H. *et al.* (2011). Dose-response relationship between alcohol consumption before and during pregnancy and the risks of low birthweight, preterm birth and small for gestational age (SGA): a systematic review and meta-analyses. *BJOG* **118**: 1411–1421.

Peacock, A., Hutchinson, D., Wilson, J. *et al.* (2018). Adherence to the caffeine intake guideline during pregnancy and birth outcomes: A prospective cohort study. *Nutrients* **10**: 319.

Pereira, K.N., Knoppka, C.K. and da Silva, J.E. (2014). Association between uric acid and severity of pre-eclampsia. *Clinical Laboratory* **60**(2): 309–314.

Pereira-da-Silva, L., Cabo, C., Moreira, A.C. *et al.* (2015). The effect of long-chain polyunsaturated fatty acids intake during pregnancy on adiposity of healthy full-term offspring at birth. *Journal of Perinatology* **35**: 177–180.

Pickens, C.M., Hogue, C.J., Howards, P.P. *et al.* (2019). The association between gestational weight gain z-score and stillbirth: a case-control study. *BMC Pregnancy and Childbirth* **19**: 451.

Pinto, T.J., Farias, D.R., Rebelo, F. *et al.* (2015). Lower inter-partum interval and unhealthy life-style factors are inversely associated with n-3 essential fatty acids changes during pregnancy: a prospective cohort with Brazilian women. *PLoS One* **10**: e0121151.

Pitiphat, W., Joshipura, K.J., Gillman, M.W. *et al.* (2008). Maternal periodontitis and adverse pregnancy outcomes. *Community Dentistry and Oral Epidemiology* **36**: 3–11.

Placek, C.D., Madhivanan, P., Hagen, E.H. (2017). Innate food aversions and culturally transmitted food taboos in pregnant women in rural southwest India: separate systems to protect the fetus? *Evolution of Human Behaviour* **38**: 714–728.

Poston, L. (2006). Endothelial dysfunction in pre-eclampsia. *Pharmacological Reports* **58**(Suppl): 69–74.

Poston, L., Briley, A.L., Seed, P.T. *et al.* (2006). Vitamins in Preeclampsia (VIP) Trial Consortium. Vitamin C and vitamin E in pregnant women at risk for pre-eclampsia (VIP trial): randomised placebo-controlled trial. *Lancet* **367**: 1145–1154.

Poston, L., Igosheva, N., Mistry, H.D. *et al.* (2011). Role of oxidative stress and antioxidant supplementation in pregnancy disorders. *American Journal of Clinical Nutrition* **94**(6 Suppl): 1980S–1985S.

Poston, L., Bell, R., Croker, H., *et al.* (2015). Effect of a behavioural intervention in obese pregnant women (the UPBEAT study): a multicentre, randomised controlled trial. *Lancet Diabetes and Endocrinology* **3**: 767–777.

Prentice, A.M. and Goldberg, G.R. (2000). Energy adaptations in human pregnancy: limits and long-term consequences. *American Journal of Clinical Nutrition* **71**: 1226S–1232S.

Rainville, A.J. (1998). Pica practices of pregnant women are associated with lower maternal hemoglobin level at delivery. *Journal of the American Dietetic Association* **98**: 293–296.

Rao, A.K., Cheng, Y.W. and Caughey, A.B. (2004). Perinatal complications among different Asian-American subgroups. *American Journal of Obstetrics and Gynecology* **194**: e39–41.

Rasmussen, M.A., Maslova, E., Halldorsson, T.I. *et al.* (2014). Characterization of dietary patterns in the Danish national birth cohort in relation to preterm birth. *PLoS One* **9**: e93644.

Reader, D.M. (2007). Medical nutrition therapy and lifestyle interventions. *Diabetes Care* **30**(Suppl 2): S188–S193.

Rhee, J., Kim, R., Kim, Y. *et al.* (2015). Maternal caffeine consumption during pregnancy and risk of low birth weight: A dose-response meta-analysis of observational studies. *PLoS One* **10**: e0132334.

Ringholm, L., Mathiesen, E.R., Kelstrup, L. *et al.* (2012). Managing type 1 diabetes mellitus in pregnancy: from planning to breastfeeding. *Nature Reviews in Endocrinology* **8**: 659–667.

Ritchie, L.D., Whaley, S.E., Spector, P. *et al.* (2010). Favorable impact of nutrition education on California

WIC families. *Journal of Nutrition Education and Behaviour* **42**: S2–S10.

Roberts, J.M. and Gammill, H.S. (2005). Preeclampsia: recent insights. *Hypertension* **46**: 1243–1249.

Roberts, J.M., Balk, J.L., Bodnar, L.M. *et al.* (2003). Nutrient involvement in preeclampsia. *Journal of Nutrition* **133**: 1684S–1692S.

Roberts, J.M., Bodnar, L.M., Lain, K.Y. *et al.* (2005). Uric acid is as important as proteinuria in identifying fetal risk in women with gestational hypertension. *Hypertension* **46**: 1263–1269.

Roselló-Soberón, M.E., Fuentes-Chaparro, L. and Casanueva, E. (2005). Twin pregnancies: eating for three? Maternal nutrition update. *Nutrition Reviews* **63**: 295–302.

Rumbold, A., Ota, E., Hori, H. *et al.* (2015). Vitamin E supplementation in pregnancy. *Cochrane Database of Systematic Reviews* **2015**(9): CD004069.

Sablok, A., Batra, A., Thariani, K. *et al.* (2015). Supplementation of vitamin D in pregnancy and its correlation with feto-maternal outcome. *Clinical Endocrinology* **83**: 536–541.

Sanders, T.A. (1999). Essential fatty acid requirements of vegetarians in pregnancy, lactation, and infancy. *American Journal of Clinical Nutrition* **70**: 555S–559S.

Santos, K.D., Patrício, P.T., Lima, T.S.V. *et al.* (2019). A pilot intervention to reduce postpartum weight retention at primary health care in Brazil. *Nutrition and Hospital* **36**: 854–861.

Sanz, M. and Kornman, K. (2013). Periodontitis and adverse pregnancy outcomes: consensus report of the Joint EFP/AAP Workshop on Periodontitis and Systemic Diseases. *Journal of Periodontology* **84**(4 Suppl): S164–S169.

Sapra, K.J., Buck Louis, G.M., Sundaram, R. *et al.* (2018). Time-varying effects of signs and symptoms on pregnancy loss <20 weeks: Findings from a preconception prospective cohort study. *Paediatric and Perinatal Epidemiology* **32**: 30–39.

Scholl, T.O. (2005). Iron status during pregnancy: setting the stage for mother and infant. *American Journal of Clinical Nutrition* **81**: 1218S–1222S.

Scholl, T.O. and Reilly, T. (2000). Anemia, iron and pregnancy outcome. *Journal of Nutrition* **130**: 443S–447S.

Schummers, L., Hutcheon, J.A., Hernandez-Diaz, S. *et al.* (2018). Association of short interpregnancy interval with pregnancy outcomes according to maternal age. *JAMA Internal Medicine* **178**: 1661–1670.

Sculley, D.V. and Langley-Evans, S.C. (2003). Periodontal disease is associated with lower antioxidant capacity in whole saliva and evidence of increased protein oxidation. *Clinical Science* **105**: 167–172.

Sebire, N.J., Jolly, M., Harris, J. *et al.* (2001). Is maternal underweight really a risk factor for adverse pregnancy outcome? A population-based study in London. *BJOG* **108**: 61–66.

Sgolastra, F., Petrucci, A., Severino, M. *et al.* (2013). Relationship between periodontitis and pre-eclampsia: a meta-analysis. *PLoS One* **8**: e71387.

Shirazian, T., Monteith, S., Friedman, F. *et al.* (2010). Lifestyle modification program decreases pregnancy weight gain in obese women. *American Journal of Perinatology* **27**(5): 411–414.

Shuffrey, L.C., Myers, M.M., Isler, J.R. *et al.* (2020). Association between prenatal exposure to alcohol and tobacco and neonatal brain activity: results from the Safe Passage Study. *JAMA Network Open* **3**: e204714.

Silverman, B.L., Metzger, B.E., Cho, N.H. *et al.* (1995). Impaired glucose tolerance in adolescent offspring of diabetic mothers: relationship to fetal hyperinsulinism. *Diabetes Care* **18**: 611–617.

Smith, C., Teng, F., Branch, E. *et al.* (2019). Maternal and perinatal morbidity and mortality associated with anemia in pregnancy. *Obstetrics and Gynecology* **134**: 1234–1244.

Sommer, C., Mørkrid, K., Jenum, A.K. *et al.* (2014). Weight gain, total fat gain and regional fat gain during pregnancy and the association with gestational diabetes: a population-based cohort study. *International Journal of Obesity* **38**: 76–81.

Spary-Kainz, U., Semlitsch, T., Rundel, S. *et al.* (2019). How many women take oral supplementation in pregnancy in Austria? Who recommended it? A cross-sectional study. *Wiener klinische Wochenschrift* **131**: 462–467.

Spohr, H.L., Willms, J. and Steinhausen, H.C. (2007). Fetal alcohol spectrum disorders in young adulthood. *Journal of Pediatrics* **150**: 175–179.

Steinmetz, A.R., Abrams, E.T., Young, S.L. (2012). Patterns of nausea, vomiting, aversions, and cravings during pregnancy on Pemba Island, Zanzibar, Tanzania. *Ecology Food and Nutrition* **51**: 418–430.

Stokes, T. (2006). The earth eaters. *Nature* **444**: 543–544.

Stråvik, M., Jonsson, K., Hartvigsson, O. *et al.* (2019). Food and nutrient intake during pregnancy in relation to maternal characteristics: results from the NICE birth cohort in Northern Sweden. *Nutrients* **11**: 1680.

Su, X.J., Huang, S.J., Li, X. *et al.* (2020). Prepregnancy overweight and obesity are associated with an increased risk of preterm birth in Chinese Women. *Obesity Facts* **13**: 237–244.

Swift *et al.* (2017)

Symington, E.A., Baumgartner, J., Malan, L. *et al.* (2019). Maternal iron-deficiency is associated with premature birth and higher birth weight despite routine antenatal iron supplementation in an urban South African setting: the NuPED prospective study. *PLoS One* **14**: e0221299.

Tan, P.C., Jacob, R., Quek, K.F. *et al.* (2007). Pregnancy outcome in hyperemesis gravidarum and the effect of laboratory clinical indicators of hyperemesis severity. *Journal of Obstetrics and Gynaecology Research* **33**: 457–464.

Thihalolipavan, S., Candalla, B.M. and Ehrlich, J. (2013). Examining pica in NYC pregnant women with elevated blood lead levels. *Maternal and Child Health Journal* **17**: 49–55.

Trofimiuk-Müldner, M., Konopka, J., Sokołowski, G. *et al.* (2020). Current iodine nutrition status in Poland (2017): is the Polish model of obligatory iodine prophylaxis able to eliminate iodine deficiency in the population? *Public Health Nutrition* **23**: 2467–2477.

Trogstad, L.I., Stoltenberg, C., Magnus, P. *et al.* (2005). Recurrence risk in hyperemesis gravidarum. *BJOG* **112**: 1641–1645.

Umer, A., Lilly, C., Hamilton, C. *et al.* (2020). Prevalence of alcohol use in late pregnancy. *Pediatric Research* **88**: 312–319.

Vandraas, K.F., Vikanes, A.V., Vangen, S. *et al.* (2013). Hyperemesis gravidarum and birth outcomes-a population-based cohort study of 2.2 million births in the Norwegian Birth Registry. *BJOG* **120**: 1654–1660.

Verberg, M.F., Gillott, D.J., Al-Fardan, N. *et al.* (2005). Hyperemesis gravidarum, a literature review. *Human Reproduction Update* **11**: 527–539.

Vikanes, Å.V., Støer, N.C., Magnus, P. *et al.* (2013). Hyperemesis gravidarum and pregnancy outcomes in the Norwegian Mother and Child Cohort: a cohort study. *BMC Pregnancy and Childbirth* **13**: 169.

Villar, J., Purwar, M., Merialdi, M. *et al.* (2009). World Health Organization multicentre randomised trial of supplementation with vitamins C and E among pregnant women at high risk for pre-eclampsia in populations of low nutritional status from developing countries. *BJOG* **116**: 780–788.

Vinding, R.K., Stokholm, J., Sevelsted, A. *et al.* (2019). Fish oil supplementation in pregnancy increases gestational age, size for gestational age, and birth weight in infants: a randomized controlled trial. *Journal of Nutrition* **149**: 628–634.

von Dadelszen, P., Firoz, T., Donnay, F. *et al.* (2012). Preeclampsia in low and middle income countries-health services lessons learned from the PRE-EMPT (PRE-eclampsia-eclampsia monitoring, prevention and treatment) project. *Journal of Obstetrics and Gynaecology Canada* **34**: 917–926.

van Wijngaarden, E., Harrington, D., Kobrosly, R. *et al.* (2014). Prenatal exposure to methylmercury and LCPUFA in relation to birth weight. *Annals of Epidemiology* **24**: 273–278.

Wainwright, P.E. (2002). Dietary essential fatty acids and brain function: a developmental perspective on mechanisms. *Proceedings of the Nutrition Society* **61**: 61–69.

Walsh, S.W. (2007). Obesity: a risk factor for preeclampsia. *Trends in Endocrinology and Metabolism* **18**: 365–370.

Wei, S.Q., Qi, H.P., Luo, Z.C. *et al.* (2013). Maternal vitamin D status and adverse pregnancy outcomes: a systematic review and meta-analysis. *Journal of Maternal Fetal and Neonatal Medicine* **26**: 889–899.

Weigel, M.M., Coe, K., Castro, N.P. *et al.* (2011). Food aversions and cravings during early pregnancy: association with nausea and vomiting. *Ecology of Food and Nutrition* **50**: 197–214.

Weile, L.K.K., Hegaard, H.K., Wu, C. *et al.* (2020). Alcohol intake in early pregnancy and spontaneous preterm birth: a cohort study. *Alcohol Clinical and Experimental Research* **44**: 511–521.

Weissgerber, T.L., Gandley, R.E., Roberts, J.M. *et al.* (2013). Haptoglobin phenotype, pre-eclampsia, and response to supplementation with vitamins C and E in pregnant women with type-1 diabetes. *BJOG* **120**: 1192–1199.

Whitaker, K.M., Baruth, M., Schlaff, R.A. *et al.* (2019). Provider advice on physical activity and nutrition in twin pregnancies: a cross-sectional electronic survey. *BMC Pregnancy and Childbirth* **19**: 418.

Whittaker, P.G., Lind, T. and Williams, J.G. (1991). Iron absorption during normal human pregnancy: a study using stable isotopes. *British Journal of Nutrition* **65**: 457–463.

Wilkinson, S.A. and McIntyre, H.D. (2012). Evaluation of the 'healthy start to pregnancy' early antenatal health promotion workshop: a randomized controlled trial. *BMC Pregnancy and Childbirth* **12**: 131.

Wilkinson, S.A., van der Pligt, P., Gibbons, K.S. *et al.* (2015). Trial for reducing weight retention in New Mums: a randomised controlled trial evaluating a low intensity, postpartum weight management programme. *Journal of Human Nutrition and Dietetics* **28**(Suppl 1): 15–28.

Williams, P.J. and Broughton Pipkin, F. (2011). The genetics of pre-eclampsia and other hypertensive disorders of pregnancy. *Best Practice in Research in Clinical Obstetrics and Gynaecology* **25**: 405–417.

Woon, F.C., Chin, Y.S., Ismail, I.H. *et al.* (2019). Vitamin D deficiency during pregnancy and its associated factors among third trimester Malaysian pregnant women. *PLoS One* **14**: e0216439.

Workicho, A., Belachew, T., Argaw, A. *et al.* (2020). Maternal nutritional status mediates the association between maternal age and birth outcomes. *Maternal and Child Nutrition* **16**: e13015.

World Health Organization. (2018). WHO recommendation: calcium supplementation during pregnancy for prevention of pre-eclampsia and its complications. Geneva: World Health Organization. https://apps.who.int/iris/handle/10665/277235 (accessed 3 April 2021).

Wu, Y., Xiong, X., Fraser, W.D. *et al.* (2012). Association of uric acid with progression to preeclampsia and development of adverse conditions in gestational hypertensive pregnancies. *American Journal of Hypertension* **25**: 711–717.

Xu, N. and Zhang, W. (2020). PTX3 Gene 3'UTR polymorphism and its interaction with environmental factors are correlated with the risk of preeclampsia in a Chinese Han population. *Medicine (Baltimore)* **99**: e18740.

Yao, R., Park, B.Y., Foster, S.E. *et al.* (2017). The association between gestational weight gain and risk of stillbirth: a population-based cohort study *Annals of Epidemiology* **27**: 638–644.

Yao, R., Schuh, B.L., Caughey, A.B. (2019). The risk of perinatal mortality with each week of expectant management in obese pregnancies. *Journal of Maternal Fetal and Neonatal Medicine* **32**: 434–441.

Yeh, J. and Shelton, J.A. (2007). Association of pre-pregnancy maternal body mass and maternal weight gain to newborn outcomes in twin pregnancies. *Acta Obstetrica et Gynecologica Scandinavica* **86**: 1051–1057.

Yifu, P., Lei, Y., Yujin, G. *et al.* (2020). Shortened postpartum magnesium sulfate treatment vs traditional 24h for severe preeclampsia: a systematic review and meta-analysis of randomized trials. *Hypertension in Pregnancy* **39**: 186–195.

Young, S.L., Goodman, D., Farag, T.H. *et al.* (2007). Geophagia is not associated with Trichuris or hookworm transmission in Zanzibar, Tanzania. *Transactions of the Royal Society of Tropical Medicine* **101**: 766–772.

Yu, C.K.H., Teoh, T.G. and Robinson, S. (2006). Obesity in pregnancy. *BJOG* **113**: 1117–1125.

Zeng, S., Cheng, X., Chen, R. *et al.* (2020) Low level of vitamin D is a risk factor for the occurrence of early and late onset pre-eclampsia in pregnant women. *Clinical Laboratory* **66**: 10.7754

Zhang, B., Shang, S., Li, S. *et al.* (2020). Maternal folic acid supplementation and more prominent birth weight gain in twin birth compared with singleton birth: a cross-sectional study in northwest China. *Public Health Nutrition* **23**: 2973–2982.

Zhao, L., Li, X., Liu, G. *et al.* (2019). The association of maternal diabetes with attention deficit and hyperactivity disorder in offspring: a meta-analysis. *Neuropsychiatric Disease and Treatment* **15**: 675–684.

Zhou, J., Zhao, X., Wang, Z. *et al.* (2012). Combination of lipids and uric acid in mid-second trimester can be used to predict adverse pregnancy outcomes. *Journal of Maternal Fetal and Neonatal Medicine* **25**: 2633–2638.

Additional reading

If you would like to find out more about the material discussed in this chapter, the following sources may be of interest.

Lammi-Keefe, C.J., Couch, S.C. and Kirwan, JP. (eds) (2019). *Handbook of Nutrition and Pregnancy*. Totowa, NJ: Humana Press.

Vinciguerra, M. and Cordero Sanchez, P. (eds) (2020). *Molecular Nutrition: Mother and Infant*. Cambridge, MA: Academic Press.

CHAPTER 4

Fetal nutrition and disease in later life

LEARNING OBJECTIVES

This chapter will enable the reader to:
- Understand the adaptive nature of fetal development and the capacity of the fetal organs and tissues to respond to changes in the maternal environment.
- Define what is meant by the terms fetal or nutritional programming and outline the basis of the developmental origins of health and disease hypothesis.
- Describe the association between risk factors operating in fetal life and disease during adulthood.
- Discuss the epidemiological evidence that suggests that maternal nutrition during pregnancy may programme the risk of major disease later in life.
- Demonstrate an awareness of the limitations of epidemiology as a tool for exploring nutritional programming of disease.
- Give an overview of the evidence obtained from experimental models that shows the biological plausibility of the nutritional programming concept.
- Discuss the candidate mechanisms that have been proposed to explain how maternal undernutrition might programme disease in the developing fetus.
- Show an awareness of the epigenetic mechanisms through which gene expression is regulated and describe how these processes might define the functions of cells, tissues and organs.
- Discuss the ways in which variation in the individual response to food arises beyond the genetic level.
- Discuss the potential application of understanding of nutritional programming in designing future public health interventions or personalized nutrition strategies to prevent coronary heart disease, obesity and type 2 diabetes.

4.1 Introduction

Chapter 3 outlined the importance of nutrition during pregnancy from the perspective of maintaining the health of the pregnant woman and ensuring the safe delivery of her infant. It is now clear that nutrition during pregnancy is also important in determining the long-term health and wellbeing of the developing fetus. This concept lies at the core of the idea that health and disease and the individual response to food at all stages of life are the product of cumulative experiences across the lifespan. This chapter focuses on the evidence that under- or overnutrition in early life can exert powerful effects, termed 'programming', on the development of organs and systems, and that these programming effects are an important risk factor for disease. The chapter reviews some of the proposed mechanisms that link nutrition during fetal life to diseases such as coronary heart disease and diabetes in the older adult.

4.2 The developmental origins of adult disease

4.2.1 The concept of programming

The term programming describes the process through which exposure to environmental stimuli or insults during critical phases of development brings about permanent changes to the physiology or metabolism of the organism. A dramatic example of programming at work is provided by the mechanisms that determine sex in crocodilians. Alligators and crocodiles lack sex chromosomes. Their eggs are laid into heaped mounds within which exists a temperature gradient. At most temperatures within the nest, the embryos will develop into females, while within a very specific range of 2–3°C, the embryos are programmed to become males (Figure 4.1). These effects are seen because the temperature of the egg determines the expression of genes responsible for the synthesis of the sex steroids, which then govern the physiological development of these reptiles.

Nutrition, Health and Disease: A Lifespan Approach, Third Edition. Simon Langley-Evans.
© 2021 John Wiley & Sons Ltd. Published 2021 by John Wiley & Sons Ltd.
Companion website: www.wiley.com/go/langleyevans/lifespan3e

This is clearly a programming response under the definition provided earlier, since the stimulus is temperature, the critical phase of development lies within the embryonic period and the effect of the exposure is permanent.

Within mammalian systems, programming is a feature of the plasticity of cell lines during embryonic

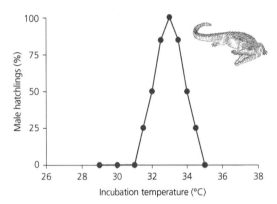

Figure 4.1 While genetics sets the basis for organisms to develop, cellular plasticity allows development to respond to environmental factors. In alligators and crocodiles, this extends to environmental determination of something as critical as biological sex. The temperature at which eggs are incubated governs the activity of enzymes that set the hormonal scenario in which the embryo develops. Males develop only within a narrow range of incubation temperatures.

and fetal life. Plasticity refers to the ability of cells and tissues to adapt their differentiation and maturation programmes in response to their current environment. In some types of cell, this adaptive capacity remains present throughout life but in most cases is a feature of the embryonic and fetal stages. The developing organism has populations of progenitor cells that have the capacity to differentiate into mature cell types (Figure 4.2). Progenitors can only develop into target cells related to their particular lineage and may remain present in adult tissues to enable tissue repair. In contrast, stem cells are able to either replicate themselves or develop into a range of different cell types in response to growth factor or cytokine signals. Their plasticity enables them to form variable cell types in response to the prevailing environment. Embryonic stem cells are termed pluripotent as their plasticity confers the capacity to differentiate into any cell type. These cells are present only in embryonic and fetal life. These are the critical developmental phases that are of greatest interest in the context of nutrition and human health and disease.

The capacity to programme mammalian systems through early life stimuli can be demonstrated just as dramatically as the example of temperature-dependent sex determination in reptiles. Treatment of newborn female rats with testosterone in the first few days of life impacts upon their lifelong reproductive function. Regions of the hypothalamus that

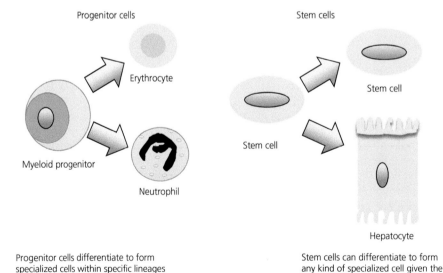

Figure 4.2 Progenitor cells and stem cells have the property of plasticity whereby growth factor or cytokine signals can trigger a differentiation response or cell division. The fates of progenitor cells are limited to specific lineages of cells within a tissue or system, but embryonic stem cells are pluripotent and, in response to cues during development, can give rise to any cell type.

control the reproductive axis and archetypal female reproductive behaviours are remodelled to resemble the male brain and the female rats are rendered sterile (Arai and Gorski, 1968). The critical period in which this androgenizing treatment is effective is relatively short but the effects are permanent.

There is also evidence that programming by the environment is a normal feature of human physiology. The Japanese military made the discovery during the Second World War that the number of sweat glands in humans is set soon after birth and cannot then be further adjusted. Individuals born in cooler climates activate a smaller number of sweat glands than individuals born in warmer climates. Thus, the response to the prevailing environment during the early postnatal period brings about permanent changes to physiology that allow the individual born in a warm climate to be optimally adapted for life in that climate. The individual from a cold climate will cope less well with the heat.

4.2.2 Fetal programming and human disease

4.2.2.1 Fetal growth

The capacity of the developing mammal to respond to environmental cues or physiological insults in the manner described earlier suggests something profound and unexpected about the nature of development. For decades, we have believed that development is essentially a gene-led process and that activation and switching off of the expression of genes, in well-ordered sequences, brings about the normal growth and development of organisms, from the fertilized egg to the adult offspring. The concepts of developmental plasticity and programming would suggest that the environment can change the profile of genes that are expressed at any given stage of development and, in the case of adult stem cells, throughout life. In other words, the genes do not necessarily lead the process of development and instead can follow the signals from the environment (which in mammals is the mother) that indicate the availability of nutrients, the presence of stressors and the need to adapt accordingly.

The impact of the environment on apparently genetically determined processes could be simply observed by looking at the effects of maternal factors upon fetal growth. The growth trajectory of a fetus is determined by the genes inherited from both the mother and the father, but evolution has provided mechanisms through which the genetically determined growth rate can be constrained. Classic experiments using embryo transfers in horses and cattle show that the size of the mother is a primary factor governing fetal growth. The Shetland pony is a small breed of horse, standing at no more than 10 hands (around 107 cm), while the Shire horse stands at an impressive 18 hands (180 cm). The foals of each of these horses are of a size commensurate with their breed. When Shetland mares carry the foals resulting from Shire horse–Shetland pony crosses, the genetically large offspring are born at a size similar to the pure Shetland. This form of constraint is in the interest of maternal survival, as carrying a fetus that will become too large to pass through the birth canal is likely to prove fatal to mother and offspring.

Constraint of growth also occurs in response to other characteristics of mothers. A whole range of factors that signal underprivilege or other indicators of a less than optimal environment are associated with lower weights at birth among human babies. One of the strongest predictors of the weight of a baby at birth is the socioeconomic class of the mother. In a study of 300 pregnant women from Northampton (Figure 4.3), average weights at birth were 400 g lower in babies of women from social class V (unemployed) than in babies of women from social class I (professionals; Langley-Evans and Langley-Evans, 2003). Social class is a crude indicator of many different factors including family income, nutritional status, access to healthcare services, smoking and other health behaviours. Several of these factors are known to influence fetal growth in their own right. Maternal smoking during pregnancy, for example, restricts fetal growth and increases risk of low birth weight and premature birth. The same risks are associated with maternal infection and severe maternal distress during pregnancy. Smits *et al.* (2006) studied 1885 Dutch

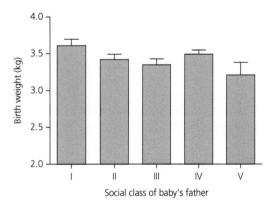

Figure 4.3 Effect of socioeconomic status on birth weight. Social class: I, professionals; II, clerical workers; III, skilled manual or non-manual workers; IV, unskilled workers; V, unemployed.

women who were pregnant at the time of the 9/11 terrorist attacks on the World Trade Center. Compared with women giving birth one year later, babies of this cohort were smaller, supporting the hypothesis that psychological stress can impact upon growth and development.

4.2.2.2 Nutrition and the constraint of growth

The ability of maternal nutrition related factors to constrain fetal growth is an area of some controversy. In populations exposed to famine, it is simple to demonstrate that there is a detrimental impact on fetal growth. The effects are, however, often remarkably small. In the winter of 1944–1945, an area of western Holland was subject to a famine of approximately six months' duration as the occupying Nazi forces blocked delivery of rations in reprisal for strike action among Dutch rail workers. At the height of the famine, the adult ration delivered only 500–600 kcal/day. Because of the duration of the famine, some pregnant women were affected over the final stages of pregnancy, while others were undernourished in early pregnancy. Birth weights among babies affected by famine in late gestation were approximately 250 g lower than those of babies born before or conceived after the famine (Roseboom *et al.*, 2001). Surprisingly, the babies caught by famine in the first trimester of gestation were heavier at birth than the Dutch norm for that period.

Women living in rural areas of the Gambia are subject to seasonal variation in nutritional status, which reflects variation in climate. During the dry season, agriculture is relatively easy as the soil is light and easy to work. Crop growth is good and conditions for food storage are favourable. Thus, at this time, women are relatively well nourished. During the lengthy wet season, however, the women lose 4–5 kg of weight due to a relative scarcity of food, because of the inability to keep food stores dry and the difficulty of working the fields and growing viable crops (Moore *et al.*, 1999). The variation in maternal nutritional status between these seasons is reflected in infant birth weights, which are on average 200 g lighter in the wet season than in the dry. Providing women with modest supplements of energy during the wet season has been shown to abolish this difference in birth weight (Figure 4.4).

Among well-nourished populations, simple measures of maternal intake tend to be only weakly related to babies' birth weights or other markers of fetal growth. Mathews *et al.* (1999) studied pregnant women living in Portsmouth and found that there were no significant associations between

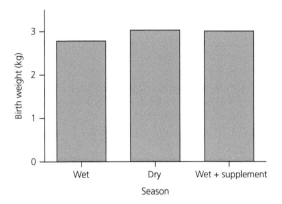

Figure 4.4 Seasonal variation in birth weight among children born in the Gambia. Women are poorly nourished in the wet season and give birth to smaller babies than in the dry season. Supplementation of the diet with energy (431 kcal/day) in the wet season removed the seasonal difference in birth weight, showing that it was related to nutritional status. *Source:* based on Prentice *et al.* (1983).

babies' weights at birth and maternal intakes of any nutrient. Also, in a UK population, Langley-Evans and Langley-Evans (2003) found that while energy and protein intake in the first trimester of pregnancy were not predictive of later birth weight, the mothers of babies who were born smaller had lower intakes of iron (Figure 4.5). Godfrey *et al.* (1996) reported that birth weights of babies were related to maternal intakes of protein in late gestation (low protein diets were associated with lower birth weights) and maternal sucrose intakes in early gestation (high sucrose intakes were associated with lower birth weights). Sharma *et al.* (2018) reported small increases in birth weight associated with greater intakes of fat and carbohydrate in the first trimester of pregnancy. Birth weight was also marginally higher with greater intakes of glucose and lactose in the second trimester. A positive association between sugar intake in early pregnancy and birth weight was also reported by Günther *et al.* (2019). Brei *et al.* (2018) noted greater birth weight with higher intakes of monounsaturated fatty acid in the first trimester and no significant associations between birth weight and overall energy intake or macronutrients in the third trimester.

A number of studies have considered maternal dietary patterns, rather than intakes of specific nutrients, and these studies have suggested that a healthier dietary pattern (high in fruit and vegetables, whole grains, lean protein sources and low-fat dairy produce) is associated with greater birth weight (Günther *et al.*, 2019). Like studies of specific macro- or micronutrients in relation to weight at

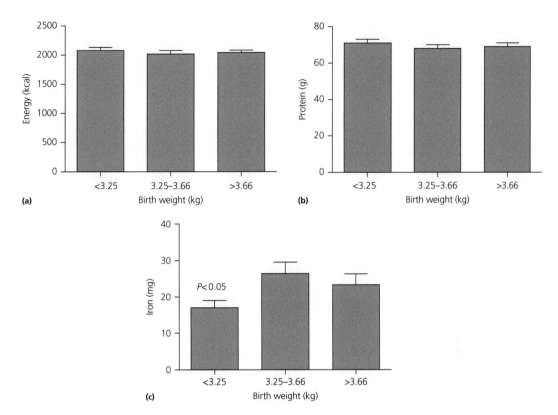

Figure 4.5 The relationship between maternal nutrient intake and birth weight. In a study of 300 pregnant women, the eventual birth weights of their children were not related to energy (a), protein (b), or other macronutrients in the first trimester of pregnancy. Among the micronutrients, only iron intake (c) was associated with weight at birth.

birth, these studies of dietary pattern are prone to inconsistent and inconclusive findings (Chia *et al.* 2019). The lack of clear and consistent effects of maternal nutrient intakes upon babies' birth weights is unsurprising, as the delivery of nutrients to the fetus to drive growth depends on more than just maternal intakes of those nutrients (Figure 4.6). Well-nourished women will generally have adequate reserves of nutrients and can therefore maintain delivery of most substrates to the fetal tissues even if their intakes are compromised in the short to medium term. Fetal nutrition will also depend upon the ability of the placenta to supply substrates, and this in turn may be influenced by maternal adaptations to pregnancy, nutritional factors and hormonal signals.

4.2.2.3 Fetal growth, health and disease
Constraint of fetal growth leading to a lower weight at birth is an indicator that the developing fetus is adapting to aspects of the maternal environment. Given the evidence presented so far, showing that fetal growth can respond to maternal nutritional signals and that events in early life can programme

developing organs and tissues, it is reasonable to assert that maternal nutrition can also affect how mature organs subsequently function and therefore programme aspects of physiology and metabolism, which ultimately determine risk of major disease.

The rate of fetal growth is likely to be set at a very early stage in gestation and could be partly determined by the nutrition of the mother before pregnancy. The availability of plentiful maternal stores may allow the genetically large fetus to get off to a rapid initial growth (Harding, 2004). The rapidly growing fetus may be more vulnerable to undernutrition later on in pregnancy, while a fetus that has been following a slower growth trajectory throughout earlier gestation may be able to maintain this rate of growth even in the face of a nutrient shortage (Figure 4.7).

Some of the first evidence of a possible association between early life nutrition and disease came from simple studies that set out to explore the north–south divide in health noted in England and Wales. In the 1980s, there was a profound difference in risk of coronary heart disease death between the south-eastern corner of England and

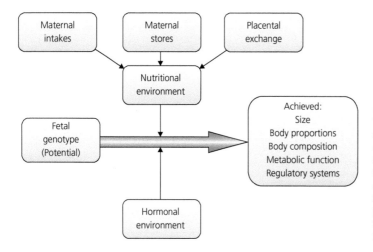

Figure 4.6 Influences on fetal growth. The growth trajectory of the fetus is determined by the genotype. Genetically determined growth rates may be constrained by influences from the mother or placenta. These can act directly on the fetal tissues (e.g. maternal hormones crossing the placenta) or indirectly by modifying the range or concentration of nutrients reaching the fetal tissues.

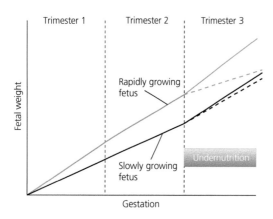

Figure 4.7 Growth is more likely to be constrained in rapidly growing fetuses. Growth of the fetus is primarily set by the genetic potential of the individual. Factors such as maternal undernutrition can constrain this genetic growth rate. The effects of constraint will be greater where growth and the demand for nutrients and oxygen are high. In this example, the slowly growing fetus achieves approximately the same eventual birth weight as the undernourished rapidly growing fetus, irrespective of nutritional status.

the industrialized regions of northern England and South Wales. David Barker and his colleagues were able to demonstrate that there was a robust association between 1970s coronary mortality rates in the different regions and infant death rates some 60 years earlier (Barker and Osmond, 1986). Those parts of the country with high infant mortality early in the twentieth century were the same regions with high coronary death rates. Further investigation of the death certificates of over two million Britons showed that place of birth was a strong predictor of death from coronary heart disease, with greatest risk associated with birth in the industrial north (Bradford, Halifax, Huddersfield, Preston), and lowest risk associated with birth in the south and southeast (East Sussex, West Sussex, Isle of Wight). Most importantly, this risk was independent of subsequent migration, so individuals born in Bradford would retain their greater likelihood of coronary heart disease death later in life, even if they lived out their adult years in Sussex (Osmond et al., 1990). The simplest interpretation of these studies is that adverse factors, such as poor maternal nutrition, during fetal development either led to the death of the infant or prompted irreversible physiological adaptations that allowed survival but led to greater risk of cardiovascular disease (CVD) later in life. Such observations were the main spark for Barker's proposal of the developmental origins of adult disease hypothesis (Barker, 1998).

The developmental origins of health and disease hypothesis explicitly advances the idea that any form of adverse environment encountered in early life can elicit adaptive responses that modify the future health of the individual. While a range of adverse factors could be responsible for the developmental programming of health and disease, maternal nutrition was proposed as the main factor that would determine the nature of fetal development (Figure 4.8). The proposal of nutrition as the primary driver of programming stemmed from the fact that the epidemiological evidence suggesting programming of human disease highlighted impaired fetal growth as a predictor of heart disease and diabetes. As can be seen in the following sections, this evidence mostly came from studies of groups of people

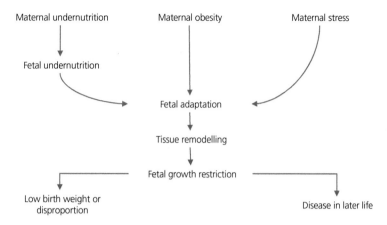

Figure 4.8 The developmental origins of health and disease hypothesis. Maternal undernutrition promotes fetal undernutrition, which in turn will slow fetal growth rates. The relationship between fetal undernutrition and disease in later life may be directly the result of fetal adaptations to undernutrition or may be related to the restriction of fetal growth and organ development.

born in Britain early in the twentieth century, a period where undernutrition was rife among young adult women.

4.3 Evidence linking maternal nutrition to disease in later life

4.3.1 Epidemiology

4.3.1.1 Association of disease with birth anthropometry

A full exploration of the possible programming relationship between maternal diet and disease in later life would require detailed records of many aspects of maternal diet and lifestyle during pregnancy and long-term follow-up of children into late adulthood. This is not a realistic possibility for most researchers. The alternative approach involves locating adults for whom some indicator of prenatal exposure to putative risk factors is available and then relating these exposure indicators to disease patterns. This is called a retrospective cohort study. Historically, the only data that were reliably recorded about pregnancy outcomes were some simple anthropometric measures of infants, such as birth weight, length at birth and head circumference. These measurements give an imprecise indicator of nutritional influences. As described earlier, undernutrition can constrain growth and reduce birth weight. It is also suggested that the nutritional constraint of birth weight may be greater than that of linear growth, leading to the birth of a baby who is relatively thin (lightweight in relation to body length; Godfrey, 2001).

A unique set of records from the county of Hertfordshire provided the basis of the first major epidemiological study to consider relationships between birth anthropometry and disease in later life. Records from 16 000 men and women born in Hertfordshire between 1911 and 1930 were traced. It was found that while mortality rates for all causes were unrelated to size at birth or in infancy, both lower birth weight and lower body weight at one year were predictive of increased CVD mortality (Barker *et al.*, 1989). By following up individuals from this cohort who were still living in the county, researchers showed that low weight at birth also predicted risk factors for CVD, including blood pressure, type 2 diabetes and the insulin resistance syndrome (syndrome X) (Hales *et al.*, 1991; Barker *et al.*, 1993a). Infants who weighed less than 5.5 lbs at birth (2.5 kg) were twice as likely to die from coronary heart disease, six and a half times more likely to develop type 2 diabetes and 18 times more likely to develop syndrome X than individuals who weighed more than 9.5 lbs (4.3 kg). The Hertfordshire study and many similar studies from all over the world showed that low weight at birth was a significant predictor of disease 60–70 years later and supported the concept that maternal undernutrition may programme disease processes (Figure 4.9).

It became clear from a study of a cohort of men and women born in Sheffield that body proportions at birth were also significant predictors of CVD risk (Figure 4.10). Among 1586 men born in Sheffield between 1907 and 1923, CVD death rates were not only related to birth weight, but they also rose significantly with decreasing ponderal index (Barker *et al.*, 1993b). The latter (weight/height, kg/m³) is a marker of relative thinness (low ponderal index) or fatness (high ponderal index) at birth. Ponderal index at birth was also a significant predictor of blood pressure. These data therefore showed that babies who were born small and thin were at greater risk of disease in later life. The US Nurses' Health Study collected data on birth weight by self-report from 70 297 women and found that among full-term singletons, after adjustment for adult body mass index (BMI), risk of coronary heart disease and

stroke were both related to weight at birth (Curhan *et al.*, 1996). A lower weight at birth increased risk of coronary heart disease (relative risk estimate 0.85 per kg increase in birth weight) and stroke (relative risk estimate 0.85 per kg increase in birth weight) and was associated with higher blood pressure in adult life. Table 4.1 summarizes observed relationships between anthropometry at birth and later disease and disease risk factors.

Evidence of associations between characteristics at birth and risk factors for major disease can also be shown in studies of children. Bavdekar *et al.* (1999) studied eight-year-old children in India and found

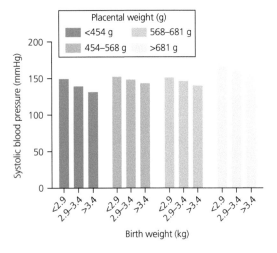

Figure 4.9 Blood pressure in 50-year-old men and women grouped by weight at birth and placental weight. For any birth weight class, blood pressure was higher as placental weight increased. For any placental weight class, a lower weight at birth was associated with higher blood pressure. *Source:* Reproduced with permission from Barker (1998). © Elsevier.

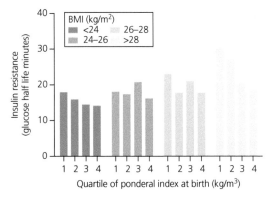

Figure 4.10 Insulin resistance in 50-year-old men and women grouped by ponderal index at birth (PI) and body mass index (BMI) at age 50. For any PI class, insulin resistance was higher as adult BMI increased. For any adult BMI class, a thinness at birth was associated with greater insulin resistance. Quartiles of PI are: (1) <20.6 kg/m³, (2) 20.6–22.3 kg/m³, (3) 22.3–25 kg/m³ and (4) >25 kg/m³. *Source:* Reproduced with permission from Barker (1998). © Elsevier.

Table 4.1 Associations between infant anthropometry at birth and later disease.

Anthropometric indicator	Measurement	Associated disorder in later life
Lower birth weight	Weight (kg)	High blood pressure Metabolic syndrome Type 2 diabetes Coronary heart disease death Stroke death
Thinness at birth	Weight (kg)/body length (cm)³	High blood pressure Metabolic syndrome Type 2 diabetes Coronary heart disease death
Larger abdomen	Abdominal circumference (cm)	Dyslipidaemia Coronary heart disease death
Small head size	Head circumference (cm)	Atopy
Disproportionately large head	Head circumference (cm)/birth weight (kg) *or* head circumference (cm)/body length (cm)	High blood pressure Coronary heart disease death

that lower weight at birth was associated with lower sensitivity to insulin and impaired glucose tolerance. In effect, these young children whose birth weight was lower were already on the road to type 2 diabetes. This suggests that the programming influences of fetal life impact metabolism and physiology immediately after birth and do not depend on ageing to be expressed.

The most powerful cohort studies to assess possible programming of CVD and diabetes in humans have emerged from investigations of two populations born in Helsinki (1924–1933 and 1933–1944). Eriksson *et al.* (1999) found that birth weight was inversely associated with risk of both coronary heart disease and stroke-related mortality. Among men, a low ponderal index at birth was also related to risk of coronary heart disease death if BMI was high in childhood. The most important aspect of the Helsinki 1933–1944 cohort was that the babies had been subject to serial measures of weight and height until age 12. Studies of this cohort showed that low birth weight was a predictor of coronary heart disease events, type 2 diabetes and metabolic syndrome and again demonstrated that relative thinness at birth (low ponderal index) and relative fatness in childhood (greater BMI) were associated with risk of these conditions.

An increasing body of evidence from these large cohorts has begun to consider whether there is any interaction between factors that influence fetal growth rates and influences on postnatal growth. For example, it is of interest to know whether the fate of the low birth weight baby differs depending on how they are fed and how they grow during childhood. Where studies were able to look at postnatal as well as prenatal growth, it is apparent that a rapid gain from birth to adulthood was a risk in addition to prenatal growth restriction. This could be an indicator that the two observations (pre- and postnatal growth) represented independent risk factors, that the most severely constrained babies are subject to postnatal catch-up growth and this is a marker of CVD risk, or that there is a genuine interaction of pre- and early postnatal factors in programming. The Helsinki data suggest the latter, as the fate of individuals with the most rapid rates of infant growth differed depending on their size at birth. Those born small and growing most rapidly in infancy had highest risk of CVD, while those who were larger at birth had lower CVD risk if weight gain was rapid in infancy. The fact that the small infant at birth who remained small throughout infancy had no increased risk of adult CVD argues that the pre- and postnatal interaction is of prime importance in cardiovascular programming. Figure 4.10 reinforces

the importance of the interaction between fetal growth and weight gain in later life. Among 50-year-old men and women, risk of insulin resistance was greatest in those of higher BMI in adulthood. However, at any adult BMI classification, there was also a relationship between insulin resistance and ponderal index at birth. The greatest risk of insulin resistance was observed with relative thinness at birth (low ponderal index) and relative fatness (higher BMI) in adulthood.

4.3.1.2 Maternal nutrition and later disease

The aforementioned studies are limited in that they are only able to report associations between disease states and anthropometric measurements at birth. The latter are only weak markers of the nutritional environment encountered by the fetus during critical periods of development. The Dutch famine, described in Section 4.2.2.2, has been useful in extending the developmental origins hypothesis since it provides an easily accessible population whose mothers were subject to a brief period of food restriction. Follow-up of the Dutch famine babies showed that their health status was poor relative to their contemporaries whose mothers had not been affected by the famine (Table 4.2). Exposure to famine in early gestation was associated with greater prevalence of coronary heart disease, with raised circulating lipids, with raised concentrations of blood clotting factors and with more obesity compared with those not exposed to the famine (Roseboom *et al.*, 2001). Exposure to the famine during mid-gestation was associated with microalbuminuria, an indicator of impaired kidney function. Exposure to famine during late gestation was associated with disorders of glucose metabolism that lead to type 2 diabetes.

Similar support for there being an association between maternal nutritional status and disease in later life has been provided by studies of children in Jamaica and the United States. A small-scale study of Jamaican boys aged 10–11 years demonstrated that their blood pressures were related to markers of undernutrition in their mothers during pregnancy (Godfrey *et al.*, 1994). The boys whose mothers had the lowest circulating haemoglobin concentrations (indicating low iron status) and lowest triceps skinfold thicknesses (indicating low body fat reserves) had the highest blood pressures.

Prospective cohort studies have sought to assess relationships between maternal factors and offspring health. The only large cohort in Europe to date has been the Southampton Women's Survey, which recruited 12 583 non-pregnant women aged 20–34 years. From this sample, a total of 3158 babies were

Table 4.2 Fetal exposure to the Dutch Famine of 1944–1945 is associated with disease in later life.

Disease state/risk factors	Developmental stage when exposed to famine		
	Early gestation	Mid-gestation	Late gestation
Breast cancer	✓	–	–
Coronary heart disease	✓	–	–
Dyslipidaemia*	✓	–	–
Glucose intolerance	✓	✓	✓
Increased clotting factors	✓	–	–
Microalbuminuria†	–	✓	–
Obesity‡	✓	–	–
Obstructive airway disease	–	✓	–

✓ indicates that exposure to famine during a key developmental stage of development is associated with disease or disease risk factors in middle age.
* Increased concentrations of LDL-cholesterol and triglycerides.
† Increased excretion of protein in the urine is an indicator of renal disease.
‡ Obesity was more prevalent in women, but not men, exposed to family in early gestation.

born, with full assessment of maternal diet and lifestyle before, during and after pregnancy. The babies were followed up at one, seven and nine years of age. The survey has reported a number of outcomes which are consistent with nutritional programming during fetal development, although as yet the children are far too young to properly investigate the conclusions drawn from retrospective cohorts in relation to cardiovascular and metabolic diseases. Crozier *et al.* (2010) reported that children of women who gained excessive weight in pregnancy had greater fat mass at birth, four and six years. Childhood obesity was related to rates of childhood growth (Norris *et al.*, 2020). Van Lee *et al.* (2019) found that fatness at birth was associated with maternal choline concentrations in pregnancy, but the association was no longer seen at age five. Maternal consumption of n-3 LCPUFA was associated with aortic stiffness at nine years of age, suggesting that greater consumption of oily fish in pregnancy may protect babies against cardiovascular disease in later life (Bryant *et al.*, 2015). A similar prospective study from the United States, Project Viva, has demonstrated that greater maternal adherence to a healthy Mediterranean dietary pattern in pregnancy was associated with lower BMI, skinfold measures and blood pressure in seven-year-old children (Chatzi *et al.*, 2017). Project Viva also showed lower risk of childhood obesity in children of mothers with higher intake of n-3 LCPUFA in pregnancy (Donahue *et al.*, 2011). Taken together, the Southampton Women's Survey and Project Viva indicate that higher quality nutrition in pregnancy is related to better health indicators in children. Further findings from these cohorts, obtained as the offspring age, will be of great interest. Other prospective cohorts such as the Singapore Growing Up in Singapore Towards Healthy Outcomes (Soh *et al.*, 2014) study will add further to our understanding of programming by maternal nutrition.

4.3.1.3 Maternal obesity and later disease

Chapter 3 gave an overview of the many negative effects of maternal overweight and obesity on pregnancy and neonatal outcomes. It is also clear that maternal obesity has a long-term programming effect on developing fetuses and is adverse health outcomes in the child (Catalano and Ehrenberg, 2006). Some of the earliest evidence for the link between maternal BMI and risk of overweight and obesity in the child came from a large epidemiological study conducted by Parsons *et al.* (2001), who followed up over 10 000 individuals from the Hertfordshire cohort. A J-shaped relationship was noted between birth weight and BMI at age 33 in both men and women, meaning that those individuals who were both small and heavier at birth had a higher BMI, and were thus at higher risk of overweight, in adulthood. This relationship between birth weight and adult BMI was almost entirely explained by maternal BMI, but was not influenced by other factors, including paternal BMI or smoking.

A number of other large cohort studies show a similar J-shaped relationship between birth weight and adult BMI, such that adult BMI is increased slightly in individuals of low birth weight, but that heavier babies have a greatly elevated prevalence of overweight and obesity in adolescence and young adulthood. The results of following 7981 girls and 6900 boys who were part of the Growing up Today Study at 9–14 years of age, for example, indicated that the odds ratio for adolescent overweight was

1.4 (95% confidence interval, CI, 1.2–1.6) for each kilogram increment in birth weight (Gillman *et al.*, 2003). The majority of follow-up studies support the suggestion that parental obesity, in particular maternal obesity, is a significant risk factor for future obesity risk independent of birth weight. Infants born to obese mothers were shown by Whitaker *et al.* (1997) to be twice as likely to be obese by two years of age compared with infants of mothers who were not obese, and the prevalence of childhood obesity (BMI >95th percentile) in two-, three- and four-year-old children born to mothers with obesity was between 2.4 and 2.7 times that of children of mothers whose BMI was in the normal range.

Importantly, maternal obesity in pregnancy appears to programme metabolic function in developing fetuses. Impaired metabolic functions appear to be driven by an increased accumulation of body fat in utero. Catalano and Ehrenberg (2003) and Catalano *et al.* (2009) established that the higher birth weight in infants of mothers with obesity was largely due to a greater accumulation of body fat. Such infants also had higher insulin resistance at birth, as measured by the homeostasis model assessment–insulin resistance index and this was also directly related to neonatal adiposity (Catalano *et al.*, 2009).

4.3.2 Criticisms of the programming hypothesis

The compelling epidemiological findings described earlier have major implications for our understanding of how disease processes are initiated and for public health policy across the world. If nutritional programming has a genuine influence on human disease, then interventions designed to prevent disease must be targeted at pregnant women, for the benefit of their children, as well as being aimed at the adults whose lifestyles may increase risk of obesity and related disorders. The developmental origins hypothesis would suggest that altering patterns of disease in populations may be the equivalent of trying to turn around an oil tanker, as effective public health strategies could take decades to come to fruition.

Given the profound implications for public health, it is right that the developmental origins hypothesis should be subjected to close scrutiny and critique. The epidemiology underpinning the hypothesis has been criticized on several different levels. Importantly, most of the epidemiology in this area has focused on measuring disease outcomes in adults aged 50–80 and then attempting to relate these outcomes retrospectively to proxy markers of maternal nutrition from many decades previously. The quality of the data on exposure is therefore very poor and it is relatively easy to invoke the influences of confounding factors that are either not adjusted for (e.g. maternal physical activity, maternal infection, childhood infection, quality of the infant diet in the postnatal period, adult lifestyle factors) or only crudely adjusted for (e.g. social class). Bartley *et al.* (1994) showed how important social class could be in confounding the birth weight–disease association. Their study showed that individuals born into a poor family tended to be of lower weight at birth. Most individuals born into a family of lower socioeconomic class tended to remain in that lower class when they were adults. It is well established that being of lower socioeconomic status is a risk factor for CVD, and thus the birth weight–CVD association could be purely an influence of poverty. There are also studies that do not fit with the hypothesis. For example, Matthes *et al.* (1994) studied 330 adolescents and found that there was no difference in blood pressure between those who were lighter than 3 kg at birth and those who were 3 kg or heavier at birth. Similarly, Falkner *et al.* (1998) found no elevation in blood pressure in young adults who were of low birth weight.

Most epidemiological studies that have examined the maternal diet–later disease association have relied upon birth weight or other proportions at birth as a proxy for maternal nutritional status. This is problematic since, as described earlier, maternal nutrient intakes have only minor influences on fetal growth rates compared with some other factors. Studies of the wartime famines in Holland or the Soviet Union have been widely reported as providing evidence from 'natural experiments' in which we can be sure that the babies born at those times were subject to undernutrition. While they have yielded interesting findings, these studies are subject to important criticisms. During wartime, birth rates can fall dramatically and so it may be that the women having children at these times were in some way not representative of the whole population. Wartime is stressful and maternal stress could programme long-term effects independently of nutrition. It is also apparent that there were ways around rationing and a black market in foodstuffs may have relieved some of the hardships of pregnant women in at least the Dutch famine.

The most potent criticism of the epidemiological studies showing associations between infant birth weights and disease risk indicators in later life has come from the work of Huxley *et al.* (2002). This group performed a meta-analysis of all studies that had considered the association between birth weight and blood pressure in adulthood. Generally, in epidemiology, it is expected that studies with the most subjects give the most reliable and robust findings. Huxley *et al.* (2002) found that the strongest influences of birth weight on blood pressure were reported in small-scale studies, while large cohort studies found the weakest associations. It was concluded that the birth weight–blood pressure association was partly a product of publication bias (in which small studies showing an effect are prioritized by journal editors over small studies showing no effect) and reflected random error, selective emphasis of particular results, methodological flaws and confounding factors. It is worth noting, however, that other meta-analyses are more supportive of the developmental origins hypothesis. Whincup *et al.* (2008) found that for every kilogram higher weight at birth, risk of type 2 diabetes decreased by 23%. Low birth weight was shown by White *et al.* (2009) to increase risk of chronic kidney disease (odds ratio, OR, 1.73) and end-stage renal disease (OR 1.58). The meta-analysis of Schellong *et al.* (2012) proved counterintuitive as high birth weight rather than low birth weight was associated with greater risk of adult overweight (OR 1.66).

The criticisms described earlier are inevitable products of the complexity of any likely relationship between nutritional exposures in fetal life and disease outcomes that may not manifest for 60–70 years. It is questionable whether epidemiological approaches have the capacity to investigate these questions at all. Studies such as the Hertfordshire study, which was so influential in promoting interest in developmental programming as a risk factor in human disease, were already no longer representative of influences at work in the modern population, at the time at which they were published. The nutritional and social influences on fetal development operative in the period 1910–1930 were clearly vastly different to those operative in 1990. As alluded to earlier, maternal obesity is now the principal nutritional challenge experienced during fetal life, as opposed to the undernutrition that was prevalent early in the twentieth century. It is possible that the disease consequences that will be observed in 2050 will differ from those noted by Barker and colleagues in the elderly Hertfordshire men and women. It is critical, therefore, that there are studies in this field that can establish the biological plausibility of programming as a risk factor for disease. It is very important to identify the influences of different patterns of diet (e.g. overnutrition, as well as undernutrition) upon development and disease and to begin to describe the mechanisms through which programming occurs.

4.3.3 Experimental studies

To perform a study in humans that could adequately test the developmental origins of health and disease hypothesis would require prospective study of women before and during pregnancy, with follow-ups of their children for 50–60 years. Although this is challenging in terms of human resources and cost, several continuing cohort studies aim to examine the links between early life factors and health. Project Viva (Donahue *et al.*, 2011) recruited 2128 women and their babies between 1999 and 2002 for long-term follow-up. The Millennium cohort in the UK recruited 19 000 babies born between 2000 and 2001 who are followed up at approximately two-year intervals. The Southampton Women's Study is the largest European prospective cohort focused upon early life nutrition and later outcomes, with 3156 children born between 1998 and 2007 in the cohort following prospective recruitment of 12 583 women aged 20–34 years (Inskip *et al.*, 2006). However, significant insight into the early life antecedents of diseases associated with ageing is not expected from these cohorts for decades. It is not ethically acceptable to manipulate the diets of pregnant women to attempt to influence the future health of their offspring, potentially inducing major disease states. There is, therefore, little alternative to using appropriate animal models to explore the relationship between maternal diet and disease (see Research Highlight 4.1).

Many different animal models have been developed for this purpose, and these will be described below (Figure 4.11). Researchers have focused primarily on rodents (rats and mice) for such studies. This is because these species are simple to breed, it is straightforward to modify their diets in pregnancy, gestation is short (rat 22 days, mouse 18 days) and their offspring grow to adulthood very quickly (overall lifespan is around 2 years). There are disadvantages associated with these species, however. The main difference between rodents and humans is that rodents deliver litters of offspring (typically 10–15 pups in the rat) and these offspring are born very immature. Guinea pigs provide an alternative as although these still produce litters of offspring (3–6 pups), gestation is long (68 days), the placenta is more similar to that of the human and the offspring are born at a similar level of maturity to the human infant. The sheep is a broadly favoured species of fetal physiologists, primarily because of the long gestation (147 days) and the fact that the fetus is of similar size to a human (3.5–4 kg). However, as the sheep is a ruminant, the ability to manipulate diet in pregnancy is very limited.

Research Highlight 4.1 Animal models of early life programming by nutrition.

Animal models have played a vital role in uncovering the processes which link maternal nutritional status during pregnancy to disease of ageing. As discussed in Chapter 1 (Figure 1.16) research based on animal models is considered to be at the bottom of the hierarchy of research evidence for human health and disease. Why then has the nutritional programming field of research been so heavily dependent upon such approaches?

The study of early life programming is challenging both ethically and practically. It is not, for example, feasible or ethical to perform a randomized controlled trial of diet in pregnancy that could result in development of life-threatening disease in the offspring as they age. Similarly, there is not a feasible means of invasively sampling developing embryos or fetal tissues, or of obtaining later samples other than blood or other bodily fluids from offspring, which greatly limits capacity to do mechanistic studies. Observational epidemiology in this area either requires researchers to consider retrospective cohorts, with many associated problems of inadequate dietary exposure data and confounding, or to conduct prospective cohort studies which will have to end before disease develops in the participants or will have to run for so long that the results will have little relevance by the time they are available.

Animals are not the only possible alternatives to studying humans and for many areas of medical science in vitro studies are of tremendous utility. Nutritional programming studies again pose a unique challenge as they must effectively consider how a signal of maternal nutritional status passes from mother to fetus and then determine how this impacts differently on many different cell types in multiple tissues and at different developmental stages. Most in vitro studies can at best look at the responses and interactions of two cell types and current technology cannot model the complexity of the problem under study.

Animal models of nutritional programming allow researchers to control maternal diet composition and observe the impact on the health and longevity of relatively short-lived species. Any tissue in mother, fetus, offspring or placenta can be obtained for mechanistic investigation. This approach has been critical for demonstrating that a link between variation in a mother's diet and the health of her adult offspring in biologically plausible. It has also paved the way for determining how programming occurs (McMullen and Mostyn, 2009). It is critical, however, for researchers to appreciate the limitations of their findings and to design their experiments carefully so that their choice of animal species and dietary change is appropriate to test their research hypothesis.

Researchers who work with animals are pressed by the organizations that fund them and the publishers who disseminate their work to follow the three Rs principles (replacement, refinement and reduction), which aim to improve animal welfare and the quality of science (Burden et al., 2015). At the heart of this aim is the need to use no more animals than are required to deliver reliable results, and to make use of the optimal techniques in the most relevant model species. Despite widespread endorsement of the three Rs principles, many researchers give insufficient thought to the choice of model and the relevance of their work to human health and clinical outcomes (Veening-Griffioen et al., 2020).

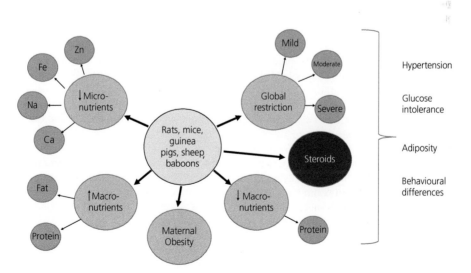

Figure 4.11 Researchers considering the developmental origins of health and disease hypothesis have used a diverse range of animal species and different types of nutritional insult. All models show the same general outcomes with maternal nutrition influencing physiological and metabolic outcomes.

Using these varied species, researchers have attempted to model the developmental origins hypothesis in different ways. Many have sought to simply replicate the relationship between fetal growth restriction and later outcomes. Poore *et al.* (2002) exploited the natural variability in birth weight among litters of piglets and showed that birth weight was inversely associated with blood pressure, just as in humans. This approach is unusual and the relationship is more generally explored by limiting food intake of the pregnant mother and therefore restricting intakes of all macro- and micro-nutrients (global undernutrition). Some groups take a more drastic approach and retard fetal growth by surgically placing a ligature around the uterine artery to limit the supply of blood and nutrients. Persson and Jansson (1992) showed, using this approach, that growth restriction of the guinea pig fetus resulted in hypertension later in life. Other researchers have chosen to look beyond the birth weight–disease association and model the effects of specific nutrients in the diet. This allows investigation of the long-term consequences of either nutritional deficit or excess.

4.3.3.1 Global undernutrition

Restriction of overall food intake during pregnancy has a range of different effects that are dependent upon the severity of the restriction imposed and upon the animal species. Woodall *et al. et al.* (1996) reported that feeding pregnant rats only 30% of their normal daily rations led to major restriction of the growth of their fetuses. As adults, these low birth weight offspring exhibited high blood pressure and profound obesity. The latter seemed to be caused by an increase in the appetite of the animals and a reduction in their levels of physical activity. Holemans *et al.* (1999) also worked with pregnant rats and fed 50% of normal rations, but only in the second half of pregnancy. Under these conditions, the offspring did not develop high blood pressure but, as adults, did display abnormalities of cardiovascular function. In the sheep, feeding 50% of nutrient requirements during pregnancy has a number of effects upon the cardiovascular function and metabolic state of the adult lambs. The prenatally nutrient-restricted lamb is generally fatter and has higher blood pressure than a lamb from a well-fed mother, by the age of three years (Gardner *et al.*, 2007).

Even mild restriction of maternal food intake in pregnancy can programme the offspring. In the rat, feeding 70% of ad libitum intake produced pups that became hypertensive as adults (Ozaki *et al.*, 2001). Similarly, in guinea pigs, reducing maternal food intake by just 15% was sufficient to programme

hypertension and raised blood lipids in the adult off-spring (Kind *et al.*, 2002). When pregnant sheep were fed 85% of requirements over the first 70 days of gestation, their fetuses showed altered cardiovascular function at the end of gestation (Hawkins *et al.*, 2000).

4.3.3.2 Micronutrients

Iron deficiency anaemia is the most common nutrient deficiency disorder in the world and particularly impacts upon women during pregnancy. The normal physiological adaptation to pregnancy involves a major expansion of blood volume and, typically, the plasma volume expansion outstrips the production of new red cells and haemoglobin. As a result, blood haemoglobin concentrations fall. Although this sign of iron deficiency may be regarded as a normal part of pregnancy, more severe anaemia is associated with poor pregnancy outcomes. It is estimated that two thirds of pregnant women will develop some degree of iron deficiency in the course of their pregnancy (see Section 3.3.2). In the pregnant rat, iron deficiency anaemia can be shown to programme fetal development (Gambling *et al.*, 2003). The iron-deficient rat embryo has an abnormally enlarged heart and as an adult will have high blood pressure, suggesting that iron plays a key role in the normal development of the cardiovascular system.

Maternal intakes of calcium are of considerable interest in the programming context. Suboptimal intakes of calcium are relatively common among women of childbearing age, particularly younger women and adolescents. Gillman *et al.* (2004) showed that increasing intakes of calcium from supplements during pregnancy could lower blood pressure in young children. In rats, the relationship between maternal calcium intake and offspring blood pressure is complex. Rats, whose mothers were fed a calcium-deficient diet, had blood pressures that were 12 mmHg higher than seen in the offspring of rats fed a control diet (Bergel and Belizan, 2002). However, high consumption of calcium in the maternal diet also elevated blood pressures in the offspring, suggesting a U-shaped relationship between calcium intake and later outcomes.

Sodium intake is a major determinant of blood pressure in adults, and there is great concern at the high levels of intake seen within the modern western diet (see Section 8.4.4.3.6). There have been few studies that have considered the potential for variation in the sodium content of the diet to exert programming effects in utero. Battista *et al.* (2002) interestingly showed that a low-sodium diet fed to rats in the last week of their pregnancies induced fetal growth restriction and high blood pressure in their offspring.

4.3.3.3 Macronutrients

Protein restriction is one of the mostly widely studied manipulations of the maternal diet in animals. Although protein deficiency per se is relatively rare in most populations of the world, the degree of variation in protein intake both within and between populations is substantial. In the UK, for example, intakes in pregnancy tend to be lower in women of lower socioeconomic status and in younger mothers. Five to ten per cent of the population may consume protein at less than the 51 g/day reference nutrient intake for pregnancy (Langley-Evans *et al.*, 2003). On a global scale, access to protein is a significant issue for almost two thirds of the population, with women in developing countries often subsisting on lower-quality plant protein sources (Figure 4.12).

There is an extensive literature reporting the programming effects of feeding a low-protein diet during rat pregnancy. Relatively mild manipulation of protein intake produces subtle variations in the growth of the offspring, which undergo a late gestation restriction of growth, particularly affecting the development of the truncal organs such as the lungs and kidneys (Langley- Evans *et al.*, 1996a). Although of low to normal birth weight, rats exposed to protein restriction in fetal life develop raised blood pressure by three to four weeks of age, and this hypertension persists into adult life (Langley-Evans *et al.*, 1994; Langley-Evans and

Jackson, 1995). In the postnatal period, these animals have an accelerated progression towards renal failure and their lifespan is significantly shorter than that of rats exposed to a protein-replete diet in fetal life (Aihie Sayer *et al.*, 2001).

The offspring of rats fed low-protein diets in pregnancy exhibit a number of age-related disorders that make this an interesting model to study in the context of the metabolic syndrome in humans. Typically, humans become more insulin resistant as they age and develop type 2 diabetes as a consequence. Rats exposed to protein restriction in fetal life are relatively lean in early adult life and show increased sensitivity to insulin. As they age, however, insulin resistance begins to appear and with this the animals develop raised blood lipid profiles and deposit large amounts of fat in their livers (Erhuma *et al.*, 2007).

An excess of protein in the diet is also a major issue in the diets of populations living in the westernized nations. In parts of Europe and the United States, it is not uncommon for women to consume 120 g protein per day, which is more than double the UK reference nutrient intake (Langley- Evans *et al.*, 1996a). Daenzer *et al.* (2002) considered the potential programming effects of high-protein diets in pregnant rats. Offspring of rats fed a 40% protein diet were shown to be more prone to obesity through reduced total energy expenditure.

In human populations throughout the world, one of the major nutritional concerns is the consumption of diets containing excessive amounts of energy derived from fat and sugar. Rodent studies suggest that such a dietary pattern in pregnancy may programme the later blood pressure and metabolic functions of the resulting offspring. Maternal overfeeding, generally with high-fat diets, has similar programming effects in both rats and mice (Samuelsson *et al.*, 2008; Shankar *et al.*, 2008) with elevated blood pressure, impaired glucose tolerance and dyslipidaemia. Feeding rats a cafeteria diet (a varying menu of highly palatable human foods) prior to pregnancy to induce obesity can impact upon the metabolic function of their later offspring, with changes in glucose homeostasis (Akyol *et al.*, 2012). Sophisticated studies with the capacity to distinguish the effects of maternal obesity in pregnancy and lactation (which generally occur together) have shown that obesity in pregnancy favours improved insulin sensitivity in the offspring when they are young adults. In contrast, being suckled by a mother who is obese programmes obesity and insulin resistance (George *et al.*, 2019a, 2019b). Obesity has also been shown to have a greater effect in lactation than pregnancy with respect to programming offspring feeding

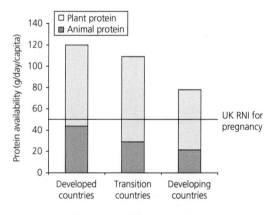

Figure 4.12 Global protein availability statistics. *Source:* data extracted from 2004 United Nations Food and Agriculture Organization food balance sheets. Food balance methods only determine the protein available (i.e. produced through agriculture or imported) per head of population. Actual consumption will be below the figures shown and highly variable within each region (e.g. affluent vs poor, urban vs rural). Sixty-five per cent of the world population are likely to consume protein at less than the UK reference nutrient intake and are therefore at risk of low-protein intake during pregnancy. Many in developing countries rely on lower-quality plant protein sources. RNI, reference nutrient intake.

behaviour and learning ability in rats (Wright *et al.*, 2011, Wright *et al.*, 2014).

The most remarkable aspect of all of the animal studies described earlier is the fact that very diverse nutritional manipulations in pregnancy (ranging from severe global undernutrition to an energy-rich, junk-food diet) in a diverse range of species (including rodents and ruminants) can produce very similar effects in the offspring (typically high blood pressure, glucose intolerance and obesity; Figure 4.11). The commonality of the responses to diverse dietary insults suggests that programming is driven by a small number of common mechanisms, any of which might be initiated by a maternal signal that the nutritional environment is not optimal. Understanding of those mechanisms is of major importance if the developmental origins hypothesis is ever to have any significant impact upon the way in which public health problems related to nutrition are treated or prevented.

4.4 Mechanistic basis of fetal programming

4.4.1 Thrifty phenotypes and genotypes

Metabolic 'thrift' is defined as the possession of metabolic and physiological characteristics that ensure the most efficient and effective use of substrates. Neel (1962) first proposed this concept, suggesting that in the early evolution of the human species, regular exposure to food shortages would favour the survival of those that carried thrifty genes and that the population would therefore have evolved to store fat during times of plenty and use that resource during periods of famine. Clearly, a thrifty genotype would no longer be an advantage in modern society, and the mismatch between our current westernized lifestyle and the environment that humans have experienced through 99.9% of their history could be invoked as an explanation for modern trends in obesity, CVD and diabetes.

Thrifty genes could influence many aspects of the acquisition and processing of nutrients, and many different candidate genes that confer thrift have been proposed (Breier *et al.*, 2004). These include genes that control feeding behaviour, such as leptin and the melanocortin receptor; genes that are involved in metabolic regulation, such as peroxisome proliferator-activated receptor γ and genes that play a role in insulin signalling and other signal transduction pathways. Hattersley and Tooke (1999) have proposed that thrifty genotypes could entirely explain the observed association between weight at birth and diabetes in later life. Insulin is an important driver of fetal growth, and so genetic defects of

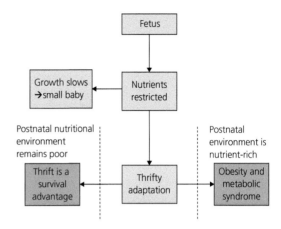

Figure 4.13 The thrifty phenotype hypothesis.
Source: based on Hales and Barker (2001).

the insulin axis, which would ultimately promote diabetes, might also be associated with fetal growth restriction. Mutations of the glucokinase gene are associated with both maturity onset diabetes and low birth weight in this way. Arguments in favour of a thrifty genotype driving the development of disease are weakened by the fact that while the metabolic diseases (obesity, type 2 diabetes) are very common in westernized society, mutations of the candidate genes that are proven to be associated with disease are extremely rare.

Thrift, however, remains an important consideration in the diet–disease relationship and comes to the fore in the nutritional programming area. Hales and Barker (1992) first proposed the thrifty phenotype hypothesis (Figure 4.13). This suggests that the developing fetus exposed to suboptimal nutrition undergoes adaptations to key metabolic tissues such as the liver and pancreas. Primarily, these enable the fetus to maximize the resources that are available during that phase of development. However, as programming events are permanent, the thrift that is acquired at the time of undernutrition will remain through to adult life. For our hunter-gatherer ancestors, this would provide the same survival advantage as the thrifty genotype proposed by Neel (1962). In the modern world, some thrifty individuals would be born into an environment where food shortages still occur and hence would benefit from their fetal experience. However, should the individual programmed to be thrifty be born into an environment where food is plentiful, the thrift would drive excessive fat gain and the development of the associated disease states.

Hales and Barker (1992) proposed several examples of the thrifty phenotype in action. Most of these focused upon populations where it has been shown that rapid changes from a traditional to a westernized diet have been accompanied by soaring rates of diabetes. The prevalence rate for type 2 diabetes in the population of the Pacific island of Nauru is among the highest in the world. Prior to the Second World War, this population was habitually undernourished, but industrial development since the 1940s sparked an epidemic of diabetes.

Observations of twins tend to support the thrifty phenotype hypothesis rather than the concept of a thrifty genotype. Studies of twin pairs (mono- and dizygotic) in which one twin but not the other suffered from diabetes (Poulsen *et al.*, 1997; Bo *et al.*, 2000) showed that insulin resistance, raised circulating triglycerides and cholesterol were more common in the twin with the lower birth weight. Given that in each case the twins would have very similar or identical genotypes, these findings suggest that fetal growth constraint, perhaps driven by unequal distribution of nutritional resources from the mother, programmed the diabetes.

As many countries around the world acquire greater economic stability and wealth, their populations generally undergo a nutritional transition, moving from a diet rich in complex carbohydrates and low in animal fats and meat to an energy-dense, westernized diet. The thrifty phenotype hypothesis would predict that in such countries, for example, India, China and Brazil, generations of undernutrition impacting upon pregnant women and their offspring would drive high rates of obesity and diabetes that exceed those seen in the West, where affluent lifestyles have been the norm for several generations. In support of this hypothesis, it is noted that between 1985 and 2010, the prevalence of childhood obesity increased 40-fold in China, with the greatest increase observed in seven- to nine-year-olds (Song *et al.*, 2013). Among boys, the prevalence of obesity more than doubled between 2000 and 2010.

4.4.2 Mismatched environments

Gluckman and Hanson (2004) have proposed that the thrifty phenotype is just one aspect of a broader phenomenon, which they describe as the 'predictive adaptive response'. This is perhaps better considered as the mismatch between the environments experienced during the developmental period and later life. The concept of 'thrift' is clearly applicable to the handling of energy substrates and metabolic disorders, but does not cover the full gamut of conditions that are programmed by undernutrition. For example, there is a body of evidence that suggests that humans who were of lower weight at birth have a lower complement of nephrons in their kidneys (Hinchliffe *et al.*, 1992). The nephrons are the

functional units of the kidney and are responsible for the filtration of the blood and production of urine. Individuals with fewer nephrons are more prone to kidney disease and high blood pressure in later life. If nephron number is programmed in fetal development, this does not indicate a thrifty phenotype. This is more suggestive of an adaptation related to immediate survival of hostile environments that becomes maladaptive if the challenges in the adult environment are grossly different.

When the supply of nutrients to the fetus is restricted or when the passage of hormones from mother to fetus is indicative of stress, the pregnancy may be aborted or the fetus may undergo adaptations to its physiology that ensure immediate survival. Often, these adaptations will relate to a prioritizing of valuable nutrients and resources away from systems that are less critical for fetal survival (e.g. the lungs and kidneys, whose functions are met by the placenta) towards more critical systems such as the brain and circulatory system. This ability to adapt, due to the plasticity of fetal tissues, is clearly advantageous. Disease will only stem from this adaptive response if the new physiological make-up is inappropriate for the environment subsequently encountered by the individual. In the case of the kidney with fewer nephrons, there would be no adverse consequences unless the individual habitually consumed a diet rich in protein or sodium, necessitating greater renal function to process the load. On this basis, the responses that we refer to as programming may be considered favourable if the nutritional environment encountered during fetal life is persistent. Like the concept of thrift, a biological response that optimizes development for particular conditions will be advantageous only until those conditions no longer exist.

4.4.3 Tissue remodelling

The thrifty phenotype and mismatch hypotheses are merely conceptual frameworks and do not actually explain the biological processes that link maternal undernutrition, fetal physiology and later disease. One of the simplest mechanisms that can explain these phenomena invokes the process of tissue remodelling. Changes to the numbers of cells or the type of cells present within a tissue would reshape the morphology of that tissue and could have profound effects upon organ function.

The remodelling of organ structure could occur due to disruption of cell proliferation or differentiation at different developmental stages (Figure 4.14). In simple terms, all tissues and organs are derived from small populations of embryonic progenitor cell lines (Figure 4.2). During early embryonic development,

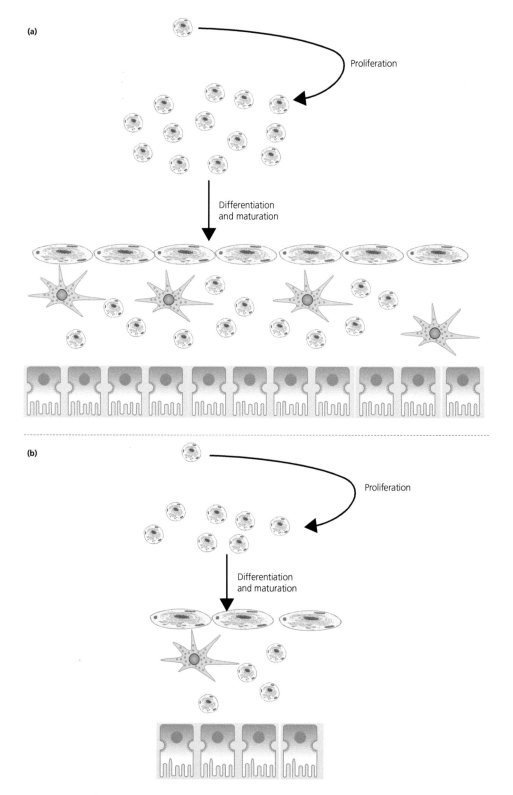

Figure 4.14 Tissue remodelling is an important link between early nutrition and later physiological function. Normal development of tissues and organs is driven by waves of cell proliferation, differentiation and maturation. This leads to formation of specialist structures with multiple cell types. The numbers of these functional units determines gene expression profiles, hormone secretion, responses to hormones, transport functions and cellular integrity. The way in which the tissue develops is therefore critical to the maintenance of homeostasis in response to future environment changes and ageing. (a) Normal development of a tissue element. (b) If proliferation and/or differentiation phases are impaired then the tissue will have fewer functional units and this cannot be recovered once the developmental stage has passed.

these cell lines proliferate, increasing the size of the embryo and early structures. In later fetal periods, they differentiate into specialized cell types, bringing about the maturation of the organs. A lack of nutrients or a disruption of normal endocrine signals during these developmental stages can alter tissue structure, leaving irreversible consequences.

There are many animal studies which demonstrate that tissue remodelling is a consequence of maternal undernutrition in pregnancy, but the kidney is the only organ for which the available evidence supports the view that this is a mechanism associated with human disease (see Research Highlight 4.2). Studies of rats exposed to maternal low-protein diets during fetal development show that this dietary manipulation results in the offspring developing a pancreas with reduced numbers of islets, which are smaller and less effectively vascularized than in control animals (Snoeck *et al.*, 1990). This has a major impact upon insulin production and hence glucose homeostasis at the whole-body level (Dahri *et al.*, 1991). Similarly, fetal and neonatal undernutrition in the rat alters the size, neuronal density and types of neurone present within the key appetite centres of the hypothalamus (Plagemann *et al.*, 2001).

Modifying the numbers and types of cells present within a tissue will have a range of consequences. It is easy to envisage how such changes might impact upon specialized functions that are dependent upon certain structures, as in the case of the kidney. Alterations to the profile of cell types present within a tissue may also modify the capacity of a tissue to produce or respond to hormones, up- or downregulate essential genes expressed within a tissue or interfere with cell–cell signalling pathways. Some of these changes may have very localized effects, simply impacting upon the function of a particular tissue, but others could disrupt whole-body physiology and metabolic regulation. For example, remodelling of a brain region such as the hypothalamus (Plagemann *et al.*, 2001) has the potential to disrupt most endocrine axes and hence the function of almost all physiological and metabolic systems.

4.4.4 Endocrine imbalance

The most widely recognized function of the placenta is to permit the exchange of nutrients, gases and waste products between mother and fetus. It should also be appreciated that there are critical endocrine signals that pass between placenta and fetus and between mother and placenta. These regulate

---

Research Highlight 4.2 Fetal programming of nephron number: evidence for programming driven by tissue remodelling.

The function of the kidney is to filter the blood, remove waste products and reabsorb nutrients. The kidney also plays a critical role in regulating the blood plasma volume and hence blood pressure. The basic functional unit responsible for renal capacity is the nephron. In humans, there is tremendous variation in nephron number and while the average complement is one million nephrons per kidney, nephron number may be a low as 300 000 (Brenner *et al.*, 1988). As all nephrons are formed before birth, the long-term function of the kidney can be determined by prenatal factors that influence nephrogenesis, and the number of nephrons present at birth must last throughout life. As nephrons are progressively lost with ageing due to infections, injury and hyperglycaemia, a lower nephron number at birth may predispose to impairment of renal function and high blood pressure with ageing (Kanzaki *et al.*, 2015).

Observations of human nephron numbers determined from samples taken at autopsy show that, in both babies and adults, nephron numbers are strongly related to weight at birth (Beech *et al.*, 2000; Hughson *et al.*, 2003; Koike *et al.*, 2017). Individuals with hypertension and chronic kidney disease tend to have fewer nephrons than healthy subjects (Luyckx and Brenner, 2020). Follow-up of individuals born in Helsinki between 1924 and 1944 showed that chronic kidney disease was more prevalent in those born at a lower birth weight (Eriksson *et al.*, 2018). There is therefore a strong body of epidemiological evidence to suggest that the setting of nephron number in fetal life plays a role in determining lifelong kidney function and risk of disease.

In rodents, nephrogenesis is not complete at birth and continues for 10 days after delivery. However, studies show that nephron numbers are acutely sensitive to variation in maternal nutrition. Feeding a low-protein diet (Langley-Evans *et al.*, 1999), an iron-deficient diet (Swali *et al.*, 2011) or a cafeteria diet during rat pregnancy reduces nephron numbers in the resulting offspring by between 30% and 40%. Similarly, maternal undernutrition in sheep results in reduced nephron numbers in lambs (Gopalakrishnan *et al.*, 2005). Fetal exposure to maternal undernutrition in rats is associated with high blood pressure and impaired kidney function (Joles *et al.*, 2010). As such animals age, they develop chronic kidney disease and in male rats exposed to low-protein diets in utero, this is the major cause of death (Langley-Evans and Sculley, 2006).

It is clear therefore that the intrauterine environment plays a key role in remodelling the fetal kidney and that the effects of this determine long-term health and disease. The fact that a deficit in the number of functional units in the tissue cannot be retrieved after birth, provides a clear indication of how the remodelling effects of adverse maternal environments become irreversible.

aspects of fetal development and also control the partitioning of nutrients to deliver the balance between maternal, placental and fetal requirements (Power and Tardif, 2005). There are hormones of placental origin, which are involved in the maintenance of pregnancy (e.g. progesterone), the preparation of the breasts for lactation (e.g. human chorionic somatomammotrophin) and the determination of the timing of labour (e.g. corticotrophin-releasing hormone). Other hormones may move from mother to fetus and these exchanges require tight regulation to avoid inappropriate fetal responses.

The glucocorticoids are steroid hormones that have a wide range of different functions. Classically, they act to maintain blood glucose concentrations, generally opposing the effects of insulin (Table 4.3).

Table 4.3 The classical actions of glucocorticoids.

System	Action
Metabolic	Inhibition of glucose uptake by extra-hepatic tissues
	Stimulation of hepatic gluconeogenesis
	Stimulation of lipolysis
	Mobilization of amino acids from extra-hepatic tissues
Physiological	Suppression of inflammatory responses
	Inhibition of bone formation
	Regulation of fluid balance
	Mediator of stress responses
	Control of feeding behaviour

They are also important stress hormones and have immunosuppressive effects. Most, although not all, the functions of glucocorticoids are mediated through their binding to the glucocorticoid receptor. As it is a classical nuclear receptor transcription factor (Figure 4.15), the glucocorticoid receptor is able to bind to glucocorticoid response elements within gene promoters and activate transcription of many different genes. Glucocorticoids are steroid hormones and are therefore able to cross cell membranes through passive diffusion. In the context of maternal–fetal exchange across the placenta, this is potentially problematic as, without any barrier mechanism, the hormones should be able to move freely between the mother and the fetus and could therefore upregulate fetal gene expression at inappropriate stages of development.

There is, however, a protective mechanism that should prevent this movement from occurring. Placental tissue expresses the enzyme 11β-hydroxysteroid dehydrogenase-2 (11βHSD2), which converts active glucocorticoids (e.g. cortisol in humans, corticosterone in rats) to forms that lack physiological activity (e.g. cortisone in humans, 11-dehydrocorticosterone in rats). 11βHSD2, therefore, acts as a 'gatekeeper' enzyme that limits the movement of active glucocorticoids into the fetal circulation (Figure 4.16). Indeed, there is a major gradient of glucocorticoids across the placenta, with maternal concentrations maintained at 100- to 1000-fold greater than in the fetus. This allows the fetal

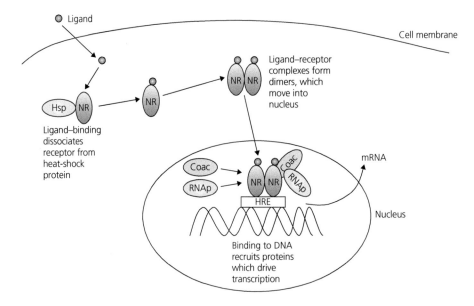

Figure 4.15 The mode of action of nuclear receptors. Nuclear receptors (NR) are typically located in the cytosol associated with heat shock proteins (Hsp). On binding ligand, the ligand–receptor complex forms dimers which bind to hormone response elements (HRE) on DNA, where they promote transcription. Coac, coactivator; RNAp, RNA polymerase.

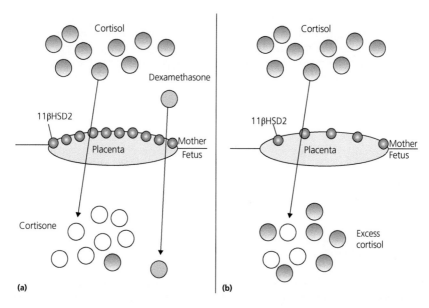

Figure 4.16 Placental 11β-hydroxysteroid dehydrogenase (11βHSD2) acts as a barrier to the movement of active glucocorticoids between mother and fetus. (a) Normal gatekeeper functions of 11βHSD2 convert active cortisol to inactive cortisone and hence protect fetal tissues from hormones of maternal origin. Only synthetic glucocorticoids such as dexamethasone may pass across the placenta unchanged. (b) In the undernourished mother, expression of 11βHSD2 in placenta is diminished and hence the fetal tissues are overexposed to active glucocorticoids.

hypothalamic–pituitary–adrenal axis to develop free of maternal influences and also ensures that maternal hormones do not interfere with the normal developmentally regulated patterns of gene expression within fetal tissues.

The consequences of excessive fetal glucocorticoid exposure are well documented. Glucocorticoids have the effect of restricting growth but promoting cellular differentiation, producing a smaller fetus with more mature organs. Synthetic glucocorticoids, which are only weakly metabolized by 11βHSD2, such as dexamethasone, are used clinically to enhance the maturation of the lungs of babies whose mothers are going into premature labour. Benediktsson *et al.* (1993) administered dexamethasone to pregnant rats throughout gestation and then assessed the impact of this treatment on their offspring. The rats exposed to prenatal steroids were smaller at birth, as expected, and as adults they had elevated blood pressure. This suggested that glucocorticoids, like maternal undernutrition, could programme long-term health and wellbeing. The involvement of 11βHSD2 in this glucocorticoid programming was confirmed by treating pregnant rats with carbenoxolone, which is an inhibitor of 11βHSD2 activity. Offspring from such pregnancies also had raised blood pressure as adults (Langley-Evans, 1997).

Clues to a role for 11βHSD2 in programming in human pregnancy have emerged from studies of pregnant women and their children in Finland. In Finland, salmiakki is a much-enjoyed food produced by treating liquorice extract with ammonium chloride to the liquorice extract. The characteristic flavour and sweetness of liquorice is due to glycyrrhizin, which is an inhibitor of 11βHSD. Strandberg *et al.* (2001, 2002) reported that consuming glycyrrhizin at more than 500 mg per week significantly shortened the length of gestation and increased the risk of preterm birth by twofold compared with consumption at less than 250 mg per week. The children of women who consumed salmiakki while pregnant exhibit signs that cognitive and behavioural functions have been programmed. Eight-year-olds with high fetal exposure were 2.6 times more likely to have attention deficit hyperactivity disorder and were more aggressive and more likely to break rules at school (Räikkönen *et al.*, 2009). When exposed to a social stress test, the children of high liquorice consumers had an exaggerated release of cortisol (Räikkönen *et al.*, 2010). This suggests that the liquorice exposure and the resulting greater exposure to maternal glucocorticoid associated with 11βHSD inhibition had a programming effect upon the developing hypothalamic–pituitary–adrenal axis. As this endocrine system plays a major role in homeostasis, effects upon metabolic and physiological function would be expected in these children as they age.

While this glucocorticoid-driven mechanism of programming may seem unrelated to nutritional programming, the two processes may be linked. In humans, lower expression or activity of 11βHSD2 is associated with lower birth weight and greater degrees of illness in premature infants (Kajantie *et al.*, 2006). McTernan *et al.* (2001) reported that 11βHSD2 mRNA expression in the placenta was lower in pregnancies complicated by intrauterine growth restriction. Most importantly, however, in rats, maternal protein restriction results in a lower activity of placental 11βHSD2, and this suggests that nutritional factors can alter the capacity of the placenta to protect the fetal tissues from maternal hormone signals (Langley-Evans *et al.*, 1996b). These hormone signals may provide the mechanistic link between undernutrition and long-term ill health. Indeed, treating pregnant rats fed a low-protein diet with a drug that inhibits synthesis of corticosterone prevented their offspring from developing high blood pressure.

There is, therefore, a body of evidence to suggest that undernutrition reduces the capacity of the placenta to maintain the maternal–fetal gradient of glucocorticoid concentrations. Overexposure to steroids of maternal origin will impact on tissue development and programme disease. It is relatively simple to see how this mechanism could trigger tissue remodelling, as the glucocorticoids would curtail proliferation of cells and promote differentiation. This is just one maternal–fetal hormone exchange that has been examined in the context of fetal programming. There are likely to be other such influences that are, as yet, unidentified.

4.4.5 Nutrient–gene interactions
4.4.5.1 Polymorphisms in humans
It is clear from epidemiological studies that the developmental programming phenomenon involves interactions of early life factors with the genome. Peroxisome proliferator-activated receptor γ2 (PPAR-γ2) is a ligand-dependent transcription factor that is predominantly expressed in adipose tissue where it regulates fat and energy metabolism. The PPAR-γ2 gene has a polymorphic region within exon B, and individuals may carry either an alanine coding or proline coding allele of the gene depending on their pro12ala genotype. Eriksson *et al.* (2002b) studied the relationship between this polymorphism, birth anthropometry and risk of type 2 diabetes in cohorts of men and women born in Helsinki between 1924 and 1933. The Ala12 allele was shown to be associated with markers of lower diabetes risk in these individuals, but the beneficial effect of the polymorphism was seen only in individuals who had been of lower weight at birth. Low birth weight individuals with the Pro12 gene variant were at greater risk of diabetes, hypertension and raised blood lipids, suggesting that a single genotype can give rise to different phenotypes due to variation in early life experience and variation in the quality of early life nutrition. Similar studies in a Chinese population found that there were associations between common variants of the zinc transporter SLC30A8, the transcription factor TCF7L2 and the potassium channel KCNQ1 and glucose metabolism. These associations were modified by weight at birth, such that impaired metabolism was seen with gene variants only when birth weight was below 3kg (Zhang *et al.*, 2015).

These examples are supportive of the idea that genetically determined risk of disease is modified by maternal diet or other factors that operate during fetal development and also impact on growth. However, an increasing volume of work suggests that the relationship between birth weight and disease in later life is wholly determined by genetics and is not evidence of developmental programming. A number of reports show that single nucleotide polymorphisms that are known to increase disease risk as also associated with lower birth weight. For example, the T677T variant of methylene tetrahydrofolate reductase, which is well known as a risk factor for coronary heart disease (see Section 1.3.2), was found to be associated with both low birth weight and elevated fasting insulin concentrations in 14-year-old children (Frelut *et al.*, 2010). Huang *et al.* (2019) analyzed data from 49 different studies and concluded that genetic predisposition to lower birth weight was also related to increased risk of type 2 diabetes. This may indicate an integrated mechanism linking fetal growth to later disease, or the low birth weight and diabetes may be parallel outcomes associated with particular genetic variants.

Analysis of data from over 300 000 individuals showed that the relationship between blood pressure and birth weight was entirely explained by genetic factors (Warrington *et al.*, 2019). Gene variants associated with lower weight at birth also associated with hypertension. Thus, a developmental programming explanation for the epidemiological observations between size and shape at birth and later disease, as described earlier in this chapter, may be called into question. However, it can be argued that the associations of disease with lower birth weight were only ever crude indicators of important maternal influences on fetal development and that they are no longer the most important evidence that programming determines the health and wellbeing across the lifespan. Data emerging from prospective cohorts (see Section 4.3.1.2) shows that maternal dietary patterns during pregnancy influence metabolic and cardiovascular functions in children (Bryant *et al.* 2015; Chatzi *et al.*, 2017; van Lee *et al.*, 2019). These observations and the extensive body of evidence from the Dutch Hunger Winter argue strongly for developmental programming of human disease.

Animal studies, which are free of confounding factors and where genetic variation is minimal, also convincingly demonstrate programming by nutrition. In most animal models, the impact of maternal diet on metabolic, renal or cardiovascular outcomes occurs in the absence of reduced birth weight. Importantly, nutritional programming has now been demonstrated in non-human primates, which makes it certain that the same processes will operate in humans. Young adult baboons exposed to 30% maternal food restriction in fetal life exhibited premature ageing of the heart, consistent with poor cardiovascular health (Kuo *et al.*, 2017). The same protocol altered function of the critical hypothalamic–pituitary–adrenal axis (Li *et al.*, 2017).

4.4.5.2 Gene expression in animals

The animal studies of programming outlined earlier consistently show that even brief periods of maternal undernutrition have the capacity to impact upon development of major organs (kidney, heart, liver, brain, adipose tissue, skeletal muscle). These changes are associated with disease processes. It is attractive to attempt to explore the mechanistic basis of programming by looking for changes in the expression of genes, proteins and pathways in the affected tissues of adult animals. This would be expected to give insight into the linkage between the fetal nutritional exposure and the physiological or metabolic consequences in the adult.

Many researchers have taken the approach of looking for differences in the expression of genes and proteins in older animals, comparing those exposed to a maternal nutrition insult in fetal life with unexposed controls. There are now thousands of reports in the literature which detail such differences. It is a mistake, however, to assume that the difference in expression of gene X, protein Y, or pathway Z in an aged animal explains how the animal's physiological or metabolic functions were programmed by diet in fetal life. Any observed differences are just as likely to be a consequence of the aged physiological state induced by maternal diet as they are to play a mechanistic role in programming. For example, aged offspring of rats fed a low-protein diet in pregnancy develop hepatosteatosis and show overexpression of genes and proteins associated with hepatic lipogenesis (Erhuma *et al.*, 2007). However, as young animals, the expression of the very same genes is suppressed in comparison with offspring of rats fed a control diet. This tells us that these genes cannot explain the programming mechanism. If experiments had only examined gene expression in older animals, incorrect conclusions could be drawn.

The gene expression changes that occur at the time of the maternal nutritional insult are of much greater interest, as these will show the true primary responses to nutrition that set in train the effects that ultimately lead to disease in later life. Under- or overnutrition during embryonic and fetal development could trigger a series of events, such as tissue remodelling or less effective regulation of hormone exchange across the placental barrier, that in turn have the long-term programming effect on fetal physiology. These primary nutrient–gene interactions may be difficult to observe as they may be transient. An insult in early life, which may be experienced for only a few hours or days, but which impacts on cell proliferation or differentiation during a critical phase of organ development, could have long-term consequences (Figure 4.17). In the case of the kidney, for example (see Research Highlight 4.2), a brief impairment of nephrogenesis might result in a 10% decline in nephron number at birth. Functionally, this would have no consequence until age-related loss of nephrons resulted in the organ no longer being able to maintain physiological function.

4.4.6 Epigenetic regulation

The gene expression patterns described earlier have often been found to represent permanent changes in the level of transcription of specific genes in specific tissues. For such patterns to persist throughout the lifespan of an animal, there must be mechanisms that preserve the cellular memory of the events that occurred in early life. Stable changes in the expression of genes can reasonably be attributed to changes in DNA methylation induced by maternal nutritional stimuli. DNA methylation is a potent suppressor of gene expression, either through blocking access of transcriptional machinery to the chromatin structure surrounding specific gene promoters or through interference with the binding of transcription factors to DNA (Figure 4.18). Around the time of embryo implantation, the majority of the genome is unmethylated, and this naïve state is remodelled as a normal element of development. The differentiation of tissues is accompanied by the

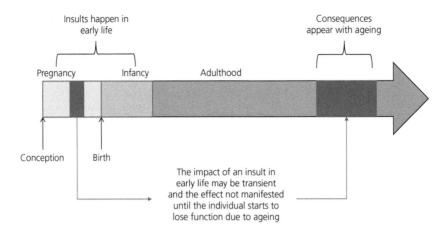

Figure 4.17 Maternal dietary factors influence fetal development during short windows of time. These may last for days or even hours. Insults during this time may have a permanent impact but are difficult to detect. Outcomes such as low birth weight may be crude indicators that changes to cells, tissues and organs, including tissue remodelling, have taken place. Observing an effect of maternal diet on gene expression in adulthood does not indicate that the change is a causal factor in the programming mechanism. It is far more likely to be a response to tissue remodelling and a part of the programmed phenotype.

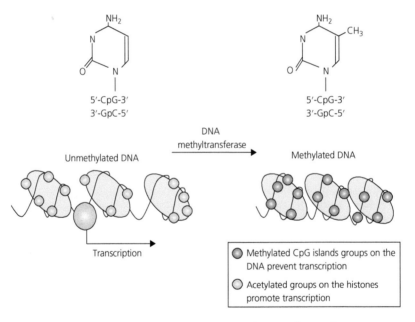

Figure 4.18 DNA methylation and histone acetylation are epigenetic mechanisms that regulate gene transcription. CpG islands in DNA may be methylated or unmethylated. In the unmethylated state, the histone proteins associated with the DNA tend to be acetylated and the DNA is less tightly coiled. Transcription factors and transcription machinery can access gene promoters and hence the unmethylated genes can be expressed. Methylation leads to deacetylation of histones and prevents transcription.

methylation and silencing of unrequired genes. A series of DNA methyltransferases (DNMT) are responsible for establishing and maintaining the patterns of DNA methylation within cells (Bird, 2002). DNMT1 is important during development, as it maintains the DNA methylation pattern when DNA replicates during cell division. This is essential for normal development; mice deficient for this gene die in utero. The other DNMT (DNMT3L, DNMT3a and DNMT3b), which are only expressed in the embryo, are responsible for de novo DNA methylation. DNA methylation patterns have been shown to be stably inherited and may therefore allow phenotypic traits, acquired as a result of nutritional

Table 4.4 Epigenetic regulation of gene expression.

Epigenetic mechanism	Effect
DNA methylation	Methylation of cytosine bases alters the interaction of DNA with transcriptional apparatus to silence gene expression. Effect is preserved when cells go through division.
Histone modification	Histone proteins H2A, H2B, H3 and H4 can be modified, altering the interaction of DNA with transcriptional apparatus. Acetylation of proteins increases expression, but methylation can both increase expression and silence expression dependent on type of amino acid residue that is methylated.
RNA-based regulation	Long and short non-coding RNA strands can silence expression by altering chromatin structure.

Epigenetic regulation is a process through which the same genotype in an organism can produce different patterns of gene transcription in different cell types and at different life stages.

programming, to be passed on to subsequent offspring. Thus, a brief period of undernutrition during embryonic, fetal or even early postnatal development may irreversibly modify DNA methylation in a manner that compromises normal physiology and metabolism. In addition to DNA methylation, modifications to the histone proteins which associate with DNA in chromosomes allow for epigenetic regulation (Table 4.4).

Epigenetic changes initiated by features of maternal nutritional status are believed to play an important role in the developmental programming of disease (Burdge *et al.*, 2007). The extensive resetting of DNA methylation marks during the embryonic and fetal period makes this process sensitive to the effects of under- or overnutrition. A wide range of evidence now points to methylation as both a biomarker and mechanism of nutritional programming. For example, differences in methylation were found at the insulin-like growth factor-2 locus between individuals exposed to the Dutch famine and their unexposed siblings (Heijmans *et al.*, 2008). In the same cohort, DNA methylation patterns differed between exposed individuals and controls subjects and were associated with variations in adult BMI but not glucose or lipid concentrations in circulation (Tobi *et al.*, 2018). Investigations of the consequences of the Great Chinese Famine yield similar findings. The famine, which lasted from 1959 to 1961, resulted in the deaths of tens of millions of people from starvation. Individuals exposed in utero have been shown to have greater abdominal

circumference as adults, and differential methylation of the insulin receptor gene appears to associate with this greater adiposity (Wang *et al.*, 2020).

In addition to observations of methylation differences following perinatal famine exposure, more direct measures of maternal nutritional status in human pregnancy and epigenetic regulation in offspring have been reported, but with mixed findings. Poor vitamin D status in pregnancy was found to lower weight at birth, but result in greater weight gain up to three years of age. This was not associated with epigenetic changes in a cluster of nine genes that regulate fetal growth (Benjamin Neelon *et al.*, 2018). A meta-analysis of 19 cohorts found that DNA methylation changes were causally involved in the relationship between maternal BMI and later outcomes for offspring, but only 8 of 9044 gene loci that were investigated showed methylation differences (Sharp *et al.*, 2017).

There is good evidence from animal models of undernutrition during fetal life that maternal diet can alter the epigenome, particularly DNA methylation, and this may establish changes in gene expression that permanently modify tissue structure or reset the responses to dietary and age-related challenges that occur later in life (Lillycrop *et al.*, 2007; Sinclair *et al.*, 2007; Bogdarina *et al.*, 2010; Altobelli *et al.*, 2013). Exposure to high-fat diets has also been shown to alter DNA methylation and histone marks in rodents, non-human primates and humans, with the brain being particularly sensitive to dietary influences (Jacobsen *et al.*, 2012; Seki *et al.*, 2012; Carlin *et al.*, 2013; Langie *et al.*, 2013).

Changes to the epigenome are likely to have a number of effects upon later health and wellbeing. Ultimately, the state of the epigenome determines whether genes are to be expressed or silenced. Epigenetic memory of transient nutritional exposures will determine how genes are expressed in response to further environmental challenges. The state of the epigenome is not entirely stable throughout life and so further nutritional or other influences will modify the memory or imprint of early life events. As epigenetic drift occurs, patterns of gene expression within tissues can change and this change has been linked to certain cancers and Alzheimer's disease. The nature of age-related drift may be partly mediated by early life events and the state of the epigenome in infancy.

Further interest in the role of epigenetic factors in determining fetal development and long-term health and disease risk has been sparked by observations which suggest that paternal diet has a programming effect in addition to maternal diet (see Research Highlight 4.3). As the father contributes

Research Highlight 4.3 The contribution of paternal diet to long-term health and wellbeing.

Evidence from epidemiology and experimental studies has shown that the developing fetus is acutely sensitive to variation in the quality of the maternal diet and metabolic status, and that both under- and overnutrition can programme long-term risk of disease. An even more remarkable series of observations suggests that the quality of the paternal diet may also be a key factor, despite the fact that fathers contribute no more than sperm to the embryonic and fetal environment.

The first observation of a paternal effect was reported by Ng et al., (2010), who noted that the female offspring of male rats fed a high-fat diet had abnormal pancreatic function. These offspring were glucose intolerant and the less healthy phenotype could be transmitted to a subsequent generation. Watkins and Sinclair (2014) fed male mice a low-protein diet for seven weeks prior to mating. The adult offspring of these matings were glucose intolerant, fatter and showed evidence of vascular dysfunction. Further studies showed that paternal protein restriction impacted upon fetal growth and, in particular, the attainment of bone mineral density (Watkins et al., 2017).

The mechanism which enables paternal nutritional status to influence fetal development is unclear. Sperm delivers genetic material, with accompanying epigenetic markers to the egg. The epigenetic markers comprise DNA methylation sites and small non-coding RNAs. These epigenetic markers are rapidly erased after fertilization occurs and it is not known how such transient signals can become integrated into the embryo and influence development (Galan et al. 2020). Seminal fluid is an often overlooked element of male ejaculate. The composition of seminal fluid partly determines the environment in which fertilization takes place and regulates the maternal response to fertilization by altering the inflammatory environment which drives embryo implantation (Robertson, 2007). When male mice were fed a low-protein diet, the epigenetic marks on sperm DNA were greatly altered (Watkins et al., 2018) but the cytokine concentrations in seminal plasma were unchanged. Further studies are needed to elucidate quite how the nutrition of males can impact on the long-term health and wellbeing of their offspring.

only sperm to the environment in which embryonic and fetal development takes place, non-genetic factors present in the sperm themselves, or in seminal fluid, must provide the essential signal of paternal nutritional status.

4.5 Implications of the developmental origins hypothesis

4.5.1 Public health interventions
The importance of developmental programming as a risk factor for human disease is currently difficult to estimate. There are, however, some interesting indicators that suggest it may be appropriate to target pregnancy for major health interventions. Depending on age, blood pressure differences between individuals weighing 2.5 kg at birth might be expected to be up to 5 mmHg higher than those who were a kilogram heavier (Barker, 1998). This is a negligible blood pressure difference for an individual, but if blood pressures were to decline by 5 mmHg across the whole population of the UK, there would be 50 000 fewer deaths from CVD. Developing public health interventions that can prevent adverse nutritional programming or offset some of the effects of prenatal nutrition may therefore be worthy of consideration.

For achievement of such goals, there are many possible options that could be considered. The simplest might be to improve the general advice given to pregnant women regarding the quality of their diets. However, more research would be required to determine what might constitute the optimal diet for fetal development. The possibility of using drugs in early life to counteract programming effects of undernutrition was explored by Sherman and Langley-Evans (2000). Pregnant rats were fed control or low-protein diets. Their offspring were then either untreated or administered losartan, an antihypertensive drug, while still being suckled by their mothers. When blood pressure was determined in the adult offspring, while untreated offspring of low-protein fed mothers had raised blood pressure, as expected, those treated with losartan had normal blood pressure (Figure 4.19). This suggests that postnatal interventions could be designed to overcome the intrauterine effects of nutrition.

Early intervention with drugs to prevent disease would carry many practical and ethical problems. There would be a high risk of adverse effects as well as the intended benefits, and the range of disease states that appear programmed would necessitate a major expansion of the pharmacological arsenal. The development of personalized nutrition advice is a highly desirable alternative. Personalized nutrition is a strategy whereby individuals are given advice about diet, physical activity and lifestyle based upon their genotype for particular traits associated with disease and other characteristics. Our growing knowledge of early life programming mechanisms and the interaction of early life factors and genotype could be used to formulate personalized nutrition approaches based upon the

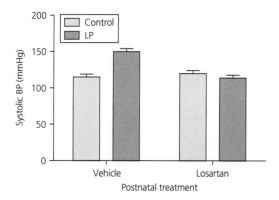

Figure 4.19 Postnatal treatment with antihypertensive drugs reverse programming effects of maternal undernutrition. Pregnant rats were fed control or low-protein diets in pregnancy. On giving birth, all animals were fed the same diet, but half the litters from each group were treated with losartan, an antagonist of the angiotensin II AT1 receptor for two weeks. Blood pressure was measured eight weeks later. Blood pressure of offspring from untreated rats fed a low-protein diet was elevated compared with controls, but the low protein-exposed rats treated with losartan had normal blood pressure. *Source:* data from Sherman and Langley-Evans (2000).

developmental origins hypothesis. Personalized nutrition could be used to target pregnant women to optimize the health of their children, or any individual could be given advice based upon a range of factors including genotype and characteristics at birth. Novel approaches to disease prevention will emerge by developing our understanding of how disease is determined through the early life interactions of genotype, epigenetics and the maternal environment (Figure 4.20).

4.5.2 Transgenerational transmission of disease risk

It is suggested that the programming influences of the fetal period upon disease in later life become apparent when there is a mismatch between the prenatal and postnatal environment. This is essentially the basis of the thrifty phenotype hypothesis. Babies whose growth was restricted by adverse factors during their fetal growth tend to exhibit catch-up growth in the postnatal period, that is, they grow more rapidly to achieve their genetic potential once the influence of maternal factors is withdrawn. There is good evidence to demonstrate

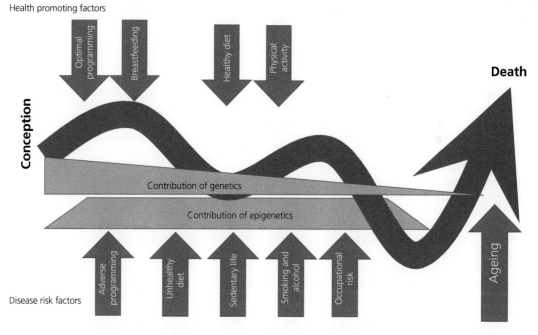

Figure 4.20 Life is a journey from conception to death and throughout that journey physiological and metabolic systems must respond to influences in the environment. In the early stages of life, genetic factors play the major role in determining how the individual responds to the environment and these genetic factors will be modified by fetal programming and tissue remodelling. With ageing, the significance genetics declines and the influence of epigenetics will become greater as epigenetic regulation plays a role in determining the response disease-promoting factors such as unhealthy diet or sedentary lifestyle. At every stage of life, the way in which the body responds to the environment will be shaped by earlier responses, so events such as fetal programming exposures, encountering infections, gaining or losing weight all have a cumulative effect over their life course.

that this rapid catch-up growth following prenatal growth restriction is one of the strongest predictors of the metabolic syndrome (Eriksson *et al.*, 2002a).

In populations that are undergoing economic and nutritional transition from poor to relatively affluent status (e.g. India, China, South Africa), the mismatch of early life influences and the adult diet and lifestyle might therefore be expected to drive an explosion of obesity, type 2 diabetes and CVD. The rapid improvements in maternal nutrition and health that will accompany the nutritional transition in such countries might be expected to lessen the importance of nutritional programming as a contributor to the overall disease burden. However, it is argued that programming could have effects that extend across several generations. The consequences of deficits in maternal nutrition in pregnancy might ultimately be transmitted to grandchildren. This means that across the globe, nutritional and economic transition may represent a sharp decline in malnutrition-related disease to be followed by half a century of unavoidable metabolic disease.

Pembrey (1996) proposed that such an inter-generational feedforward control loop exists, linking the growth and health of an individual with the nutrition of their grandparents. This form of control would be likely to involve some epigenetic marking of genes, with these markers then passed on to subsequent generations. The outcome of such imprinting would be very long-term health consequences for populations that are exposed to either undernutrition or overnutrition at some stage in their history. The complexity of the epidemiological studies that would be necessary to investigate intergenerational programming in human populations largely precludes such work. However, there are some examples that do appear to support the hypothesis advanced by Pembrey. Studies of individuals exposed to the acute but severe famine in wartime Holland indicate that undernutrition of women during pregnancy influenced the nutrition of their daughters, and this subsequently had an impact upon the birth weight of their grandchildren. Intergenerational effects are not necessarily the product of disturbances in maternal nutrition. Bygren *et al.* (2001) reported that the grandchildren of men who were overfed in the prepubertal growth period had a significantly shorter lifespan.

Intergenerational programming by nutritional insults in fetal life has been noted in studies of animals. Beach *et al.* (1982) assessed immune function in the offspring of mice fed a zinc-deficient diet in pregnancy. This nutritional manipulation in fetal

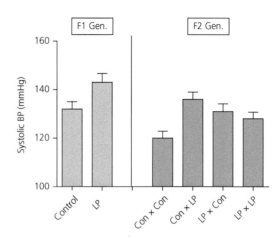

Figure 4.21 Programming of blood pressure across generations. Pregnant rats were fed control (Con) or low-protein (LP) diets in pregnancy. On giving birth, all animals were fed the same diet and when adult the offspring were mated to produce four separate crosses (control male × control female, control male × LP female, LP male × control female, LP male × LP female). Blood pressures of first-generation (F1) and second-generation (F2) offspring were measured at eight weeks of age. *Source:* data from Harrison and Langley-Evans (2009).

life led to severe immunosuppression in the adult offspring. Surprisingly, even though zinc status was normalized at the end of the original pregnancies, the impact on the immune system persisted into a third generation before resolving. The feeding of a low-protein diet in rat pregnancy produced high blood pressure in the adult offspring (Figure 4.21). When these adults were mated in all possible combinations of males and females from different dietary backgrounds, the next generation of adults were found to have higher blood pressure if they had at least one parent exposed to undernutrition as a fetus (Harrison and Langley-Evans, 2009). Drake *et al.* (2005) reported that the treatment of pregnant rats with dexamethasone in pregnancy, an intervention known to restrict fetal growth and programme hypertension and glucose intolerance in the offspring, produced effects on glucose homeostasis that persisted for two generations.

The main explanation of how programmed traits can be passed on to second or third generation is that the original nutritional insult initiates heritable epigenetic changes to DNA at specific gene loci, as described in Section 4.4.6, and evidence is beginning to emerge to suggest that this is the case. There are, however, other mechanisms that could explain intergenerational programming effects of undernutrition that are specifically transmitted via the maternal line. Rather than genomic imprinting playing a critical role, physiological or endocrine disturbances in mothers, particularly in the response to the challenge of pregnancy, may lead to programming responses in their offspring. For example, undernutrition during fetal life will induce insulin resistance and eventually type 2 diabetes in the resultant adult individual. In women, this will make gestational diabetes more likely to occur, which generally produces an overgrown baby. These babies are more likely to gain excess weight in childhood and adolescence and will themselves be more likely to become diabetic. Studies of rats fed low-protein diets in pregnancy and lactation show that this is in fact the case and that modification of pancreatic function during fetal life has effects that persist for several generations (Reusens and Remacle, 2001).

SUMMARY

- Programming is the process through which exposure of the developing fetus to an insult or stimulus at a critical stage of development can permanently alter physiology and metabolism.
- Exposure to undernutrition or overnutrition in early life is a risk factor for major disease states in adulthood.
- Epidemiological studies show that anthropometric measures associated with poor nutrition in fetal life, such as lower birth weight or thinness at birth, predict later risk of coronary heart disease and type 2 diabetes.
- Rapid catch-up growth in infancy following fetal growth restriction increases the disease risk associated with a poor maternal diet in pregnancy.
- Animal studies show that restricted intakes or excessive intakes of a variety of macro- and micronutrients in pregnancy programme obesity, glucose intolerance and high blood pressure in the developing fetus.
- Discovery of the mechanisms through which programming occurs will be an important first step in planning future public health interventions that may target pregnancy as a period for preventing major diseases of adulthood.
- Candidate mechanisms that have been proposed to explain the association between maternal nutrition and disease in the offspring include disturbance of maternal–fetal hormone exchange across the placenta, specific nutrient–gene interactions that impact on tissue development and disruption of epigenetic regulation of gene expression.

References

Aihie Sayer, A., Dunn, R., Langley-Evans, S. *et al.* (2001). Prenatal exposure to a maternal low protein diet shortens life span in rats. *Gerontology* **47**: 9–14.

Akyol, A., McMullen, S. and Langley-Evans, S.C. (2012). Glucose intolerance associated with early-life exposure to maternal cafeteria feeding is dependent upon post-weaning diet. *British Journal of Nutrition* **107**: 964–978.

Altobelli, G., Bogdarina, I., Stupka, E. *et al.* (2013). Genomewide methylation and gene expression changes in newborn rats following maternal protein restriction and reversal by folic acid. *PLoS One* **8**: e82989.

Arai, Y. and Gorski, R.A. (1968). Critical exposure time for androgenization of the developing hypothalamus in the female rat. *Endocrinology* **82**: 1010–1014.

Barker, D.J. and Osmond, C. (1986). Infant mortality, childhood nutrition, and ischaemic heart disease in England and Wales. *Lancet* **1**: 1077–1081.

Barker, D.J., Hales, C.N., Fall, C.H. *et al.* (1993a). Type 2 (non-insulin-dependent) diabetes mellitus, hypertension and hyperlipidaemia (syndrome X): relation to reduced fetal growth. *Diabetologia* **36**: 62–67.

Barker, D.J., Osmond, C., Simmonds, S.J. *et al.* (1993b). The relation of small head circumference and thinness at birth to death from cardiovascular disease in adult life. *British Medical Journal* **306**: 422–426.

Barker, D.J., Winter, P.D., Osmond, C. *et al.* (1989). Weight in infancy and death from ischaemic heart disease. *Lancet* **2**: 577–580.

Barker, D.J.P. (1998). *Mothers, Babies and Health in Later Life*. Edinburgh: Churchill Livingstone.

Bartley, M., Power, C., Blane, D. *et al.* (1994). Birth weight and later socioeconomic disadvantage: evidence from the 1958 British cohort study. *British Medical Journal* **309**: 1475–1478.

Battista, M.C., Oligny, L.L., St-Louis, J. *et al.* (2002). Intrauterine growth restriction in rats is associated with hypertension and renal dysfunction in adulthood. *American Journal of Physiology* **283**, E124–E131.

Bavdekar, A., Yajnik, C.S., Fall, C.H. *et al.* (1999). Insulin resistance syndrome in 8-year-old Indian children: small at birth, big at 8 years, or both? *Diabetes* **48**: 2422–2429.

Beach, R.S., Gershwin, M.E. and Hurley, L.S. (1982). Gestational zinc deprivation in mice: persistence of immunodeficiency for three generations. *Science* **218**: 469–471.

Beech, D.J., Sibbons, P.D., Howard, C.V., van Velzen, D. (2000). Renal developmental delay expressed by reduced glomerular number and its association with growth retardation in victims of sudden infant death syndrome and in "normal" infants. *Pediatric Development and Pathology* **3**: 450–454.

Benediktsson, R., Lindsay, R.S., Noble, J. *et al.* (1993). Glucocorticoid exposure in utero: new model for adult hypertension. *Lancet* **341**: 339–341.

Benjamin Neelon, S.E., White, A.J., Vidal, A.C. *et al.* (2018). Maternal vitamin D, DNA methylation at imprint regulatory regions and offspring weight at birth, 1 year and 3 years. *International Journal of Obesity* **42**: 587–593.

Bergel, E. and Belizan, J.M. (2002). A deficient maternal calcium intake during pregnancy increases blood pressure of the offspring in adult rats. *BJOG* **109**: 540–545.

Bird, A. (2002). DNA methylation patterns and epigenetic memory. *Genes and Development* **16**: 6–21.

Bo, S., Cavallo-Perin, P., Scaglione, L. *et al.* (2000). Low birth weight and metabolic abnormalities in twins with increased susceptibility to type 2 diabetes mellitus. *Diabetic Medicine* **17**: 365–370.

Bogdarina, I., Haase, A., Langley-Evans, S. *et al.* (2010). Glucocorticoid effects on the programming of AT1b angiotensin receptor gene methylation and expression in the rat. *PLoS One* **5**: e9237.

Brei, C., Stecher, L., Meyer, D.M. *et al.* (2018). Impact of dietary macronutrient intake during early and late gestation on offspring body composition at birth, 1, 3, and 5 years of age. *Nutrients* **10**: 579.

Breier, B.H., Krechowec, S.O. and Vickers, M.H. (2004). Maternal nutrition in pregnancy and adiposity in offspring. In: *Fetal Nutrition and Adult Disease* (ed. S.C. Langley-Evans), 211–234. Wallingford: CABI Publishing.

Brenner, B.M., Garcia, D.L. and Anderson, S. (1988). Glomeruli and blood pressure: less of one, more the other? *American Journal of Hypertension* **1**: 335–347.

Bryant, J., Hanson, M., Peebles, C. *et al.* (2015). Higher oily fish consumption in late pregnancy is associated with reduced aortic stiffness in the child at age 9 years. *Circulation Research* **116**: 1202–1205.

Burden, N., Chapman, K., Sewell, F. and Robinson, V. (2015). Pioneering better science through the 3Rs: an introduction to the national centre for the replacement, refinement, and reduction of animals in research (NC3Rs). *Journal of the American Association for Laboratory Animal Science* **54**: 198–208.

Burdge, G.C., Hanson, M.A., Slater-Jefferies, J.L. *et al.* (2007). Epigenetic regulation of transcription: a mechanism for inducing variations in phenotype (fetal programming) by differences in nutrition during early life? *British Journal of Nutrition* **97**(6): 1036–1046.

Bygren, L.O., Kaati, G. and Edvinsson, S. (2001). Longevity determined by paternal ancestors' nutrition during their slow growth period. *Acta Biotheoretica* **49**: 53–59.

Carlin, J., George, R. and Reyes, T.M. (2013). Methyl donor supplementation blocks the adverse effects of maternal high fat diet on offspring physiology. *PLoS One* **8**: e63549.

Catalano, P.M. (2003). Obesity and pregnancy: the propagation of a viscous cycle? *Journal of Clinical Endocrinology and Metabolism* **88**: 3505–3506.

Catalano, P.M. and Ehrenberg, H.M. (2006). The short and long term implications of maternal obesity on the mother and her offspring. *International Journal of Obstetrics and Gynaecology* **113**: 1126–1133.

Catalano, P.M., Presley, L., Minium, J. and Hauguel-de Mouzon, S. (2009). Fetuses of obese mothers develop insulin resistance in utero. *Diabetes Care* **32**: 1076–1080.

Chatzi, L., Rifas-Shiman S.L., Georgiou, V. *et al.* (2017). Adherence to the Mediterranean diet during pregnancy and offspring adiposity and cardiometabolic traits in childhood. *Pediatric Obesity* **12**: 47–56.

Chia, A.R., Chen, L.W., Lai, J.S. *et al.* (2019). Maternal dietary patterns and birth outcomes: a systematic review and meta-analysis. *Advances in Nutrition* **10**: 685–695.

Crozier, S.R., Inskip, H.M., Godfrey K.M. *et al.* (2010). Weight gain in pregnancy and childhood body composition: findings from the Southampton Women's Survey. *American Journal of Clinical Nutrition* **91**: 1745–1751.

Curhan, G.C., Chertow, G.M., Willett, W.C. *et al.* (1996). Birth weight and adult hypertension and obesity in women. *Circulation* **94**: 1310–1315.

Daenzer, M., Ortmann, S., Klaus, S. *et al.* (2002). Prenatal high protein exposure decreases energy expenditure and increases adiposity in young rats. *Journal of Nutrition* **132**: 142–144.

Dahri, S., Snoeck, A., Reusens-Billen, B. *et al.* (1991). Islet function in offspring of mothers on low-protein diet during gestation. *Diabetes* **40**(Suppl 2): 115–120.

Donahue, S.M., Rifas-Shiman, S.L., Gold, D.R. *et al.* (2011). Prenatal fatty acid status and child adiposity at age 3 y: results from a US pregnancy cohort. *American Journal of Clinical Nutrition* **93**: 780–788.

Drake, A.J., Walker, B.R. and Seckl, J.R. (2005). Intergenerational consequences of fetal programming by in utero exposure to glucocorticoids in rats. *American Journal of Physiology* **288**: R34–R38.

Erhuma, A., Salter, A.M., Sculley, D.V. *et al.* (2007). Prenatal exposure to a low-protein diet programs disordered regulation of lipid metabolism in the aging rat. *American Journal of Physiology* **292**: E1702–E1714.

Eriksson, J.G., Forsen, T., Tuomilehto, J. *et al.* (1999). Catch-up growth in childhood and death from coronary heart disease: longitudinal study. *BMJ* **318**: 427–431.

Eriksson, J.G., Forsen, T., Tuomilehto, J. *et al.* (2002a). Effects of size at birth and childhood growth on the insulin resistance syndrome in elderly individuals. *Diabetologia*, **45**, 342–348.

Eriksson, J.G., Lindi, V., Uusitupa, M. *et al.* (2002b). The effects of the Pro12Ala polymorphism of the peroxisome proliferator-activated receptor-gamma2 gene on insulin sensitivity and insulin metabolism interact with size at birth. *Diabetes* **51**: 2321–2324.

Eriksson, J.G., Salonen, M.K., Kajantie, E. and Osmond, C. (2018). Prenatal growth and CKD in older adults: Longitudinal findings from the Helsinki Birth Cohort Study, 1924–1944. *American Journal of Kidney Disease* **71**: 20–26.

Falkner, B., Hulman, S. and Kushner, H. (1998). Birth weight versus childhood growth as determinants of adult blood pressure. *Hypertension* **31**: 145–150.

Frelut, M.L., Nicolas, J.P., Guilland, J.C. and de Courcy, G.P. (2011). Methylenetetrahydrofolate reductase 677 C->T polymorphism: a link between birth weight and insulin resistance in obese adolescents. *International Journal of Pediatric Obesity* **6**: e312–e317.

Gambling, L., Dunford, S., Wallace, D.I. *et al.* (2003). Iron deficiency during pregnancy affects postnatal blood pressure in the rat. *Journal of Physiology* **552**: 603–610.

Galan, C., Krykbaeva, M. and Rando, O.J. (2020). Early life lessons: The lasting effects of germline epigenetic information on organismal development. *Molecular Metabolism* **38**: 100924.

Gardner, D.S., Bell, R.C. and Symonds, M.E. (2007). Fetal mechanisms that lead to later hypertension. *Current Drug Targets* **8**: 894–905.

George, G., Draycott, S.A.V., Muir, R. *et al.* (2019a). The impact of exposure to cafeteria diet during pregnancy or lactation on offspring growth and adiposity before weaning. *Scientific Reports* **9**: 14173.

George, G., Draycott, S.A.V., Muir, R. *et al.* (2019b). Exposure to maternal obesity during suckling outweighs in utero exposure in programming for post-weaning adiposity and insulin resistance in rats. *Scientific Reports* **9**: 10134.

Gillman MW, Rifas-Shiman S, Berkey C.S. *et al.* (2003). Maternal gestational diabetes, birth weight, and adolescent obesity. *Pediatrics* 111: e221–226.

Gillman, M.W., Rifas-Shiman, S.L., Kleinman, K.P. *et al.* (2004). Maternal calcium intake and offspring blood pressure. *Circulation* **110**: 1990–1995.

Gluckman, P.D. and Hanson, M.A. (2004). Living with the past: evolution, development, and patterns of disease. *Science* **305**: 1733–1736.

Godfrey, K.M. (2001). The 'gold standard' for optimal fetal growth and development. *Journal of Pediatric Endocrinology and Metabolism* **14**(Suppl 6): 1507–1513.

Godfrey, K.M., Forrester, T., Barker, D.J. *et al.* (1994). Maternal nutritional status in pregnancy and blood pressure in childhood. *BJOG* **101**: 398–403.

Godfrey, K.M., Robinson, S., Barker, D.J. *et al.* (1996). Maternal nutrition in early and late pregnancy in relation to placental and fetal growth. *BMJ* **312**: 410–414.

Gopalakrishnan, G.S., Gardner, D.S., Dandrea. J. *et al.* (2005). Influence of maternal pre-pregnancy body composition and diet during early-mid pregnancy on cardiovascular function and nephron number in juvenile sheep. *British Journal of Nutrition* **94**: 938–947.

Günther, J., Hoffmann, J., Spies, M. *et al.* (2019). Associations between the prenatal diet and neonatal outcomes-A secondary analysis of the cluster-randomised GeliS trial. *Nutrients* **11**: 1889.

Hales, C.N. and Barker, D.J. (2001). The thrifty phenotype hypothesis. *British Medical Bulletin* **60**: 5–20.

Hales, C.N. and Barker, D.J. (1992). Type 2 (non-insulin-dependent) diabetes mellitus: the thrifty phenotype hypothesis. *Diabetologia* **35**: 595–601.

Hales, C.N., Barker, D.J., Clark, P.M. *et al.* (1991). Fetal and infant growth and impaired glucose tolerance at age 64. *BMJ* **303**: 1019–1022.

Harding, J. (2004). Nutritional basis for the fetal origins of adult disease, in *Fetal Nutrition and Adult Disease* (ed S.C. Langley-Evans), 21–54. Wallingford: CABI.

Harrison, M. and Langley-Evans, S.C. (2009). Intergenerational programming of impaired nephrogenesis and hypertension in rats following maternal protein restriction during pregnancy. *British Journal of Nutrition* **101**: 1020–1030.

Hattersley, A.T. and Tooke, J.E. (1999). The fetal insulin hypothesis: an alternative explanation of the association of low birth weight with diabetes and vascular disease. *Lancet* **353**: 1789–1792.

Hawkins, P., Steyn, C., Ozaki, T. *et al.* (2000). Effect of maternal undernutrition in early gestation on ovine fetal blood pressure and cardiovascular reflexes. *American Journal of Physiology* **279**: R340–R348.

Heijmans, B.T., Tobi, E.W., Stein, A.D. *et al.* (2008). Persistent epigenetic differences associated with prenatal exposure to famine in humans. *Proceedings of the National Academy of Sciences of the United States of America* **105**: 17046–17049.

Hinchliffe, S.A., Lynch, M.R., Sargent, P.H. *et al.* (1992). The effect of intrauterine growth retardation on the development of renal nephrons. *BJOG* **99**: 296–301.

Holemans, K., Gerber, R., Meurrens, K. *et al.* (1999). Maternal food restriction in the second half of pregnancy affects vascular function but not blood pressure of rat female offspring. *British Journal of Nutrition* **81**: 73–79.

Huang, T., Wang, T., Zheng, Y. *et al.* (2019). Association of birth weight with type 2 diabetes and glycemic traits: A Mendelian randomization study. *JAMA Network Open* **2**: e1910915.

Hughson, M., Farris, A.B., Douglas-Denton, R. *et al.* (2003). Glomerular number and size in autopsy kidneys: the relationship to birth weight. *Kidney International* **63**: 2113–2122.

Huxley, R., Neil, A. and Collins, R. (2002). Unravelling the fetal origins hypothesis: is there really an inverse association between birth weight and subsequent blood pressure? *Lancet* **360**: 659–665.

Inskip, H.M., Godfrey, K.M., Robinson, S.M. *et al.* (2006). Cohort profile: the Southampton Women's Survey. *International Journal of Epidemiology* **35**(1): 42–48.

Jacobsen, S.C., Brøns, C., Bork-Jensen, J. *et al.* (2012). Effects of short-term high-fat overfeeding on genome-wide DNA methylation in the skeletal muscle of healthy young men. *Diabetologia* **55**(12): 3341–3349.

Joles, J.A., Sculley, D.V. and Langley-Evans, S.C. (2010). Proteinuria in aging rats due to low-protein diet during mid-gestation. *Journal of the Developmental Origins of Health and Disease* **1**: 75–83.

Kajantie, E., Dunkel, L., Turpeinen, U. *et al.* (2006). Placental 11beta-HSD2 activity, early postnatal clinical course, and adrenal function in extremely low birth weight infants. *Pediatric Research* **59**: 575–578.

Kanzaki, G., Tsuboi, N., Haruhara, K. *et al.* (2015). Factors associated with a vicious cycle involving a low nephron number, hypertension and chronic kidney disease. *Hypertension Research* **38**: 633–641.

Kind, K.L., Simonetta, G., Clifton, P.M. *et al.* (2002). Effect of maternal feed restriction on blood pressure in the adult guinea pig. *Experimental Physiology* **87**: 469–477.

Koike, K., Ikezumi, Y., Tsuboi, N. *et al.* (2017). Glomerular density and volume in renal biopsy specimens of children with proteinuria relative to preterm birth and gestational age. *Clinical Journal of the American Society of Nephrology* 12: 585–590.

Kuo, A.H., Li, C., Kuo, A.H., Li, C., Huber, H.F. *et al.* (2017). Maternal nutrient restriction during pregnancy and lactation leads to impaired right ventricular function in young adult baboons. *Journal of Physiology* **595**: 4245–4260.

Langie, S.A., Achterfeldt, S., Gorniak, J.P. *et al.* (2013). Maternal folate depletion and high-fat feeding from weaning affects DNA methylation and DNA repair in brain of adult offspring. *FASEB Journal* **27**: 3323–3334.

Langley-Evans, S.C. (1997). Maternal carbenoxolone treatment lowers birth weight and induces hypertension in the offspring of rats fed a protein-replete diet. *Clinical Science* **93**: 423–429.

Langley-Evans, S.C. and Jackson, A.A. (1995). Captopril normalises systolic blood pressure in rats with hypertension induced by fetal exposure to maternal low protein diets. *Comparative Biochemistry and Physiology* **110**: 223–228.

Langley-Evans, A.J. and Langley-Evans, S.C. (2003). Relationship between maternal nutrient intakes in early and late pregnancy and infants weight and proportions at birth: prospective cohort study. *Journal of the Royal Society for the Promotion of Health*, **123**: 210–216.

Langley-Evans, S.C., Sculley, D.V. (2006). The association between birthweight and longevity in the rat is complex and modulated by maternal protein intake during fetal life. *FEBS Letters* **580**: 4150–4153.

Langley-Evans, S.C., Gardner, D.S. and Jackson, A.A. (1996a). Association of disproportionate growth of fetal rats in late gestation with raised systolic blood pressure in later life. *Journal of Reproduction and Fertility* **106**: 307–312.

Langley-Evans, S.C., Phillips, G.J., Benediktsson, R. *et al.* (1996b). Protein intake in pregnancy, placental glucocorticoid metabolism and the programming of hypertension in the rat. *Placenta* **17**: 169–172.

Langley-Evans, S.C., Phillips, G.J. and Jackson, A.A. (1994). In utero exposure to maternal low protein diets induces hypertension in weanling rats, independently of maternal blood pressure changes. *Clinical Nutrition* **13**: 319–324.

Langley-Evans, S.C., Langley-Evans, A.J. and Marchand, M.C. (2003). Nutritional programming of blood pressure and renal morphology. *Archives of Physiology and Biochemistry* **111**: 8–16.

Langley-Evans, S.C., Welham, S.J. and Jackson, A.A. (1999). Fetal exposure to a maternal low protein diet impairs nephrogenesis and promotes hypertension in the rat. *Life Science* **64**: 965–974.

Li, C., Jenkins, S., Mattern, V. *et al.* (2017). Effect of moderate, 30 percent global maternal nutrient reduction on fetal and postnatal baboon phenotype. *Journal of Medical Primatology* **46**: 293–303.

Lillycrop, K.A., Slater-Jefferies, J.L., Hanson, M.A. *et al.* (2007). Induction of altered epigenetic regulation of the hepatic glucocorticoid receptor in the offspring of rats fed a proteinrestricted diet during pregnancy suggests that reduced DNA methyltransferase-1 expression is involved in impaired DNA methylation and changes in histone modifications. *British Journal of Nutrition* **97**: 1064–1073.

Luyckx, V.A. and Brenner, B.M. (2020). Clinical consequences of developmental programming of low nephron number. *Anatomical Record* **303**: 2613–2631.

Mathews, F., Yudkin, P. and Neil, A. (1999). Influence of maternal nutrition on outcome of pregnancy: prospective cohort study. *BMJ* **319**: 339–343.

Matthes, J.W., Lewis, P.A., Davies, D.P. *et al.* (1994). Relation between birth weight at term and systolic blood pressure in adolescence. *BMJ* **308**: 1074–1077.

McMullen, S. and Mostyn, A. (2009). Animal models for the study of the developmental origins of health and disease. *Proceedings of the Nutrition Society* **68**: 306–320.

McTernan, C.L., Draper, N., Nicholson, H. *et al.* (2001). Reduced placental 11beta-hydroxysteroid dehydrogenase type 2 mRNA levels in human pregnancies complicated by intrauterine growth restriction: an analysis of possible mechanisms. *Journal of Clinical Endocrinology and Metabolism* **86**: 4979–4983.

Moore, S.E., Cole, T.J., Collinson, A.C. *et al.* (1999). Prenatal or early postnatal events predict infectious deaths in young adulthood in rural Africa. *International Journal of Epidemiology* **28**: 1088–1095.

Neel, J.V. (1962). Diabetes mellitus: a 'thrifty' genotype rendered detrimental by 'progress'? *American Journal of Human Genetics*, **14**, 353–362.

Ng, S.F., Lin, R.C., Laybutt, D.R. *et al.* (2010). Chronic high-fat diet in fathers programs β-cell dysfunction in female rat offspring. *Nature* **467**: 963–966.

Norris, T., Crozier, S.R., Cameron, N. *et al.* (2020). Fetal growth does not modify the relationship of infant weight gain with childhood adiposity and blood pressure in the Southampton Women's Survey. *Annals of Human Biology* **47**: 150–158.

Osmond, C., Barker, D.J. and Slattery, J.M. (1990). Risk of death from cardiovascular disease and chronic bronchitis determined by place of birth in England and Wales. *Journal of Epidemiology and Community Health* **44**: 139–141.

Ozaki, T., Nishina, H., Hanson, M.A. *et al.* (2001). Dietary restriction in pregnant rats causes gender-related hypertension and vascular dysfunction in offspring. *Journal of Physiology* **530**: 141–152.

Parsons T.J., Power, C. and Manor O. (2001). Fetal and early life growth and body mass index from birth to early adulthood in 1958 British cohort: longitudinal study. *BMJ* 323: 1331–1335.

Pembrey, M. (1996). Imprinting and transgenerational modulation of gene expression; human growth as a model. *Acta Geneticae Medicae et Gemellologiae* **45**: 111–125.

Persson, E. and Jansson, T. (1992). Low birth weight is associated with elevated adult blood pressure in the chronically catheterized guinea-pig. *Acta Physiology Scandinavia* **145**: 195–196.

Plagemann, A., Harder, T., Rake, A. *et al.* (2001). Hypothalamic nuclei are malformed in weanling offspring of low protein malnourished rat dams. *Journal of Nutrition* **130**: 2582–2589.

Poore, K.R., Forhead, A.J., Gardner, D.S. *et al.* (2002). The effects of birth weight on basal cardiovascular function in pigs at 3 months of age. *Journal of Physiology* **539**: 969–978.

Poulsen, P., Vaag, A.A., Kyvik, K.O. *et al.* (1997). Low birth weight is associated with NIDDM in discordant monozygotic and dizygotic twin pairs. *Diabetologia* **40**: 439–446.

Power, M.L. and Tardif, S.D. (2005). Maternal nutrition and metabolic control of pregnancy. In: *Birth, Distress and Disease: Placenta–Brain interactions.* (ed. M.L. Power and J. Schulkin), 88–113. Cambridge: Cambridge University Press.

Prentice, A.M., Whitehead, R.G., Watkinson, M. *et al.* (1983). Prenatal dietary supplementation of African women and birth-weight. *Lancet* **321**: 489–492.

Räikkönen, K., Pesonen, A.K., Heinonen, K. *et al.* (2009). Maternal licorice consumption and detrimental cognitive and psychiatric outcomes in children. *American Journal of Epidemiology* **170**: 1137–1146.

Räikkönen, K., Seckl, J.R., Heinonen, K. *et al.* (2010). Maternal prenatal licorice consumption alters hypothalamic-pituitary-adrenocortical axis function in children. *Psychoneuroendocrinology* **35**: 1587–1593.

Reusens, B. and Remacle, C. (2001). Intergenerational effect of an adverse intrauterine environment on perturbation of glucose metabolism. *Twin Research* **4**: 406–11.

Robertson, S.A. (2007). Seminal fluid signaling in the female reproductive tract: lessons from rodents and pigs. *Journal of Animal Science* **85**: E36–E44.

Roseboom, T.J., Van Der Meulen, J.H., Ravelli, A.C. *et al.* (2001). Effects of prenatal exposure to the Dutch famine on adult disease in later life: an overview. *Molecular and Cellular Endocrinology* **185**: 93–98.

Samuelsson, A.M., Matthews, P.A., Argenton, M. *et al.* (2008). Diet-induced obesity in female mice leads to offspring hyperphagia, adiposity, hypertension, and insulin resistance: a novel murine model of developmental programming. *Hypertension* **51**: 383–392.

Schellong, K., Schulz, S., Harder, T. *et al.* (2012). Birth weight and long-term overweight risk: systematic review and a meta-analysis including 643,902 persons from 66 studies and 26 countries globally. *PLoS One* **7**: e47776.

Seki, Y., Williams, L., Vuguin, P.M. *et al.* (2012). Minireview: Epigenetic programming of diabetes and obesity: animal models. *Endocrinology* **153**: 1031–1038.

Shankar, K., Harrell, A., Liu, X. *et al.* (2008). Maternal obesity at conception programs obesity in the offspring. *American Journal of Physiology* **294**: R528–R538.

Sharma, S.S., Greenwood, D.C., Simpson, N.A.B. and Cade, J.E. (2018). Is dietary macronutrient composition during pregnancy associated with offspring birth weight? An observational study. *British Journal of Nutrition* **119**: 330–339.

Sharp G.C., Salas, L.A., Monnereau, C. *et al.* (2017). Maternal BMI at the start of pregnancy and offspring epigenome-wide DNA methylation: findings from the pregnancy and childhood epigenetics (PACE) consortium. *Human Molecular Genetics* **26**: 4067–4085.

Sherman, R.C. and Langley-Evans, S.C. (2000). Antihypertensive treatment in early postnatal life modulates prenatal dietary influences upon blood pressure in the rat. *Clinical Science* **98**: 269–275.

Sinclair, K.D., Allegrucci, C., Singh, R. *et al.* (2007). DNA methylation, insulin resistance, and blood pressure in offspring determined by maternal periconceptional B vitamin and methionine status. *Proceedings of the National Academy of Sciences of the United States of America* **104**: 19351–19356.

Smits, L., Krabbendam, L., de Bie, R. *et al.* (2006). Lower birth weight of Dutch neonates who were in utero at the time of the 9/11 attacks. *Journal of Psychosomatic Research* **61**: 715–717.

Snoeck, A., Remacle, C., Reusens, B. *et al.* (1990). Effect of a low protein diet during pregnancy on the fetal rat endocrine pancreas. *Biology of the Neonate* **57**: 107–118.

Soh, S.E., Chong, Y.S., Kwek, K. *et al.* (2014). Insights from the Growing Up in Singapore Towards Healthy Outcomes (GUSTO) cohort study. *Annals of Nutrition and Metabolism* **64**: 218–225.

Song, Y., Wang, H.J., Ma, J. *et al.* (2013). Secular trends of obesity prevalence in urban Chinese children from 1985 to 2010: gender disparity. *PLoS One* **8**: e53069.

Strandberg, T.E., Järvenpää, A.L., Vanhanen, H. *et al.* (2001). Birth outcome in relation to licorice consumption during pregnancy. *American Journal of Epidemiology* **153**: 1085–1088.

Strandberg, T.E., Andersson, S., Järvenpää, A.L. *et al.* (2002). Preterm birth and licorice consumption during pregnancy. *American Journal of Epidemiology* **156**: 803–805.

Swali, A., McMullen, S., Hayes, H. *et al.* (2011). Cell cycle regulation and cytoskeletal remodelling are critical processes in the nutritional programming of embryonic development. *PLoS One* **6**: e23189.

Tobi, E.W., van den Heuvel, J., Zwaan, B.J. *et al.* (2018). Selective survival of embryos can explain DNA methylation signatures of adverse prenatal environments. *Cell Reports* **25**: 2660–2667.

van Lee, L., Crozier, S.R., Aris, I.M. *et al.* (2019). Prospective associations of maternal choline status with offspring body composition in the first 5 years of life in two large mother-offspring cohorts: the Southampton Women's Survey cohort and the Growing Up in Singapore Towards healthy Outcomes cohort. *International Journal of Epidemiology* **48**: 433–444.

Veening-Griffioen, D.H., Ferreira G.S., Boon, W.P.C. *et al.* (2020). Tradition, not science, is the basis of animal model selection in translational and applied research. *ALTEX* **38**: 49–62.

Wang, Z., Song, J., Li, C. *et al.* (2020). DNA methylation of the INSR gene as a mediator of the association between prenatal exposure to famine and adulthood waist circumference. *Scientific Reports* **10**: 12212.

Warrington, N.M., Beaumont, R.N., Horikoshi M. *et al.* (2019). Maternal and fetal genetic effects on birth weight and their relevance to cardio-metabolic risk factors. *Nature Genetics* **51**: 804–814.

Watkins, A.J. and Sinclair, K.D. (2014). Paternal low protein diet affects adult offspring cardiovascular and metabolic function in mice. *American Journal of Physiology* **306**: H1444–1452.

Watkins, A.J., Sirovica, S., Stokes, B. *et al.* (2017). Paternal low protein diet programs preimplantation embryo gene expression, fetal growth and skeletal development in mice. *Biochimica Biophysica Acta* **1863**: 1371–1381.

Watkins, A.J., Dias, I., Tsuro, H. *et al.* (2018). Paternal diet programs offspring health through sperm- and seminal plasma-specific pathways in mice. *Proceedings of the National Academy of Sciences of the United States of America* **115**: 10064–10069.

Whincup, P.H., Kaye, S.J., Owen, C.G. *et al.* (2008). Birth weight and risk of type 2 diabetes: a systematic review. *Journal of the American Medical Association* **300**: 2886–2897.

Whitaker, R.C., Wright, J.A., Pepe, M.S. *et al.* (1997). Predicting obesity in young adulthood from childhood and parental obesity. *New England Journal of Medicine* 337: 869–873.

White, S.L., Perkovic, V., Cass, A. *et al.* (2009). Is low birth weight an antecedent of CKD in later life? A systematic review of observational studies. *American Journal of Kidney Disease* **54**: 248–261.

Woodall, S.M., Johnston, B.M., Breier, B.H. *et al.* (1996). Chronic maternal undernutrition in the rat leads to delayed postnatal growth and elevated blood pressure of offspring. *Pediatric Research* **40**: 438–443.

Wright, T., Langley-Evans, S.C., Voigt, J.P. (2011). The impact of maternal cafeteria diet on anxiety-related behaviour and exploration in the offspring. *Physiology and Behaviour* **103**: 164–172.

Wright, T.M., King, M.V., Davey, W.G. *et al.* (2014). Impact of cafeteria feeding during lactation in the rat on novel object discrimination in the offspring. *British Journal of Nutrition* **112**: 1933–1937.

Zhang, Y., Xiao, X., Zhang, Z. *et al.* (2015). Role of high-risk variants in the development of impaired glucose metabolism was modified by birth weight in Han Chinese. *Diabetes and Metabolism Research Reviews* **31**: 790–795.

Additional reading

If you would like to find out more about the material discussed in this chapter, the following sources may be of interest.

Patel, V.B., Preedy, V.R. and Rajendram, R. (eds) (2017). *Diet, Nutrition and Fetal Programming From Womb to Adulthood*. Cham: Humana Press.

Vaiserman A. (2019). *Early Life Origins of Ageing and Longevity*. Health, Ageing and Logevity, Volume 9. Cham: Springer.

Vinciguerra, M. and Cordero Sanchez, P. (eds) (2020). *Molecular Nutrition: Mother and infant*. London: Academic Press.

CHAPTER 5

Lactation and infant feeding

LEARNING OBJECTIVES

This chapter will enable the reader to:
- Describe the anatomy of the human breast and the synthesis of milk within mammary alveolar tissue.
- Demonstrate an understanding of the endocrine control of lactation.
- Discuss the extra nutrient demands that are imposed by lactation and the maternal dietary changes that may be required to meet those demands.
- Critically review the evidence that breastfeeding is beneficial for the health and wellbeing of mothers and their infants.
- Critically review global advice to exclusively breastfeed for six months.
- Describe trends in infant feeding behaviours seen in developed countries and discuss the global strategies that have been developed to promote breastfeeding.
- Discuss current guidance on breastfeeding and HIV infection.
- Discuss the composition of infant formula milks and describe the need for specialized formulas for premature babies and infants with food allergies and intolerances.

5.1 Introduction

The period of early infancy and the provision of nutrients in an optimal balance are critical for the immediate health and wellbeing of the child. It is also becoming clear that events that occur during this phase of development can also have a major impact upon the long-term physiology, metabolism and disease risk of the individual (Chapter 4). There are different strategies available for feeding infants in the first four to six months of life, and these include breastfeeding, bottle-feeding an artificial formula and a mixed approach using both breast and formula milks. The health of both the infant and the mother is best served by exclusive breastfeeding. This chapter reviews the processes through which human milk is produced and why breastfeeding is optimal for health and development. The chapter also describes the composition of formula milks and how these can be shaped to meet the varying demands of life stage and special clinical circumstances.

5.2 The physiology of lactation

5.2.1 Anatomy of the breast

The anatomy of the human mammary gland is shown in Figure 5.1. The breast is a major site of fat deposition, particularly during pregnancy, when high levels of oestrogen promote storage in preparation for later lactation. This fat underlies the skin of the breast and provides protection for the ducts and alveolar structures that are required for milk production. There are four key structures within the breast to be aware of in the context of lactation.

5.2.1.1 The nipple and areola

The nipples are surrounded by a dark pigmented region termed the areola. Both structures contain smooth muscle cells that will contract when mechanically stimulated, allowing the nipple to stiffen. This is essential to allow the suckling baby to grip the nipple and to take the whole of the area into its mouth (see Section 5.2.1.5). The nipple and areola also have structures called Montgomery's

Nutrition, Health and Disease: A Lifespan Approach, Third Edition. Simon Langley-Evans.
© 2021 John Wiley & Sons Ltd. Published 2021 by John Wiley & Sons Ltd.
Companion website: www.wiley.com/go/langleyevans/lifespan3e

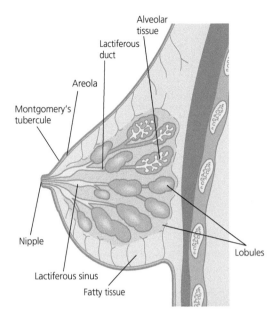

Alveolar tissue

Lactiferous duct

Areola

Montgomery's tubercule

Nipple

Lactiferous sinus

Fatty tissue

Lobules

Figure 5.1 The anatomy of the human breast. The breast comprises 10–12 lobules, each containing mammary alveolar tissue with associated lactiferous ducts. The ducts terminate at the lactiferous sinuses that discharge via the nipple.

tubercles, which are sebaceous glands that produce lubricants during suckling.

5.2.1.2 The lactiferous ducts
Each breast has 15–20 lobes in which the machinery for production of milk develops. Within each lobe lies a lactiferous duct that links the milk-producing tissues to the nipple where milk is released.

5.2.1.3 The lactiferous sinuses
The lactiferous sinuses lie at the nipple end of each duct. These sinuses provide some limited capacity for storage of milk between feeds but, more importantly, they are lined with contractile myoepithelial cells that have the role of ejecting milk from the nipple when the baby suckles.

5.2.1.4 The alveolar cells
The mammary alveoli are the site of milk synthesis. The key cells in these structures are the epithelial cells, which form a single layer around the alveolar lumen that drains into the lactiferous duct. Alveolar epithelial cells are polar in nature, meaning that there are specialized organelles on the basal side (the side of the cell in contact with the vascular system) and on the apical side (the side of the cell in contact with the alveolar lumen). This reflects the function of these cells, which requires uptake of nutrients from the blood and secretion of milk. The apical side of the cells

is therefore packed with secretory structures (Golgi apparatus, secretory vesicles and fat droplets).

5.2.1.5 The rooting reflex
Successful suckling requires that the baby correctly takes the nipple into the mouth and stimulates the nerve endings that lie beneath the areola. To achieve this correct latching-on, the human infant is born with an innate response called the rooting reflex. All newborn babies will turn their heads towards anything that strokes their cheek or mouth and open the mouth. Thus, brushing the cheek with the nipple will cause the baby to take it into the mouth and initiate suckling. The nipple is drawn up to the palate, and the tongue and palate then squeeze together to draw milk from the sinuses. The baby then starts the actual milking action, which involves a tongue movement from areola to nipple. These movements are instinctively coordinated with breathing and swallowing.

5.2.2 Synthesis of milk
The average composition of mature human milk is shown in Table 5.1. Generally speaking, women will produce 750–800 ml of milk per day at the peak of lactation and, within this milk, approximately 50% of the energy will be delivered as fat and 40% as carbohydrate. Carbohydrate is primarily delivered in the form of lactose and fats as triacylglycerols.

Table 5.1 The composition of human milk (selected nutrients).

	Units per 100 g milk		
	Colostrum	Transitional milk	Mature milk
Energy (kcal)	56.0	67.0	69.0
Protein (g)	2.0	1.5	1.3
Protein (% energy)	14.0	9.0	8.0
Fat (total, g)	2.6	3.7	4.1
Fat (% energy)	42.0	51.0	53.0
Carbohydrate (g)	6.6	6.9	7.2
Carbohydrate (% energy)	44.0	40.0	39.0
Calcium (mg)	28.0	25.0	34.0
Phosphorus (mg)	14.0	16.0	15.0
Sodium (mg)	47.0	30.0	15.0
Zinc (mg)	0.6	0.3	0.3
Riboflavin (mg)	0.03	0.03	0.03
Nicotinic acid (mg)	0.8	0.6	0.7
Vitamin B6 (µg)	Trace	Trace	0.01
Folate (µg)	2.0	3.0	5.0
Vitamin C (mg)	7.0	6.0	4.0
Vitamin A (µg)	177.5	91.2	62.0

Source: Data from Holland *et al.* (1991).

Table 5.2 Non-nutritive components of breast milk.

Class of bioactive agent	Specific forms in human milk
Hormones	Somatotrophin
	Calcitonin
	Ghrelin
	Adiponectin
	Leptin
Cells	Macrophages
	Stem cells
Cytokines	Interkeukin-6, -7, -8, -10
	Interferon γ
	Transforming growth factor β
	Tumour necrosis factor α
Chemokines	Granulocyte colony-stimulating factor
	Macrophage migration inhibitory factor
Anti-microbial agents	Mucins
	Lactoferrin
	Lactadherin
Immunoglobulins	Immunoglobulin-A, -G, -M
	Epidermal growth factor
	Vascular endothelial growth factor
	Nerve growth factor
	Insulin-like growth factors
Growth factors	Erythropoetin

Protein comprises casein and whey proteins (α-lactalbumin, lactoferrin).

The true composition of human milk is highly complex, as there are a number of non-nutritional components in addition to the basic nutritional requirements of the infant (Table 5.2). There is also a wide variation in composition between women and between breasts within the same woman. Some of this variation may be explained by the differences in quality of maternal diet and maternal body composition and stores. Human milk changes in composition at different stages across the full lactation period, with time of day and within the course of a feed. There are also known relationships between milk composition and maternal dietary intake.

The concentration of protein remains relatively stable in milk, irrespective of maternal nutrition (Lönnerdal, 1986). Similarly, milk lactose content does not appear to be strongly influenced by changes in dietary intakes (Smilowitz et al., 2013). Breast milk fat concentrations are, however, closely related to habitual maternal intakes as they are derived from a combination of maternal stores, dietary intake and de novo synthesis (Koletzko, 2016). Dietary trans-fatty acid and polyunsaturated fatty acids (PUFA) profiles in milk correlate strongly with maternal intake (Samur et al., 2009, Jonsson et al., 2016).

5.2.2.1 Foremilk and hindmilk

The first milk to be released during a feed is called the foremilk. Once the full letdown of milk occurs (see the following text), hindmilk is released. Foremilk tends to be less concentrated than hindmilk and may serve primarily to meet the thirst of the infant and provide some instant satisfaction of the desire to feed. The foremilk is lower in fat content and richer in lactose than the hindmilk and is therefore less energy and nutrient dense. As the hindmilk provides more of the energy requirements of the infant, it is important for the breast to be suckled for a lengthy period at each feed, rather than adopt the strategy of allowing the infant to suckle for only a few minutes on each breast at each feed.

5.2.2.2 Time of day

Several studies have documented that the composition of human milk varies during the course of the day. Lubetzky et al. (2006) reported that in mothers of premature infants who were expressing milk for their babies, the fat content of the milk was greater in the evening than in the morning. Similarly, Mitoulas et al. (2003) found that the fatty acid composition of milk from mothers of full-term infants varied over the day, with generally more fat produced in the evenings. The dynamic quality of milk composition may be explained by the diurnal variation in nutrient reserves of the mother or possibly by endocrine factors. Concentrations of macronutrients follow a general pattern of increase through the course of a day (Figure 5.2).

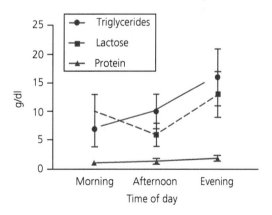

Figure 5.2 The composition of human milk varies across the course of a day. Milk samples were collected at hourly intervals from nine women in the first three months of lactation. Data are shown as averages in the morning (0800–1200 hours), afternoon (1200–1600 hours) and evening (1600–2000 hours). *Source:* Ward and Langley-Evans (unpublished data).

5.2.2.3 Course of lactation

The greatest variation in milk composition is associated with the developmental stage of the infant (Table 5.1). Mothers of premature babies produce milk that differs in composition to mothers of full-term babies. Preterm milk contains greater concentrations of protein, non-protein nitrogen, arachidonic acid and docosahexaenoic acid (DHA; Kovacs *et al.*, 2005).

The first secretions of the mammary gland following the birth of the baby are called colostrum. Colostrum is a thick, sticky, yellowish fluid produced in small quantities (around 100 ml/day). Because of the low quantity produced, it has long been believed that colostrum has little nutritive function and that it is instead a protective secretion that minimizes the infants' risk of infection and promotes maturation of the gut. Colostrum has a low content of lactose and fat and has a protein concentration that is considerably greater than in mature milk (Table 5.1). Most of the proteins in colostrum are protective factors, the principal elements being secretory immunoglobulin A (IgA) and lactoferrin. Colostrum is also rich in retinol.

Between three and seven days postpartum, the mammary gland switches from the production of colostrum to the synthesis of transitional milk. This milk is produced in a larger volume and has a lower protein and sodium content than colostrum. Lactose and fat concentrations are more similar to mature milk. Mature milk will be secreted from around 14 days postpartum.

A growing literature demonstrates that the composition of mature milk depends on a number of factors, including the age and size of the infant. Milk produced by mothers of preterm babies differs from that of mothers with full-term babies. Preterm milk is richer in protein and fat and has a greater energy content (Mills *et al.*, 2019). These differences are greater if the infant is also small for gestational age. The composition of preterm milk is less stable as babies age. Wei *et al.* (2019) reported that the phospholipid content increased with age, while this was not the case with full-term milk. As lactation proceeds, the carbohydrate content remains stable but the concentrations of fat, protein and some micronutrients (sodium, zinc, potassium and selenium) decline across the first six to seven months (Mills *et al.*, 2019; Sabatier *et al.*, 2019). Beyond this point, milk becomes more enriched and in women who continue to feed their infants beyond 18 months, the protein and lactoferrin concentrations increase significantly (Czosnykowska-Lukacka *et al.*, 2019).

5.2.2.4 Synthesis of carbohydrates

The primary carbohydrate within milk is lactose, which comprises approximately 80% of the total carbohydrate load. The remaining carbohydrate is in the form of oligosaccharides that are believed to have an immunoprotective role. Oligosaccharides escape digestion within the small intestine and pass to the colon, where they act as prebiotics. Prebiotic compounds provide substrates for the growth of bacteria within the colon. Maintaining a healthy population of *Lactobacillus* and *Bifidobacterium* species appears to reduce the risk of infection with diarrhoea-causing species.

Lactose is synthesized from glucose in the polar alveolar epithelial cells (Figure 5.3). Galactose is primarily synthesized de novo from glucose, although some galactose will be taken up from the maternal diet. Lactose is synthesized from glucose and galactose through the action of lactose synthetase, which is a multi-enzyme complex comprising galactosyltransferase and α-lactalbumin. Galactosyltransferase is expressed in the mammary glands during pregnancy, but as there is little α-lactalbumin, the mature complex cannot be formed.

Lactose synthesis occurs within the Golgi apparatus on the apical side of the alveolar epithelial cell. Lactose is packaged into secretory vesicles and because of the high osmolality of the disaccharide, the vesicles take up water and electrolytes such as potassium and sodium. Lactose synthesis is therefore responsible for generating the fluid portion of the milk. Secretory vesicles and their contents are discharged into the alveolar lumen by exocytosis.

5.2.2.5 Origins of milk fats

Milk contains fat in the form of emulsified droplets that consist of a mixture of triacylglycerides, diacylglycerides, monoacylglycerides, free fatty acids, cholesterol and phospholipids. Ninety-eight per cent of the fat is in the form of triacylglycerides. Lipid droplets are formed within the alveolar epithelial cells as lipids that are derived from maternal circulation or from de novo synthesis coalesce and migrate towards the apical side of the cell. The droplets are eliminated from the cells by exocytosis and, in this process, a small portion of the apical cell membrane is lost. This will therefore deliver some maternal phospholipids and cell membrane proteins into the milk (Figure 5.3). Glycerol for the synthesis of triacylglycerides is derived from the maternal circulation. This, together with the longer-chain fatty acids (16 or more carbon chain), is cleaved from triacylglycerides by the action of lipoprotein lipase in the mammary capillaries. As these fatty acids are derived from the

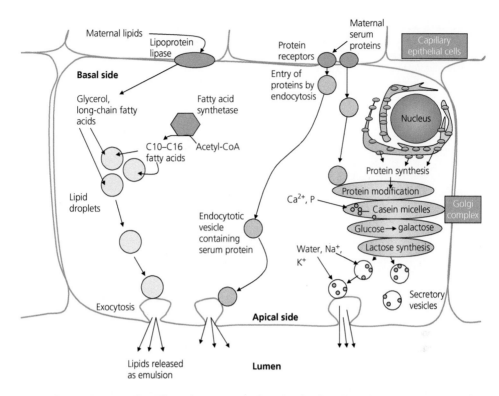

Figure 5.3 Synthesis of human milk. Milk synthesis occurs in the polar alveolar cells of the mammary tissue. Substrates for milk production are either synthesized de novo within the cytoplasm and Golgi complexes of the alveolar cell or are imported from the maternal circulation through endocytotic uptake on the basal side of the cell. Lipid droplets and maternal circulation-derived proteins are discharged to the alveolar lumen by exocytosis. Lactose, casein micelles, water and micronutrients are secreted to the lumen from the Golgi apparatus.

maternal diet, the composition of breast milk will therefore reflect the composition of the fats consumed by the mother. Shorter-chain fatty acids are synthesized within the cytosol of the alveolar cells. Acetyl-CoA, which is generated from the citric acid cycle in the mitochondria, is transported to the cytosol via the acetyl-group shuttle. Carboxylation generates malonyl-CoA, which is the substrate for the fatty acid synthetase complex, which progressively conjugates two carbon units up to C16 palmitic acid. Fatty acids of C10–C16 length synthesized in this manner will be incorporated into milk fat.

5.2.2.6 Milk proteins

Human milk contains a broad array of proteins, many of which have non-nutritive functions. In addition to the major milk proteins, casein, α-lactalbumin and β-lactoglobulin, which are synthesized de novo within the mammary epithelial cells, there are proteins that are derived from the maternal circulation. These include secretory IgA, lactoferrin, antiviral agents, enzymes and growth factors

(insulin-like growth factor 1, mammary-derived growth factor, insulin and nerve growth factor). IgA that is secreted into milk will reflect the antigen exposures of the mother and serves to protect the infant from gastrointestinal infection and to prime the neonatal immune system. Lactoferrin is an iron-binding protein that minimizes risk of infection of the infant gut by removing iron that could be used as a bacterial substrate.

Bloodborne proteins, including IgA, generally enter the alveolar cells from the basal side through passive mechanisms (Figure 5.3). Endocytotic vesicles will either deliver the proteins to the Golgi complex for packaging into the same secretory vesicles which deliver lactose and water to the lumen or will move across to the apical side of the cell and discharge the proteins through exocytosis. Proteins that are synthesized de novo within the alveolar cells are transported to the Golgi complex for posttranslational modification and secretion. Casein (of which there are $\alpha_s 1$, $\alpha_s 2$, β and κ forms), for example, is combined with calcium and phosphate

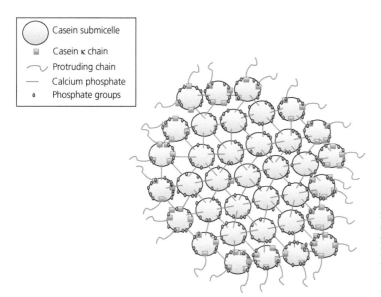

- ○ Casein submicelle
- ▪ Casein κ chain
- ∿ Protruding chain
- — Calcium phosphate
- ๐ Phosphate groups

Figure 5.4 The structure of a casein micelle. Micelles bind and transport calcium and phosphate in milk. The internal submicelles comprise hydrophobic α and β caseins, while those on the external surface of the structures incorporate hydrophilic κ casein chains.

to form a complex micelle structure (Figure 5.4). Hydrophobic α and β caseins form the core of these spherical structures with hydrophilic κ casein on the external surface (Phadungath, 2005). These casein micelles not only give milk many of its physical characteristics (e.g. the white colour) but also have an important biological function. Micelles carry large amounts of highly insoluble calcium phosphate in a liquid form. They then form a clot in the neonatal stomach, which increases the efficiency of absorption of these minerals. Micelles also deliver citrate, electrolytes and digestive enzymes such as lipase.

5.2.3 Endocrine control of lactation

Once established, lactation is under the control of a cascade of hormones of hypothalamic and pituitary origin. However, the actions of sex steroids produced during pregnancy and endocrine factors produced from the placenta are also critical in stimulating the maturation of the breast tissue and ensuring that milk production does not occur until after the birth of the infant.

5.2.3.1 The breast during pregnancy

The mammary glands are extremely sensitive to the actions of the sex steroids, oestrogen and progesterone. The development of the breast is primarily driven by these hormones and occurs in a number of distinct stages. The early stages occur during puberty in direct response to the rising concentrations of oestrogen and progesterone that occur at

this time. The actions of these hormones produce the structures shown in Figure 5.1. However, the full functional differentiation of the breast tissue does not occur until pregnancy. With the establishment of pregnancy, the breast undergoes extensive changes that are an essential preparation for feeding the baby after delivery. Oestrogen acts, together with growth hormone, to stimulate elongation of the lactiferous ducts. Progesterone and prolactin trigger alveologenesis where, essentially, new ducts are formed, branching off from the ducts formed during pubertal breast development, and new alveolar tissue is laid down around these ducts. While oestrogen and progesterone will be produced from the placenta, prolactin is a product of the anterior pituitary.

The main function of prolactin is to stimulate secretion of milk but, during pregnancy, the high circulating concentrations of progesterone and oestrogen inhibit this process. However, prolactin and the placentally derived human chorionic somatomammotropin are still able to act on alveolar cells to stimulate the maturation of the enzyme systems that will be required for milk production. Genes that encode human milk proteins have been shown to be expressed from mid-gestation, and this expression is under the control of prolactin.

5.2.3.2 Established lactation

After delivery of the baby, concentrations of progesterone and oestrogen fall rapidly and inhibition of the effect of prolactin on alveolar cells is lifted. Lactation is now principally governed by prolactin and the posterior pituitary hormone oxytocin. These hormones are produced in a coordinated manner which ensures that milk synthesis and release are coupled together (Figure 5.5).

The suckling of the baby provides stimulation to the mechanoreceptors located in the nipple. This sends nerve signals to the hypothalamus, which then coordinates the response. The hypothalamus releases prolactin-releasing hormone, which stimulates secretion of prolactin. Prolactin acts on the alveolar epithelial cells of the breast and milk is

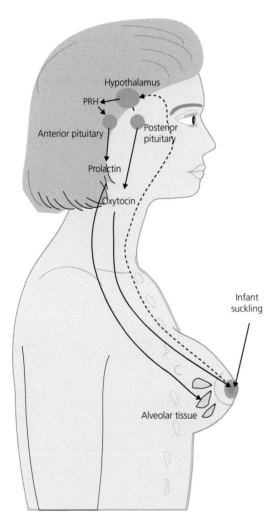

released into the alveolar lumen. Simultaneously, the synthesis of more milk is activated. Secretion of oxytocin by the posterior pituitary is stimulated by nerve impulses from the hypothalamus. Oxytocin acts on the myoepithelial cells surrounding the alveolar lumen and contractions move milk into the ducts, where further contractions forcibly eject the milk from the nipple (Figure 5.5). The ejection of milk should, in a correctly latched baby, lead to the transfer of milk directly to the throat of the baby. As a result, the baby does not need to suck, but simply to stimulate the nipple through action of their gums. This suckling 'technique' is markedly different from that required by a bottle-fed baby, which has to suck the teat to access the milk.

The coordinated secretion of prolactin and oxytocin is called the letdown reflex. In new mothers, letdown will be triggered solely by the mechanical stimulation of the nipples, but in women who have a well-established lactation or who have previously breastfed a baby, letdown can be triggered by other cues, such as the sound of a baby crying. The coupling of milk synthesis and release means that lactation is a demand-led process. Essentially, the more a baby suckles at the breast, the greater the stimulation of prolactin secretion and the more milk will be produced. This important principle lies at the heart of the advice to breastfeeding women to feed on demand. While bottle-fed babies are usually fed to a strict (usually four-hourly) schedule, breastfed babies need to control the feeding schedule to ensure that the supply is sufficient to meet their requirements.

In the very early stages of lactation, the baby will receive only small amounts of colostrum, which will not satisfy hunger. As a result, the baby may suckle 12–18 times in a 24-hour period. This gruelling period for the new mother serves to establish a good supply of milk once the inhibition of prolactin effect is lifted. Within a few weeks, a more predictable pattern of feeding (6–10 feeds per day) will develop and the breasts will produce sufficient milk to satiate the baby, which in the process develops the capacity to regulate its own food intake. During phases of more rapid growth, the baby will suckle more to obtain the extra energy and nutrients required, and the stimulus to the breasts will increase milk production accordingly. This is sometimes referred to as cluster feeding.

5.2.3.3 The breast after weaning

Once lactation has ended, the stimulation of mammary tissue by prolactin comes to an end. Remarkably, the remodelling of the breast tissue that occurred during pregnancy is then largely

Figure 5.5 The neuroendocrine control of lactation. Milk letdown is stimulated by activation of mechanoreceptors in the nipple. The hypothalamus coordinates the response to stimulation, involving oxytocin and prolactin, thereby ensuring that milk synthesis and release occur simultaneously. PRH, prolactin-releasing hormone.

reversed, as the milk production apparatus is essentially dismantled and reconstructed for any subsequent pregnancies. This process, termed involution, involves apoptosis of the epithelial cells of the mammary alveoli and recruitment of inflammatory cells to the breast tissue. Most of the new ducts and alveolar tissue are removed in this process, and the breasts enter a resting phase. Only the myoepithelial cells of the ducts and some secretory cells are retained, with the bulk of the alveolar tissue laid down in pregnancy replaced by fibrous tissue. At the end of reproductive life, complete involution occurs and the breast structure returns to the prepregnancy state.

During involution, the composition of human milk undergoes a change (Table 5.1). If weaning is gradual rather than abrupt, then this will impact upon the delivery of nutrients to the infant. Involutional milk is lower in lactose content but is richer in protein, fat and sodium. The composition changes occur because retention of unused milk in the breast forces apart tight cell junctions, allowing flow of extracellular fluids containing non-milk proteins and electrolytes into the ducts.

5.2.4 Maintenance of lactation

The demand-led nature of lactation means that it can be maintained for as long as the baby is suckled. In most westernized countries, breastfeeding beyond 9–12 months is an unusual behaviour, but in many other societies, prolonged breastfeeding (sometimes up to three years) is relatively commonplace. In such circumstances, the demand-led nature of the process means that women can maintain production of around 500 ml milk per day. Similarly, women who are feeding twins will produce twice as much milk as women feeding a singleton baby, as milk production matches demand. Lactation will come to an end only when the stimulus of suckling is withdrawn for 7–14 days. This results in a cessation of prolactin secretion and subsequently the cessation of milk production and breast involution.

Lactation is remarkably robust and even malnourished women appear able to maintain successful breastfeeding. Prentice et al. (1994) noted that extreme malnutrition (famine or near-famine conditions) is the only state in which milk production will be significantly impaired. There is no detectable relationship between the body mass index (BMI) of the mother and the volume or composition of the milk she produces. Very thin women (BMI <18.5 kg/m^2) appear capable of maintaining normal lactational performance.

There are circumstances where it may be necessary to temporarily avoid suckling the baby but maintain the lactation. Such a situation may arise if the woman requires a short period of medical treatment with drugs that are excreted into breast milk. This can be achieved through artificial withdrawal of milk from the breast using a breast pump. This process is termed expressing. In circumstances where the milk may be a hazard to the infant, an artificial formula can be used and the expressed breast milk discarded until safe to resume feeding. In circumstances where the baby is unable to feed, for example, due to prematurity, ill health or surgery, expressed milk can be safely stored and given from a cup, spoon or bottle, or mixed with solids at a later date.

5.2.5 Nutritional demands of lactation

Lactation is a highly demanding state for the mother, and there are undoubted increases in requirements for a broad range of nutrients while breastfeeding continues. However, with the exception of protein and energy, the exact nature of the altered requirements is generally poorly understood, and it is difficult to conclude whether lactating women need to make significant changes to the quality of their diet. Table 5.3 shows the increments for lactation that are added to UK reference nutrient intakes. For many nutrients, these levels of intake are likely to be met comfortably within the normal diets of women in westernized countries.

The micronutrient composition of human milk is relatively constant. Studies of women in developing countries where micronutrient deficiencies are endemic show that milk composition is most affected by maternal deficiencies of the water-soluble

Table 5.3 UK reference nutrient intakes (RNI) for lactating women.

Nutrient	UK RNI for lactation* (Lactation increment)	Estimated intake for UK women[†] mean (standard deviation)
Protein (g/day)	45.0 (+11)	63.7 (16.6)
Riboflavin (mg/day)	1.11 (+0.5)	1.6 (0.6)
Vitamin B12 (µg/day)	1.5 (+0.5)	4.8 (2.7)
Folate	200 (+60)	251 (90)
Vitamin C (mg/day)	40 (+30)	109 (63–160)
Vitamin A (µg/day)	600 (+350)	671 (633)
Calcium (mg/day)	800 (+550)	777 (268)
Magnesium (mg/day)	270 (+50)	229 (70)
Zinc (mg/day)	7.0 (+6.0)	7.4 (2.1)
Copper (mg/day)	1.2 (+0.3)	1.03 (0.38)

Sources: Department of Health (1991), Henderson et al. (2002).
* For the first 4–6 months of lactation.
[†] Non-pregnant, non-lactating women.
RNI, reference nutrient intake.

vitamins, thiamine, riboflavin, vitamin C, vitamin B6 and vitamin B12. Marginal maternal deficiency of these factors will limit milk concentrations, but supplementation restores milk vitamin content. With respect to folic acid and all the minerals, very severe maternal deficiency has to occur before any appreciable decline in milk concentrations is observed. Variation in maternal intake of fat-soluble vitamins has less impact on milk composition, as to some extent there is a reserve of these nutrients in adipose tissue. Maternal vitamin A status is, however, to some extent reflected in milk. Protection of milk composition against variation in maternal intake is achieved through mobilization of maternal reserves. For example, if intakes are less than optimal, calcium will be released from the skeleton to maintain milk calcium concentrations. Nakamori *et al.* (2009) reported that milk concentrations of iron, zinc and copper among undernourished Vietnamese women in the sixth to twelfth months of lactation, were not correlated with either maternal intake or maternal serum concentrations.

Dijkhuizen *et al.* (2001) studied mother–infant pairs in Java and found that the micronutrient deficiencies (vitamin A deficiency, iron-deficiency anaemia) observed in the mothers tended also to occur in their children. However, this was not well explained by the micronutrient composition of breast milk. Only 13% of variation in milk retinol and 24% of variation in milk β-carotene were explained by variation in maternal plasma concentrations. Compromised accumulation of infant reserves during fetal development or use of weaning diets low in these nutrients would be a much greater risk factor for infant deficiency. A study of Nepalese women and babies found that although maternal intakes and breast milk concentrations of n-3 PUFA were low, the red blood cell concentrations of docosahexaenoic acid were higher than in their mothers (Henjum *et al.*, 2018). This would suggest that infants can compensate for some aspects of maternal undernutrition through improved absorption from breast milk.

The energy requirements for lactation are extremely high, and over the first six months of lactation, a woman will need to mobilize approximately 115 000 kcal (481 MJ) for milk production. These figures are calculated on the basis that human milk has an energy content of around 0.67 kcal/g, that the conversion of maternal energy to milk energy is around 80% and that women will secrete around 750 ml milk per day. Thus, the energy cost of lactation is around 640 kcal (2.7 MJ) per day in the first six months of lactation, declining to around 510 kcal (2.1 MJ) per day beyond six months.

Most of the extra energy requirement will need to be derived from increasing energy intake within the maternal diet. Although some studies have suggested that there are metabolic adaptations to conserve energy, the balance of opinion is that resting metabolic rate and thermogenesis do not change in lactation. Physical activity levels tend to be lower in women in the first four to six weeks after childbirth, but energy savings achieved through a sedentary lifestyle are unlikely to have much impact on availability of energy for lactation. Most women will lose around 2 kg body weight per month during lactation, and this provides around 150 kcal per day for milk production. It is suggested therefore that women require approximately 500 kcal (2.1 MJ) per day extra within the diet to meet requirements during lactation.

The protein content of milk varies with the stage of lactation (colostrum contains 30 g protein/l, while mature milk has 8–9 g/l). It is estimated that women require an extra 11 g protein per day over the first six months of lactation, falling to 8 g per day for more prolonged breastfeeding to meet this demand. In developed countries, most women consume protein well in excess of this requirement and would not need to alter diet during lactation (Table 5.2). Studies of animals suggest that the protein content of the maternal diet has an influence upon the quantity and quality of milk produced, but it is not clear whether this is also true of humans. Generally, a higher protein intake is believed to increase milk volume, but variation in protein intake within normal ranges does not appear to alter milk composition. Some studies have shown that short-term reductions in maternal protein intake decrease milk protein and non-protein nitrogen content, but it is unclear whether longer-term reductions in protein intake have the same effect.

5.3 The advantages of breastfeeding

5.3.1 Advantages for the mother
5.3.1.1 Convenience and cost
Breastfeeding an infant carries a number of advantages for the mother, which encompass both the ease of childrearing and her short- and long-term health (Table 5.4). The most obvious advantage is the convenience of being able to feed the baby on demand, at any time and in any place, without the need for special preparation. Moreover, breastfeeding costs nothing, in contrast to formula feeding, which carries the cost of bottles, teats, sterilizing equipment and, of course, the infant formula itself.

Table 5.4 The health benefits of breastfeeding for women and their babies.

Group	Benefits
Women	Promotes uterine recovery
	Reduced risk of postpartum haemorrhage
	Delayed menstruation promotes recovery of iron stores
	Delayed menstruation may be contraceptive
	Reduced anxiety and better emotional bond with baby
	Lower risk of breast cancer
	Lower risk of endometrial and ovarian cancer
	Improved bone mass and reduced risk of osteoporosis
Babies	Priming of the immune system and reduced infection risk
	Lower risk of sudden infant death syndrome
	Less constipation and improved gastrointestinal function
	Reduced risk of childhood leukaemia
	Lower risk of type 1 diabetes
	Better IQ, developmental scores and behavioural traits in childhood
	Lower risk of childhood obesity
	Reduced atopy in children with a family history of allergy

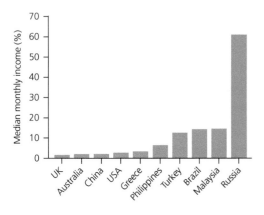

Figure 5.6 The cost of formula feeding. Data show the cost of one month's supply of powdered milk for a two- to three-month infant, as a proportion of the median monthly income for a single person. Increasingly, milk is purchased ready made up, which increases costs. In developed countries use of formula is greater in families on incomes below the median. For the UK, one month of supply would use approximately 3.5% of the income of a single person on the minimum wage.

The costs of formula can make up a significant proportion of the median monthly income of people in some countries (Figure 5.6). At the low end of the cost spectrum, a typical infant milk formula in the UK, for example, is likely to cost a family £6 (US$10) per week (2020), which for a lower-income family is still a significant investment. Milk voucher schemes exist to assist with this cost in some countries but are often unclaimed by parents.

5.3.1.2 Bond with infant

Breastfeeding helps to develop the emotional bond between the mother and baby. The act of feeding involves close physical contact and eye contact (termed mutual gazing), which is suggested to increase the quality of the mother–child relationship. Oxytocin secretion associated with the letdown reflex has the effect of reducing anxiety through increasing activity of the parasympathetic nervous system. This helps the mother to develop the emotional bond with her child and promotes her sensitivity to the needs of the infant.

5.3.1.3 Recovery from pregnancy

Breastfeeding aids the maternal recovery from pregnancy in a number of ways. Primarily, the early initiation of feeding promotes the involution of the uterus and reduces the risk that the mother will suffer a postpartum haemorrhage, as the uterus is a target for actions of oxytocin. Endocrine factors that control lactation also delay the onset of reproductive cycling, and this means that women who breastfeed will have a longer delay before resumption of their normal periods. Suckling inhibits the production of follicle-stimulating hormone and luteinizing hormone from the anterior pituitary. This lactational amenorrhoea confers two benefits. First, reduced blood losses help to preserve iron stores and hence lead to a more rapid recovery of normal iron status after pregnancy. Second, lactational amenorrhoea acts as a natural form of contraception. In populations where other forms of contraception are not readily available, this approach (which is estimated to be 90% effective in women fully breastfeeding for six months) helps to space out pregnancies. This has a number of benefits for maternal health, allowing full recovery between successive pregnancies, and in turn reduces the likelihood of children being of low birth weight and hence at greater risk of neonatal mortality.

Pregnancy is associated with extensive deposition of fat reserves that are primarily intended for mobilization during lactation to meet the energy requirements of milk production. It has been widely assumed therefore that breastfeeding will promote a more rapid loss of weight gained during pregnancy because of the high energy expenditure associated with lactation. The evidence base which considers the effect of breastfeeding on postpartum weight loss is complex and difficult to interpret, as a result of confounding. Many studies fail to control for the important influence of gestational weight gain, prepregnancy weight and lifestyle factors on post-partum weight loss, and as a result studies in this area often generate conflicting outcomes. For example, Lopez-Olmedo et al. (2016) found that women who exclusively breastfed for three months lost 4 kg more than women who did not breastfeed, while a study of women who were obese who had been diagnosed with gestational diabetes found that breastfeeding improved their insulin sensitivity without promoting weight loss (Yasuhi et al., 2019).

To see the possible benefit of breastfeeding for maternal weight loss, it may be necessary to follow women for longer after giving birth. Tahir et al. (2019) found that by five to six months postpartum, women who had maintained breastfeeding for more than three months had lost more weight than those who stopped feeding between one and three months into lactation. The systematic review of He et al. (2015) also found that breastfeeding had a small but significant benefit for postpartum weight loss. This became apparent between three and six months postpartum and exclusive breastfeeding led to 0.96 kg (range 0.53–1.40 kg) greater weight loss

than that achieved by women who formula-fed their babies.

5.3.1.4 Long-term health
Lactation carries a number of benefits for women in the longer term, with some evidence that it provides protection against several types of cancer and osteoporosis. As described in Research Highlight 5.1, the case for the role of breastfeeding in reducing the risk of cancer is compelling.

A number of studies have evaluated the impact of lactation upon maternal bone health. Milk production places heavy demands for calcium, and it is estimated that 200–225 mg calcium per day is transferred from mother to infant via breast milk. Over a period of a six-month lactation, this equates to an additional calcium requirement of between 35 and 40 g. Bone is a dynamic tissue and acts as a reserve for calcium that can be readily released in order to support the lactation. This results in changes in the level of bone mineral present within the maternal skeleton. This can be measured using the technique of dual x-ray absorptiometry, which determines the amount of bone mineral present per unit area of skeleton (bone mineral density, BMD). Typically,

Research Highlight 5.1 Breastfeeding and lifelong risk of cancer.

There is now compelling evidence to suggest that breastfeeding is protective against long-term risk of cancer in women, with benefits seen for a number of specific tumour sites and types. For some cancers, including breast cancer, risk is significantly reduced by having a child. This makes it challenging to dissect out the relative benefits of breastfeeding and pregnancy. For breast cancer, the Collaborative Group on Hormonal Factors in Breast Cancer (2002) examined data from 47 studies covering 50 302 women with breast cancer and 96 973 controls. They showed that cancer risk fell by 7% for every birth and that each year of breastfeeding independently reduced risk by 4.3%. A long-term follow-up of the US Nurses' Health Study from the 1970s showed that the benefits of breastfeeding depended on tumour type. Women who had breastfed were less likely to develop oestrogen receptor-negative breast tumours, but not oestrogen receptor-positive tumours (Fortner et al., 2019). John et al. (2018) reported that women who had never breastfed but had given birth were markedly more at risk of triple negative (negative for oestrogen receptor, progesterone receptor and human epidermal growth factors receptor-2) breast cancer (OR 2.02, 95% CI 1.12–3.63). This greater risk was seen only for women under the age of 50 years. A meta-analysis of 65 studies found that the risk of breast cancer in women who had exclusively breastfed children was lower than in those who had never breastfed and that breastfeeding was protective for both pre- and post-menopausal women (OR 0.72, 95% CI 0.58–0.90; Unar-Manguia et al., 2017). In women at very high risk of breast cancer due to mutation of the *BRCA1* gene, breastfeeding reduced risk by 32%, although no protection was observed for carriers of mutated *BRCA2* (Kotsopoulos et al., 2012).

The protective mechanism for breastfeeding has not yet been established. Animal studies have suggested that the acceleration involution of the breast that occurs if lactation is not established is associated with inflammatory processes which promote tumour formation. It is also likely that the protection derives from the suppression of menstrual cycles, which will also contribute to reduced risk of other gynaecological cancers, including ovarian and endometrial tumours. For endometrial cancer, although the very large European Prospective Investigation into Cancer (302 618 women) found no protective effect of breastfeeding (Dossus et al., 2010), other studies are more suggestive. Salazar-Martinez et al. (1999) found a 60% reduction in endometrial cancer risk when comparing women who had breastfed children with those who had never breastfed. A meta-analysis of 3 cohort studies and 14 case–control studies suggested that any breastfeeding had a protective effect on endometrial cancer (OR 0.89, 95% CI 0.81–0.98) and that longer duration (up to nine months) conferred increased protection (Jordan et al., 2017). Meta-analysis also showed significant protective effects of breastfeeding against ovarian and thyroid cancers (Sung et al., 2016; Yi et al., 2016). For ovarian cancer, more episodes of breastfeeding across the fertile years enhanced benefits. While breastfeeding one child reduced risk by 22%, breastfeeding three or more children reduced ovarian cancer risk by 51% (Modugno et al., 2019).

lactation for a period of six months results in loss of around 4–6% of BMD, with most losses coming from the spine and hip (Karlsson *et al.*, 2005). This loss of bone mineral occurs despite the fact that most lactating women reduce their intakes of alcohol and caffeine, which are known to exert negative influences on BMD. It is probably driven by low levels of oestrogen, resulting from suppression of the hypothalamic–pituitary–ovarian axis.

With these negative influences of lactation upon the skeleton, it is clearly important to evaluate whether breastfeeding is associated with long-term risk of osteoporosis, a disease associated with increased risk of bone fracture in older adults. A number of studies have shown that there are no long-term negative impacts of breastfeeding upon fracture risk. Crandall *et al.* (2017) followed up 93676 post-menopausal women and found that their lifetime history of breastfeeding was not related to hip fracture risk. Bjornerem *et al.*, (2011) found that breastfeeding was actually protective and among a population of 4681 post-menopausal women the risk of hip fracture was markedly lower in those who had breastfed at some point compared with those who had not (hazard ratio 0.50, 95% confidence interval, CI, 0.32–0.78).

While there is little evidence that breastfeeding for up to one year has a negative impact on future fracture risk, prolonged breastfeeding may reduce BMD. Among South Korean women breastfeeding for more than 24 months was associated with lower BMD at the lumbar spine and femoral neck (hip; Lee, 2019). Similar findings were reported in a Chinese population, but the negative impact of breastfeeding disappeared when the analysis corrected for confounding factors (Yan *et al.*, 2019). A meta-analysis from Chowdhury *et al.* (2015) found no evidence of a significant association between breastfeeding and BMD in the longer term.

The lack of evidence of increased osteoporosis risk associated with lactation in most women is explained by the fact that BMD is fully recovered once the infant is weaned and lactation ends. Most studies show that all bone mineral lost during lactation is replaced within 12–18 months of giving birth. A number of adaptive mechanisms appear to conserve calcium and promote remineralization, of which the most important is an increase in the capacity to absorb calcium from the diet. Bioavailability of calcium (i.e. the proportion of dietary intake that is taken up across the gut) in non-lactating women is approximately 25–30%. This increases with lactation to 32–52% but to an extent that reflects habitual intake. In a study of well-nourished US women, using radioisotope tracers, Ritchie *et al.*

(1998) showed that early lactation was not associated with a significant increase in calcium absorption, but that renal losses of calcium were reduced to around half of prepregnancy levels. This renal conservation was maintained at five months past the resumption of reproductive cycling.

5.3.2 Advantages for the infant

As described earlier in this chapter, the composition of human milk changes with the stage of infant development, across the day and across the course of a feed. These compositional changes and the robust nature of milk production, which ensures that nutrient content is maintained even by relatively poorly nourished mothers, guarantee that the nutrient availability for the infant is optimal. This aspect of breastfeeding can clearly be viewed from a teleological perspective, as ensuring that there are health advantages for the infant in the short term (Table 5.4). Similarly, from what is known about early life influences on long-term health and well-being (Chapter 4), it is reasonable to propose that breastfeeding will confer lifelong benefits.

5.3.2.1 Immunoprotection

In the short term, one of the most important advantages for the infant is derived from the immunoprotective factors that are present in milk and that are indirectly associated with the process of breastfeeding (Table 5.2). Among the developing countries, in particular, where hygiene and sanitation standards may be poor, the major hazards to infants are diarrhoeal infections and infections of the respiratory tract. Many factors contribute to risk of potentially fatal infectious disease in low-income settings, including unsafe water supply and storage methods, poor household hygiene and close exposure of infants to livestock and their droppings (Mbae *et al.*, 2020).

Breastfeeding is demonstrably protective. Among Ethiopian infants, initiation of breastfeeding within one hour of birth significantly lowered the prevalence of diarrhoea and respiratory infections up to the age of two years (Ahmed *et al.*, 2020). Exclusive breastfeeding was particularly protective in reducing the risk of diarrhoea (odds ratio, OR, 0.61, 95% CI 0.39–0.65). Similarly, Pakistani six-month-olds suffered less diarrhoea and fewer acute respiratory infections and fevers if exclusively breastfed (Saeed *et al.*, 2020).

In Vietnamese infants, the early introduction of formula feed or prelacteal feeding (compensating for the gap between delivery and establishment of lactation by feeding water, honey, fruit juices or formula), was associated with greater risk of hospitalization due to diarrhoea in the first six months of life. Formula feeding increased risk of diarrhoeal infections (OR 1.50 95% CI 1.02–2.21; Nguyen *et al.*, 2020). A survey of infant deaths in East African countries found that initiation of breastfeeding was associated with a 32% reduction in mortality over the first year (Agho *et al.*, 2010). Babies who were not exclusively breastfed in the first month were almost four times more likely to die before 28 days of age.

A large proportion of this protective effect can be attributed to the presence of immunoglobulins, lactoferrin, B lymphocytes, complement proteins and macrophages in human milk. These factors provide the capacity to actively combat infection and also bind out substrates that may be beneficial for bacterial growth. Breastfeeding is also protective against gastrointestinal infection, as provision of human milk ensures that fluids consumed by the infant are clean and free of contaminating factors. Poor sterilization of bottle-feeding equipment or the use of infected water supplies for formula preparation are avoidable causes of infection.

5.3.2.2 Sudden infant death

The term sudden infant death syndrome (SIDS) describes the sudden unexplained death of an infant under one year of age. Risk of SIDS is increased by parental smoking and alcohol use and by placing infants to sleep on their stomachs. Some studies have suggested that SIDS is more prevalent in formula-fed infants than in breastfed infants. Alm *et al.* (2002) examined 244 cases of SIDS from Scandinavia. After careful adjustment for potential confounding factors, it was found that short-duration breastfeeding (less than four weeks) was associated with 5.1-fold increased risk of SIDS, compared with breastfeeding for longer than 15 weeks. Similarly, Ford *et al.* (1993) reported that risk of SIDS was almost doubled in non-breastfed infants compared with those who were breastfed. A meta-analysis by Ip *et al.* (2007) concluded that breastfeeding reduced SIDS risk by 36%. Hauck *et al.* (2011) later confirmed the benefits of breastfeeding, with their analysis showing that any breastfeeding and exclusive breastfeeding for up to two months reduced the risk of SIDS by 62% and 73%, respectively. The possible explanation for the reduction in risk associated with breastfeeding could be a reduction in the occurrence of respiratory infections.

Advocacy of breastfeeding to reduce risk of SIDS creates an ethical dilemma. Risk of SIDS is increased by the practice of bed sharing (in which the baby sleeps with the parents). As bed sharing facilitates the establishment of breastfeeding, parents are faced with potentially contradictory advice about infant feeding and sleeping arrangements. There is some concern that parents may receive mixed messages relating to SIDS that will ultimately discourage breastfeeding.

5.3.2.3 Cognitive development

The last trimester of pregnancy and the first two years of life are the most rapid stage of brain development in humans. The brain increases in size from around 350 g at birth to 1100 g at 12 months of age. This rapid growth makes the brain vulnerable to adverse environments during this time, including undernutrition. Grantham-McGregor and colleagues (1991) showed in a group of Jamaican infants with stunted growth that a combination of nutritional supplements and stimulation through play increased developmental scores. This, like most other studies of this kind, indicated that the main effects of nutrition upon brain development were on the development of locomotor abilities. This is in keeping with the idea that rather than overall brain growth being vulnerable to undernutrition, it is specific brain functions that may suffer if nutrition is less than optimal.

As described in Research Highlight 5.2, investigating the impact of breastfeeding on the cognitive development of infants is problematic, but the balance of opinion is that breastfeeding is beneficial for brain development, There are numerous reports that longer duration breastfeeding is associated with better cognitive ability and fewer behavioural problems (Boucher *et al.*, 2017; Lenehan *et al.*, 2020). Guzzardi *et al.* (2020) reported that exclusive breastfeeding was associated with enhanced locomotor ability at two years of age and hearing and language ability between two and five years in girls. The benefits of breastfeeding may be assumed to be solely derived from factors associated with milk composition, but a follow-up of children from the Growing Up in Singapore cohort suggested that other factors may be involved (Pang *et al.*, 2020). Children who were fed human milk from a bottle or were breastfed performed better than formula-fed infants in cognitive tests at age 2 and 4.5 years. However, the infants who were given human milk from a bottle performed less well in tests of memory than those fully nursed by their mothers. Physical contact between mothers and infants may therefore have benefits additional to milk factors, perhaps through reduction of infant stress. Early stress in rodents is known to have permanent behavioural effects.

It is argued that most of the observed differences in behavioural and developmental outcomes noted between infants fed human milk and those fed

Research Highlight 5.2 Breastfeeding and intelligence quotient

Human intelligence is challenging to measure quantitatively, but a number of approaches may be taken for research purposes. These may include assessment of school performance, scores on specific standardized tests of memory, reading or verbal reasoning, and the standardized intelligence quotient (IQ). All such tests need to be validated for the population and age group under study. Intelligence by such measures is found to be strongly determined by the family environment in which individuals grow up and heritable factors. The latter may include genetics but, perhaps more importantly, parental involvement in activities which help the cognitive development of children will also be a component of this apparently heritable effect (Flensborg-Madsen et al., 2020).

The nature of the factors which determine IQ make the study of associations between breastfeeding and intelligence particularly difficult. Socioeconomic status, maternal and paternal intelligence, sex and birth order are all powerful confounders of any observed relationship. For example, in developed countries prolonged breastfeeding is a characteristic of better educated, wealthier women, so any relationship between infant feeding and later IQ is likely to be a product of a generally more supportive and advantageous learning environment. A number of studies have suggested that breastfeeding does have a positive impact on intelligence in the infant. Foroushani et al. (2010) reported that breastfeeding for longer was associated with infants achieving developmental milestones at an earlier age and better scores on tests of memory and reading in adults. Ten-year-olds who were predominantly breastfed for six months or longer, performed better in mathematics, reading and spelling in standardized tests (Oddy et al., 2011). Tests of IQ in children suggest higher scores at ages five and seven years in those who had been breastfed (Jedrychowksi et al., 2012; Strøm et al., 2019). It is suggested that these associations may result from greater supply of LC-PUFA during critical phases of brain development (Hartwig et al., 2019).

Although such reports are compelling, these findings are not universal. For example, Bernard et al. (2017) found that IQ was markedly higher in children who had been ever breastfed compared with never breastfed. This effect was no longer significant after adjustment for confounding factors. A small systematic review and meta-analysis which suggested a clear benefit of breastfeeding in development of intelligence (Horta et al., 2015) was poorly analysed and ignored clear publication bias (Ritchie, 2017). A much larger systematic review of 84 studies found that 45 reported a positive association between breastfeeding and measures of intelligence, of which 12 were of low quality (Walfisch et al., 2013). With the very strong influence of confounding factors, it seems that the only way to resolve the question of whether breastfeeding benefits intelligence would be to conduct a large observational study with the capacity to compare breastfed and never breastfed siblings.

formula milk are explained by the provision of particular fatty acids. In terms of composition, the brain is around 60% lipid and, in particular, it is rich in long-chain PUFA, arachidonic acid and DHA. Lipids become concentrated in the cell membranes of non-myelinated cells of the brain and in the retina and accumulate during the rapid phase of brain growth. DHA has been shown to be critical for the normal development of a number of visual and mental functions (Carlson et al., 1994). Extrapolation from animal studies suggests that over the first six months of life, infants accumulate high quantities of DHA of which approximately 50% will be incorporated into the brain (Cunnane et al., 2000).

DHA is not widely found in the diet; it is chiefly derived from fish oils. It can be synthesized from α-linolenic acid via a series of desaturase- and elongase-catalysed reactions, but it is generally considered that this pathway cannot support the high demand of the infant brain for this fatty acid. Thus, the delivery of DHA in a presynthesized form in breast milk may represent a significant advantage during the brain growth spurt. The DHA content of human milk varies considerably and generally reflects the maternal diet. Studies have shown that supplementation of women with fish oils can boost

DHA excretion in their milk. Typically, DHA constitutes 0.3–0.4% of the fatty acids present in human milk.

In the past, infant formula used in bottle-feeding contained negligible amounts of DHA, but many formula manufacturers now include long-chain fatty acids derived from egg, and these milks contain DHA at a level around 0.2% of total fatty acids. A number of international expert groups have published recommendations for optimal levels of DHA and arachidonic acid supplementation in term infant formula. Recommendations of 0.2–0.4% fatty acids for DHA and 0.35–0.7% fatty acids for arachidonic acid are based on the median worldwide range of concentrations of these fatty acids in breast milk. Given the contribution of long-chain n-3 fatty acids to brain development, is it suggested that increasing intakes may be of long-term benefit for development, especially in preterm infants who miss the last gestation surge in transfer of these fatty acids across the placenta. However, the case for supplementing infants either through formula or breast milk via their mothers to boost cognition is not fully established. A number of studies suggest some limited possibility of short-lived benefits. Enriching standard formula with DHA and arachidonic acid improved the visual acuity of infants at one year old (Birch *et al.*, 2007). Similarly, supplementing preterm formula with LC-PUFA was associated with better scores on tests of verbal intelligence quotient (IQ) and vocabulary in five-year-olds (Colombo *et al.*, 2013). However, a similar approach had no cognitive benefits for nine-year-olds who had been born preterm (Isaacs *et al.*, 2011). Similarly, Collins *et al.* (2015) observed no benefit of supplementing preterm infants with DHA when followed up at seven years. Meldrum *et al.* (2020) performed a trial of fish oils (DHA 250 mg, EPA 60 mg per day) for six months in breastfed infants and found no difference in cognitive or behavioural markers at six years of age. A meta-analysis of 38 randomized controlled trials of n-3 fatty acid supplementation of infants or mothers found some evidence of improvements in psychomotor and visual development, but no impact on IQ (Shulkin *et al.*, 2018).

5.3.2.4 Obesity

Some controversy surrounds claims that breastfeeding is protective against the development of obesity in childhood. The rising prevalence of overweight and obesity among children across the globe has prompted interest in the possible contribution of early life nutrition to this problem. In many developed countries, the beginning of an upward trend in childhood overweight coincided with widespread rejection of breastfeeding. Gaining a definitive view of whether breastfeeding is protective against childhood obesity is challenging. Inconsistencies in the methods used for breastfeeding data collection, definitions of breastfeeding and confounding factors that inevitably arise in such research make interpretation of research findings difficult. For example, women who are better educated and wealthier are more likely to breastfeed their infants and are more likely to have children that consume a healthy diet and exercise, hence avoiding obesity.

Arenz *et al.* (2004) performed a systematic review of the literature published between 1966 and 2003 to address the possible association between breastfeeding and childhood obesity. The meta-analysis associated with this review incorporated data from nine studies including 69 000 participants, aged 3–26 years. Breastfeeding was found to significantly reduce the risk of childhood obesity with an adjusted odds ratio of 0.78 (95% CI 0.71–0.85). In four of the nine studies, duration of breastfeeding was shown to be an important factor. Similar findings emerged from the systematic review of Weng *et al.* (2012), who found that the risk of childhood overweight was lower in breastfed compared with non-breastfed individuals

(OR 0.85; 95% CI 0.75–0.99). A number of other systematic reviews conclude that breastfeeding is protective (Lefebvre and John, 2014; Hess *et al.*, 2015) but all acknowledge that higher-quality research that adequately controls for confounding factors is required to fully address the issue.

A number of putative mechanisms have been suggested to explain a potential protective effect of breastfeeding. First, it is noted that formula-feeding leads to an earlier adiposity rebound (see Chapter 6). Early adiposity rebound is predictive of obesity later in life. Another explanation of a protective effect relates to the fact that breastfeeding is demand led and the infant controls energy intake. With formula-feeding, loss of infant control over intake causes the normal hypothalamic regulators of appetite to develop in a way that favours excess intake in the longer term. Furthermore, formula-fed infants have higher plasma insulin concentrations than breastfed infants. This favours early deposition of fat and an increase in fat cell number. Protection against obesity may also be attributable to the composition of human milk, which include the presence of bioactive factors that maintain a pattern of growth that favours a leaner body mass. The lower ratio of n-3 to n-6 fatty acids in formula milk compared with human milk promotes adipose tissue development.

5.3.2.5 Atopy

It has been suggested that breastfeeding may have an influence on the development of allergies in children, which will most commonly manifest as either atopic dermatitis (allergic eczema) or asthma. The main reasoning here is that formula feeding generally involves exposure of the infant to cow's milk proteins at an early stage of development. Allergies to cow's milk proteins are among the most common food allergies noted in children, but while using modified hydrolysed formulas (Section 5.6.4) reduces risk of allergy to cow's milk protein compared with standard formulas in high-risk infants, there is no robust evidence that breastfeeding is protective (de Silva *et al.*, 2014). Clearly, breastfeeding prevents this early exposure and sensitization but could also be beneficial since human milk provides passive immunity and promotes the development of the infant immune system. However, it is also clear that proteins and peptides can cross from the maternal circulation into milk, and so some argue that breastfeeding could increase risk of allergic sensitization by exposing the infant to allergens consumed by the mother. One study has shown that β-lactoglobulin from cows' milk is detectable in breast milk for up to seven days after the mother ingested it (Matangkasombut *et al.*, 2017).

Some groups have argued that women who show allergic tendencies themselves should restrict intakes of dairy products, nuts and other common food allergens while breastfeeding to lower risk in their children, but the evidence base suggests that this is neither necessary nor effective (de Silva *et al.*, 2014). A growing literature is also suggesting that early and frequent exposure to small amounts of antigens may be beneficial in preventing food allergies. However, Kelly *et al.* (2019) found that providing supplemental formula in the first few days of breastfeeding increased the risk of cows' milk protein allergy by 16-fold compared with infants who were never breastfed.

Atopy, a tendency to develop allergies, is strongly associated with genetic components, and the impact of breastfeeding on risk of atopic symptoms (atopic dermatitis, allergic rhinitis and wheezing) varies between children that have a family history of atopy and those who do not. Results are generally conflicting between studies and while some suggest that breastfeeding is protective, this is not a universal observation. Harvey *et al.* (2020) followed children of mothers with asthma over the first year of life. Breastfeeding for six months reduced the risk of wheezing in the infants by 40% when compared with infants who were formula fed. Among children of women with a history of allergic asthma, breastfeeding for 13 weeks or more reduced prevalence of atopic dermatitis by 40% (Kerkhof *et al.* 2003).

In children with no atopic heredity, there is no clear evidence that breastfeeding has either a beneficial or detrimental effect on risk of atopic dermatitis. However, Kramer *et al.* (2001), to date the only group to carry out a randomized controlled trial comparing breastfeeding with formula feeding, reported a 46% decrease in risk of atopic dermatitis when children were exclusively breastfed for three months. Observational studies tend not to support this observation. Although Kotecha *et al.* (2019) reported a 33% reduction in wheezing among 11-year-old children of the UK Millennium Cohort who had been breastfed, the systematic review of Güngör *et al.* (2019) could find no evidence that breastfeeding provided protection against wheezing, atopic dermatitis or allergic rhinitis. Many of the reported benefits of breastfeeding upon risk of atopy may be explained by confounding factors (Matheson *et al.*, 2012). The development of allergies is, for example, strongly related to respiratory infections in infancy. It is well established that breastfeeding reduces the prevalence of such infections. It is increasingly recognized that the gastrointestinal microbiome plays a pivotal role in development of food allergies. Galazzo *et al.* (2020) found that there were differences in the faecal microbiome of atopic and non-atopic infants and concluded that some bacteria genera and families may be protective (for example the *Lachinospiraceae*). Populations of bacteria in the gut may shift markedly with dietary stimuli in infancy, including cessation of breastfeeding and introduction of other foods.

5.3.2.6 Milk contaminants

Earlier in this chapter, the hazard of serious infection resulting from the preparation of formula milk using unsafe water sources was described. There are other forms of milk contamination which are avoided by infants being breastfed. Powdered milk formula may be contaminated in other ways during preparation. For example, the transfer of microbes from hand to utensils and then to milk was reported in a study from South Korea (Cho *et al.*, 2019), and poor hand hygiene among caregivers can be an issue in any setting. There are periodic episodes of microbial contamination of formula milk powder in factories. In 2017, a French manufacturer was forced to recall its milk globally because of a salmonella infection at source.

In addition to pathogens in formula milk, there are reports that environmental contaminants are found in milk formula, but below toxic levels. These include plasticizers, pesticides, flame retardants and heavy metals (Lehmann *et al.*, 2018). Most notoriously, in 2008, a Chinese formula manufacturer deliberately added melamine to milk powder to disguise the low protein content of the product. Six babies died and 54 000 were hospitalized as a consequence.

Breastfeeding clearly provides protection against most of these hazards but does not ensure that infants are not exposed to contaminants. The metabolic processes which have evolved to eliminate xenobiotics from the body include excretion of modified forms into breast milk. Breast milk therefore, like formula, contains low levels of environmental contaminants, including heavy metals (Lehmann *et al.*, 2018). Alcohol will appear in milk when women who are lactating consume it, with the peak level appearing in milk between 30 and 90 minutes after drinking. Caffeine is also eliminated in milk, but intakes below 300 mg per day are considered safe. Approximately 1% of the dose of medications will pass into breast milk following maternal consumption. Most are safe to use but some should be avoided, such as codeine. The pharmacokinetics of all prescription and over-the-counter medicines are well understood and breastfeeding women should read drug information literature or seek advice before taking any medication. In some cases, medication and breastfeeding are incompatible due to drugs passing into milk at levels that cannot be safely metabolized by the infant liver (e.g. chemotherapy agents used in cancer treatment) so breastfeeding will not be possible.

5.3.3 Recommendation to breastfeed for six months

In 1990, participants at a World Health Organization (WHO)/Unicef policymakers' meeting on breastfeeding produced the Innocenti Declaration. This was in recognition of the fact that breastfeeding provides optimal infant nutrition and carries significant benefits for the health of infants and their mothers. The declaration set out a number of global goals and operational targets. The central aims were:

- To ensure optimal maternal and child health, all women should be enabled to practise exclusive breastfeeding for four to six months.
- To reinforce a breastfeeding culture and defend this against development of a bottle-feeding culture.
- To increase confidence of women in their ability to breastfeed.
- To ensure that women are adequately nourished. The declaration called upon all governments to take effective steps to centrally coordinate breastfeeding promotion and enact legislation to protect the rights of women to breastfeed. International organizations were called upon to develop action plans to promote and support breastfeeding and to support national governments in delivering breastfeeding policies.

The main outcome of the Innocenti Declaration was the establishment of a global policy for the promotion of breastfeeding. At the heart of this is the WHO/Unicef recommendation that infants should be exclusively breastfed for the first six months of life. The benefits of such a policy for infant and maternal health are clear, particularly in the developing countries. The most important advantage is the reduction in the risk of gastrointestinal infection, which is a major killer of infants. Globally, diarrhoeal disease is a cause of up to two million deaths among under-fives each year.

While the overwhelming benefits of exclusive breastfeeding for six months outweigh potential hazards in most developing countries, there are some suggestions that four to six months might be a more appropriate guideline in developed countries. In fact, not all countries have adopted the WHO advice, and while the UK and Australia are among those that have, the majority of European countries and the United States have alternative guidance.

The WHO recommendations were largely based upon the systematic review of Kramer and Kakuma originally published in 2002, which had evaluated the impact of exclusive breastfeeding upon maternal and infant health. This showed clear benefits in terms of infant growth, maternal recovery of iron stores postpartum and, most importantly, a reduction in infection among infants. The relevance of the WHO recommendations for developing countries where infectious disease is the driver of high infant mortality is not disputed.

For developed countries, where the morbidity and mortality associated with infection are controlled through other means, there are important concerns about the appropriateness of the guidance to exclusively breastfeed for six months (Fewtrell, 2011). The main concern is that exclusive breastfeeding may not be adequate to meet nutrient requirements for a full six months. Iron deficiency is the major issue as human milk is a poor source of iron and infants must rely on stores accrued before birth. Chantry et al. (2007) reported that, among US infants exclusively breastfed for more than six months, there was a 10% prevalence of iron-deficiency anaemia compared with 2.3% among children exclusively breastfed for four months or up to six months. Iron-deficiency anaemia in infants is associated with irreversible deficits in motor, cognitive and social development (Lozoff and Georgieff, 2006; Algarín et al., 2013), and this risk of deficiency must be carefully weighed against the immune benefits of breastfeeding.

An update of the Kramer and Kakuma (2012) review concluded that there were no deficits in infant growth associated with six months of exclusive breastfeeding in either developed or developing countries. Risk of iron deficiency was confined to developing countries, where the iron stores accrued by the infant in utero may be compromised by poor maternal iron status. Breastfeeding with iron supplementation may therefore be an effective strategy for preventing iron deficiency in infants who are exclusively breastfed. Wells et al. (2012) conducted a randomized controlled trial in Iceland, in which infants were randomized to either four- or six-months of exclusive breastfeeding. In keeping with the Kramer and Kakuma (2012) evidence, the study found no deficits in infant growth, body composition or energy intake associated with a longer duration of exclusive breastfeeding.

Another concern relates to coeliac disease, which is an autoimmune disorder resulting in inflammation of the gastrointestinal tract if gluten is consumed. There is some evidence that there is an optimal time frame for exposure of the gastrointestinal tract to allergens such as gluten. If exclusive breastfeeding is maintained for longer than that time period, then allergic sensitization may be more likely. Olsson *et al.* (2008) reported that, in Sweden, a change of advice to introduce gluten to infants at six months rather than four months resulted in an increase in incidence of early-onset coeliac disease.

5.4 Trends in breastfeeding behaviour

Despite the clear evidence that breastfeeding is the best infant feeding option for the health of both the mother and her infant, the majority of babies in developed countries are bottle-fed with artificial formula preparations. The WHO recommends that all babies are exclusively breastfed until six months of age to maximize the benefits for the infant. However, in the United States and most European countries, exclusive breastfeeding is an activity pursued by a very small minority of women and formula-feeding or a mixed feeding regimen is the norm.

Understanding the literature on breastfeeding trends and breastfeeding in relation to health can often be confusing, due to the different terms used to describe and define approaches to infant feeding. Table 5.5 provides an overview of some of these terms. Looking at trends over time or making comparisons between countries is particularly difficult due to variation in these definitions. Considering global trends in infant feeding, Unicef estimates that 97.6% of babies born in low-income countries are ever breastfed and that this figure is markedly lower in high-income countries (78.8%). The best rates of ever breastfeeding in the developed countries are seen in Sweden, Oman and Uruguay, where initiation of breastfeeding is almost universal (Unicef, 2019). In general, the rates of breastfeeding have been increasing across the western world over the past two to three decades, as women increasingly become aware of the positive impact it has on the development of their babies. However, in some countries, the significant increase has come from a very low base, so breastfeeding rates remain low. In the United States, for example, a mere 25% of babies born in 1970 were ever breastfed, rising to 77% by 2009. In 2017, 84.1% of new mothers in the United States initiated breastfeeding, but with tremendous variation between states. The highest initiation rates were seen in Minnesota (95.3%) and Idaho (94.6%) and the lowest in Alabama (69%) and Louisiana (66.2%; Centers for Disease Control and Prevention 2020).

In the UK, increases in the rates of breastfeeding were noted from a low base in the mid- 1970s

Table 5.5 Definitions of breastfeeding behaviour.

Term	Definition
Breastfeeding*	Process of feeding baby human milk either directly from the breast or in expressed[†] form
Ever breastfed	Infant has been breastfed on at least one occasion
Exclusive breastfeeding	Infant has only ever been fed with breast milk. No other liquids or solids have been introduced, with the exception of vitamin and mineral supplements
Predominant breastfeeding	Infant has mainly been breastfed but may have consumed water, fruit juices, teas or oral rehydration fluids
Full breastfeeding	Includes both exclusive and predominant breastfeeding behaviour
Bottle-feeding[‡]	Process of feeding baby liquid or semi-solid foods via a bottle with a teat. Generally, this refers to feeding a cow's milk-derived substitute to human milk
Mixed feeding	Process through which an infant is nourished through a combination of breastfeeding and bottle-feeding
Complementary feeding	The infant is nourished through a combination of breastfeeding and solid or semi-solid foods

* Successful breastfeeding is generally baby led. Baby is fed on demand rather than to a timed schedule.
[†] Expressing refers to the technique of manually drawing milk off the breast for feeding via a bottle, spoon or cup, or through mixing with solid foods.
[‡] Bottle-fed babies are generally fed to a timed schedule, for example, one bottle every four hours.

through to the 1980s, taking the overall numbers of babies who were ever breastfed to around 65% of the population. Since then, considerable progress has been made in the promotion of breastfeeding, and the 2010 Office for National Statistics Infant Feeding Survey (McAndrew *et al.*, 2012) found that 81% of British babies were ever breastfed (Figure 5.7). Since the 2010 Infant Feeding Survey, monitoring of breastfeeding has been devolved to the four UK nations and all report a decline in breastfeeding initiation over the subsequent decade (England 74%; Scotland 64% ever breastfed in 2017). Like the United States, Britain sees variation related to ethnicity (over 95% of non-white women initiate breastfeeding) and social class (90% of women in managerial and professional occupations breastfeed). There is also a tremendous regional variation and, despite large increases in breastfeeding rates in Wales, Scotland and Northern Ireland in recent years (Figure 5.7), these countries within the UK have always lagged behind England in terms of uptake of breastfeeding.

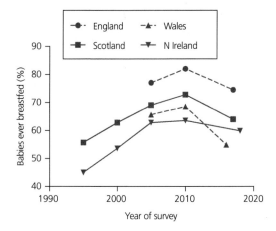

Figure 5.7 Breastfeeding trends in the UK from 1995 to 2020.

The UK has some of the lowest breastfeeding initiation rates in Europe, with the exception of Ireland and Belgium. Initiation is near universal in Sweden, Germany and Norway, and strong breastfeeding cultures are noted in Spain, Italy, Denmark and Switzerland (Theurich *et al.*, 2019).

While trends in the initiation of breastfeeding are encouraging, exclusive breastfeeding for six months as recommended by the WHO is considerably less commonplace (Figure 5.8). Exclusive breastfeeding rates are highest in low-income countries where a lack of access to clean water and suitable alternatives leads women to rely on breastfeeding for their babies. However, even in the impoverished regions of the world, up to half of women will choose to introduce other foods to their babies before six months. In developed countries, the strongest engagement with advice to exclusively breastfeed is often in those where initiation rates are highest. In the United States, approximately 26% of mothers exclusively breastfeed to six months (Centers for Disease Control and Prevention, 2020). In Europe, 39% of Dutch, 28% of Spanish and 28% of Belgian infants are exclusively breastfed for six months (Theurich *et al.*, 2019). In the UK, fewer than 1% of mothers follow this advice.

While across Europe breastfeeding is initiated by 70–98% of women, the dropout rate is very high and, as noted previously, the numbers of infants who are exclusively breastfed to six months of age are typically low. Figure 5.9 shows the fall-off in the

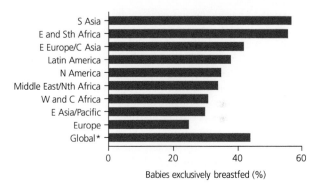

Figure 5.8 Global prevalence of exclusive breastfeeding for five months (2018–2020). *Source:* Unicef.

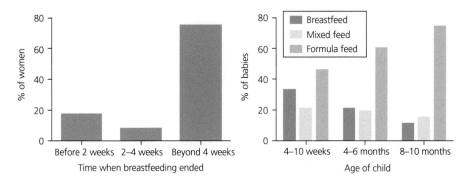

Figure 5.9 Attrition among breastfeeding women is high in the UK. A significant proportion (25%) of breastfeeding women give up within the first four weeks. By 4–10 weeks after birth, only 33% of babies are solely breastfed. *Source:* McAndrew *et al.* (2012).

number of breastfed infants in the UK (McAndrew *et al.*, 2012). It can be clearly seen that of the women who initiate breastfeeding at birth of their babies, more than 25% will give up within the first four weeks, with especially high attrition in the first two weeks. Two thirds of mothers will switch to formula or mixed feeding within 10 weeks, and only 20% will maintain breastfeeding to 4–6 months. Evidence of high dropout is seen across all developed countries. In the United States, 20% of babies whose mothers initiate breastfeeding will be given formula within two days of birth, for example (Centers for Disease Control and Prevention, 2020). Some European countries have cultures which support women in breastfeeding for longer (Theurich *et al.*, 2019) and over 50% of infants receive some breastmilk for up to six months in Belgium, Germany, the Netherlands, Norway, Spain, Sweden and Switzerland. The observation that large numbers of women initiate breastfeeding but switch to formula or mixed feeding approaches provides a clue to the fact that breastfeeding can be difficult for women to sustain unless they are well supported in doing so.

5.4.1 Reasons why women do not breastfeed

Unless they have been impacted by trauma to the breast tissue or have rare endocrine disorders, all women are physically able to breastfeed, yet throughout developed regions of the world, maintaining breastfeeding rates is a struggle for public health agencies. In considering why bottle-feeding is the preferred infant feeding method for the majority of women in developed countries, we need to consider two sets of factors, summarized in Figure 5.10. The first are the factors that prevent women from initiating breastfeeding in the first place (largely cultural factors), and the second group of factors are those that lead women to give up breastfeeding at some stage in the first six months (problems with technique, stress and infections).

5.4.1.1 Cultural factors

Most of the factors that women cite as important in leading them to choose formula-feeding in preference to breastfeeding are socially and culturally related. For example, in the United States, the 2005 Women's Health Survey found that Hispanic women were most likely to breastfeed, while non-Hispanic black women were least likely. In European studies, the women who are least likely to breastfeed are younger mothers, women with low educational attainment and women from a lower-income family. Figure 5.11 shows data from a survey of

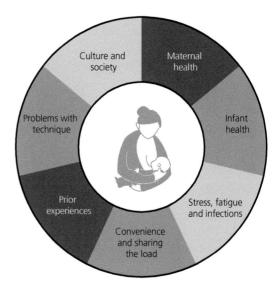

Figure 5.10 A number of factors contribute to women making the choice to not breastfeed and to abandoning the practice early. Cultural and societal factors, previous poor experience and the desire to share the load may lead women to select formula feeding initially. Health issues for mothers and babies, stress and fatigue and difficulties with breastfeeding techniques can all lead to a switch to formula feeding.

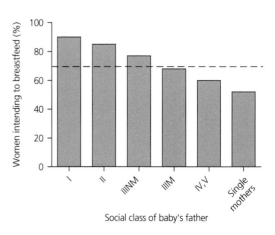

Figure 5.11 Socioeconomic factors are a strong determinant of breastfeeding behaviour. Three hundred pregnant women from Northampton were interviewed regarding their breastfeeding intentions in the 32nd week of pregnancy (Langley-Evans and Langley-Evans, 2003). The dotted line shows the proportion of women in the UK who would be expected to breastfeed (Hamlyn *et al.*, 2002). Social class I, professionals; II, clerical workers; IIINM, skilled non-manual workers; IIIM, skilled manual workers; IV, partly skilled workers; V, unskilled workers.

300 women from Northampton, who were surveyed in the final trimester of pregnancy. The data show that among higher social classes, the intention to breastfeed was indicated by a number of women that were well above the national average, while only 50–60% of single mothers and women of lower socioeconomic class indicated that they would breastfeed their babies.

These behaviours almost certainly arise from women's perception of the social acceptability of breastfeeding. Women who choose not to breastfeed may do so because of embarrassment at breastfeeding in public, as in the western world the breast is perceived as a sexual object. The attitudes of their partners may also shape this viewpoint. Although mothers in the UK, Australia and most of the United States are protected by law when breastfeeding in public places, experiences of negative comments while feeding and non-compliance with the law discourages and reduces confidence of women who do so (Brown, 2017). Boyer (2012) described how women always feel that they must be discrete when breastfeeding outside their own home, and that public spaces do not feel safe. There are countless instances of women being asked to leave restaurants or other establishments if they breastfeed or being asked to feed their babies in the toilets, out of view.

Women may also need to return to work early after delivery, and patterns of breastfeeding can easily be seen to reflect the financial support offered by governments to support parents. Countries such as Slovenia and Denmark where up to one year of maternal leave at full pay can be taken see initiation of breastfeeding in approximately 97% of mothers. Similarly, in Slovakia and Austria where up to three years of fully paid leave is available, around 90% of women will breastfeed. Lower uptake of breastfeeding is noted where there are less liberal arrangements. In the UK, for example, statutory maternity leave is less generous (6 weeks at 90% of full pay, 33 weeks at a lower rate and 13 weeks unpaid) and women of lower socioeconomic class, for example, may not be able to afford an extended period of leave after having their babies.

Women who have previously breastfed and had a negative experience are also disinclined to repeat the process. Some women also report that they would like to share feeding of their baby with other family members and thereby spread the burden of childcare. The experience of members of the extended family is of major importance, and women will often take advice from and mirror the behaviours of their mothers. In some cultures, this influence can produce quite extreme feeding practices. In some parts of Canada, including Newfoundland, breastfeeding rates are very low (around 40% initiate breastfeeding), and there is a tradition of feeding babies evaporated or condensed cow's milk, which is passed on from mothers to daughters and through social networks (Matthews *et al.*, 1998). Although this practice, based on saving money, has been suggested to cause harm to infants because of the high associated protein and solute loads, it remains prevalent among aboriginal groups and low-income families.

Societal attitudes which reduce maternal confidence in breastfeeding are evident in television, film and printed media (Brown, 2017). While these media typically portray formula feeding as normal, accessible and unproblematic, breastfeeding is stereotypically portrayed as difficult, sexual or comical. Austen *et al.* (2016) explored the attitudes of young women and found that although they valued breastfeeding and intended to do so, they viewed it as 'something to be done, but not seen'. More visibility of the population to normalized breastfeeding images may help to overcome the apprehension that women may feel about being seen to be breastfeeding.

5.4.1.2 Technique, infection and stress

Successful breastfeeding requires a good technique, and problems with establishing this technique and in overcoming the difficulties of the first few days of lactation account for the very high dropout in the first weeks after birth. Latching the baby on to the nipple correctly is something that has to be learned by all women. Incorrect latching-on such that the baby grips solely the nipple, rather than taking the whole of the areola into the mouth, will lead to soreness and, in the worst cases, blistering and bleeding of the nipple tissue. Even with correct technique and with experience of previous breastfeeding, the early days of feeding are likely to be uncomfortable and hence some women will look for alternatives. Breast engorgement may also lead women to give up breastfeeding. After two to three days beyond birth, the decline in production of the sex steroids lifts the inhibitory effect upon prolactin stimulus of milk synthesis. The breasts begin to produce mature milk in large quantities due to the high level of stimulation from the baby over the preceding days. The breasts become large, hard and painful, and it can be difficult to continue feeding. As this engorgement generally coincides with an emotional low that is also associated with falling progesterone and oestrogen concentrations, women are liable to give up feeding at this point.

Breast engorgement and sore or bleeding nipples do not preclude maintaining breastfeeding for women who are prepared to work through the difficult early days. With an engorged breast, the solution is to manually express milk to soften the breast tissue sufficiently for the baby to be able to suckle and drain off the engorgement, which will pass within a few days. Sore nipples can be treated with ointments and by exposing to the air between feeds to promote healing.

Other problems that can arise with breastfeeding, at any time, can also be debilitating and discourage further maintenance of feeding. These include infection of the nipple with *Candida albicans* and mastitis. The latter arises either through infection of damaged nipples or due to breast engorgement or blockage of ducts. Mastitis due to infection can produce severe flu-like symptoms and requires treatment with a suitable antibiotic to resolve it. Mastitis due to non-infective causes is generally a consequence of the breast not being fully drained at each feed. This can promote localized infections, and so the breast needs to be manually drained through massage, and relief from symptoms can be gained through cooling with wet towels, ice packs or even cabbage leaves.

While these physical problems account for much of the early drop-off in breastfeeding rates, the decision to stop feeding after the first few weeks is generally because women perceive that they are producing insufficient milk (Colin and Scott, 2002). Due to lactation being a demand-led process, it is highly unlikely that the capacity to produce milk will be genuinely outstripped by infant requirements in the first four to six months of life. Agostoni *et al.* (1999) clearly showed that, in fact, over the first six months of life, exclusively breastfed babies grew faster than formula-fed babies. However, many women perceive unsettled behaviour in their children or episodes of cluster feeding as a sign of hunger and may start to introduce solid foods or formula top-up feeds in addition to breastfeeding or cease breastfeeding completely in response. Stress related to feeding the infant, or the inevitable fatigue associated with a 24-hour demand-feeding schedule, can inhibit the letdown reflex and hence interfere with successful lactation.

5.4.2 Promoting breastfeeding

Across Europe, Australasia and North America, there is an active support for the aims of the Innocenti Declaration, and there are a number of organizations and initiatives that aim to promote breastfeeding and provide support for breastfeeding mothers. The most important development on a global scale is the Unicef Baby Friendly Hospital Initiative (BFHI). This worldwide programme of the WHO and Unicef was launched in 1992 to encourage maternity hospitals

Table 5.6 Ten steps to successful breastfeeding.

No.	Step
	Facilities providing maternity services and care for newborn infants should:
1	Have a written breastfeeding policy that is routinely communicated to all healthcare staff
2	Train all healthcare staff in skills necessary to implement this policy
3	Inform all pregnant women about the benefits and management of breastfeeding
4	Help mothers in initiating breastfeeding within half an hour of birth
5	Show mothers how to breastfeed and how to maintain lactation if separated from their infants
6	Give newborn infants no food or drink other than breast milk, unless medically indicated
7	Practise rooming-in (mothers and infants to remain together at all times)
8	Encourage breastfeeding on demand
9	Give no artificial teats or pacifiers to breastfeeding infants
10	Foster the establishment of breastfeeding support groups and refer mothers to them on discharge from the hospital

Source: WHO/Unicef (1989).

to implement the 10 steps to successful breastfeeding (Table 5.6) and to practice in accordance with the International Code of Marketing of Breastmilk Substitutes, which seeks to limit the promotion of formula milks to mothers.

The BFHI is coordinated in individual countries by local organizations. The attainment of sufficiently high standards to gain baby-friendly status and the implementation of the BFHI seven-point plan are relatively low across the world and there is considerable variation across the world in terms of coverage (Figure 5.12). Globally, less than 10% of babies are born in BFHI hospitals and only 25% of countries have attained BFHI accreditation in 50% or more of their hospitals and maternity units. Sweden was an early adopter and, by 1998, all 65 maternity hospitals in the country had full accreditation. The UK is noted for low engagement of mothers with breastfeeding and particularly exclusive breastfeeding, so initiatives to promote the practice are a critical element of public health strategies. In Scotland and Northern Ireland, all babies born in hospitals are born in BFHI accredited units (Wales 78%, England 58%). Universities can also receive accreditation and in the UK 47% of midwifery and 15% of health visitor training is accredited. Barriers to BFHI accreditation in UK hospitals include a lack of willingness among local health authorities to prioritize

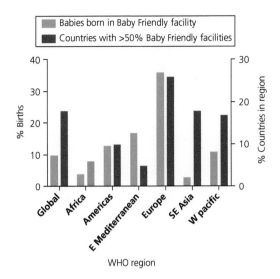

Figure 5.12 Globally, a minority of babies are born in baby-friendly hospitals. Most industrialized nations lag behind developing countries in ensuring the Baby Friendly Hospital Initiative standards. *Source:* Unicef (2019).

breastfeeding. It is reported that staff in units can be resistant to implementation and women giving birth in BFHI-accredited units can feel that these environments promote unrealistic expectations of breastfeeding (Fallon *et al.*, 2019). In particular, a lack of guidance on how to formula feed safely or discussion of alternatives to breastfeeding can lead to guilty emotions among women who choose not to breastfeed.

BFHI standards provide a clear benefit in terms of increasing uptake of advice to breastfeed. Numerous studies show that babies born in a BFHI hospital are more likely to be breastfed. For example, 83.5% of Belgian mothers intended to breastfeed on discharge from BFHI units, compared with 72.4% leaving units that were not accredited (Robert *et al.*, 2019). Kivlighan *et al.* (2020) reported significant increases in breastfeeding among hard-to-reach rural communities in the USA with BFHI exposure. However, while the BFHI is highly successful in terms of getting women to initiate breastfeeding, the support is too short to sustain through the challenges of the feeding beyond the first few days (Bartington *et al.*, 2006; Hawkins *et al.*, 2014).

BFHI promotes and supports breastfeeding through national health services and may therefore be effective only in the first few days of breastfeeding when women are in close contact with midwives. Other organizations exist to provide support and encouragement outside the healthcare setting. The UK has a national breastfeeding helpline operated by the Breastfeeding Network, enabling women experiencing difficulties to seek telephone support from experienced breastfeeding mothers. The La Leche League (international) and the National Childbirth Trust (UK) are charitable organizations that can be easily accessed by women requiring support. Both organizations are involved in training of health professionals and providing peer counsellors who can give practical advice and moral support to breastfeeding mothers in difficulty.

Just as social networks can strongly influence the initial decision on whether to breastfeed or bottle-feed, peer support groups can be very important in helping women to continue breastfeeding and overcome the challenges faced in the early weeks. The Australian RUBY (Ringing Up about Breastfeeding) trial compared usual postpartum care of first-time mothers with telephone-based support from a peer volunteer, which began 24–48 hours after hospital discharge and continued for up to six months (Forster *et al.*, 2019). Infants of women who received the telephone peer support were more likely to still be breastfeeding at six months (OR 1.10, 95% CI 1.02–1.18). Similarly, a Spanish programme of peer support through a web-based platform led to greatly enhanced rates of exclusive breastfeeding at three months (OR 2.65, 95% CI 1.21–5.78) and six months (OR 3.30, 95% CI 1.52–7.17; Gonzalez-Darias *et al.*, 2020). One-to-one informal peer support in addition to more formal antenatal education is an effective way of promoting breastfeeding initiation among low-income women (Dyson *et al.*, 2014). Continuing that support into the postnatal period also reduces the risk that breastfeeding will be discontinued by approximately 30% (Kaunonen *et al.*, 2012; Sudfeld *et al.*, 2012). Personal, one-to-one interactions with experienced breastfeeding mothers can enable new mothers to persist through provision of emotional support, encouragement and practical advice on common problems. Regan and Brown (2019) reported that women particularly value online groups to provide such support, as they are available around the clock and are less daunting than attending face-to-face sessions.

5.5 Situations in which breastfeeding is not advised

There may be circumstances in which breastfeeding is not advised, as to do so would put the infant at risk. This may occur due to maternal exposure to toxic agents that are excreted in the milk, for example, heavy metals, or through maternal usage of prescription or non-prescription drugs that might have a negative impact on the infant. Drugs and other exogenous organic chemicals, perhaps encountered in the workplace, undergo a two-phase metabolism in the liver. Phase I metabolism comprises oxidation, reduction or hydrolytic reactions catalysed by the cytochrome P450 system, yielding stable products that are targets for phase II metabolism. This consists of conjugation with either glucuronide, sulphonate or amino acids. The conjugated products are then excreted, and in lactating women, excretion into breast milk is one route of disposal. The pharmacokinetics of all prescription drugs are well characterized, and women will be advised accordingly if it is necessary to administer a drug likely to appear in the milk in this way.

There are also a number of inborn errors of metabolism that may make breastfeeding inadvisable or difficult to pursue (Figure 5.13). Galactosaemia is an inherited disorder in which individuals lack the enzyme galactose-1-phosphate uridyl transferase. This occurs in approximately 1 in 45 000 live births in the UK. In the absence of this enzyme, galactose will accumulate, which leads to extensive damage in the liver and kidney. Individuals with galactosaemia therefore have to restrict galactose consumption throughout life but even with restrictive diets, there are many long-term complications that cannot be avoided. Clearly, as lactose is metabolized to glucose and galactose, consumption of human or normal formula milk is impossible, and infants with galactosaemia cannot be breastfed. There are galactose-free formulas available for use in this situation.

It has been widely supposed that most inborn errors of metabolism may preclude breastfeeding, but this need not be the case if mothers want to confer some of the health benefits of human milk upon their children. There are two approaches that can be taken to achieve this. First, expressed milk mixed with other required ingredients can be fed via a bottle. Second, infants can be breastfed on demand but pre-fed with specialized formula to limit intake. Phenylketonuria (PKU) provides a good example of the possibilities of the latter approach.

Infants with PKU lack the enzyme phenylalanine hydroxylase and as a result have to restrict

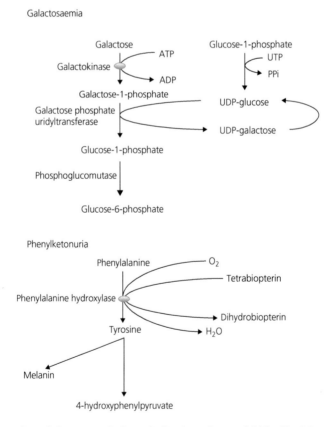

Figure 5.13 Inborn errors of metabolism can make breastfeeding hazardous to child health. Galactosaemia and phenylketonuria necessitate the feeding of special infant formulas.

intake of phenylalanine (Figure 5.13). Human milk has a relatively low content of phenylalanine. Some mothers feed their infants weighed quantities of expressed milk to regulate phenylalanine intake. More commonly, women will breastfeed but begin each feed by giving a measured amount of a phenylalanine formula, following up with breastfeeding until the infant is satiated. Another possible approach is to adopt a mixed feeding schedule in which infants are alternately breastfed and bottle-fed with low-phenylalanine formula.

There are situations where breastfeeding can increase the risk of transmission of disease from mother to infant, either through direct passage of infective organisms via the milk (e.g. HIV) or through the close contact between baby and infected mother (e.g. tuberculosis). The ideal protocols for dealing with these situations will depend upon other factors in the maternal–infant environment but could involve the use of an alternative to breastfeeding. HIV infection of the infant during breastfeeding occurs due to movement of virus in maternal milk into the infant circulation through uptake at points in the mouth, throat or intestine where the integrity of the mucosal cells lining the digestive tract is compromised (e.g. due to ulcers or inflammation). The most likely cause of a breakdown in the mucosal integrity is the introduction of solid foods. In developed countries maternal infection with HIV should be regarded as a firm contraindication for breastfeeding. Free access to clean, safe water and an inexpensive supply of formula means that all risk of vertical transmission of HIV (from mother to infant) can be completely eliminated. Women who are HIV positive are advised not to breastfeed regardless of their use of anti-retroviral therapies (ART) or the magnitude of their viral load (American Academy of Pediatrics, 2013).

In developing countries, the advice is very different, as the risks associated with insecure supplies of formula and unsanitary conditions for preparation of feeds, are greater than the risk of vertical HIV transmission via milk, particularly if mothers are supported with ART. WHO updated its guidance for women who are HIV positive in developing countries in 2010 (World Health Organization, 2010). These guidelines were further reviewed and updated in 2016. WHO recommends that women should either exclusively formula feed or breastfeed for a minimum of 12 months alongside the use of antiretroviral drugs. ART can be provided either to the infant (option A) or to the mother (option B+). Breastfeeding and ART should be used only in situations where diarrhoeal disease and malnutrition

are a major cause of infant mortality, with formula preferred if it is safe, feasible and affordable to do so.

The clear concern about formula feeding is that children are vulnerable to malnutrition if families cannot afford or access formula and to infection if clean water supplies to make up formula are not secured. Some women also feel that their feeding choices will identify them as being HIV positive, and thus, their feeding behaviour effectively stigmatizes them. Fear of this and uncertain access to formula milk leads some women to take a mixed feeding approach (Coutsoudis *et al.*, 2008). The WHO update (World Health Organization, 2016) indicated that while exclusive breastfeeding is optimal, mixed feeding supported by ART remains the better option compared with no breastfeeding. Ideally, breastfeeding should be maintained for up to 24 months, but shorter periods carry less risk than never initiating breastfeeding. As discussed in Research Highlight 5.3, while governments in regions where HIV is endemic are supportive of the option B+ strategy, progress in delivering successful prevention of maternal-to-child transmission is limited.

Tuberculosis is becoming increasingly common on a global scale and in many areas occurs alongside HIV infection. In the past, it was common practice to separate women with tuberculosis from their infants to prevent cross infection but in developing countries this would tend to increase infant death rates due to loss of the immunoprotective effects of breast milk. It is now recognized that the best way to prevent tuberculosis infection of infants is to immunize the infant, treat the disease in the mother and maintain exclusive breastfeeding for six months, if compatible with management of HIV. In the absence of HIV, women with tuberculosis should continue breastfeeding with complementary foods for up to two years.

5.6 Alternatives to breastfeeding

The evidence that breastfeeding carries both short- and long-term health benefits for both mother and infant is overwhelming. However, for the vast majority of infants born in developed countries, feeding will be largely based upon the use of artificial milk formulas fed via a bottle. The main benefit of this approach to feeding is that it reduces the dependency of the infant upon the mother as the main carer and allows closer bonding with other family members. Formula feeding is also clearly advantageous to women who need to return to work early after the delivery of their baby.

As described previously, there are some hazards and drawbacks associated with formula feeding that

Research Highlight 5.3 The challenge of preventing mother-to-child transmission of HIV.

The United Nations has set a global goal of eliminating the mother-to-child transmission of HIV. Shifting the behaviour of mothers in developing countries away from previous advice to formula feed if HIV infected towards exclusive breastfeeding supported by ART is a critical element of achieving that goal. Implementation of prevention of mother-to-child transmission programmes is the responsibility of national governments. The success of such programmes will depend on: a) being able to identify infected women and at-risk children through reliable HIV testing; b) detecting cases early enough to prevent transmission in pregnancy and labour; c) ensuring that the supply of ART to mothers and infants is secure and affordable and; d) reducing the loss of mothers to long-term follow-up. HIV is most prevalent in Sub-Saharan Africa where healthcare systems struggle to manage these factors, especially when mothers and infants live in rural communities.

Since the introduction of WHO guidelines in 2010, rates of exclusive breastfeeding supported with ART have improved markedly, for example increasing from 0% to 46% in Senegal between 2010 and 2015 (Gueye *et al.*, 2019). Coverage is far from universal, however. Where breastfeeding with ART can be accomplished, HIV-free survival of infants over the first two years of life is better than where infants of HIV-infected women are formula-fed (Chikhungu *et al.*, 2016). The WHO protocol substantially reduces risk of HIV transmission, but in many cases the ART support ends when the infant is six months old, reducing efficacy (Bispo *et al.*, 2017).

Successful prevention of mother-to-child transmission, like breastfeeding in developed countries, is assisted by the provision of support to facilitate exclusive breastfeeding. For example, in the Democratic Republic of Congo, HIV-infected women who received support at delivery of their babies were more likely to be breastfeeding at six weeks, but even then, 31% of women had switched to formula (Mpody *et al.*, 2019). A lack of support can be a major reason for non-adherence to guidelines. In Ethiopia, women were less likely to breastfeed if giving birth at home, or if they needed to return to work quickly (Ayele *et al.*, 20219). Among South African women with HIV, non-adherence to guidelines was more likely in those aged 16–24 or over 34 years (Larsen *et al.*, 2019) and in some communities the exclusive formula feeding rate was found to be as high as 70%, driven by fear of HIV infection of the child (Remmert *et al.*, 2020).

The stigma of HIV infection is powerful in Sub-Saharan Africa and many women may not disclose their HIV status, even to their spouse. Studies from Ethiopia (Belay and Wubneh, 2019) and South Africa (Larsen *et al.*, 2019) indicate that non-disclosure is a factor associated with non-adherence to the guideline to breastfeed with ART. Yapa *et al.* (2020) reported that HIV prevalence was 47% in a sample of 1693 South African women. Although the women living with HIV were more knowledgeable on correct feeding recommendations for their infants than non-infected women, a greater proportion of this group chose to formula feed. If they are to be successful, prevention of mother-to-child transmission programmes therefore face a major challenge in overcoming powerful cultural beliefs, stigma about HIV, the lack of paid maternity leave and family pressures.

may make it an inappropriate choice for families on low incomes and for women in developing countries where a clean water supply cannot be guaranteed. It should also be appreciated that formula feeding can increase the risk of allergic sensitization to cow's milk protein and can be hazardous if feeds are not prepared according to manufacturers' instructions. Under-concentrating milk formula (i.e. adding less milk powder per unit volume) is a strategy that may be adopted by families on low incomes, to make the formula last longer, which can lead to infant malnutrition. Overconcentration of the formula (i.e. adding too much milk powder per unit volume) can lead to dehydration of the infant, as more water will have to be excreted to deal with the ingested protein and electrolytes.

There is a huge array of different milk formulas available to consumers. They vary little in their composition as there are strict regulations that limit the capacity of manufacturers to alter formula constituents. As described in the following text, however, there are formulas designed for specific situations, and formulas may vary in composition to deliver an optimal balance of nutrients according to the developmental stage of the infant.

5.6.1 Cow's milk formulas

Most infant formulas are based on cow's milk, modified to produce a composition that is more similar to the average composition of human milk. Unmodified cow's milk should not be given to infants below the age of 12 months, although it can be mixed with solids as part of complementary feeding before this time. Unmodified cow's milk would promote the development of nutrient deficiencies in infants as it is low in vitamin C, vitamin E, essential fatty acids and iron. Iron deficiency would also be promoted as adverse reactions to components of cow's milk would promote blood loss in the digestive tract. Importantly, the high nitrogen, calcium, phosphorus, sodium, potassium and chloride content of cow's milk would promote dehydration as water would be required to excrete the excess solute load.

Figure 5.14 shows a comparison of the macronutrient and micronutrient composition of human,

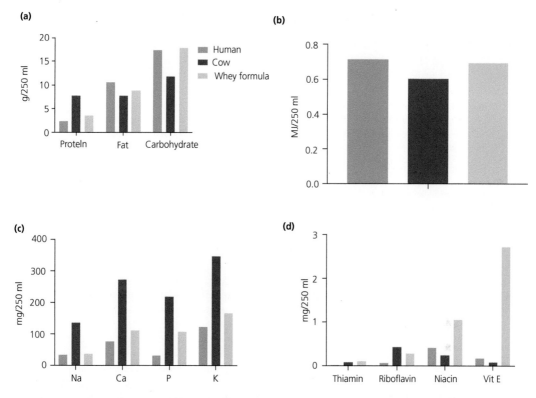

Figure 5.14 Comparison of the compositions of milks from humans and cows, alongside a typical infant formula. (a) Macronutrients; (b) Energy; (c) Minerals; (d) Vitamins.

cow's and a typical formula milk. Cow's milk contains almost threefold more protein than human milk and has a lower sugar content, and so the main modifications made during formula production include processing to remove protein and the addition of lactose. Many of the raw materials used in the production of infant formulas are actually waste products from other areas of the dairy industry and, generally, the starting material for formula production is not whole, unmodified milk. The processing to remove protein may involve a variety of steps including evaporation, condensation and hydrolysis, and other components of the cow's milk will be lost along the way. Much of the whey protein that is included in formula milks is discarded during cheese manufacture and, when added to formula mixes, will consist of demineralized, fat-free whey protein (Jost *et al.*, 1999). All infant formulas will contain vegetable oils added to attain the required total fat content. Between 25% and 75% of fats in formulas may be of vegetable origin, and this will clearly impact upon the overall fatty acid composition of the formula.

It is a relatively simple process for manufacturers to add vitamins and minerals to achieve optimal concentrations and, indeed, this is necessary if processing demineralizes the raw materials that comprise the basis of the formula. For many micronutrients, this addition will need to take into account the bioavailability of the nutrient from the formula milk matrix (Figure 5.14). This is exemplified by iron, which in human milk is present in the highly absorbed haem form but in formula milk, it is in the non-haem form. It is therefore necessary to add iron to cow's milk formula at a concentration many times greater than seen in either human milk or the cow's milk from which the formula is derived.

5.6.1.1 Milk stages and follow-on milk

In the processing of cow's milk to produce formula, it becomes possible to manipulate the casein/whey ratio of the proteins in the milk. Unmodified cow's milk has a casein/whey ratio of 80 : 20, which is markedly different to human milk where the ratio is 40 : 60. Most manufacturers take advantage of the ability to alter this ratio to market separate first-stage and second-stage milks. First-stage milks are whey-rich products and have a casein/whey ratio that mimics mature human milk. Second-stage milks provide the 80 : 20 ratio seen in cow's milk and are proposed to be more difficult to digest within the infant gut but to have a more satiating effect on infant appetite.

It is suggested that feeding a whey-rich formula may have a number of benefits for the infant. The predominant whey proteins in infant formulas derived from cow's milk are β-lactoglobulin and α-lactalbumin. β-Lactoglobulin is not found in human milk, but α-lactalbumin is the dominant whey protein consumed by breastfed infants. Some formulas are manufactured to contain a level of α-lactalbumin that is similar to human milk. It is suggested that these enriched formulas may aid in the neurodevelopment of infants as they increase circulating concentrations of tryptophan, an amino acid that plays an important role in brain development (Lien, 2003). Other whey proteins that are present in whey-rich formulas may provide some antimicrobial protection for infants. Lactoferrin, for example, has been shown in animal studies to have immune system priming actions and may therefore help the maturation of the cellular immunity of infants. The lactoferricin B fragment of bovine lactoferrin, which is generated during digestion within the stomach (Kuwata *et al.*, 1998), has been shown to have the capacity to damage cell membranes and inhibit growth of a number of food-borne pathogens, including *Salmonella*, *Listeria* and *Campylobacter* species.

The progression from whey-rich to casein-rich formulas is not an absolute necessity. Feeding casein-rich formula at an earlier age would do no harm, and the whey-rich formulation can sustain the nutritional requirements of an infant up to six months of age. At six months, however, it is advisable for parents to switch formula and introduce a follow-on (stage 3) milk to their infant. Follow-on milks derived from cow's milk are less modified than the milks produced for younger infants and therefore contain more protein and minerals to meet the increasing demands of the infant past six months. Follow-on milks are used as a mixer during weaning or as a drink during complementary feeding.

5.6.2 Preterm formulas

Approximately 6% of all infants born in the UK are born prematurely (less than 38 weeks of gestation). The infants at greatest risk of significant morbidity are those born before 32 weeks of gestation, who make up around one third of all preterm deliveries. This latter group of preterm infants poses a number of problems from a nutritional point of view, as they have high demands for nutrients and yet cannot be fed by conventional means.

As seen in earlier chapters of this book, the organs develop and mature at differing rates. Organs and systems that mature relatively late in gestation are those which will be least mature in a preterm infant. Lung immaturity leads to life-threatening complications that significantly raise nutrient demands due to the need for mechanical ventilation. Immaturity of the digestive system poses considerable problems in terms of feeding strategies. Before 32 weeks of gestation, the infant lacks the rooting reflex and so is unable to breastfeed. The digestive system is so underdeveloped that the stomach capacity is only around 3 ml for a 1.5-kg infant, and this clearly limits the quantity of food that can be taken via the enteral route. The gut is also functionally immature and lacks effective peristalsis and the key enzymes and other factors required for digestion.

The last stages of gestation are normally a time when the fetus acquires nutrients for storage from the mother. In terms of energy, for example, the full-term 40-week infant has fat reserves of approximately 450 g (4530 kcal, 18.98 MJ), whereas a 26-week infant has a meagre 20 g fat (320 kcal, 1.34 MJ). The nutritional status of preterm infants is therefore often poor at earlier stages of their clinical management, as they have low intakes of nutrients, low reserves and high demands associated with trauma and their high growth rate (human body weight normally doubles between 28 and 40 weeks of gestation).

Strategies for feeding preterm infants will depend upon their size and their gestational age. For infants born prior to 34 weeks, normal bottle-feeding or breastfeeding is not possible, and the infant will need artificial feeding using a tube via the enteral route (a nasogastric tube carries milk directly to the stomach) or using a parenteral feeding (intravenous feeding of nutrients in the simplest form, e.g. free fatty acids, glucose and amino acids) protocol. Human milk may be fed to older preterm babies via a tube. Ideally, this is milk expressed by the baby's own mother, which will have a composition suited to the stage of development. Mothers of preterm infants are reported to produce a more energy-dense milk with a greater protein, fat and sodium content than mothers of full-term infants. Feeding human milk conveys the immunological benefits to the infant, but does carry some risk. Osteopenia of prematurity is a condition of bone in which bone mineralization is compromised. This can arise due to the low calcium and phosphate content of human milk. Thus, when human milk is used as the basis of enteral feeding for premature babies, it is mixed with fortifiers to increase the vitamin and mineral content (Schanler, 1995).

Where preterm infants are fed with formula milk, it is inappropriate to use a normal full-term formula as the nutrient density is insufficient to meet demands. Given the lower capacity of the

Table 5.7 Comparison of full-term and preterm infant formula composition (selected nutrients).

Nutrient	Formula content/100 ml reconstituted milk	
	Term formula	Preterm formula
Energy (kcal)	70.0	70.0
Protein (g)	1.5	1.9
Calcium (mg)	48.0	120.0
Phosphate (mg)	35.0	59.0
Iron (mg)	1.2	1.2
Sodium (mg)	20.0	30.0
Vitamin A (µg retinol equivalents)	100.0	350.0
Vitamin D (µg)	1.0	3.0
Vitamin C (mg)	5.8	24.0

premature gut and raised nutrient demands, most constituents are needed at greater concentrations than in term formula. Preterm formulas are based upon β-lactoglobulin as the protein source and are hence whey rich. Owing to the functional immaturity of the gut, the fat and sugar components are delivered as mixtures that are more easily digested and which do not overwhelm the existing enzyme systems. Sugars are provided as a mixture of lactose and glucose polymers, while fats are provided as a mixture of long-chain and medium-chain triglycerides. Table 5.7 shows a comparison of the nutrient composition of preterm and full-term formulas, highlighting their differing nutrient density.

5.6.3 Soy formulas

Some infants are intolerant of cow's milk-derived formulas, which is usually because of lactose intolerance, and may therefore require a lactose-free alternative. Soy formulas are produced from isolated soy protein and provide sugar as glucose rather than lactose. Originally, soy-based formulas were developed for infants with cow's milk protein allergy, but as the proteins in these formulas cross-react with cow's milk protein to a large extent, infants allergic to cow's milk are highly likely to respond to soy formulas in the same way. Soy formulas should not be confused with standard soy milk. They should only be used on medical advice, and there are some concerns that there are implications for the development of the reproductive tract and fertility in male babies exposed to phytoestrogens in soy formulas.

5.6.4 Hydrolysed protein and amino acid-based formulas

Cow's milk protein allergy is the most common food allergy seen in children. The only effective treatment

is the exclusion of all dairy produce from the diet, and this means that for formula-fed infants, specialized products must be introduced. Soy formula is generally inappropriate, as described previously, and approximately 50% of all children who are allergic to cow's milk will be allergic to soy formula. A systematic review of the literature found that in children with a family history of atopy, feeding a soy formula also increased risk of soy protein allergy by twofold compared with feeding standard formula (Osborn and Sinn, 2006). This suggests that soy formulas would not be the ideal choice of feed for infants at risk of allergies.

The alternative is to feed infants with either extensively hydrolysed protein or amino acid-based formulas. Hydrolysed protein formulas are generally based upon the whey fraction of cow's milk, with the major proteins hydrolysed to smaller peptides that are less allergenic than the native proteins. Extensively hydrolysed protein formulas do not prevent the development of allergies, but are an effective treatment for managing children with established cow's milk protein allergy. Amino acid-based formulas play the same role and are formulations that are free of intact proteins and peptides, instead providing all nitrogen in the form of isolated amino acids. Not all infants are able to tolerate hydrolysed protein formulas. Niggemann et al. (2001) suggested that children with intolerance or allergy to cow's milk had better growth rates when fed amino acid-based formula compared with hydrolysed proteins. An Australian consensus panel (Kemp et al., 2008) recommended that, on diagnosis of cow's milk protein allergy, children under the age of six months should be fed extensively hydrolysed formula with amino acid formula reserved for infants with more severe allergy or other complications. Taylor et al. (2012) found that there were no major differences in clinical outcomes between amino acid formulas and extensively hydrolysed formulas and that the hydrolysed formula was the more cost-effective option.

5.6.5 Other formulas

Formula milks based upon sheep or goat's milk may be promoted as an alternative to cow's milk formula, the argument being that consumption of such milks would reduce risk of allergy to cow's milk protein. The milk proteins of sheep and goats are very similar to those of cows and so this argument is fatuous. Milk from sheep or goats provides an inadequate supply of folic acid, iron and vitamins A, D and C, and so formulas from these sources should not be given to infants. Infant formulas and follow-on formulas based on sheep or goat milk have not been approved for use in

Europe, but full-fat sheep or goat's milks can be used for preparing sauces that are used in complementary feeds from six months of age. Zhou *et al.* (2014), however, carried out a double-blind randomized controlled trial of a goat formula compared with standard formula in term infants. There were no differences in infant growth, occurrence of allergy or dermatitis or serious adverse health outcomes. This suggests that concerns about safety may be unfounded, but further trials would be required.

SUMMARY

- Mammary alveoli are the sites of milk synthesis. This process involves de novo synthesis of lactose, fatty acids and proteins.
- Human milk production is under endocrine control through actions of prolactin and oxytocin. Hypothalamic integration of the secretion of these hormones ensures that milk supply meets infant demand.
- Lactation increases maternal demand for energy, protein and micronutrients.
- Breastfeeding confers health benefits upon lactating women, including a more rapid recovery from childbirth, suppression of reproductive cycling and protection against breast and ovarian cancers.
- Breastfeeding delivers immunoprotective factors to the infant, in addition to nutrients, in an optimal formulation. Immunoprotective cells and proteins reduce the risk of gastrointestinal and respiratory tract infections.
- Breastfeeding is associated with lower risk of SIDS, childhood obesity and allergies in susceptible infants. The delivery of docosahexaenoic acid in human milk is believed to enhance infant brain development.
- WHO recommends that infants are exclusively breastfed for the first six months of life. The only exceptions to this are where children have inborn errors of metabolism or where mothers are HIV positive.
- Despite the advantages of breastfeeding for mothers and infants, the majority of infants in developed countries do not experience the recommended six months of exclusive breastfeeding. The decision to use alternative feeding methods is largely shaped by social and cultural factors.
- Promotion of breastfeeding through initiatives such as the Baby Friendly Hospital Initiative contributes to greater initial rates of breastfeeding. Peer support interventions help women to maintain breastfeeding beyond the early weeks.
- Infant formulas are generally manufactured using modified by-products of the dairy industry. Their composition mimics average human milk and must comply with strict legislation.
- Specialized infant formulas are used for the feeding of preterm infants and infants with confirmed allergies or intolerance to cow's milk.

References

Agho, K.E., Ezeh, O.K., Ferdous, A.J. *et al.* (2010). Factors associated with under-5 mortality in three disadvantaged East African districts. *International Health* **12**: 417–428.

Agostoni, C., Grandi, F., Gianni, M.L. *et al.* (1999). Growth patterns of breast fed and formula fed infants in the first 12 months of life: an Italian study. *Archives of Disease in Childhood*,**81**: 395–399.

Ahmed, K.Y., Page, A., Arora, A. and Ogbo, F.A. (2020). Associations between infant and young child feeding practices and acute respiratory infection and diarrhoea in Ethiopia: a propensity score matching approach. *Plos One* **15**: e0230978.

Algarín, C., Nelson, C.A., Peirano, P. *et al.* (2013). Iron-deficiency anemia in infancy and poorer cognitive inhibitory control at age 10 years. *Developmental Medicine and Child Neurology* **55**: 453–458.

Alm, B., Wennergren, G., Norvenius, S.G. *et al.* (2002). Breast feeding and the sudden infant death syndrome in Scandinavia 1992–1995. *Archives Disease in Childhood* **86**: 400–402.

American Academy of Pediatrics. (2013). Infant feeding and transmission of human immunodeficiency virus in the United States. *Pediatrics* **131**: 391–396.

Arenz, S., Ruckerl, R., Koletzko, B. *et al.* (2004). Breast-feeding and childhood obesity: a systematic review. *International Journal of Obesity* **28**: 1247–1256.

Austen, E.L., Dignam, J. and Hauf, P. (2016). Using breastfeeding images to promote breastfeeding among young adults. *Health Psychology Open* **3**(2): doi:10.1177/2055102916671015.

Ayele, A.A., Seid, K.A. and Muhammed, O.S. (2019). Determinants of none-exclusive breast feeding practice among HIV positive women at selected Health Institutions in Ethiopia: case control study. *BMC Research Note*s **12**: 400.

Bartington, S., Griffiths, L.J., Tate, A.R. *et al.* (2006). Are breastfeeding rates higher among mothers delivering in Baby Friendly accredited maternity units in the UK? *International Journal of Epidemiology* **35**, 1178–1186.

Belay, G.M. and Wubneh, C.A. (2019). Infant feeding practices of HIV positive mothers and its association with counseling and HIV disclosure Status in Ethiopia: A systematic review and meta-analysis. *AIDS Research and Treatment* **2019**: 3862098.

Bernard, J.Y., Armand, M., Peyre, H. *et al.* (2017). Breastfeeding, polyunsaturated fatty acid levels in colostrum and child intelligence quotient at age 5–6 Years. *Journal of Pediatrics* **183**: 43–50.

Birch, E.E., Garfield, S., Castañeda, Y. *et al.* (2007). Visual acuity and cognitive outcomes at 4 years of age in a double-blind, randomized trial of long-chain polyunsaturated fatty acid-supplemented infant formula. *Early Human Development* **83**: 279–284.

Bispo, S., Chikhungu, L., Rollins, N. *et al.* (2017). Postnatal HIV transmission in breastfed infants of HIV-infected women on ART: a systematic review and meta-analysis. *Journal of the International AIDS Society* **20**: 21251.

Bjørnerem, A., Ahmed, L.A., Jørgensen, L. *et al.* (2011). Breastfeeding protects against hip fracture in postmenopausal women: the Tromsø study. *Journal of Bone and Mineral Research* **26**: 2843–50.

Boucher, O., Julvez, J., Guxens, M. *et al.* (2017). Association between breastfeeding duration and cognitive development, autistic traits and ADHD symptoms: a multicenter study in Spain. *Pediatric Research* **81**: 434–442.

Boyer, K. (2012). Affect, corporeality and the limits of belonging: breastfeeding in public in the contemporary UK. *Health and Place* **18**: 552–560.

Brown, A. (2017). Breastfeeding as a public health responsibility: a review of the evidence. *Journal of Human Nutrition and Dietetics* **30**: 759–770.

Carlson, S.E., Werkman, S.H., Peeples, J.M. *et al.* (1994). Long-chain fatty acids and early visual and cognitive development of preterm infants. *European Journal of Clinical Nutrition*, **48**(Suppl 2): S27–S30.

Centers for Disease Control and Prevention. (2020). Breastfeeding Report Card, United States 2020. https://www.cdc.gov/breastfeeding/data/reportcard.htm (accessed 6 April 2021).

Chantry, C.J., Howard, C.R. and Auinger, P. (2007). Full breastfeeding duration and risk for iron deficiency in U.S. infants. *Breastfeeding Medicine* **2**: 63–73.

Chikhungu, L.C., Bispo, S., Rollins, N. *et al.* (2016). HIV-free survival at 12–24 months in breastfed infants of HIV-infected women on antiretroviral treatment. *Tropical Medicine and Internal Health* **21**: 820–828.

Cho, T.J., Hwang, J.Y., Kim, H.W. *et al.* (2019). Underestimated Risks of Infantile Infectious Disease from the Caregiver's Typical Handling Practices of Infant Formula. *Scientific Reports* **9**: 9799.

Chowdhury, R., Sinha, B., Sankar, M.J. *et al.* (2015). Breastfeeding and maternal health outcomes: a systematic review and meta-analysis. *Acta Paediatrica* **104**: 96–113.

Colin, W.B. and Scott, J.A. (2002). Breast-feeding: reasons for starting, reasons for stopping and problems along the way. *Breastfeeding Reviews* **10**: 13–19.

Collaborative Group on Hormonal Factors in Breast Cancer (2002). Breast cancer and breast-feeding: collaborative reanalysis of individual data from 47 epidemiological studies in 30 countries, including 50 302 women with breast cancer and 96 973 women without the disease. *Lancet* **360**: 187–195.

Collins, C.T., Gibson, R.A., Anderson, P.J. *et al.* (2015). Neurodevelopmental outcomes at 7 years' corrected age in preterm infants who were fed high-dose docosahexaenoic acid to term equivalent: a follow-up of a randomised controlled trial. *British Medical Journal Open* **5**: e007314.

Colombo, J., Carlson, S.E., Cheatham, C.L. *et al.* (2013). Long-term effects of LCPUFA supplementation on childhood cognitive outcomes. *American Journal of Clinical Nutrition* **98**: 403–412.

Coutsoudis, A., Coovadia, H.M. and Wilfert, C.M. (2008). HIV, Infant feeding and more perils for poor people: new WHO guidelines encourage review of formula milk practices. *Bulletin of the World Health Organization* **86**: 210–214.

Crandall, C.J., Liu, J., Cauley, J. *et al.* (2017). Associations of Parity, Breastfeeding, and Fractures in the Women's Health Observational Study. *Obstetrics and Gynecology* **130**: 171–180.

Cunnane, S.C., Francescutti, V., Brenna, J.T. *et al.* (2000). Breast-fed infants achieve a higher rate of brain and whole body docosahexaenoate accumulation than formula-fed infants not consuming dietary docosahexaenoate. *Lipids* **35**: 105–111.

Czosnykowska-Łukacka, M., Orczyk-Pawiłowicz, M., Broers, B. and Królak-Olejnik, B. (2019). Lactoferrin in human milk of prolonged lactation. *Nutrients* **11**: 2350.

Department of Health. (1991). *Dietary Reference Values for Food Energy and Nutrients for the United Kingdom*. London: Stationery Office.

de Silva, D., Geromi, M., Halken, S. *et al.* (2014). Primary prevention of food allergy in children and adults: systematic review. *Allergy* **69**: 581–589.

Dijkhuizen, M.A., Wieringa, F.T., West, C.E. *et al.* (2001). Concurrent micronutrient deficiencies in lactating mothers and their infants in Indonesia. *American Journal of Clinical Nutrition* **73**: 786–791.

Dossus, L., Allen, N., Kaaks, R. *et al.* (2010). Reproductive risk factors and endometrial cancer: the European Prospective Investigation into Cancer and Nutrition. *International Journal of Cancer* **127**: 442–451.

Dyson, L., McCormick, F.M. and Renfrew, M.J. (2014). Interventions for promoting the initiation of breastfeeding. *São Paulo Medical Journal* **132**: 68.

Fallon, V.M., Harrold, J.A. and Chisholm, A. (2019). The impact of the UK Baby Friendly Initiative on maternal and infant health outcomes: a mixed-methods systematic review. *Maternal and Child Nutrition* **15**: e12778.

Fewtrell, M.S. (2011). The evidence for public health recommendations on infant feeding. *Early Human Development* **87**: 715–721.

Flensborg-Madsen, T., Falgreen Eriksen, H.L. and Mortensen, E.L. (2020). Early life predictors of intelligence in young adulthood and middle age. *PLoS One* **15**: e0228144.

Ford, R.P., Taylor, B.J., Mitchell, E.A. *et al.* (1993). Breastfeeding and the risk of sudden infant death syndrome. *International Journal of Epidemiology* **22**: 885–890.

Forster, D.A., McLardie-Hore, F.E., McLachlan, H.L. *et al.* (2019). Proactive peer (mother-to-mother) breastfeeding support by telephone (ringing up about breastfeeding early [RUBY]): a multicentre, unblinded, randomised controlled trial. *EClinicalMedicine* **8**: 20–28.

Fortner, R.T., Sisti, J., Chai, B. *et al.* (2019). Parity, breastfeeding, and breast cancer risk by hormone receptor status and molecular phenotype: results from the Nurses' Health Studies. *Breast Cancer Research* **21**: 40.

Foroushani, A.R., Mohammad, K., Mahmoodi, M. and Siassi, F. (2010). Effect of breastfeeding on cognitive performance in a British birth cohort. *East Mediterranean Health Journal* **16**: 202–208.

Galazzo, G., van Best, N., Bervoets, L. *et al.* (2020). Development of the microbiota and associations with birth mode, diet, and atopic disorders in a longitudinal analysis of stool samples, collected from infancy through early childhood. *Gastroenterology* **158**: 1584–1596.

Guzzardi, M.A., Granziera, F., Sanguinetti, E. *et al.* (2020). Exclusive breastfeeding predicts higher hearing-language development in girls of preschool age. *Nutrients* **12**: 2320.

Gonzalez-Darias, A., Diaz-Gomez, N.M. *et al.* (2020). Supporting a first-time mother: assessment of success of a breastfeeding promotion programme. *Midwifery* **85**: 102687.

Grantham-McGregor, S.M., Powell, C.A., Walker, S.P. *et al.* (1991). Nutritional supplementation, psychosocial stimulation, and mental development of stunted children: the Jamaican study. *Lancet* **338**: 1–5.

Gueye, S.B., Diop-Ndiaye, H., Diouf, O. *et al.* (2019). Effectiveness of the prevention of HIV mother -to-child transmission (PMTCT) program via early infant diagnosis (EID) data in Senegal. *PLoS One* **14**: e0215941.

Güngör, D., Nadaud, P., LaPergola, C.C. *et al.* (2019). Infant milk-feeding practices and food allergies, allergic rhinitis, atopic dermatitis, and asthma throughout the life span: a systematic review. *American Journal of Clinical Nutrition* **109**: 772S–799S.

Hamlyn, B., Brooker, S., Oleinikova, K. *et al.* (2002). *Infant Feeding 2000*. London: Department of Health.

Hartwig, F.P., Davies, N.M., Horta, B.L. *et al.* (2019). Effect modification of FADS2 polymorphisms on the association between breastfeeding and intelligence: results from a collaborative meta-analysis. *International Journal of Epidemiology* **48**: 45–57.

Harvey, S.M., Murphy, V.E., Gibson, P.G. *et al.* (2020). Maternal asthma, breastfeeding, and respiratory outcomes in the first year of life. *Pediatric Pulmonology* **55**: 1690–1696.

Hauck, F.R., Thompson, J.M., Tanabe, K.O. *et al.* (2011). Breastfeeding and reduced risk of sudden infant death syndrome: a meta-analysis. *Pediatrics* **128**: 103–110.

Hawkins, S.S., Stern, A.D., Baum, C.F. *et al.* (2014). Compliance with the Baby-Friendly Hospital Initiative and impact on breastfeeding rates. *Archives of Disease in Childhood* **99**: F138–F143.

He, X., Zhu, M., Hu, C. *et al.* (2015). Breast-feeding and postpartum weight retention: a systematic review and meta-analysis. *Public Health Nutrition* **18**: 3308–3316.

Henderson, L., Gregory, J. and Swan, G. (2002). *National Diet and Nutrition Survey: Adults Aged 19–64 Years*. London: Office for National Statistics.

Henjum, S., Lie, Ø., Ulak, M. *et al.* (2018). Erythrocyte fatty acid composition of Nepal breast-fed infants. *European Journal of Nutrition* **57**: 1003–1013.

Hess, C., Ofei, A. and Mincher, A (2015). Breastfeeding and childhood obesity among African Americans: a systematic review. *American Journal of Maternal and Child Nursing* **40**: 313–319.

Holland, B., Welch, A.A., Unwin, I.D. *et al.* (1991). *McCance and Widdowson's The Composition of Foods*, 5th ed. Cambridge: Royal Society of Chemistry.

Horta, B.L., Loret de Mola, C. and Victora, C.G (2015). Breastfeeding and intelligence: a systematic review and meta-analysis. *Acta Paediatrica* **104**: 14–19.

Ip, S., Chung, M., Raman, G. *et al.* (2007). Breastfeeding and maternal and infant health outcomes in developed countries. *Evidence Report/Technology Assessment* **153**: 1–186.

Isaacs *et al.* (2011).

Jedrychowski, W., Perera, F. and Jankowski, J. (2012). Effect of exclusive breastfeeding on the development of children's cognitive function in the Krakow prospective birth cohort study. *European Journal of Pediatrics* **171**: 151–158.

John, E.M., Hines, L.M., Phipps, A.I. *et al.* (2018). Reproductive history, breast-feeding and risk of triple negative breast cancer: the Breast Cancer Etiology in Minorities (BEM) study. *International Journal of Cancer* **142**: 2273–2285.

Jonsson, K., Barman, M., Moberg, S. *et al.* (2016). Fat intake and breast milk fatty acid composition in farming and nonfarming women and allergy development in the offspring. *Pediatric Research* **79**: 114–123.

Jordan, S.J., Na, R., Johnatty, S.E. *et al.* (2017). Breastfeeding and endometrial cancer risk: an analysis from the Epidemiology of Endometrial Cancer Consortium. *Obstetrics and Gynecology* **129**: 1059–1067.

Jost, R., Maire, J.-C., Maynard, F. *et al.* (1999). Aspects of whey protein usage in infant nutrition, a brief review. *International Journal of Food Science and Technology* **34**: 533–542.

Karlsson, M.K., Ahlborg, H.G. and Karlsson, C. (2005). Maternity and bone density. *Acta Orthopaedica* **76**: 2–13.

Kaunonen, M., Hannula, L. and Tarkka, M.T. (2012). A systematic review of peer support interventions for breastfeeding. *Journal of Clinical Nursing* **21**: 1943–1954.

Kelly, E., DunnGalvin, G., Murphy, B.P., Hourihane, J.O'B. (2019). Formula supplementation remains a risk for cow's milk allergy in breast-fed infants. *Pediatric Allergy and Immunology* **30**: 810–816.

Kemp, A.S., Hill, D.J., Allen, K.J. *et al.* (2008). Guidelines for the use of infant formulas to treat cows milk protein allergy: an Australian consensus panel opinion. *Medical Journal of Australia* **188**: 109–112.

Kerkhof, M., Koopman, L.P., van Strien, R.T. *et al.* (2003). Risk factors for atopic dermatitis in infants at high risk of allergy: the PIAMA study. *Clinical and Experimental Allergy* **33**: 1336–1341.

Kivlighan, K.T., Murray-Krezan, C., Schwartz, T. *et al.* (2020). Improved breastfeeding duration with Baby Friendly Hospital Initiative implementation in a diverse and underserved population. *Birth* **47**: 135–143.

Koletzko, B. (2016). Human milk lipids. *Annals of Nutrition and Metabolism* **69**(Suppl 2): 28–40.

Kotecha, S.J., Watkins, W.J., Lowe, J. *et al.* (2019). Comparison of the associations of early-life factors on wheezing phenotypes in preterm-born children and term-born children. *American Journal of Epidemiology* **188**: 527–536.

Kotsopoulos, J., Lubinski, J., Salmena, L. *et al.* (2012). Breastfeeding and the risk of breast cancer in BRCA1 and BRCA2 mutation carriers. *Breast Cancer Research* **14**: R42.

Kovacs, A., Funke, S., Marosvolgyi, T. *et al.* (2005). Fatty acids in early human milk after preterm and full-term delivery. *Journal of Pediatric Gastroenterology and Nutrition* **41**: 454–459.

Kramer, M.S. and Kakuma, R. (2002). Optimal duration of exclusive breastfeeding. *Cochrane Database of Systematic Reviews* (1): CD003517.

Kramer, M.S. and Kakuma, R. (2012). Optimal duration of exclusive breastfeeding. *Cochrane Database of Systematic Reviews* (8): CD003517.

Kramer, M.S., Chalmers, B., Hodnett, E.D. *et al.* (2001). Promotion of breast-feeding intervention trial (PROBIT): a randomized trial in the Republic of Belarus. *JAMA* **285**: 413–420.

Kuwata, H., Yip, T.T., Yamauchi, K. *et al.* (1998). The survival of ingested lactoferrin in the gastrointestinal tract of adult mice. *Biochemical Journal* **334**: 321–323.

Langley-Evans, A.J. and Langley-Evans, S.C. (2003). Relationship between maternal nutrient intakes in early and late pregnancy and infants weight and proportions at birth: prospective cohort study. *Journal of the Royal Society for the Promotion of Health* **123**: 210–216.

Larsen, A., Magasana, V., Dinh, T.H. *et al.* (2019). Longitudinal adherence to maternal antiretroviral therapy and infant Nevirapine prophylaxis from 6 weeks to 18 months postpartum amongst a cohort of mothers and infants in South Africa. *BMC Infectious Disease* **19**(Suppl 1): 789.

Lee, E.N. (2019). Effects of parity and breastfeeding duration on bone density in postmenopausal women. *Asian Nursing Research* **13**: 161–167.

Lefebvre, C.M. and John, R.M. (2014). The effect of breastfeeding on childhood overweight and obesity: a systematic review of the literature. *Journal of the American Association of Nurse Practitioners* **26**: 386–401

Lehmann, G.M., LaKind, J.S., Davis, M.H. *et al.* (2018). Environmental Chemicals in Breast Milk and Formula: Exposure and Risk Assessment Implications. *Environmental Health Perspectives* **126**: 96001.

Lien, E.L. (2003). Infant formulas with increased concentrations of α-lactalbumin. *American Journal of Clinical Nutrition* **77**(Suppl): 1555S–1558S.

Lenehan, S.M., Boylan, G.B., Livingstone, V. *et al.* (2020). The impact of short-term predominate breastfeeding on cognitive outcome at 5 years. *Acta Paediatrica* **109**: 982–988.

Lönnerdal, B. (1986). Effects of maternal dietary intake on human milk composition. *Journal of Nutrition* **116**: 499–513.

López-Olmedo, N., Hernández-Cordero, S., Neufeld, L.M. *et al.* (2016). The associations of maternal weight change with breastfeeding, diet and physical activity during the postpartum period. *Maternal and Child Health Journal* **20**: 270–280.

Lozoff, B. and Georgieff, M.K. (2006). Iron deficiency and brain development. *Seminars in Paediatric Neurology* **13**: 158–165.

Lubetzky, R., Littner, Y., Mimouni, F.B. *et al.* (2006). Circadian variations in fat content of expressed breast milk from mothers of preterm infants. *Journal of the American College of Nutrition* **25**: 151–154.

Matangkasombut, P., Padungpak, S., Thaloengsok, S. *et al.* (2017). Detection of β-lactoglobulin in human breastmilk 7 days after cow milk ingestion. *Paediatrics and International Child Health* **37**: 199–203.

Matheson, M.C., Allen, K.J. and Tang, M.L. (2012). Understanding the evidence for and against the role of breastfeeding in allergy prevention. *Clinical and Experimental Allergy* **42**: 827–851.

Matthews, K., Webber, K., McKim, E. *et al.* (1998). Maternal infant-feeding decisions: reasons and influences. *Canadian Journal of Nursing Research* **30**: 177–198.

Mbae, C., Mwangi, M., Gitau, N. *et al.* (2020). Factors associated with occurrence of salmonellosis among children living in Mukuru slum, an urban informal settlement in Kenya. *BMC Infectious Disease* **20**: 422.

McAndrew, F., Thompson, J., Fellows, L. *et al.* (2012). *Infant Feeding Survey 2010*. Leeds: Health and Social Care Information Centre.

Meldrum, S.J., Heaton, A.E., Foster, J.K. *et al.* (2020). Do infants of breast-feeding mothers benefit from additional long-chain PUFA from fish oil? A 6-year follow-up. *British Journal of Nutrition* **124**: 701–708.

Mills, L., Coulter, L., Savage, E. and Modi, N. (2019). Macronutrient content of donor milk from a regional human milk bank: variation with donor mother-infant characteristics. *British Journal of Nutrition* **122**: 1155–1167.

Mitoulas, L.R., Gurrin, L.C., Doherty, D.A. *et al.* (2003). Infant intake of fatty acids from human milk over the first year of lactation. *British Journal of Nutrition* **90**: 979–986.

Mpody, C., Reline, T., Ravelomanana, N.L.R. *et al.* (2019). Breastfeeding support offered at delivery is associated with higher prevalence of exclusive breastfeeding at 6 weeks postpartum among hiv exposed infants: a cross-sectional analysis. *Maternal and Child Health Journal* **23**: 1308–1316.

Modugno, F., Goughnour, S.L., Wallack, D. *et al.* (2019). Breastfeeding factors and risk of epithelial ovarian cancer. *Gynecology and Oncology* **153**: 116–122.

Nakamori, M., Ninh, N.X. and Isomura, H. (2009). Nutritional status of lactating mothers and their breast milk concentration of iron, zinc and copper in rural Vietnam *Journal of Nutritional Science and Vitaminology* **55**: 338–345.

Nguyen, P., Binns, C.W., Ha, A.V.V. *et al,* (2020). Prelacteal and early formula feeding increase risk of infant hospitalisation: a prospective cohort study. *Archives of Disease in Childhood* **105**: 122–126.

Niggemann, B., Binder, C., Dupont, C. *et al.* (2001). Prospective, controlled, multi-center study on the effect of an amino-acid-based formula in infants with cow's milk allergy/intolerance and atopic dermatitis. *Pediatric Allergy and Immunology* **12**: 78–82.

Oddy, W.H., Robinson, M., Kendall, G.E. *et al.* (2011). Breastfeeding and early child development: a prospective cohort study. *Acta Paediatrica* **100**: 992–999.

Olsson, C., Hernell, O., Hörnell, A. *et al.* (2008). Difference in celiac disease risk between Swedish birth cohorts suggests an opportunity for primary prevention. *Pediatrics* **122**: 528–534.

Osborn, D.A. and Sinn, J. (2006). Soy formula for prevention of allergy and food intolerance in infants. *Cochrane Database of Systematic Reviews* (4): CD003741.

Pang, W.W., Tan, P.T., Cai, S. *et al.* (2020). Nutrients or nursing? Understanding how breast milk feeding affects child cognition. *European Journal of Nutrition* **59**: 609–619.

Phadungath, C. (2005). Casein micelle structure: a concise review. *Songklanakarin Journal of Science and Technology* **27**: 201–212.

Prentice, A.M., Goldberg, G.R. and Prentice, A. (1994). Body mass index and lactation performance. *European Journal of Clinical Nutrition*, **48**(Suppl 3): S78–S86.

Regan, S. and Brown, A. (2019). Experiences of online breastfeeding support: Support and reassurance versus judgement and misinformation. *Maternal and Child Nutrition* **15**: e12874.

Remmert, J.E., Mosery, N., Goodman, G. *et al.* (2020). Breastfeeding practices among women living with HIV in KwaZulu-Natal, South Africa: an observational study. *Maternal and Child Health Journal* **24**: 127–134.

Ritchie, S.J. (2017). Publication bias in a recent meta-analysis on breastfeeding and IQ. *Acta Paediatrica* **106**: 345.

Ritchie, L.D., Fung, E.B., Halloran, B.P. *et al.* (1998). A longitudinal study of calcium homeostasis during human pregnancy and lactation and after resumption of menses. *American Journal of Clinical Nutrition* **67**: 693–701.

Robert, E., Michaud-Létourneau, I., Dramaix-Wilmet, M. *et al.* (2019). A comparison of exclusive breastfeeding in Belgian maternity facilities with and without Baby Friendly Hospital status. *Maternal and Child Nutrition* **15**: e12845.

Sabatier, M., Garcia-Rodenas, C.L., Castro, C.A. *et al.* (2019). Longitudinal changes of mineral concentrations in preterm and term human milk from lactating Swiss women. *Nutrients* **11**: 1855.

Saeed, O.B., Haile, Z.T., Chertok, I.A. (2020). Association between exclusive breastfeeding and infant health outcomes in Pakistan. *Journal of Pediatric Nursing* **50**: e62–e68.

Salazar-Martinez, E., Lazcano-Ponce, E.C., Gonzalez Lira-Lira, G. *et al.* (1999). Reproductive factors of ovarian and endometrial cancer risk in a high fertility population in Mexico. *Cancer Research* **59**: 3658–3662.

Samur, G., Topcu, A., Turan, S. (2009). Trans fatty acids and fatty acid composition of mature breast milk in turkish women and their association with maternal diets. *Lipids* **44**: 405–13.

Schanler, R.J. (1995). Suitability of human milk for the low-birthweight infant. *Clinics in Perinatology* **22**: 207–222.

Shulkin, M., Pimpin, L., Bellinger, D. *et al.* (2018). n-3 Fatty acid supplementation in mothers, preterm infants, and term infants and childhood psychomotor and visual development: a systematic review and meta-analysis. *Journal of Nutrition* **148**: 409–418.

Smilowitz, J.T., O'Sullivan, A., Barile, D. *et al.* (2013). The human milk metabolome reveals diverse oligosaccharide profiles. *Journal of Nutrition* **143**: 1709–1718.

Strøm, M., Mortensen, E.L., Kesmodel, U.S. *et al.* (2019). Is breast feeding associated with offspring IQ at age 5? Findings from prospective cohort: Lifestyle During Pregnancy Study. *BMJ Open* **9**: e023134.

Sudfeld, C.R., Fawzi, W.W. and Lahariya, C. (2012). Peer support and exclusive breastfeeding duration in low and middle-income countries: a systematic review and meta-analysis. *PLoS One* **7**: e45143.

Sung, H.K., Ma, S.H., Choi, J.Y. *et al.* (2016). The effect of breastfeeding duration and parity on the risk of epithelial ovarian cancer: a systematic review and meta-analysis. *Journal of Preventive Medicine and Public Health* **49**: 349–366.

Tahir, M.J., Haapala, J.L., Foster, L.P. *et al.* (2019). Association of full breastfeeding duration with postpartum weight retention in a cohort of predominantly breastfeeding women. *Nutrients* **11**: 938.

Taylor, R.R., Sladkevicius, E., Panca, M. *et al.* (2012). Cost-effectiveness of using an extensively hydrolysed formula compared to an amino acid formula as first-line treatment for cow milk allergy in the UK. *Pediatric Allergy and Immunology* **23**: 240–249.

Theurich, M.A., Davanzo, R., Busck-Rasmussen, M. *et al.* (2019). Breastfeeding rates and programs in Europe: a survey of 11 national breastfeeding committees and representatives. *Journal of Pediatric Gastroenterology and Nutrition* 68: 400–407.

Unar-Munguía, M., Torres-Mejía, G., Colchero, M.A. and González de Cosío, T. (2017). Breastfeeding mode and risk of breast cancer: a dose-response meta-analysis. *Journal of Human Lactation* **33**: 422–434.

Unicef (2019). Infant and young child feeding. https://data.unicef.org/topic/nutrition/infant-and-young-child-feeding (accessed 6 April 2021).

Walfisch, A., Sermer, C., Cressman, A. *et al.* (2013). Breast milk and cognitive development – the role of confounders: a systematic review. *BMJ Open* **3**: e003259.

Wang *et al.* (2012).

Wei, W., Yang, J., Yang, D. *et al.* (2019). Phospholipid composition and fat globule structure i: comparison of human milk fat from different gestational ages, lactation stages, and infant formulas. *Journal of Agriculture and Food Chemistry* **67**: 13922–13928.

Wells, J.C., Jonsdottir, O.H., Hibberd, P.L. *et al.* (2012). Randomized controlled trial of 4 compared with 6 mo of exclusive breastfeeding in Iceland: differences in breast-milk intake by stable-isotope probe. *American Journal of Clinical Nutrition* **96**: 73–79.

World Health Organization. (2016) *Guideline Updates on HIV Infant Feeding*. Geneva: WHO.

World Health Organization. (2010). *Guidelines on HIV and Infant Feeding 2010: Principles and recommendations for infant feeding in the context of HIV and a summary of evidence.* Geneva: WHO.

World Health Organization/Unicef (1989). *Protecting, Promoting and Supporting Breastfeeding: The Special Role of Maternity Services*, Geneva: WHO.

Yan, G., Huang, Y., Cao, H. *et al.* (2019). Association of breastfeeding and postmenopausal osteoporosis in Chinese women: a community-based retrospective study. *BMC Women's Health* **19**: 110.

Yaoa *et al.* (2020).

Yasuhi, I., Yamashita, H., Maeda, K. *et al.* (2019). High-intensity breastfeeding improves insulin sensitivity during early post-partum period in obese women with gestational diabetes. *Diabetes and Metabolism Research Reviews* **35**: e3127.

Yi, X., Zhu, J., Zhu, X. *et al.* (2016). Breastfeeding and thyroid cancer risk in women: a dose–response meta-analysis of epidemiological studies. *Clinical Nutrition* **35**: 1039–1046.

Zhou, S.J., Sullivan, T., Gibson, R.A. *et al.* (2014). Nutritional adequacy of goat milk infant formulas for term infants: a double-blind randomised controlled trial. *British Journal of Nutrition* **111**: 1641–1651.

Additional reading

If you would like to find out more about the material discussed in this chapter, the following sources may be of interest:

Brown, A. (2016). *Breastfeeding Uncovered: Who really decides how we feed our babies?* London: Pinter and Martin.

Brown, A and Jones, W. (2019). *A Guide to Supporting Breastfeeding for the Medical Profession.* Abingdon: Routledge.

Dobbing, J. (ed.) (2013). *Brain, Behavior and Iron in the Infant Diet.* London: Springer Verlag.

Wambach, K. and Spencer, B. (eds.) (2019). *Breastfeeding and Human Lactation.* Burlington, MA: James and Bartlett Publishers.

CHAPTER 6

Nutrition and childhood

LEARNING OBJECTIVES

This chapter will enable the reader to:
- Explain that growth is the most important physiological process determining the nutrient and energy requirements of children.
- Show an appreciation of why the requirements of children must be delivered through a nutrient-dense dietary pattern.
- Describe how infectious disease and catch-up growth can promote micronutrient deficiencies among children in developing countries.
- Discuss the importance of nutrition during infancy in establishing lifelong food preferences and the opportunities for health promotion that arise during this life stage.
- Demonstrate understanding of the key issues surrounding the weaning process, with particular emphasis on the timing of the introduction of complementary foods.
- Discuss the contribution of child poverty to both malnutrition and the occurrence of overweight in the population.
- Describe the complex drivers of malnutrition in childhood.
- Demonstrate an awareness of the double burden of malnutrition and overweight, which impacts on children in many regions of the world.
- Discuss the relationship between dietary factors and dental caries in children.
- Describe the susceptibility of children to advertising of energy-dense, nutrient-poor foods and beverages and highlight the importance of regulation of such marketing to continuing health promotion strategies.
- Show an awareness of how schools contribute to health promotion among school-age children.
- Describe global trends in childhood obesity prevalence.
- Discuss the significant contribution that genetic factors make to early-onset obesity.
- Demonstrate understanding of the contribution that the modern environment makes to obesity and overweight among children.
- Critically evaluate the evidence that suggests that childhood obesity is predictive of obesity and related disorders in adult life.
- Describe optimal strategies for the prevention and treatment of obesity in children.

6.1 Introduction

Humans are almost unique among mammalian species in that there is an extended period of growth and development between birth and adulthood. Even among our closest relatives, the great apes, where lifespan is typically 30–50 years, full maturity is achieved after just 7–13 years. Human childhood represents an important physiological and psychosocial stage of the lifespan. During this time, the individual attains full adult stature and full functional capacity of organs and systems, achieves a mature view of the world and develops independence from parents. Childhood is the phase of maximum growth, enlargement of the skeleton and remodelling of body composition. These changes are driven by surges in, and maturation of, the activities of key endocrine systems, including the somatotropic, hypothalamic–pituitary–gonadal and hypothalamic–pituitary–adrenal axes. Nutrition plays a paramount role during this time as the provision of an adequate and balanced supply of energy and nutrients is essential to maintain a normal developmental profile, to provide resistance against infectious disease and to ensure good health at later stages of life. Within this book, the childhood years have been divided into three stages: infancy, childhood and adolescence. Adolescence is discussed in Chapter 7.

Nutrition, Health and Disease: A Lifespan Approach, Third Edition. Simon Langley-Evans.
© 2021 John Wiley & Sons Ltd. Published 2021 by John Wiley & Sons Ltd.
Companion website: www.wiley.com/go/langleyevans/lifespan3e

6.2 Infancy (birth to five)

6.2.1 The key developmental milestones

Nutritional demands over the first five years of life are very much shaped by the physiological and developmental processes associated with this life stage. Achieving the physical milestones sets a relatively high demand for energy and nutrients, but the psychosocial and behavioural milestones should not be ignored, as they impact on how nutrient demands are delivered and the development of attitudes and behaviours that help to shape long-term health and wellbeing. Alongside the development of the physical systems of the body and the ability to communicate and learn about the world around them, children at this preschool stage are undergoing a radical reshaping of their dietary pattern. The infant must make the transition from the milk-only diet of the first four to six months of life to a diet that comprises solids, but which remains energy dense, and then to a pattern of food intake that more resembles that which they will follow in their adult years.

Growth is the most important physiological process for the preschool child and largely explains the high nutrient requirements of infancy. The first year of life has the most rapid growth rate of any life stage and during this period, the infant will triple their body weight and increase height by approximately 75%. Growth rates slow thereafter, but growth continues to be a major demand process (Figure 6.1). Growth rates for boys and girls are similar over the first five years.

In addition to growth, the body is undergoing a series of changes in terms of composition and proportions, together with maturation of organ systems. For example, the lungs continue to undergo the process of branching off new alveoli until the age of seven to eight years. At birth, the human head is disproportionately large in relation to the trunk and the limbs are relatively short. Over the first five years, truncal and limb growth is prioritized. Between birth and one year of age, there is considerable deposition of fat reserves, taking the proportion of the body that is fat from 14% to around 25%. Over years one to four, the absolute fat mass in the body stays relatively stable, but increasing lean body mass (from 14% of body mass at birth to 20% by age five years) results in fat proportions declining to around 20%.

Body water is repartitioned in infancy. Initially, a greater proportion of water is held in the extracellular compartment making the infant more vulnerable to dehydration. Shifting of fluid to the intracellular compartment reduces this risk in the older child.

While growth of the trunk and limbs is greatest during infancy, the brain still grows at a rapid rate at this time. Brain size doubles over the first year of life, which can be observed as an increase in head circumference. Average head circumference at birth is around 34 cm, and the first year sees an increase of 12 cm. Over the next year (age one to two), this slows to a gain of just 2 cm but, despite this, the brain increases in size by around 50% between the ages of one and five years and, by the end of this period, it is around 90% of adult size.

Changes in brain size are accompanied by profound changes in the abilities of the child. At birth, the infant is relatively helpless, and while it has well-developed sensory neurones, the motor neurones are extremely immature. Over the early years, rapid development is seen in terms of these motor systems and their integration with sensory inputs. As a result, the infant years see the acquisition of key skills such as speech, walking and the ability to interact with family members and other children. Table 6.1 summarizes some of the key developmental milestones

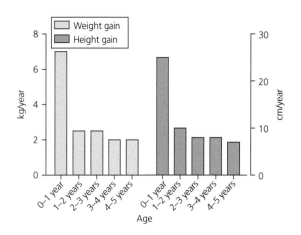

Figure 6.1 Rates of growth in preschool children.
Source: data compiled from Freeman *et al.* (1995).

Table 6.1 Developmental milestones for infants.

Age (years)	Physical changes and abilities	Psychosocial changes and food-related behaviour
0–1	Rapid growth Hand–eye coordination Sitting Crawling Convey food to mouth Eruption of teeth	Dependent on parent Good appetite Enjoys food
1–2	Walking Chewing Use of baby cup Manipulation of food items	Good appetite Enjoys food but less experimental Developing verbal communication skills
2–3	Running and jumping Fine motor skills Use of cup	Appetite slows Fluent speech Uses tantrums to influence the behaviour of others
3–4	Use of cutlery Hopping Balancing	Picky/faddy eating Develops independent food preferences
4–5	Self-feeding Adult range of dexterity	Receptive to attitudes of others Develops a circle of peers

achieved by infants. The acquisition of these new physical and social skills impacts upon the nutrition of the child, who is effectively developing a physical and psychosocial independence from their mother. Considering the supply and demand model outlined in Chapter 1, on the demand side, growth and maturation increase requirements for nutrients in relation to body size. On the supply side, there are factors such as attaining the ability to self-feed or snack, the development of preferences and attitudes about food and the interaction with adults and peers, which will all determine the quality and possibly quantity of nutrient inputs.

6.2.2 Nutrient requirements

Over the first five years of life, there is a need for a pattern of dietary intake that is both energy and nutrient dense to meet high metabolic demands. With their short stature, preschool children are unable to consume and process sufficient bulk of food to meet their needs. While in absolute terms the nutrient requirements of young children are well below those of older children and adults, on a per-body-weight basis, they can be many times higher than at the later life stages. Table 6.2 shows how energy requirements are threefold higher in infancy than in adulthood and requirements for many micronutrients are elevated to a similar extent.

One of the major challenges for delivery of nutrient requirements to this age group is to provide an appropriate balance of all nutrients, within the restrictions placed by the fact that children often have a limited range of preferred foods. Snacks are extremely important for the nutrition of younger children, as they allow the supply of nutrients to be maintained throughout the day and compensate for the limited quantity of food that can be consumed at mealtimes. Selection of snacks needs to remain focused upon nutrient rather than energy density.

During this period of life, children move through the major transitions of weaning and from a childhood dietary pattern to an adult diet. This latter transition is substantial, as the infant diet essentially delivers around 50% of energy as fat and 40% as simple sugars, with very little dietary fibre. In contrast, the adult diet should deliver no more than 35% of energy of fat and is mostly based upon bulky complex carbohydrates. Throughout this period, children need to be encouraged to experiment with a wide range of different foods, flavours and textures to establish healthy food preferences later in life.

6.2.2.1 Macronutrients and energy

As in adults, total energy expenditure in childhood is defined in terms of the resting energy expenditure plus energy expended in diet-induced thermogenesis and physical activity. For children, however, overall energy requirement is not solely defined by total energy expenditure, as there are also considerations in relation to growth and losses through urine and faeces. The latter are minor components but, compared with adults, in children they constitute a significant element of energy expenditure. Growth impacts upon energy requirements as the fat and protein deposited in growing tissue has an energy value and because energy must be expended to carry out the synthetic processes that yield new tissues (Torun, 2005).

Table 6.2 A comparison of nutrient requirements* between adults and children under the age of 5 years.

Nutrient[†]	Age			
	1–3	4–6	19–50 (male)	19–50 (female)
Energy (kcal/kg/day)	95.8	91.6	34.5	32.3
Protein (g/kg/day)	0.94	0.83	0.60	0.62
Folate (µg/kg/day)	4.0	4.21	2.02	2.50
Ascorbate (mg/kg/day)	1.6	1.12	0.29	0.36
Cobalamin (µg/kg/day)	0.032	0.039	0.017	0.021
Iron (mg/kg/day)	0.42	0.26	0.09	0.19
Zinc (mg/kg/day)	0.30	0.28	0.10	0.09
Calcium (mg/kg/day)	22.0	19.7	7.1	8.8

Data derived from UK estimated average requirements (Department of Health, 1998) and assuming body weights of 12.5 (1–3 years), 17.8 (4–6 years), 74 kg (adult male) and 60 kg (adult female).
* Selected nutrients.
[†] All figures are shown adjusted for body weight.

Over the first year of life, energy requirements are exceptionally high and can be between three and four times greater (on a per-bodyweight basis) than in adulthood. This high demand is only partly explained by the energy requirements of growth. Torun (2005) estimated the energy cost of growth for infants at around 4 kcal (17 kJ) per gram of weight gain. In a two-year-old, this would equate to around 26.4 kcal (112.2 kJ) per day, which is clearly a very minor component (around 2%) of estimated average requirement. In the neonate, the energy demand for growth is much greater but at most amounts to a third of overall energy requirement. Total energy expenditure in infants is in fact mostly related to resting energy expenditure, which increases steadily over the first five years in proportion to body weight. The smaller bodies of children compared with adults have a greater surface area to volume ratio and, as a result, more energy must be expended to maintain normal body temperature.

Children in developing countries are subject to a number of specific factors that may elevate their dietary energy requirements to a greater extent than those seen in more affluent settings. Micronutrient deficiencies are commonplace in developing countries, particularly in rural populations. If any micronutrient is limiting within the diet, then this will impact upon the efficiency of use of energy substrates and hence the capacity to meet demands for energy (Prentice and Paul, 2000). Moreover, infectious diseases are common in these communities. Disease promotes negative energy balance by increasing demand and reducing intakes. Fever has an anorectic influence; gastrointestinal infection or the presence of gastrointestinal parasites increases losses of energy and nutrients. Periods of acute infection are often followed by catch-up growth,

effectively maintaining energy requirements at a higher level over a longer period of time (Prentice and Paul, 2000). Such requirements are likely to outstrip the supply of energy from the diet, and as a result, growth will falter. Lost growth will result in either stunting (failure of linear growth) or wasting (failure to gain weight; Figure 6.2). Children in this age group are the most vulnerable to protein–energy malnutrition and associated morbidities, mortality and long-term deficits of stature, cognitive function and health.

The causes of malnutrition in children living in developing countries are complex (Figure 6.3). The immediate causes of death, stunting and wasting are inadequate supply of nutrients to meet demand and frequent exposure to infectious disease, usually gastrointestinal and respiratory infections. These immediate causes are ultimately driven by poverty and geopolitics. In many developing countries, especially those undergoing rapid economic development, the public health challenge is the management of what is termed the double burden of malnutrition, where protein–energy malnutrition and micronutrient deficiencies coexist with overweight and obesity (Figure 6.4). This can occur at the population, household or even individual level (Menon and Penalvo, 2020). For example, a child may be stunted due to early malnutrition but overweight due to subsequent overfeeding. Some households may have one or more stunted or wasted children in the family, alongside overweight children, a situation seen in more than 25% of households in Egypt, Guatemala and Azerbaijan (Popkin et al., 2020).

At the population level, the split between malnourished and overweight tends to be between rural and urban areas. In rural areas where the food system is focused on local production of a limited range of

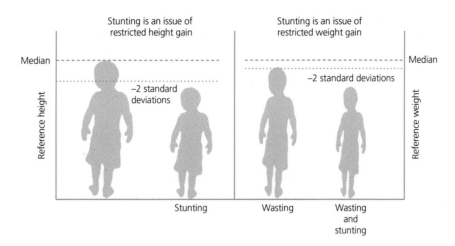

Figure 6.2 Stunting and wasting. Stunting is defined as height two standard deviations or more below the median height for age for an appropriate reference population. Wasting is defined as weight two standard deviations or more below the weight for age for an appropriate reference population.

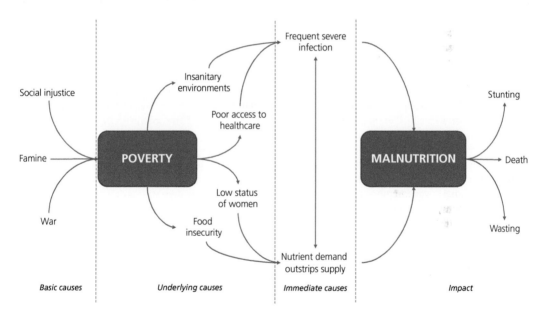

Figure 6.3 The complex causes of malnutrition. The immediate direct causes of protein–energy malnutrition or micronutrient deficiency are a failure of nutrient supply to meet demand, which can be driven by insufficient food, frequent severe infection or other metabolic traumas. The underlying causes are ultimately more complex and are associated with poverty, social injustice and geopolitical factors.

crops or subsistence farming, children are at risk of stunting and wasting due to protein–energy malnutrition and micronutrient deficiency. Public health workers then simultaneously face obesity and micronutrient deficiencies in the urban centres, where physical activity drops due to modern transport systems and intakes of energy-dense, nutrient-poor foods and sugar-sweetened beverages are high due to reliance on modern, supermarket-based food systems (Popkin *et al.*, 2020). In Ghana, for example, this pattern has resulted in a higher level of stunting in rural areas (22% compared with 15% in the urban areas), with more obesity in the urban centres (3.4% among under-fives compared with 1.9% in rural areas; Mbogori *et al.*, 2020). In the developed regions of the world, obesity and poor micronutrient status go hand in hand as the common manifestation of the double burden of child malnutrition, but with rising

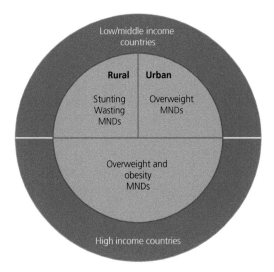

Figure 6.4 The double burden of malnutrition. Protein–energy malnutrition or micronutrient deficiencies (MNDs) can coexist with overweight and obesity in the same individual, household or population. In developing countries, this is often seen as a feature of the rural–urban divide.

levels of child poverty, stunting is not uncommon (2% prevalence in Australia, 3.5% in the United States for under-fives).

The requirements of preschool children for protein that are shown in Table 6.2, and considered in more detail in the various dietary reference value systems produced by the World Health Organization (WHO) and national governments, are estimates that are contested by some researchers in the field. Protein requirements for children have been estimated using nitrogen-balance studies, usually performed on older individuals, integrated with estimates of the nitrogen content of tissues and rates of tissue accretion. It has been noted that the actual protein intakes of breast-fed infants are below these estimates and yet growth and development are maintained. It may therefore be inferred that the estimated requirements are in excess of true values. As amino acids regulate growth and development, it is possible that consumption in excess could have negative consequences. Garlick (2006) reported the findings of potassium balance studies in young children. Potassium balance is closely correlated with nitrogen balance and, using relevant regression models, it was suggested that the average protein requirement of a six-month-old would be 1.12 g/kg body weight per day, declining to 0.74 g/kg per day by 10 years.

Provision of fat is an important consideration in the diets of preschool children as fat plays an important role in the provision of energy, maturation of

organ systems and maintenance of immune function (Butte, 2005). There are no recommendations regarding the fat intakes of children before the age of two years, but it is estimated that, at this stage, fat should be providing around 50% of total energy. It is suggested that between two and five years of age, fat should provide a minimum of 15% of dietary energy and ideally 30–40%. Including fat in the diet is important as it is the most effective means of delivering the required energy density of the infant diet. There is good evidence that restricting fat intake can impact adversely upon rates of growth. Fat may be of greater importance in some populations than in others. Children in developing countries generally expend more energy through physical activity and therefore become dependent on fat oxidation as glycogen reserves are rapidly depleted (Prentice and Paul, 2000). Immune cells preferentially use fat oxidation to provide energy for their function; so, again, children in developing countries may require more lipid for this purpose, in the face of regular infection. Essential fatty acids give rise to inflammatory mediators and therefore also make a contribution to this role. Long-chain fatty acids such as arachidonic acid and docosahexaenoic acid are required for the growth and maturation of the brain and visual apparatus. Given the rapid growth of the infant brain over the first five years, provision of sufficient essential fatty acids of the n-3 and n-6 series is a critical element of a healthy diet for infants.

6.2.2.2 Micronutrients

All vitamins and minerals are essential for the growth and wellbeing of children at this age. Infants are especially vulnerable to the development of deficiency diseases and subclinical deficiencies as they have high nutrient demands and generally low stores of micronutrients. Micronutrients can be limiting factors in the diet, causing growth faltering. Classical studies of children being treated for malnutrition in the Caribbean showed that growth of infants receiving supplemental protein and energy was heavily dependent upon adequate provision of zinc, for example.

Given the high demand for all micronutrients, this text does not focus on specific requirements in any detail and the reader is advised to consult relevant texts listing dietary reference values for more detailed information (e.g. Department of Health, 1998). However, some nutrients are noteworthy as there are either special guidelines in place or major concerns about the adequacy of their provision to infants. Calcium and vitamin D, for example, are considered important at this time as early growth and mineralization of the skeleton may boost the peak bone mass attained in early adulthood and reduce risk of osteoporosis in later life. Infants should therefore consume good sources of calcium, such as milk, and fortified sources of vitamin D.

Sodium should be restricted in the diet of infants and young children need to be taught the importance of selecting low-salt foods and not adding salt to meals, either during cooking or at the table. The Scientific Advisory Committee on Nutrition (2003) in the UK issued guidelines for salt intake in the under-fives. Their recommendation was for children under one year to consume no more than 1 g salt (400 mg sodium) per day, with this rising to 2 g salt (800 mg sodium) between two and six years.

6.2.3 Nutrient intakes and infants

The diets of young children are often quite limited in their range and can exclude foods that would actually be ideal for the delivery of the required nutrient and energy density. This limitation may be a product of children's responses to newly introduced foods, a lack of parental knowledge or the use of a limited variety of food items during weaning. The rolling programme of the UK National Diet and Nutrition Surveys has included two large studies of the diets of children (1995 and 2002) and, more recently, updates every year as part of a whole population (children and adults) time series (Public Health England, 2020). Years 7 and 8 of the rolling programme, covering 2013 to 2016, found that children aged 1.5–3 years were consuming markedly higher amounts of free sugar than the level recommended by the Scientific Advisory Committee on Nutrition (11.3% of energy compared with 5% recommendation), with the intake derived mostly through cereals, soft drinks and fruit juices (Roberts et al., 2018). Only 10% of preschool children consumed fibre at the recommended level and only 7% consumed the recommended five portions of fruit and vegetables per day. Year 8 of the survey suggested that 15% of the 1.5–3-year-old sample were consuming vitamin A below the lower reference nutrient intake compared with 6% in the previous survey; 10% of the children at this age were consuming iron at a level below the lower reference nutrient intake.

Among US preschool children, the quality of the typical diet consumed falls short of recommendations. Fox et al. (2016) examined intakes of two- to three-year-olds and found that more than 90% failed to consume sufficient whole grains and vegetables and 48% were consuming below recommendations for dairy produce. Sisson et al. (2017) found that when US children were in daycare they received more nutrient-dense meals than at home. In daycare, low-fat dairy, fruit and vegetables were favoured, while at home young children consumed more high-fat and high-sugar foods. In developing countries, the range of foods available to infants is generally considerably lower than noted for the developed countries, particularly in impoverished communities and rural areas. Even where choice is limited by overall availability, food-related behaviours of children may limit their preferences even further. Lutter and Rivera (2003) noted that among children who were undernourished and growth restricted, up to 25% of food offered was not consumed. Often, foods in these situations are low in fat and lack nutrient density. Fat is important in stimulating the appetite by virtue of its contribution to aroma, flavour and texture of food. Palatability is a particularly important determinant of food intake and choice in children.

Observations that milk is a major source of nutrients in these studies are encouraging. It is generally considered that milk should be a major staple in the diets of infants by virtue of its capacity to deliver a high proportion of required nutrients and energy, either as a drink, as a component of sauces used in cooking or added to breakfast cereals. Consuming 440 ml per day of whole milk will deliver 25–32% of daily energy requirements for a one- to four-year-old and up to 60% of protein requirement and all of the requirements for vitamin A, calcium and several B vitamins (e.g. riboflavin). To maintain energy density and intakes of fat-soluble vitamins, it is suggested that under-fives should consume whole milk but that semi-skimmed milk is acceptable for children over the age of two years. The 2015/16 UK National Diet and Nutrition Survey found that milk and dairy produce provided 25% of energy and 35% of protein intake for children aged 1.5–3 years (Roberts et al., 2018). Whole milk was the main food item in the dairy food group, consumed by this age group.

Vitamin and mineral supplements are often provided to infants by their parents and in the past have been recommended for infants who were breastfed. In a study from the United States, Briefel et al. (2006) noted that 16% of children aged four months to two years were given supplements, with a much greater proportion (31%) between the ages of one and two. Leaf (2007) highlighted UK recommendations that younger children should be supplemented with vitamin D unless consuming fortified sources. The NHS Healthy Start scheme ensures that milk and supplements are freely available for the under-fours from poor families in the UK. There are some concerns that supplements may be more likely to be provided by better educated and more affluent parents to children who do not really need them. A study from Belgium found high use of supplements among preschool children of highly educated, non-smoking parents. Although for some of this group supplements helped in achieving recommended intakes of vitamin D, intakes of other nutrients such as zinc were excessive (Huybrechts *et al.*, 2010). Among US children, the use of supplements is high and may compensate for the relatively low nutrient density of food intake. Around 20% of children up to two years of age and 45% of preschool children take supplements. As a result, there are few concerns about nutritional status in this group in the population (Bailey *et al.*, 2018; Gahche *et al.*, 2019).

6.2.4 Transition to an adult pattern of food intake

The infant years are a time of major physical and psychological development and represent an intense period of change to the diet. There are two key changes that occur between six months and the age of five. The first is the process of weaning, which generally results in the child moving from a complete dependence on milk for all nutrition to a diet that provides most nutrients from non-milk sources by the age of one year. The second is a decrease in the energy and nutrient density of the diet as the pattern of intake shifts to include foods that are lower in fat content and richer in complex carbohydrates. Accomplishing the dietary transitions of infancy should be done in such a way that the child learns dietary behaviours that will reduce risk of obesity and related disorders later in their life.

6.2.4.1 Complementary feeding

The introduction of complementary feeding (weaning) is the process through which the infant makes the transition from a milk-only diet, whether breast- or formula-fed, to a diet that contains solid foods and non-milk drinks (complementary foods). This is a key developmental milestone that exerts powerful changes in terms of functional changes to the gastrointestinal tract, the immune system and metabolic processes. From a nutritional perspective, the diversification of the diet that accompanies the introduction of complementary foods has profound effects. The weaned infant becomes exposed to a greater range of fatty acids and proteins, and these and associated micronutrients must be absorbed from a more varied food matrix. While in early infancy feeding occurs throughout the day and night, with no meal-based pattern, with the introduction of complementary foods, the infant moves to having two to three set meals per day, with snacks in between, and often ceases night feeding. This changes metabolic parameters markedly, producing bigger fluctuations in glucose and insulin concentrations between the fasted and fed states.

Complementary feeding is critical for a number of reasons. First, it is essential to ensure that the requirements of the infant for nutrients are met by the dietary supply. Milk is a poor source of certain nutrients, particularly iron, zinc, vitamin D and vitamin A, all of which are essential for the maintenance of normal growth and function. Prior to weaning, the infant, particularly if breastfed, is reliant on stores of these nutrients that were accrued in the last trimester of pregnancy. These stores are largely depleted by the age of six months. The introduction of solid foods also serves to stimulate the development of the reflexes that coordinate biting and chewing with swallowing of food. Weaning is also the transition to a dietary pattern that includes most of the normal range of foods consumed by the mature individual. This process provides a useful opportunity to promote development of food preferences and feeding behaviours that will be associated with good health later in life.

The initiation of complementary feeding can be seen as a period of vulnerability. In developing countries, the transition from sterile breast milk greatly increases vulnerability of infants to food- and water-borne infection. It can also promote malnutrition, as children from poor communities may be weaned onto low-quality foods that lack essential nutrients, or which cannot provide the necessary energy and nutrient densities. It is this latter point that has prompted the WHO to issue advice relating to weaning, which should ideally be adopted on a global scale. Essentially, parents are advised that all babies should be exclusively breastfed for the first six months of life, with no introduction of complementary foods prior to this time. At six months, nutritionally adequate complementary foods should be introduced, with continuation of breastfeeding to two years of age. This policy is likely to be highly effective in rural populations in developing countries, where access to clean water and uncontaminated foods is difficult. Later weaning reduces the likelihood of diarrhoeal disease and associated mortality and has been shown to have no detriment in terms of the growth of children. In developed countries, however, many have questioned the appropriateness of this advice, which represents a significant shift away from the long-held view that weaning after four months but no later than six months should be normal practice (Fewtrell, 2011).

The Department of Health advice to parents is essentially the same as the WHO recommendation to delay weaning until six months of age, but their guidelines suggest flexibility by wording the advice as delay until 'around six months'. It is generally thought that while a delay to six months has no significant detriment to infants it is not imperative to do so. Babies who can sit up and hold their head steady, have good hand–eye coordination, have lost the tongue thrust reflex (which expels material from the mouth to stop choking) and are growing at a rapid rate, may benefit from introduction of solids between four and six months. Babies with a family history of atopy may benefit from introduction to solids within the four- to six-month window, as this has been shown to reduce the risk of allergic sensitization to eggs and peanuts (Burgess *et al.*, 2019). Guidelines for approaching weaning are shown in Table 6.3, which highlights the recommended staged approach which takes the child from an early experience of fine textured foods in a limited range, through to what are essentially coarsely chopped versions of normal family meals over the course of six months.

With the rising prevalence of childhood obesity, there has been considerable interest in the possibility that elements of the early diet may be risk factors for adiposity in childhood. Early complementary feeding may be one such risk factor for childhood obesity. Brophy *et al.* (2009) reported that in the UK Millennium Cohort, children who had been weaned before three months of age were more likely to be obese at age five years (odds ratio, OR, for obesity 1.2, 95% confidence interval, CI, 1.02–1.5). A US study found that delaying weaning reduced the risk of childhood obesity by 0.1% for every month delay beyond four months (Hediger *et al.*, 2001). In contrast, studies of the Avon Longitudinal Study of Parents and Children (ALSPAC) and the Southampton Women's Study cohorts in the UK reported no association between age at introduction of complementary feeding and childhood obesity (Reilly *et al.*, 2005; Robinson *et al.*, 2009). Most of the literature showing effects of timing of weaning upon subsequent obesity, however, are small studies with poor adjustment for confounding effects of breastfeeding exposure, maternal education, socioeconomic status and birth weight, all of which are also related to obesity. The systematic review of Pearce *et al.* (2013) concluded that the timing of the introduction of complementary foods has no clear association with childhood obesity, although very early introduction of solid foods (four months of age or younger) may result in higher childhood body mass index (BMI).

In most developed countries, parents will begin complementary feeding earlier than six months of age. Among US infants, 55% had received solids before six months in the study of Barrera *et al.* (2018), with one third of those experiencing solids before four months. Early weaning was more common in those infants whose mother was less than 25 years of age and where breastfeeding was maintained for less than

Table 6.3 Complementary feeding stages.

	First introduction (17–26 weeks)	26–30 weeks	30–39 weeks	40–52 weeks
Foods to introduce*	Baby rice, ground oat porridge, cooked starchy vegetables, banana, cooked fruit	Meat, fish, poultry Noodles, pasta, full-fat yoghurt, custard, fromage frais, cheese, well-cooked eggs	Well-cooked shellfish, raw soft vegetables, raw soft fruit, citrus fruit	
Food preparation	Pureed with milk	Finely mashed and mixed with milk	Mashed with small lumps. Provide finger foods	Chopped, minced family foods, with finger foods
Frequency	A few teaspoons once per day	Two solid feeds per day	Three solid feeds per day	Aim for three to four servings of starchy foods and three to four servings of fruits and vegetables, with two servings of protein-rich foods per day
Foods to avoid	Foods with high salt, added salt in cooking and serving, foods with high sugar content, low-fat foods, honey, whole nuts, unpasteurized dairy products			

In the early stages of weaning, foods should be pureed or mashed mixed with either breast milk or an appropriate formula to give an easily swallowed texture and consistency. Finger foods are easily handled food items that babies can pick up and convey to the mouth, such as bite-sized pieces of fruit. This encourages biting, chewing and swallowing, together with independent feeding and developing coordination skills.

* Foods that are highly allergenic (wheat products, eggs, fish, shellfish, foods containing nuts) may be introduced at any time but should be given one at a time with a gap of 2–3 days in between to monitor for a reaction.

four months. In the UK, 75% of babies had started to be weaned before five months in a 2010 survey (Health and Social Care Information Centre, 2012), with earlier weaning being more common among socially deprived and ethnic minority families. In the UK, a level of confusion exists about the timing of weaning, as the advice given to parents has been inconsistent. As a result, many parents mistrust the advice of health professionals (Moore *et al.*, 2012) and they prefer to make use of possibly unreliable sources to make judgements about timing and pattern of introduction of complementary foods (Figure 6.5).

Complementary feeding with solids prior to four months of age is not advisable and may be detrimental to the health of the child. Prior to this age, most babies are unable to masticate and swallow solids safely and are therefore at risk of choking. Moreover, the immaturity of the kidneys and gastrointestinal tract presents a significant hazard. The introduction of solid foods increases the quantity of nitrogen and solutes delivered to the body. This can overwhelm the excretory capacity of the kidneys, promoting dehydration. The immature gut does not produce the full range of pancreatic and intestinal secretions, so solid food may remain undigested in the gut for longer periods. This can promote gastroenteritis and damage to the lining of the tract. Moreover, the immature gut is more permeable and will allow larger proteins to cross into systemic circulation. This can promote allergic sensitization.

Late weaning (i.e. beyond six months of age) may also be a cause for concern. It is more likely to be associated with certain ethnic subgroups in the population. In the UK Infant Feeding Survey 2000 (Hamlyn *et al.*, 2002), it was noted that mothers from Asian backgrounds were most likely to delay weaning. In some Muslim communities, the first stage of weaning involved a switch to whole cow's milk, accompanied by lengthy use of convenience weaning foods. In developing countries, later weaning reduces morbidity and mortality among infants but, where infectious disease is not a major issue, it is of greater concern that late-weaned infants may become malnourished due to depletion of nutrient stores.

The introduction of complementary foods should be accomplished gradually and the full process of weaning will typically take six months. Throughout that time, milk should remain a key part of the diet. Feeds of breast milk or appropriate infant formula should continue, with both later being used for drinks and mixing with solid foods. Weaning foods must be prepared to a consistency that is appropriate to the neuromuscular development of the child (Table 6.3). This means that initially foods need to be pureed and should contain no lumps that may cause choking. Over time, this should give way to mashed and finely chopped food and eventually to normal family foods. To help children become familiar with biting and chewing and the conveyance of food from hand to mouth, it is suggested that children of around six months of age should be given 'finger foods', which might be pieces of bread, rusks, biscuits, fruit or raw vegetables. The first foods during weaning have more to do with giving the baby the experience of food and portion sizes and meal frequency are not a consideration. To aid acceptance of food and to avoid these early experiences displacing nutrients from milk, solids should be offered to the child immediately after a milk feed. As described in Research Highlight 6.1 a new approach to introduction of complementary foods, termed 'baby-led weaning', is increasing in popularity. This introduces finger foods much earlier in the process.

The foods that should be used in weaning can generally be normal family foods that have been prepared to suit the stage of the child, as described earlier. A key part of the process is providing the child with a varied range of flavours, textures and aromas, as this should help with acceptance of a broad range of foods later in life. Most parents introduce new foods one at a time, to check whether any might produce an adverse reaction. The energy density of the food needs to be high (more than 4.2 kJ/g food) and the salt content should be low. If the diet does not include meat, then an alternative source of iron (generally fortified cereals) should be included.

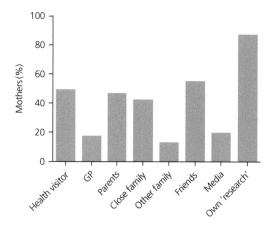

Figure 6.5 A UK survey of 474 mothers of young infants showed that the most trusted source of advice on when and how to introduced complementary foods was their 'own research', which included accessing internet articles and reading books. General practitioners (GP) were the least trusted source of information *Source:* Spray and Langley-Evans, unpublished data.

Research Highlight 6.1 Baby-led weaning and the development of appetite regulation.

The recommended approach to the introduction of solid foods is to feed babies pureed food items, generally via a spoon, gradually increasing the range of flavours and textures, so that over time the child transitions to unprocessed 'finger foods'. This is a process which is driven by parents and concern has been raised that this creates an environment where the child is pressured to eat and is not able to experiment and develop their preferences. The British nurse Gill Rapley advocated an alternative approach termed 'baby-led weaning', which has gained popularity in the UK, New Zealand and other western nations. The basis of baby-led weaning is that infants are provided with finger foods from the initiation of weaning and are given the opportunity to self-select from the same foods that the rest of the family are consuming (Gomez et al., 2020). This is proposed to enable the development of appropriate satiety mechanisms and encourage the development of motor skills. It is argued that in the longer-term the development of self-regulation around food will reduce risk of obesity.

The cross-sectional study of Brown and Lee (2011) found that mothers who took the baby-led approach did facilitate self-regulation of intake. They were less concerned about baby weight gain and did not pressure their child to eat or control the amount of food consumed. The baby-led infants had a lower prevalence of overweight than traditionally weaned children. Similarly, Townsend and Pitchford (2012) found less obesity among children who had been weaned using the baby-led method. Although apparently compelling, both of these studies suffered from sample bias as they recruited mostly breastfeeding mother–infant pairs, with high adherence to guidelines on delaying the introduction of complementary feeding to six months of age. In contrast, the randomized controlled trial of Taylor et al. (2017) found no difference in the BMI z scores of baby-led and traditionally weaned infants. In fact, the baby-led group tended to have a greater prevalence of overweight, although this was not statistically significant.

There are two possible risks associated with baby-led weaning. The first is the possibility that babies will choke on foods which are too coarse in texture or too bulky to swallow. Several studies have, however, found that there is no greater risk with baby-led compared with traditional weaning (Fangupo et al., 2016; Brown 2018). The other risk is a nutritional issue as the self-selecting baby may not choose to eat an appropriate range of foods. Cameron et al., (2013) found that baby-led weaning tended to be delayed until six months of age and so may exacerbate concerns about exhaustion of iron stores. This approach to weaning has been associated with low intakes of iron, zinc and vitamin B12 and increased intakes of total and saturated fat (Morison et al., 2016) and carbohydrates (Townsend and Pitchford, 2012).

Infants require a diet that is low in phytate to maximize the absorption of micronutrients. Foods that are at risk of being infected with pathogens, for example, unpasteurized soft cheeses, raw or only lightly cooked eggs and paté, should be avoided. The introduction of foods that are commonly associated with food allergy in children (eggs, milk, soya, wheat, peanuts) can proceed at any stage of weaning but with close and careful monitoring for reactions following first use.

There is a vast range of commercially available weaning foods. These foods certainly do not disadvantage infant growth and development and their major downside is their expense. As these foods are formulated in a way that ensures they meet with regulations on salt and provision of a balanced nutrient content, they may to some extent be superior to homemade foods used in early weaning. For example, many babies' first experience of food may be pureed fruit. This has inadequate energy and nutrient density and a better choice would be a milk-based non-wheat porridge or baby cereal. In many developing countries, the move of populations from rural to urban areas is increasing the proportion of food that is purchased rather than grown, particularly in Latin America and the Caribbean. This provides an opportunity to address some of the problems of malnutrition that are associated with weaning on to inadequate diets or with foods which are rich in phytates and goitrogens (inhibitors of iodine uptake), which impede micronutrient absorption. However, poor and rural communities remain dependent on limited food staples and inappropriate feeding decisions remain a problem. For example, McLennan (2017) reported that in the Dominican Republic and Haiti, foods made from bread and noodles, potatoes and legumes were the main items used in weaning and that there had been little change in use between 1996 and 2012. There have been numerous attempts to introduce low-cost, highly nutritious foods for weaning in developing countries (Ward and Ainsworth, 1998; Lutter et al., 2003), but these have limited success as parental choices around weaning are heavily shaped by level of education, tradition and food insecurity.

6.2.4.2 Nutrition-related problems

Infants are vulnerable to micronutrient deficiencies, which are often not detected until at an advanced stage. This vulnerability arises in part due to a lack of extensive reserves of nutrients but also due to factors that impact upon nutrient intakes, nutrient losses and the bioavailability of nutrients. Nutrient intake is most often compromised due to poverty but may also arise because children are provided with an insufficiently varied diet. For example, in many parts of the world, children will live on rice as a staple food, which is often not adequately complemented by other nutrient sources. Rice is a poor source of vitamin A and, as a consequence, vitamin A deficiency becomes rife among children in these regions. Cooking methods (e.g. boiling) or food processing that leaches nutrients from raw food ingredients may also limit the nutrient supply to children. Losses of nutrients via the kidneys or digestive tract may be a consequence of infectious disease. Infection and chronic disease processes can lead to malabsorption of micronutrients. For example, children with cystic fibrosis are vulnerable to deficiencies of fat-soluble vitamins due to the accumulation of mucous in the digestive tract. Foods that are rich in phytates, as are commonly used in weaning in some cultures, limit the bioavailability of micronutrients. In addition, short-term periods of malnutrition, for example, following repeated episodes of infection, will stimulate catch-up growth. This rapid growth may increase demands for micronutrients beyond the capacity of the diet to supply them.

6.2.4.2.1 Zinc deficiency

Zinc deficiency is difficult to detect as it has few clinical signs and biochemical assessment of zinc status is far from straightforward. It is estimated that zinc deficiency may occur in one third of the world population (Shamah and Villalpando, 2006) and in children it will impair growth, immune function and brain development. Zinc deficiency is most commonly seen in children who do not eat meat, either by virtue of cultural background or due to poverty,

and where the diet is rich in cereal fibre (containing phytic acid; Figure 6.6). Zinc deficiency can also arise as a consequence of diarrhoeal disease, which increases losses. Zinc is a major component of digestive enzymes secreted into the small intestine, and so maintaining zinc status is dependent upon reuptake from the gut. Reuptake of zinc is impaired by gastrointestinal infection. Although clinically relevant zinc deficiency is mostly seen in developing countries, low intakes of zinc during childhood are also a cause for concern in more affluent populations (Cowin and Emmett, 2007; Bates *et al.*, 2011).

Zinc is a prerequisite for growth as it is required for the synthesis of DNA during cell replication. Growth faltering is therefore the main clinical indicator of deficiency. Zinc is also essential for brain development during infancy, partly due to the need for cell division during brain growth but also because zinc is required for neurotransmitter release. There are reports that zinc deficiency may be associated with poor cognitive development, but the balance of evidence suggests that it mostly limits the motor skills of infants. Supplementation of children with zinc deficiency increases their activity and ability to explore the world, possibly increasing their ability to exploit learning opportunities in their environment (Black, 2003).

The immune function of zinc-deficient children is impaired, increasing their vulnerability to infectious diseases. Zinc deficiency is endemic in low and middle-income (developing) countries, where the main cause is inadequate intake due to limited intakes of animal produce (Gupta *et al.*, 2020). Deficiency is also driven by increased demand due to regular infection and losses and malabsorption associated

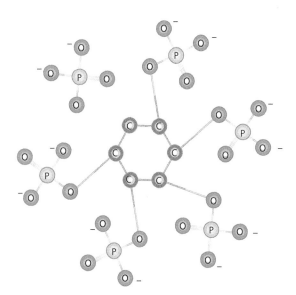

Figure 6.6 The structure of phytic acid. Phytates are found in many cereals and legumes, where they occur bound to proteins and starches. The phosphate groups of phytic acid are able to chelate cations, and as a result, phytate in the gut will reduce bioavailability of minerals such as zinc, calcium and magnesium.

with diarrhoeal disease. Globally it is estimated that 4.4% of childhood deaths and almost 4% of the overall disease burden in under-fives are directly attributable to zinc deficiency (Fischer Walker *et al.*, 2009). In countries such as the Democratic Republic of Congo, Afghanistan, India, Ethiopia and Nigeria, zinc deficiency is a factor in almost 50% of child deaths, with half of those deaths being caused by diarrhoea. Zinc deficiency is also a major cause of stunting, contributing up to 23% of the risk according to the analysis of Wessells and Brown (2012).

6.2.4.2.2 Vitamin D deficiency

Poor vitamin D status is commonplace among children, with deficiency defined as a circulating concentration of 25-hydroxy-vitamin D below 50 nmol/l and insufficiency as a concentration between 50 and 100 nmol/l. Clinically, vitamin D deficiency manifests as rickets in children who are undergoing rapid growth. Rickets is characterized by soft, malleable bones that in weightbearing locations become deformed. This gives deficient children a characteristic bow-leggedness. Rickets also causes swelling of joints and of the skull. Although easily avoided through supplementation or consumption of fortified sources, rickets and vitamin D insufficiency continues to occur in children in northern latitudes with low levels of sunlight during the winter months. The National Diet and Nutrition Survey in the UK reported that 7.5% of 1.5–3-year-olds had 25-hydroxy-vitamin D concentrations below 25 nmol/l (Bates *et al.*, 2014). High prevalence of deficiency and insufficiency are also noted in sunnier climates, with 22% deficiency reported in the Northern Territory of Australia (Dyson *et al.*, 2014) and 58.8% deficiency in the winter months in Algeria (Djennane *et al.*, 2014). Among children living in northern Italy, prevalence of vitamin D deficiency was 46% with 9% being severely deficient (Mazzoleni *et al.*, 2019). Across northern latitudes, risk is greatest in children with dark skin colour, where it is a product of low synthesis within the skin due to dark pigmentation. In the UK, while the incidence of rickets is very low overall (8 cases per 100 000 population), the incidence is markedly higher among dark-skinned children (95 per 100 000; Uday and Hogler, 2018). Herrick *et al.*, (2019) reported that non-Hispanic Black and Asian populations in the United States were at greater risk of deficiency than the white population. For some communities, low skin exposure to sunlight due to wearing of traditional clothing and the consumption of foods rich in phytate may also be a factor. Dark-skinned infants may also be prone to vitamin D deficiency due to limited transfer from their mothers. Poor vitamin D status is near universal

among Asian adults in northern countries during the winter months and, for many women, this is not fully redressed in the summer. During pregnancy, competition for vitamin D between mother and fetus may limit transfer to fetal tissues, and this may be exacerbated postnatally through low vitamin D concentrations in breast milk.

6.2.4.2.3 Iron deficiency

Iron deficiency is the most common micronutrient deficiency in children. It is rarely seen in infants under the age of four months due to accrual of iron of maternal origin in the fetal period. Beyond four months, the rapid growth of infants means that requirements for iron can often outstrip supply from breast milk and foods used in weaning. The introduction of unmodified cow's milk to the diet between 6 and 12 months of age increases the risk of iron deficiency in infants, and this may stem from gastrointestinal blood losses triggered by the presence of cow's milk proteins.

Iron deficiency anaemia in young children has a number of adverse consequences. It is more common in children from poor families and in the developed countries is most often seen in children from ethnic minorities. In the UK, for example, Asian children are most at risk as they are more likely to be weaned on to vegetarian diets (providing iron in the less well-absorbed nonheme form) or to be breastfed for an extended period. Iron deficiency slows the growth of children and increases their susceptibility to infectious disease. The mechanisms through which iron deficiency suppresses immune function are unclear and may involve effects on the metabolism of other nutrients such as vitamin A (Muñoz *et al.*, 2000). Iron-deficient children have impaired capacity to produce T cells and their phagocytes are less active. Although iron supplements can reverse these impairments of immunity, care needs to be taken in any intervention programme to support populations where deficiency is common. Iron is used by pathogens as well as host tissues. This is a particular problem in regions of the world where malaria is common (see Research Highlight 6.2).

Iron deficiency anaemia is associated with developmental delay in preschool children, as it interferes with growth of the brain. In contrast to zinc deficiency, which impacts mainly upon motor development, iron deficiency has a detrimental effect upon the capacity to learn. Parkin *et al.* (2020) reported that in one- to three-year-olds, higher serum ferritin concentrations were associated with higher cognitive function. Children with iron deficiency have low developmental scores and poor ability to process information and are less happy, more wary and

Research Highlight 6.2 Iron status and malaria: a public health challenge.

Malaria is a disease caused by infection with parasites of the *Plasmodium* family, of which *P. falciparum* is the most dangerous species. The malaria parasite is spread by mosquitoes and as a result infection is risk endemic in all tropical areas where mosquitoes thrive. Malaria is a major killer of children under the age of five years, with approximately 409 000 deaths in 2019, mostly in Africa (World Health Organization, 2021).

There is a critical relationship between the malaria parasite and iron status in the human host. On initial infection, *Plasmodium* lies dormant in the liver, but later breaks out and invades red blood cells. This enables it to evade immune defences. In the blood the organism suppresses erythropoiesis and consumes up to 80% of the haemoglobin in the erythrocytes (Moya-Avarez *et al.*, 2016). As a result, malaria is a major driver of haemolytic anaemia in children.

Iron is critical for the parasite in its development in the liver and as a substrate in the bloodstream (Moya-Avarez *et al.*, 2016) and there is good evidence that pre-existing iron deficiency anaemia can protect children from malaria. Gwamaka *et al.* (2012) found that among Tanzanian children, anaemia reduced malaria infection by 38% and deaths by 66%. Similarly, a reduced incidence of malaria (incidence risk ratio 0.70, 95% CI 0.51–0.99) was noted among iron deficient children by Nyakeriga *et al.* (2004). These observations frame a key public health challenge as neither malaria infection nor the iron deficiency anaemia which may prevent it are good outcomes for children.

Malaria can be controlled by measures to suppress the mosquito vector or drugs to attack the parasite. When these measures are used, there is evidence that iron status of children improves. Indoor spraying with insecticides (Hamel *et al.*, 2011) and intermittent treatment with antimalarial drugs (Matangila *et al.*, 2015) have been shown to reduce the population prevalence of anaemia.

As anaemia suppresses malaria and iron can aid the parasite there is some concern about whether it is safe to supplement children with iron, if they live in malarial regions. Sazawal *et al.* (2006) conducted a randomized controlled trial of iron 12.5 mg per day, folic acid and zinc 50 µg per day in over 8000 infants aged 1–35 months. The trial had to be abandoned early due to 12% greater death and 11% greater hospitalization due to malaria among the supplemented group.

In contrast Zlotkin *et al.* (2013) provided iron 12.5 mg/day as part of a micronutrient powder supplement to Ghanaian children and showed a significant reduction in malarial infection (relative risk 0.87, 95% CI 0.79–0.97). However, in contrast to the Sazawal *et al.* (2006) trial, all the children in this study were protected from mosquitoes using insecticide-treated nets at night. The Cochrane systematic review of Neuberger *et al.* (2016) found that iron supplementation increased the risk of malaria in populations where infection control measures were lacking, but was safe and reversed anaemia when insecticide-treated nets and drug therapies were available. It is therefore appropriate to tackle anaemia in children through supplementation but only when combined with effective malaria control strategies.

more dependent upon their mothers for social support (Lozoff *et al.*, 2006). Chilean children aged 5 and 10 years showed greater social reticence and had lower verbal ability if iron deficient (East *et al.*, 2019). A study of primary school children in Cambodia found that alongside stunting, iron deficiency was a significant factor in low scores on standardized tests of intelligence and reasoning ability (Perignon *et al.*, 2014). While long-term iron supplementation can overcome many of the developmental problems associated with deficiency, some consequences may be longer lasting. Congdon *et al.* (2012) reported that brain activity in 10-year-old children who had suffered from iron deficiency anaemia was different to that of children who had not, even after anaemia had been successfully treated. Changes during development may not be corrected later in life, so any functional deficits may be irreversible. A range of studies suggest that low haemoglobin concentrations between six and nine months of age may be predictive of lower IQ at ages up to nine years. Lozoff *et al.* (2013) reported that the educational achievement and some emotional and social indices remained lower in young adults who had suffered chronic iron deficiency anaemia as infants (Figure 6.7).

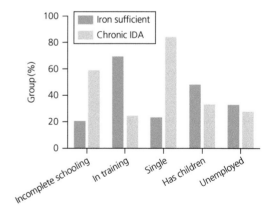

Figure 6.7 Iron deficiency anaemia has long-term effects on cognitive development and life opportunities. Costa Rican 25-year-olds who had either been chronically iron deficient (IDA) or iron insufficient in infancy were more likely to have failed to complete secondary school, were less likely to be in training during early adulthood and were more likely to be unmarried. *Source:* Lozoff *et al.* (2013).

6.2.4.2.4 Food additives and hyperactivity

While micronutrient deficiencies present a significant threat to the health and development of very young children, there is also concern that the use of food colourings, preservatives and flavourings may also impact upon wellbeing. These agents are commonly used in processed foods and especially those that are marketed at children, for example, fizzy drinks, sweets and frozen ready meals. There has been concern since the 1970s that artificial colourings, in particular, may be associated with hyperactive behaviour (i.e. impulsiveness, overactivity, poor attention span).

There is now little doubt that in some children who have a confirmed diagnosis of attention deficit hyperactivity disorder (ADHD), restriction of the diet to exclude artificial colourings and other additives can improve behaviour (Kemp, 2008). A meta-analysis by Nigg et al. (2012) suggested that 8% of children with ADHD may benefit from a restricted diet with no artificial colourings. Whether the additives have a causal role in the development of hyperactive disorders in otherwise normally behaved children is unclear. Meta-analyses show that almost all effects of additives on behaviour are restricted to children with ADHD and there is little robust evidence to suggest any impact upon the broader population (Schab and Trinh, 2004). It can be difficult to dissect out the effects of additives from other features of the diet. There is some evidence, for example, that sugar-sweetened beverages have a detrimental effect on child behaviour. Yu et al. (2016) found a dose-dependent relationship between intake of such drinks and ADHD, with 3.7-fold greater risk in children whose intake was very high. Del-Ponte et al., (2019b) reported that risk was substantially lower with a 'healthy' diet pattern. However, follow-up of the Pelotas 2004 Birth Cohort in Brazil found no association between sugar intake and ADHD (Del-Ponte et al., 2019a).

An association between non-nutritive additives and ADHD was supported by a double-blind randomized placebo trial in two groups of children aged three and nine years (McCann et al., 2007). When three-year-olds were given either a placebo or one of two mixtures of additives, children receiving a mixture of sodium benzoate, sunset yellow, carmoisine, tartrazine and Ponceau 4R exhibited more hyperactive behaviours over the subsequent week. In contrast, a randomized controlled trial of artificial colourings and sodium benzoate concluded that these agents had no impact upon behaviour in a group of eight- to nine-year-olds (Lok et al., 2013). Inconsistencies in findings may be explained by doses of artificial colourings and Stevens et al. (2014) suggest a threshold dose of 50 mg/day. The highest amounts of artificial colourings are found in beverages, sweets, ready-to-eat cereals and ready meals (Stevens et al., 2015). Beverages may be the major

source for children as they are consumed in high volumes, which is consistent with the association between sugar-sweetened beverages and ADHD reported by Yu et al. (2016).

6.2.4.2.5 Dental caries
Dental caries are the consequence of bacterial infection of the surface of the teeth. After ingestion of food, the teeth are covered in a layer of plaque, which acts as the substrate for bacterial fermentation. Some, but not all, bacterial species produce lactic acid as a product of that fermentation. The main lactic acid producer in dental plaque is *Streptococcus mutans*. Lactic acid demineralizes the tooth enamel, causing the formation of cavities, which then accumulate bacteria that further accumulate bacteria and lead to more significant erosion of the tooth surface. This will ultimately penetrate to the pulp of the tooth or to the bone. Dental caries are a serious issue in children and can impact on their teeth even before they erupt from the gums. The standard measure of caries and associated damage is delayed, missing and filled teeth (DMFT).

In 2013, 37.1% of five-year-olds and 55.5% of eight-year-olds in the UK were reported to have experienced at least one episode of tooth decay and up to 46% had active caries in their primary (milk) teeth at the time of survey (Masood et al., 2019). The risk of caries in British children was markedly higher in those from socially deprived backgrounds (OR 1.77, 95% CI 1.56–2.01). Similarly, deprivation was a major risk factor for US children, where 27.9% of under-fives and 51.2% of 6–11-year-olds had caries.

The five key factors promoting risk of caries are *S. mutans* infection, high dietary sugar intake, frequent consumption of food, low salivary flow and low fluoride status. Foods and beverages that are considered cariogenic include cakes and biscuits, white bread, flavoured milks and yoghurts, sugary breakfast cereals, jams, confectionary, ketchup, sauces and syrups and sugar-sweetened beverages. The association between sugar intake and caries in children is illustrated in Figure 6.8, which shows the direct relationship between DMFT and per capita consumption of sugar-sweetened beverages. Pitchika et al. (2020) demonstrated that consumption of sugar-sweetened beverages was greater in German 10- and 15-year-olds, with DMFT greater than 1. Among 3–10-year-olds, compared with water as the principle beverage, high consumption of sodas increased risk of caries by 69% (Samman et al. 2020). Among Scottish infants, the early introduction of high-sugar sweetened beverage intake increased DMFT by 73% compared with non-consumers (Bernabé et al., 2020).

Strategies to avoid caries in children must clearly focus on good dental hygiene and restriction of sugar

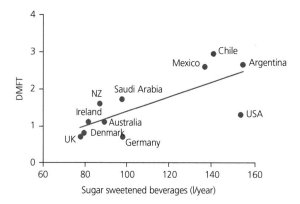

Figure 6.8 The relationship between sugar-sweetened beverage consumption and caries in children. Sugar sweetened beverage intake is shown as per capita availability for all ages. DMFT, delayed, missing and filled teeth.

consumption. Fluoride status is also an important factor. Erosion of tooth enamel is a key step in the development of caries. Enamel is composed of crystals of hydroxyapatite, $Ca_5(PO_4)_3OH$. In hydroxyapatite, the hydroxyl group can be substituted with carbonate, chloride or fluoride. The fluoridated form (fluorapatite) is more resistant to acid erosion and for this reason fluoride is beneficial in preventing caries. Improvements to fluoride status in children and adults can be achieved through fluoridated toothpastes, dental coatings or fluoridation of the water supply.

Community water fluoridation at a concentration of 1 ppm is common practice in many parts of the world. Globally approximately 400 million people benefit from community water fluoridation (Furness *et al.*, 2020), including populations in Ireland, Australia, Canada, New Zealand, the United States and the UK (only 10% of the population are covered). Despite common concerns about apparent adulteration of the water supply, fluoridation is entirely safe, with the only drawback being dental fluorosis. Fluorosis is a harmless mottling of the teeth which can occur with over-fluoridation due to combined use of fluoridated toothpaste and fluoridated water. Numerous studies show a reduction in caries among children living in areas with community water fluoridation (Pollick, 2019). For example, a 15-year follow-up of fluoridation in a Korean population found that DMFT declined from 1.5 to 0.88 in 10-year-olds and from 2.86 to 1.38 in 12-year-olds after adjustment for confounding factors (Kim *et al.*, 2019). In New Zealand, hospitalization of infants to four-year-olds for dental interventions was significantly greater in regions without community water fluoridation (incident risk ratio 1.17, 95% CI 1.06–1.29; Hobbs *et al.*, 2020). Although demonstrably effective and recommended by dental associations worldwide, plans to add fluoride to water supplies are often rejected because of unfounded population concerns.

6.2.4.3 Barriers to healthy nutrition

As described earlier, infants are vulnerable to a number of nutrition-related problems. These often arise due to a lack of parental knowledge and understanding of what constitutes a balanced diet or due to disease and other organic causes. While these nutrition-related problems are relatively uncommon in developed countries, the majority of parents express the concern that the diets their very young children consume are not healthy. This may be a misperception arising because parents do not understand that the diet that is optimal for an infant is very different to that which would be recommended for an adult. The snacks that infants depend upon are perceived as a negative element of the diet and fussy eating behaviours, which are common in infants, also cause parents a lot of concern. Although many parental worries are unfounded, modern society does impose genuine barriers to developing healthy nutrition and food-related behaviours in young children.

6.2.4.3.1 Picky eating

In developed countries, most parents of children below the age of five will readily voice concerns about the quality and quantity of nutrients in their children's diets. These are often only perceived problems and are generally not backed up by hard evidence of growth faltering or other manifestations of undernutrition. The negative perceptions of parents are explained by two common food-related behaviours in young children: food neophobia and picky eating.

Food neophobia is an inherent trait seen in most children that may well have evolved to prevent poisoning. Essentially, it involves the rejection of foods that have not been previously encountered (Dovey *et al.*, 2008). Neophobic behaviour is at a low level around the time of weaning, when children are very open to experimentation with flavours and textures, but steadily increases thereafter, reaching a peak between the ages of two and six years. It has been suggested that neophobia occurs as children are especially averse to bitter tastes. Most of the foods rejected by neophobic children are fruits and vegetables, and these often contain chemicals that have a bitter tang that is no longer perceived by the more mature adult palate. However, much of the food neophobia response appears to be based in the visual domain. In other words, children appear to reject foods that do not look right and cannot be persuaded to taste the items and confirm their negative assessment. It may well be that this rejection is based upon previous taste experience. For example, a green food (e.g. Brussels sprouts) might be tasted in early infancy and found unpleasant, and thereafter all green foods are rejected on the basis that they will be similarly unpalatable.

Most food neophobia disappears by the time the child reaches early adolescence, and repeated exposures to food items will generally result in their acceptance. Social influences are important. Acceptance of novel food items is more likely to occur if the child is in the company of a group of other people who are also consuming that food-stuff (Dovey *et al.*, 2008). At this age, this is most likely to be other family members, but as the circle of friends of the same age begins to grow, 'peer pressure' may help to bring an end to neophobic behaviours.

Food neophobia, when combined with the growing independence of the preschool child, can be a trigger for picky eating behaviours and make mealtimes an area of tension within families. Picky or faddy eating is best defined as a behaviour pattern in which a child either refuses to eat or will only eat a limited range of foods. It is perhaps best regarded as a flexing of muscle and a testing of developing powers of communication and control of the behaviour of other family members (Figure 6.9). Young children crave attention of any sort from their parents and other caregivers, and mealtimes provide an ideal opportunity to gain that attention. By refusing to eat, children can gain a response from an adult and become the centre of attention.

Picky eating behaviours are highly unpredictable and variable. Some children demonstrate a good appetite but only for a limited range of foods, while others may consume a broad range of foods but only intermittently. A food that appears to be the favourite of a child on one day may be rejected out of hand the next. Even within a mealtime, a display of temper and refusal to eat may give way to normal eating of a full portion if the child is somehow distracted. Wright *et al.* (2007) found that 8% of parents of 30-month-old children reported picky eating behaviours. The responses of the parents were often to try to mollify children by providing rewards for eating their meals and offering alternatives to the rejected food items or distract the children by providing television during mealtimes. These responses to picky eating are generally considered inappropriate as, in effect, they reward and reinforce the behaviour. An angry response accompanied by punishment is also inappropriate. The parental role in the development of picky eating is critical. Pickiness is associated with a more controlling parental feeding style, with parents often striving for a healthier diet for their children, or attempting to reduce food waste in families with low food security. Inappropriate techniques to distract from the mealtime 'performance', such as watching television while eating actually increase pickiness (Cole *et al.*, 2018). Parents beliefs and emotions play an important role in shaping children's attitudes to food (Wolstenholme *et al.*, 2019). The best approach to managing picky eating is to provide structured family mealtimes where the family gathering and the food are a pleasurable, unrestrained experience, free from negative emotions (Verhage *et al.*, 2018).

It has generally been assumed that picky eating, except in extreme forms, has little impact upon the nutritional status of infants. Children will often put

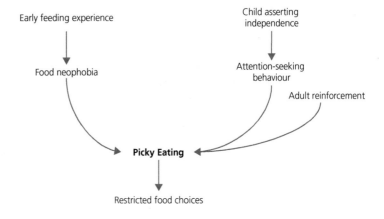

Figure 6.9 The determinants of picky eating in young children.

on a 'performance' to gain attention at one meal per day and then compensate for any lost intake through other meals and snacks throughout the rest of the day. Indeed, there is little evidence that picky eaters are more prone to growth faltering, despite their apparently limited range of preferred foods (Wright *et al.*, 2007). Children with picky eating behaviours have been observed to have lower BMI z scores, suggesting that energy intake is restricted and that pickiness may even confer protection against obesity (Fernandez *et al.*, 2020). Various reports suggest an impact on choice of food, with lower intakes of vegetables, fruit and protein sources compared with non-picky children (Brown *et al.*, 2018; Taylor *et al.*, 2019). These effects can persist for a long time, shaping food choices going into adolescence. Taylor *et al.* (2019) followed children in the large prospective ALSPAC cohort and found that those who were very picky eaters at age 3.5 years still had low intakes of certain food groups at 13 years and were high consumers of free sugar and had lower intakes of protein, fibre and some micronutrients than non-picky eaters, at age 10.

6.2.4.3.2 Poverty

The lack of progress in alleviating child poverty across the world since it was first targeted as a priority for the United Nations in the 1990s is one of the most shameful failures of society since the inception of a global, collaborative community post-Second World War. Child poverty is the primary cause of malnutrition and associated disease and child mortality. It is characterized not just by financial inequality, but by a lack of basic access to the essentials of life including safe housing, drinkable water and adequate nutrition. Unicef estimates that 663 million children live below a poverty level defined by a household income of less than US$1.90 per day and 335 million live in severe poverty (Unicef, 2020). Although children make up only one third of world population, they constitute half of those living in poverty and are more vulnerable to its effects than adults.

In 2015, the United Nations proposed the Sustainable Development Goals (United Nations, 2015). Goal 1 is to end poverty, with eradication of extreme poverty and halving of the numbers of people living in poverty by the end of 2030. This links to Goal 2, which is to end hunger, achieve food security and improve nutrition. Statistics on child poverty in 2020 suggest that the world will fail utterly to achieve such goals, particularly in the aftermath of the COVID-19 pandemic. Child poverty is endemic in developing countries and kills children. It remains rife, and is increasing, in the developed regions and in the world's richest nation (United States) one in

six children lives in poverty as defined by living in a household where the income is below the Federal Poverty Level (US$21,720 for a three-person family; Figure 6.10). Poverty follows societal inequality and reflects issues such as ethnicity. In the United States, while 1 in 11 white children live in poverty, 1 in 3 Black or Native American and 1 in 4 Hispanic children suffers the effects of low income. Poverty is heavily focused in the southern states of Mississippi, Louisiana, Alabama, Arkansas and New Mexico. Across the European Union, 23.4% of children live in at risk of poverty with a wide range from 13.1% in Slovenia to 38% in Romania (Eurostat, 2020). In the UK, 4.2 million children were in poverty in 2018–2019 (Child Poverty Action Group, 2020). Among these children, 46% were from an ethnic minority group and 44% lived in one parent families.

Poverty in developed countries has a profound impact on the quality and quantity of nutrition for young children. Although not at the life-threatening level present in low- and middle-income nations, social deprivation sees children going hungry on a daily basis. The Generation R study in the Netherlands found that children in families with a low income were twice as likely to miss out on breakfast and 2.4 times more likely to miss out on an evening meal (Wijtzes *et al.*, 2015). Similarly, Jenkins *et al.* (2015) reported that British children from poor backgrounds were more likely to have a daily breakfast that delivered 100 kcal or less. Poverty shapes parental choices about food purchasing. Cost and

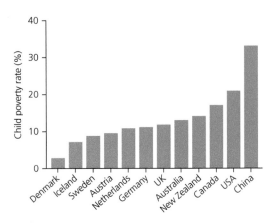

Figure 6.10 Social deprivation in children (0–17 years) from selected countries. The poverty rate is the ratio of the number of people (in a given age group) whose income falls below the poverty line; taken as half the median household income of the total population. *Source:* data from Organisation for Economic Co-operation and Development (2020).

budget efficiency influences the purchase of foods which will not be wasted, leading to more selection of palatable, ultra-processed foods in preference to perishable items (Hardcastle and Blake, 2016). Foods that are high in fat and sugar are also generally less expensive than healthier options. The Food Foundation (2018) reported that, in the UK, 47% of households with children had insufficient income to meet healthy eating guidance. Less-affluent communities also see greater densities of fast-food outlets promoting ready access to cheap, energy-dense, nutrient-poor foods. Despite generally poor micronutrient status, children living in poverty are at greater risk of overweight and obesity (Howard Wilsher *et al.*, 2016).

As described below, developed countries seek to protect children from the effects of poverty through a variety of support schemes that address food insecurity of families. However, these are often insufficient to meet the need, too restrictive or too difficult to access. As a result charitable organizations have been formed to fill a critical gap in direct provision of food. In the United States, for example, Feeding America has a network of 200 food banks and over 60 000 food pantries and meal programmes. In the UK, there are at least 1034 independent food banks (Independent Food Aid Network, 2020) and other organized networks such as the Trussel Trust, which operates more than 1200 food banks nationwide. Food banks work by obtaining donations of nonperishable foods from businesses and individuals and distributing to families in need, often through exchange of vouchers obtained from social services. Demand for food banks in the UK increased steadily through the 2010s and the 2020 COVID-19 pandemic and ensuing economic crisis increased demand dramatically. The Independent Food Aid Network (2020) reported a three-fold increase in demand at the height of the pandemic. Many of the state operated support schemes in place for children are run through schools and nurseries and as a result school holiday periods see an increase in food bank dependency (Trussel Trust, 2020).

In the UK, children living in deprivation can benefit from a number of national schemes. Where the family is in receipt of benefits (e.g. Universal Credit) school-age children can access free school meals. All children under the age of five years receive free milk (250 ml/day) at nursery or school every day and from 5–11 years the cost of milk can be subsidized. Primary schools also participate in the School Fruit and Vegetable Scheme, a government scheme that provides a piece of fruit or vegetable to all children aged four to six years. For families on state benefits in which a woman is pregnant, or

where there is a child under the age of four, Healthy Start vouchers can be claimed. These vouchers can be exchanged for vitamin supplements, milk, fruit and vegetables and pulses. Reviews of the efficacy of Healthy Start are generally positive. Scantlebury *et al.* (2018) found that families using vouchers maintained a fruit and vegetable intake equivalent to families not eligible for vouchers. While Ohly *et al.* (2017) suggested that pregnant women may use the vouchers to purchase food but use the money saved to buy other things, Griffith *et al.* (2018) did not report a similar displacement of food spend. Healthy Start vouchers increased fruit and vegetable spend, improved the nutritional quality of the average food shopping basket and were more effective than an equivalent cash benefit.

In the United States, a cash benefit is used rather than a voucher system. The US Department of Agriculture (USDA) Food and Nutrition Services operates the Special Supplemental Nutrition Program for Women, Infants and Children. The programme supports pregnant women, infants up to the age of one year and children through to five years. Eligibility for support, which includes funds for food, guidance and support with breastfeeding and healthy eating, is defined by an income that is less than 1.85 times the federal poverty level. A nutritional assessment is required to demonstrate that the family is at risk. Recipients are issued with prepaid electronic bank cards which can be used at authorized retailers.

6.2.4.3.3 The impact of advertising

The advertisement of unhealthy foods and beverages to children is a significant negative influence that works against the efforts of parents, health professionals and educators to promote the establishment of healthy eating and behaviours in children. Preschool children are avid watchers of television and are increasingly exposed to movies in cinemas and unregulated media such as the internet. For children under the age of five, there is little perception of the difference between advertisements and the actual programme content they are watching. This makes them an ideal and particularly receptive audience for the advertising of a range of items, including food and drink. Although these infants are not in direct control of food purchasing in a household, they can very effectively influence parental choices through demanding behaviour.

The budgets available to spend on advertising of food and drink are staggering and make the sums allocated for health education and health promotion pale into insignificance. The entire annual budget for the WHO to deliver all of its programmes (including COVID-19 pandemic control) in 2020/21 was

US$3.8 billion. In comparison, fast-food restaurants in the United States alone spent more than US$4.6 billion, and advertising for sugar-sweetened beverages exceeded US$1 billion. O'Dowd (2017) reported that in the UK the spend on advertising of junk (non-core, ultra-processed) foods was 27.5 times higher than the government's flagship healthy eating campaign.

As the viewing habits of children are increasingly shifting away from traditional 'live' television towards view-on-demand and internet services, food companies are expanding advertising into the digital space. The largest digital advertising markets in the world are in the United States, China and the UK, and it is estimated that children are spending an average of 15 hours per week online. Boyland *et al.* (2020) estimated that US$1.5 billion is spent on marketing to children through these media. Tan *et al.* (2018) examined the 250 most popular YouTube videos targeting children and found that they had 71 embedded advertisements for food, of which 56% were for fast food, sweets, cakes, ice cream, flavoured milks and sugar-sweetened beverages.

The investment that food companies make in advertising is not for nothing. Their marketing campaigns are highly effective in boosting brand recognition and creating positivity about their products, even when those products are recognized as unhealthy additions to the diet. Children have immature critical thinking ability and poor impulse inhibition, so are more susceptible to advertising than adults (Radeksy *et al.*, 2020). They find it difficult to resist advertising, especially if embedded in their social networks or personalized to their preferences. Boyland *et al.* (2011) showed that when 6–13-year-olds were exposed to food advertisements followed by cartoons on just two occasions, their selection of high-fat, high-sugar items increased, with children who habitually watched more television being more susceptible to this effect. Norman *et al.* (2020) found that among 7–12-year-old Australian children, advertising increased brand recognition and positive ratings of brands. In the same cohort, a randomized controlled trial in which a four-minute computer game was associated with no advertising or three different advertising approaches, found that where advertising was embedded into reward videos associated with the game, children's selection of the advertised confectionary as a post-game snack was increased (Smith *et al.*, 2020).

It is becoming clear that the preschool child is also susceptible to advertising messages and this may be more insidious due to the critical impact that this stage of life has upon future health behaviours. Goris *et al.* (2010) estimated that in the United States, as much as 40% of childhood obesity risk may be explained by exposure to food advertising. Advertisers use branding of products to increase recognition. Associating positive messages with a brand is designed to gain lifelong customers (Connor, 2006). By the age of two years, children are already able to recognize well-advertised food brands and have certain value beliefs attached to those brands (Robinson *et al.*, 2007). Two- to six-year-olds are aware of brand names and have strong recognition of logos and packaging. In an experiment with children aged between two and six years, Borzekowski and Robinson (2001) showed that when exposed to just 30 seconds of brand advertising within a 30-minute session of watching cartoons, children were up to three times more likely to choose a branded item when it was offered alongside an identical product presented in similar but unbranded packaging. Similarly, when three- to five-year-olds were offered a choice of identical foods but with one item packaged plainly and the other in McDonald's branded materials, they were up to six times more likely to choose the branded item (Robinson *et al.*, 2007). When offered branded or equivalent unbranded meals, four- to six-year-old girls consumed significantly more energy with the branded meal (732 ± 199 kcal vs 632 ± 197 kcal; Keller *et al.*, 2012). Exposure to snack food advertising can impact upon the quantity and type of foods consumed by children during television viewing, showing an immediate effect in addition to the brand-loyalty effect (Figure 6.11; Halford *et al.*, 2007).

Finding solutions to this problem will not be easy, particularly with the growth of the internet, which crosses national borders and therefore largely escapes

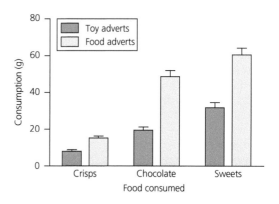

Figure 6.11 Advertising impacts the snacking habits of children. Infants were exposed to 30 minutes of cartoons with advertisements for either toys or snack foods. With free access to a range of snacks, the exposure to food adverts increased consumption. *Source:* Halford *et al.* (2007).

robust legislation. Ustjanauskas *et al.* (2014) reported that internet sites specifically aimed at children hosted 3.4 billion food advertisements, of which 84% were for foods high in fat, sugar and sodium. Given the ready acceptance of branding and logos by very young children, it may be opportune to use this high exposure to advertising messages in a positive manner; for example, branding fruits and vegetables or healthier cereals. There are some examples of this, but generally food producers and supermarkets are reluctant to interfere with their very successful marketing of less healthy, but highly profitable foods. Several studies have shown that advertising of healthy foods can increase nutritional knowledge in children but has little impact upon food choice.

Protecting children from the harmful effects of food advertising was a key priority for the WHO in its *Global Action Plan for the Prevention and Control of Non-Communicable Diseases 2013–2020* (World Health Organization, 2013). Although a few countries had already implemented some regulation in this area, the UK played a prominent role in developing policies to protect children and, in 2007, passed legislation to restrict advertising on television and digital media for which children were the main audience. Further commitment to this was expressed in 2020, with an announcement that all advertising of junk foods in television before the 9 p.m. watershed would be banned.

Other countries that have introduced similar restrictions on advertising include Mexico, Taiwan, South Korea, Chile and Sweden. Sweden banned all advertising of any kind that targets children in the 1990s, but the efficacy of this ban has reduced over time as the legislation has not kept up with marketing technology (Ó Cathaoir, 2017). Fagerberg *et al.* (2019) examined storefront and other street advertising in two areas of Stockholm and found that one third of adverts were for junk foods and that these adverts were more commonly found in the more socioeconomically deprived of the two areas. The most recent ban on advertising was introduced in Chile, where food advertising cannot be shown on television between 6 a.m. and 10 p.m. or in any television, radio or website material where the expected audience comprises more than 20% children under 14 years of age.

One of the first advertising controls was introduced in the Canadian province of Quebec in the early 1980s. This was effective in reducing sales of junk food by Can\$88m per year between 1984 and 1992 (Dhar and Baylis, 2011). This experience compares very favourably to the less draconian step of implementing a voluntary code on advertising. Spain introduced this policy, but as reported by Leon-Flandez

et al. (2017), compliance by advertisers was poor, with over 88% of adverts breaking one of more elements of the code. Effective control over the pervasive messaging to children therefore requires stricter legislation.

6.2.4.3.4 Restrictive dietary practices

Some infants may be fed diets that restrict specific foods or food groups, often because of religious, ethical or health-related beliefs held by parents, which are then incorporated into the lives of children. In most cases, these practices do not have any detrimental impact upon nutritional status or health, but careful management may be necessary to avoid problems. Hindu and Buddhist families, for example, may follow vegetarian diets, and although there are reports that infants weaned on to such diets suffer a greater incidence of iron deficiency anaemia, growth is generally maintained at a rate equivalent to omnivores. Children following vegetarian diets have been shown to maintain normal prepubertal growth patterns but only if the diet is managed to include an appropriate diversity of nutrient sources (Hackett *et al.*, 1998). Research Highlight 6.3 discusses the suitability of vegetarian diets for children in more detail. Vegan diets provide a greater challenge as they are of low energy density. To maintain growth, careful planning of diets for vegan children to include varied sources of protein (tofu, beans and meat analogues) and more energy-dense items such as avocados and vegetable oils is essential (Mangels and Messina, 2001). There are reports of vitamin B12 deficiency in vegan children, so supplements should be provided to such infants.

There are other circumstances in which parents may restrict the foods that are provided for young children with negative outcomes for growth. There are reported cases of failure to thrive in children whose parents have, in good faith, introduced a low-fat, high-fibre diet that accords with guidelines for healthy eating in adults. This is inappropriate for young children, as the bulk of food required to deliver nutrient requirements is not feasible. The introduction of adult healthy eating recommendations should be delayed until the end of the infant stage but applied flexibly. While, on average, the age of five years would be appropriate to adopt a high-fibre, low-fat diet, for slow-growing children this may be too soon and for children on a more rapid trajectory it should come earlier, but certainly not before the age of two years.

Fear of food allergies and intolerances may also prompt restrictions in children's diets. The prevalence of adverse reactions to food is estimated at 4–8% of the childhood population. Parents often mistakenly

Research Highlight 6.3   Vegetarian diet and the pre-pubescent child.

A majority of children across the world will live on a diet that is either wholly vegetarian or mostly plant based. This is often a product of poverty and food insecurity, which limits the availability of animal produce. In such scenarios, the outcomes are often unfavourable and a lack of dietary diversity drives micronutrient deficiencies and stunting. In developed countries, vegetarianism, whether complete avoidance of all animal produce (veganism) or varying degrees of meat, egg and dairy exclusion, is a lifestyle choice. This may be directed by religious adherence, ethical or environmental viewpoints or personal preferences. There are few statistics on how many children under 11 years consume a vegetarian diet, but across populations in Europe, North America and Oceania it is reasonable to assume that similar proportions of children to adults are vegetarian, and that the numbers increase markedly among adolescents. In Germany and Sweden, 10% of the population are believed to be vegetarian, while 7% of British and 5% of Americans follow a plant-based diet.

Nutritional guidelines from many countries indicate that a well-planned vegetarian or vegan diet is appropriate for children. However, such guidelines are based on surprisingly little evidence derived specifically from studies of children, and it should be appreciated that within busy families the time and knowledge needed to plan appropriate menus are likely to be lacking. Cofnas (2019) has argued that there should be concerns about the suitability of plant-based diets for children. The specific areas of concern relate to deficiencies of micronutrients such as iron and zinc due to poor bioavailability from plant material; impairments of growth due to low-energy density of foods; high intakes of phytoestrogens having a feminizing effect on boys; and impaired brain development due to poor iron status and low intakes of n-3 fatty acids. These concerns have largely been extrapolated from studies of adult vegetarians, and it is clear that there is a major lack of high-quality, contemporary research considering vegetarian children.

The available research suggests that vegetarian children grow as well as their omnivorous counterparts. Weder *et al.* (2019) considered energy and macronutrient intakes, together with anthropometric indices in vegetarian and omnivorous one- to three-year olds, and found no differences between the two groups. Similarly Yen *et al.* (2008) and Nathan *et al.* (1997) found no impact of vegetarian diet on growth. The majority of studies also find that, excluding vegans, children who are vegetarian maintain micronutrient status and only those on the most restricted diets are likely to require supplementation (Gibson *et al.*, 2014). A comparison of vitamin status between vegetarians and omnivores found no differences other than a slight deficit of vitamins D and E in the vegetarians (Laskowska-Klita *et al.*, 2011). Low vitamin D status could explain why some studies have shown lower bone mineral density in vegetarian children (Ambrozkiewicz *et al.*, 2019).

Iron and zinc are poorly absorbed from plant sources. In spite of this fact, zinc status appears to be maintained in vegetarian children (Taylor *et al.*, 2004). Although iron intake may be similar to or greater in vegetarian children, it is noted that iron deficiency anaemia is more prevalent than in omnivores (Taylor *et al.*, 2004; Gorczyca *et al.*, 2013). While intakes of fats differ between omnivores and vegetarians, with a marked difference in the n-6 : n-3 fatty acid ratio of the diet, there is little evidence of differences in circulating fatty acid profiles (Gorczyca *et al.*, 2011). The balance of evidence therefore suggests that, unless they are following a highly restrictive extreme, children following a vegetarian diet should grow and develop normally.

believe that their child has an allergy to food, and the parental report of adverse reactions is at a level three to four times above the true prevalence (Noimark and Cox, 2008). Where adverse reactions are suspected, parents may act unilaterally to remove the suspect food from the diet and in so doing exclude important sources of nutrients. Even where expert advice is given and allergy confirmed, parents may be over-zealous in the interpretation of that advice and take actions to restrict the diet without providing suitable alternative sources of nutrients and energy. This can contribute to growth faltering.

6.3 Childhood (5–13)

6.3.1 Nutrient requirements of the older child

In contrast to the earlier stages of childhood, the period between the age of five and puberty is characterized by a relative absence of nutritional problems and rapidly declining nutrient demands. Growth continues to keep nutrient requirements above those of adults, but it is striking that despite demands of growth and their larger body size, children of this age have requirements for energy and nutrients that are not grossly dissimilar to those of under-5s. Energy requirements on a per-kilogram-body-weight basis fall sharply throughout this period (Table 6.4).

While still a problem in many regions, the impact of micronutrient deficiencies upon older children is less severe. Although stunting of growth remains a significant issue, the high rates of morbidity and mortality associated with undernutrition in younger children are not seen in older age groups. This stems from more robust immune function, less vulnerability to dehydration associated with diarrhoeal disease and a longer period of time in which to accrue viable nutrient reserves. In the developed countries, the major nutritional concerns at this stage of life are overweight and obesity, which are discussed in greater detail later in this chapter.

Table 6.4 Energy requirements of children.

Age (years)	UK estimated average requirement (kcal/day)		Energy requirement (kcal/kg body weight/day)	
	Boys	Girls	Boys	Girls
3	1490	1370	97	92
5	1720	1550	88	82
7	1890	1680	78	71
9	2040	1790	69	61

Source: data from Department of Health (1998).

Children at this stage are increasing their independence from their parents and begin to hold their own strong views about food, physical activity and health. They take a greater role in the acquisition of the food that they will consume and, as they begin to experience more life outside the home through going to school, become more likely to purchase meals and snacks for their own consumption. Education about food, nutrition and health, therefore, becomes an important priority in the development of these children. By this stage of life, it is important for them to begin to follow a model along the lines of the Eatwell plate (NHS England, 2019) or similar schemes such as the US MyPlate model to develop eating habits that lower fat intake and promote consumption of starchy foods and fruits and vegetables.

6.3.2 School meals and the promotion of healthy eating

All over the world, schools provide meals for children. These are generally optional, giving children the opportunity to either bring in their own lunches from home or to purchase a cooked meal in school. While lunches brought in from home are the responsibility of parents, it is now common for schools and government agencies to provide information and advice to ensure that these meals are based upon basic principles of healthy eating. Schools, and the meals that they provide, are well placed to influence the dietary choices of children who are easily influenced, receptive to health education messages and interested in cooking and helping with food-related activities.

The meals that are provided within schools are increasingly subject to formal regulation to ensure their quality, particularly in the light of concern about rising levels of childhood obesity. These meals may be provided free of charge to children from poor backgrounds as a means of combating undernutrition. The UK provides a useful example of how legislation can be introduced to ensure that school meals fulfil

nutritional standards. In 2015, the Department for Education in England updated school meal guidelines which had been introduced across all four nations of the UK in 2006. Under the new guidance, schools which provide meals must serve high-quality meat, poultry, oily fish or non-dairy protein sources, with fruit and vegetables, bread and other cereals or potatoes. Children must be offered three different fruits and three different vegetables each week to encourage diversity in the diet. Caterers can offer no more than two portions of deep fried, battered or breaded food or pastry covered items each week. School meals and snacks must not include foods which are high in sugar, salt and fat and crisps, chocolate, sweets and sugar-sweetened beverages are not permitted. No salt can be provided for adding to food at the table (Department for Education, 2015). Comprehensive guidance on the school meal standards is provided to head teachers, school governing boards and caterers, including information on portion sizes, food groups and examples of good practice. Children whose families receive state benefits may qualify for free school lunches. These regulations apply only to government-run schools, so private schools and the rapidly growing self-governing academy sector in the UK are exempt, meaning that coverage is not universal. However, where implemented, it is reported that children increase intakes of water, vegetables and salad, fruit and starchy foods while decreasing intakes of fried starchy foods and non-fruit desserts. Overall intakes of protein, fibre and most micronutrients are increased, while energy, fat, sodium and non-milk extrinsic sugars are lower.

In 2010, the United States implemented the Healthy, Hunger-Free Kids Act, which set new nutritional standards for meals, snacks and beverages provided in schools through the National School Lunches, School Breakfast and Smart Snacks programmes (Kenney *et al.*, 2020). The School Breakfast Program and the National School Lunch Program were well-established and the new Act set new standards to increase fruit and vegetable and reduce starchy vegetable intakes. Guidelines were set for age-appropriate portion sizes and food and drink provision via school shops and vending machines. The new guidelines eliminated sugar-sweetened beverages and reduced the energy content of school foods, while increasing coverage of free and subsidized provision to children from deprived areas. Following introduction of the Act there was a decline in obesity in children of lower socioeconomic status (Kenney *et al.*, 2020) and the dietary quality of school lunches in participating schools was improved (Kinderknecht *et al.*, 2020). Under the administration of President Trump, the USDA weakened enforcement of the standards.

School meals are often just one element of a wider range of health interventions in schools, which also target physical activity and health education. Again, in the UK, the government introduced the National School Fruit and Vegetable Scheme in 2004, with the aim of providing one portion of fruit per day to school children aged between four and six years. The goal was to improve nutrient intakes and promote the five-a-day message to children. Hughes *et al.* (2012) reported that the scheme increased consumption of both fruit and vegetables, but that it was unable to overcome the impact of socioeconomic disadvantage on dietary quality. Similar schemes have been introduced in other European countries. Adoption of a school fruit and vegetable scheme in the German state of North Rhine Westphalia in 2010 was associated with an increase in fruit and vegetable consumption during the school day, with no detriment to consumption in the home environment (Methner *et al.*, 2017). A Norwegian scheme targeted to children in junior high but not primary schools was shown to increase intake of fruit by 0.36 portions per day, with no effect on vegetable intake (Hovdenak *et al.*, 2019, Øvrum and Bere, 2014). Provision of free healthy food in schools therefore appears to have a small but important impact on dietary quality for children.

6.3.3 The importance of breakfast

Breakfast is an important contributor to the overall dietary quality of children. It has been estimated that it provides between 275 and 670 kcal energy, which is delivered mostly from carbohydrate (50–72% of energy) and fat (14–40% of energy). The major breakfast foods consumed by children in developed countries are milk, fruit juices, breads and fortified cereals (Rampersaud *et al.*, 2005). Generally, breakfast will be delivering approximately 20% of daily energy intake and a greater proportion of micronutrients if based upon fortified cereals. It has an important metabolic role in that it

ends the overnight period of fasting during which glycogen stores become depleted. Breakfast induces a rise in blood glucose concentrations, which will be sustained over a longer period if the meal contains a high proportion of complex carbohydrates.

Despite its importance, breakfast is the most likely meal of the day to be missed by children. Utter *et al.* (2007) found that 3.7% of New Zealand children missed breakfast on most days and that 12.8% failed to eat it every day. These figures are similar to reports from other countries, with a prevalence of breakfast skipping of 8% in Australia and 18% in England reported by Mullan *et al.* (2014). Breakfast consumption is not universal even among very young children, with up to 5% of a sample of Dutch two- to five-year-olds missing breakfast regularly (Küpers *et al.*, 2014). Children who skip breakfast have been shown to have greater intakes of less healthy snack foods at other points in the day and often to have irregular meal patterns. Typically, their intakes of fruits and vegetables tend to be lower than seen in regular breakfast consumers. Breakfast skipping is therefore a good indicator of unhealthy food choices in children. In the study of Utter *et al.* (2007), skipping breakfast was also associated with greater BMI, consistent with other reports that although they consume less energy during the day, children who skip breakfast are more likely to be overweight (Rampersaud *et al.*, 2005). A prospective cohort study of Japanese children followed 42 663 participants from 1.5 to 12 years. Breakfast skipping was more common when the children were younger (19.3% at 4.5 years) and the behaviour declined across the follow-up period (1.9% skipped breakfast at age 11). Breakfast skipping behaviour was strongly related to parental breakfast habits. Children who skipped breakfast regularly were more likely to become overweight (OR 1.18, 95% CI 1.05–1.32), or obese (OR 2.16, 95% CI 1.55–2.99; Okada *et al.*, 2018). Although replicated in many studies (Figure 6.12), the relationship is not consistent across all age groups (Küpers *et al.*, 2014), and it is likely that breakfast skipping is an indicator of an unhealthy pattern of eating which promotes obesity rather than a causal factor in the development of obesity.

There are many reports that breakfast benefits cognitive processes and boosts performance in school. Observational studies based in school and home settings and experimental studies generally show that consumption of a breakfast that is rich in complex carbohydrate improves school attendance rates, boosts academic attainment and improves both short- and long-term memories. Liu *et al.* (2013) reported that among six-year-olds, IQ was

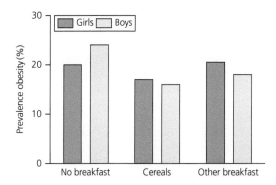

Figure 6.12 Boys who miss breakfast are more likely to be obese than those who consume a breakfast cereal or other breakfast foods on a regular basis; 9–13-year-olds in the 1999–2006 US National Health and Nutrition Examination Survey. *Source:* Deshmukh-Taskar *et al.* (2010).

higher in children who regularly consumed breakfast. Higher scores in cognitive tests were observed among 14–15-year-olds who had consumed breakfast compared with those who had not (Wesnes *et al.*, 2012). It has been argued that this result stems from the effect of breakfast upon blood glucose concentrations or possibly through modulation of neurotransmitter functions. A study by Brindal *et al.* (2012) could find no evidence of an effect of blood glucose, with no difference in cognitive function in 12-year-olds who were fed breakfasts where protein was replaced by carbohydrate sources with differing glycaemic index. A US study randomized schools to receive either an intervention in which breakfast foods were made more accessible or a control state where delivery of the intervention was delayed by a year. Children (aged 13–14 years) in the intervention arm showed no improvement in academic achievement at 3 or 18 months from the start of the intervention. Interestingly, the children of lower socioeconomic status in the control arm showed significant improvements in achievement when they eventually received the intervention (Hearst *et al.*, 2019). Ells *et al.* (2008) suggest that reports of improved cognitive performance should be treated with caution, as experiments are mostly performed in small cohorts of children and over short periods. Studies that are based in school breakfast clubs may be confounded by the social benefits of eating breakfast with peers and in younger children by poverty and family lifestyle.

The provision of breakfast in schools is seen as an important tool for dietary intervention to improve the quality of children's diets. As missing breakfast is a behaviour that is more common in socially deprived children from low-income families, provision of breakfast in schools may be a useful approach to target this population group (Moore *et al.*, 2007). The USDA oversees the School Breakfast Program, which is a major initiative to assist children from poor social backgrounds across the United States. The School Breakfast Program served 2.4 billion breakfasts and had a coverage of 14.57 million children in 2018. Participating schools must serve breakfasts that meet the Federal nutrition standards and must offer free or reduced price breakfasts to all eligible children, but breakfasts are available for purchase for children from all backgrounds. Eligibility for free breakfasts depends on family circumstances but, as a baseline, children qualify if family income is less than 130% of the Federal poverty level. The programme provides a breakfast based upon 240 ml milk, 120 ml fruit or vegetable juice, one slice of bread or an alternative and 28 g of meat or an alternative (Kennedy and Davis, 1998). This provides one quarter of the recommended daily amount for energy and a significant proportion of requirements for other nutrients. Evaluations of this scheme have shown that it improves the nutrient intakes of participants and has benefits for school attendance and performance.

In schools where breakfast clubs and other schemes along the lines of the USDA School Breakfast Program are operating, there is a major opportunity for health promotion and to make improvements to the quality of diets consumed by children. The USDA scheme, for example, engages schools with resources on healthy snacks and school wellness policies. Children participating in breakfast schemes may also consume lunch within school. A high proportion of daily food intake can therefore be managed and planned to fit well with health priorities. The importance of effective school-based interventions is further explored in Section 6.4.5.

6.4 Obesity in children

6.4.1 The rising prevalence of obesity
Obesity and overweight are a major health concern at all points across the lifespan. Chapter 8 sets out in detail the evidence that the prevalence of overweight and obesity in adults increased by twofold between 1990 and 2000 in the developed countries and is increasing at an alarming rate all across the world. The prevalence of obesity in childhood is also increasing rapidly in all parts of the world, and this may be of greater significance in terms of the future public health burden.

One of the challenges in following trends in childhood obesity over time is the often very different definitions that have been used in surveys and research papers over recent decades. In adults, BMI cut-off values can be simply applied (25 kg/m² for overweight, 30 kg/m² for obesity), and although there are many concerns about the accuracy of BMI in predicting body fatness and the suitability of these standard cut-offs for all ethnic groups, this gives a reasonable estimate of population-wide overweight and obesity rates. In children, BMI varies with age and in a nonlinear manner, so simple cut-off values are inappropriate (Figure 6.13). Instead, clinicians and researchers make reference to centile charts for BMI to define obesity. Typically, clinical reports are more stringent and define obesity as having BMI above the 98th centile (i.e. the BMI of the child is in the top 2% for the population at that age). Research reports using data collected prior to 2002 tended to define overweight as BMI above the 90th centile and obesity above the 95th centile. In an attempt to provide a standard classification to be applied globally, the International Obesity Taskforce (now the World Obesity Federation) suggested that the centile value at any given age should be projected forward to age 18 and then the cut-offs of 25 kg/m² for overweight and 30 kg/m² for obesity applied. On this basis, obese children lie just above the 98th centile for BMI and overweight is defined as just above the 90th centile.

There is a wealth of evidence to suggest that the prevalence of obesity has increased at a similar rate to that seen in adults over recent decades. It is estimated that, globally, in 2019 there were 158 million obese children aged between 5 and 19 years (World Obesity Federation, 2019), and the the World Obesity Federation projects that by 2030 this figure will have reached 254 million. The prevalence of obesity in children has more than doubled since the 1970s and this increase has been observed in all regions of the world.

Evidence from the UK suggests that a rapid rate of increase in prevalence of obesity occurred over the 1990s, with a near doubling, reported in the under-fives and a two- to threefold increase reported in 4–11-year-olds (Bundred *et al.*, 2001; Chinn and Rona, 2001). Rudolf *et al.* (2001) showed that in 9–11-year-olds, obesity prevalence had increased by fourfold over the period 1975–2000. The annual National Child Measurement Programme, which measures the height and weight of children entering school (aged four to five years) and as they leave primary school (aged 10–11 years), found that in 2019, 9.7 of children aged 4–5 years and 20.2% of those aged 10–11 years were obese (Public Health England, 2019). For the younger boys, there was evidence of a slight decrease in obesity over the preceding five years, but for girls and the older children the prevalence of obesity and excess weight was increasing. A 50% increase in prevalence of severe obesity occurred among British children between 2007 and 2019. These assessments focus on BMI rather than other measures of obesity. Griffiths *et al.* (2013) followed a cohort of nearly 700 British children from ages 11 to 12 for five years. Over this period, the prevalence of obesity as assessed by BMI decreased, but measures of waist circumference suggest that the children, and in particular the girls, increased central adiposity dramatically across the study. This implies that estimates of obesity that suggest a levelling off of prevalence may be missing changes in the prevalence of central obesity.

The trends for increasing prevalence of obesity that have been noted in the UK are typical of all of the developed countries. Analysis of the 1976–1980, 2003–2004 and 2009–2010 National Health and Nutrition Examination Survey studies from the United States indicates that among 6- to 11-year-olds, obesity prevalence increased from 7% to 18%, while for 12- to 19-year-olds, the increase was from 5% to 21% over the same period. There was some levelling off in child obesity rates in the United States from 2015, but disparities between white, black and Hispanic populations have continued to grow (Anderson *et al.*, 2019).

Globally, the highest prevalence of obesity in five- to nine-year-olds is observed in the Pacific region (Cook Islands, Nauru, Palau, all over 40%

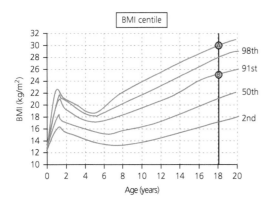

Figure 6.13 Body mass index (BMI) centiles. The most robust definitions of overweight and obesity are based upon tracking the current BMI centile of any child under the age of 18 years through to the BMI value for that centile at age 18. Standard BMI cut-offs of 25 and 30 kg/m² for overweight and obesity, respectively, can then be applied. On this basis, a child following the centile marked A on the chart would be defined as obese, while a child following the centile marked B would be defined as overweight. *Source:* data compiled from Cole *et al.* (1995). This chart is shown for illustrative purposes only and is not for clinical use.

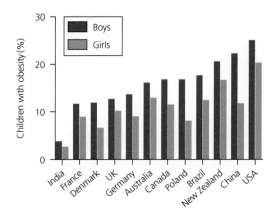

Figure 6.14 Prevalence of obesity in childhood in selected countries. *Source:* data from World Obesity Federation (2019).

obesity; Tuvalu, Marshall Islands, over 35%). In developed countries, the United States and New Zealand have the highest rates of childhood obesity (Figure 6.14), and in Europe the countries with the highest levels of obesity are in the east of the region (Poland, Bulgaria, Ukraine). The lowest rates of childhood obesity are seen in the most impoverished nations of Africa (Ethiopia, Chad, Burkina Faso, all less than 2.5%) and Asia (Nepal, India, approximately 3.5%; World Obesity Federation, 2019).

6.4.2 The causes of obesity in childhood

On a simplistic level, the causes of obesity at any age are obvious. Obesity represents the excess accumulation of body fat as a consequence of positive energy balance. In other words, the amount of energy consumed is in excess of requirement for metabolic and physiological processes. To put this another way, childhood obesity is the product of excess food intake and insufficient energy expenditure through physical activity. This explanation is, however, a superficial viewpoint and is unhelpful, as it serves to perpetuate the false idea that all obese children are greedy and lazy.

Obesity is multifactorial in origin and represents an interaction between a genetic predisposition and the environment. Obesity can be generated without gross imbalances of energy supply and demand. A habitual positive energy balance of just 10–20 kcal/day can result in a significant accumulation of excess body fat over a period of a few years. It is generally argued that the modern obesity 'epidemic' that afflicts children is a consequence of the mismatch between the biological evolution of humans and the technological revolution of recent times. This 'discordance hypothesis' suggests that early

humans evolved for subsistence on a food supply that was insecure and where considerable amounts of energy had to be expended in order to gain access to food, either through hunting or foraging. As a result, the human genome evolved to favour efficient energy storage. The modern environment is at odds with this biological background and daily consumption of energy-rich foods, with low energy expenditure through activity (Eaton *et al.*, 1988; Hill and Peters, 1998). It is proposed that obesity genes carried by many humans achieve their expression in the 'obesogenic' environment that has been constructed through social and technological changes.

Obesity-promoting genes may play an important role in determining risk of childhood obesity. It is estimated that 33–50% of the risk to any individual is derived from genetic inheritance. In a powerful analysis, Wardle *et al.* (2008) studied twins aged 8–11 years, a study therefore free of many confounding influences seen in earlier studies of adult twins, and noted that 77% of the variation in BMI and waist circumference could be explained by genetic factors. Given that many monogenic causes of obesity are likely to be of early onset, they may contribute significantly to observed levels of childhood obesity. Despite the major influence of genetic factors, it has to be recognized that the modern obesity crisis has developed over the past 20–30 years and that the human gene pool will have been relatively stable for tens of thousands of years. The overwhelming view of researchers in the field is that environmental factors explain current trends.

6.4.2.1 Physical activity

Physical activity is seen as an important element of normal healthy development and provides protection against weight gain and related disorders later in life while promoting bone mineralization and optimal growth. Some points in childhood appear to be more important than others in terms of the health gain associated with activity, for example, the preschool years and the later stages of adolescence. This may be because these are stages at which attitudes to exercise are shaped, therefore influencing activity levels at future life stages. Physical activity levels often decline with age, reflecting patterns of play in children, which often change from free, unstructured and active games (e.g. spontaneous games of chase and tag) to a more regimented sports-based pattern in early adolescence (Must and Tybor, 2005).

Declining levels of physical activity are seen as a major contributor to obesity in children. The modern environment encourages low levels of physical activity in children for a number of reasons. Modern transport networks discourage walking or cycling, and many parents will choose to drive their children to school and other activities by car even over relatively short distances. This may be due to concerns about children's safety when out and about but may also be a product of the fact that driving is easier and faster and a simpler way to integrate children's activities into busy family life. Within schools, the prioritization of academic subjects and testing over time spent in physical education, sport, dance and other more active subjects has led to a progressive fall in levels of physical activity within the working week. Alternative activities outside school can be difficult for some children to access due to cost, location or a general lack of availability.

The flip side of the coin in consideration of declining physical activity is the increase in the amount of time spent on sedentary activities. These are generally leisure activities that involve little more than the resting level of energy expenditure. In developed countries, children spend four to six hours per day either watching television or using computers and games consoles. Exceeding a recommended maximum of two hours per day sedentary screen time is the norm for children in most developed countries (Figure 6.15). Screen watching is now the preferred leisure activity of most children and is favoured by many parents as they keep the child in a safe and controlled environment.

Although physical activity is seen as a key contributor to obesity risk in children, it is difficult to quantify the extent of that risk with any certainty. Within populations, levels of physical activity are extremely variable and it is highly problematic to quantify actual energy expenditure through activity, using validated methods (Rennie et al., 2006). Most of the literature is therefore based upon indirect and subjective measurements (e.g. self-report of the hours spent watching television). Moreover, cross-sectional studies that attempt to examine relationships between activity and obesity are confounded by the fact that causality cannot be shown. In general, overweight and obese children will be less active than their lean counterparts as they find physical activity and sport more difficult and less enjoyable (Must and Tybor, 2005).

Despite these methodological issues, from the available information, it seems likely that leisure inactivity is a critical component of the modern obesogenic environment that is driving childhood obesity. Prospective studies that have considered how childhood BMI changes over time are related to activity levels consistently show strong negative associations between the two variables. A systematic review of 235 studies, which included 1.66 million children from 71 countries, concluded that higher levels of television watching were associated with greater body fatness, with unfavourable cardiometabolic risk indicators (Carson et al., 2016). While a more robust analysis, which used only gold-standard data collected using accelerometers to determine the activity of children, found no significant association of sedentary time with metabolic syndrome (Renninger et al., 2020), it is clear that interventions which target a reduction in sedentary time are effective in reducing overweight. A meta-analysis of such interventions found that they reduce BMI of children by an average of 0.15 kg/m² (95% CI–0.23 to –0.08 kg/m²; Wu et al., 2016). A 10-minute per day increase in moderate to vigorous physical activity reduced risk of metabolic syndrome in children (Renninger et al., 2020).

Sedentary time spent watching television may be doubly insidious as it not only limits physical activity but also increases consumption of snacks and sugar-sweetened beverages. As discussed earlier in this chapter, food advertising to children during sedentary time is a major issue. Emond et al. (2019) noted that child-targeted advertising of McDonalds fast food increased intake by almost twofold in three- to five-year-olds whose parents were not regular consumers of fast foods. The meta-analysis of Russell et al. (2019) showed that exposure of children to food advertising on television increased energy intake by an average of 60 kcal/day. The effect of advertising was greater in children who were overweight or obese (additional 102 kcal/day, 95% CI 32.38–171.76 kcal/day).

6.4.2.2 Food intake

From the aforementioned discussion, it should be clear that energy expenditure through physical activity among children has declined markedly over

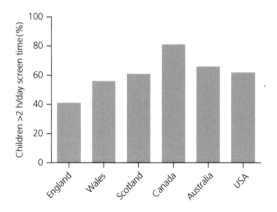

Figure 6.15 Children's daily exposure to television or other screen-based activities.

recent decades. James (2008a) highlighted the fact that this has impacted particularly heavily on the rapidly developing countries such as China and India. In China, changes in technology and increasing use of motorized transport mean that energy requirements for children are markedly lower than they were 40 years ago. Whereas in the past children were engaged in work-related activities for much of their time, modernization and urbanization may have reduced energy requirements by 200 kcal/ day. Alongside these shifts in activity levels, the nature of the diet has undergone a revolution in almost all parts of the world, producing an increase in energy intakes and energy density of foodstuffs. Analyses of the China Health and Nutrition Surveys indicate that shifts in dietary pattern have occurred alongside the increase in prevalence of childhood overweight and obesity. Adair *et al.* (2014) found that overweight was associated with the protein density of the diet (OR for overweight 1.65, 95% CI 1.26–2.17 comparing high and low protein density). Liu *et al.* (2018) identified two dietary patterns among Chinese 6–17-year-olds. Among those children following a westernized pattern (cakes, sugar-sweetened beverages, snacks, red meat, fruit and nuts) rather than a traditional diet, BMI was greater (0.57 kg/m^2, 95% CI 0.4–0.85 kg/m^2) and the risk of obesity was significantly increased (OR 1.49, 95% CI 1.21–1.84). Similarly, in India, where the prevalence of obesity is increasing, there are reports of rising prevalence of westernized non-core foods in school aged children (Ranjani *et al.*, 2016; Gupta *et al.*, 2019). The modern environment simultaneously promotes reduced energy expenditure and increased consumption.

Studies that have sought to establish the links between dietary intakes and obesity in children have generally produced inconclusive results and at best indicate weak relationships between specific dietary factors and obesity in childhood. For example, Guillaume *et al.* (1998) found no association between energy intake from fat and body fatness in 6–12-year-olds. Similarly, Maffeis *et al.* (1998) could find no association between body fatness and intakes of macronutrients in children. Robertson *et al.* (1999) considered fatness using a comprehensive series of skinfold measurements and showed that children with more body fat had higher intakes of energy, but not of any specific macronutrient. Reilly *et al.* (2005) found no contribution of dietary factors to difference in risk of overweight among seven-year-old children, even when comparing children with an established preference for a diet rich in chocolate, crisps and sugar-sweetened beverages with those whose diets were rich in complex carbohydrates and protein.

There are major challenges in attempting such studies, and this may be responsible for the lack of consistency in the literature. Confounding factors first need to be taken into account, including body weight at birth and parental BMI. Moreover, as individuals of greater weight require more energy to maintain that weight, studies are best performed using a longitudinal design to monitor the associations between dietary factors and weight or fat gain over a period of time. Obtaining accurate measurements of dietary intake is difficult at any stage of life but is particularly difficult in children and their parents, who may fail to recall and fully record their intakes. As described in Section 6.4.1, even the anthropometric classification of overweight and obesity is far from straightforward.

Magarey *et al.* (2001) used robust methods to avoid the pitfalls identified earlier, in a study of 2–15-year-old Australian children. However, no clear influence of macronutrient intake upon BMI or body fatness measured using skinfolds could be identified. In contrast, Skinner *et al.* (2004) found associations between macronutrient intakes and change in BMI between two months and eight years of age. Regular assessment of dietary intake using weighed records and 24-hour maternal recall allowed determination of longitudinal patterns of protein, carbohydrate and fat consumption, alongside changes in BMI. Protein and fat intakes were positively associated with BMI, while carbohydrate intake was negatively associated. Surprisingly, total energy intake was not predictive of BMI. BMI at eight years was most strongly related to BMI at age two and the timing of the adiposity rebound (Figure 6.16), indicating that factors in early infancy may be critical in setting the risk of overweight and obesity and reinforcing the importance of infant feeding methods in this context (see Research Highlight 6.2).

While the macronutrient composition of the diet cannot be strongly related to body fatness in children, there is clear evidence that meal patterns, portion sizes and the energy density of foods consumed play an important role in determining risk of overweight and obesity. Dubois *et al.* (2008), for example, considered energy and macronutrient intakes in a cohort of Canadian children. These children were divided into a group who consumed breakfast on a daily basis (90% of the study population) and those who missed breakfast on at least one day each week (10% of population). Those who skipped breakfast had different overall dietary patterns to the breakfast consumers. They consumed more energy in total, consumed less protein and energy from protein and ate a greater number of carbohydrate-rich

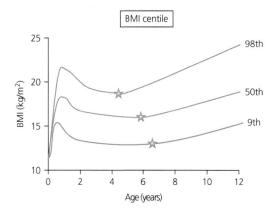

BMI centile

Figure 6.16 The adiposity rebound. In early childhood, the weight gain of children outstrips their height gain, and as a result, body mass index (BMI) rises rapidly. Beyond the first year of life, height gain tends to exceed weight gain and so BMI declines. Between the ages of 4 and 8 years, BMI begins to increase again and this point is termed the adiposity rebound. Having an earlier adiposity rebound appears to be predictive of obesity in childhood, and it can be clearly seen on the graph that for children on a higher BMI centile, the rebound (marked by the stars) occurs at an earlier age. Earlier adiposity rebound is noted in formula-fed compared with breastfed infants.

snacks. Risk of overweight among the children skipping breakfast was increased by 2.27-fold (95% CI 1.33–3.88). The study could not discount the fact that breakfast skipping could be a marker for other confounding factors, such as sedentary behaviour, but nonetheless showed how patterns of intake within the day could influence body fatness. While in the reference group BMI was unrelated to intakes at specific points in the day, in children who skipped breakfast, consumption of over 700 kcal at lunchtime was a predictor of overweight. This suggests that meal frequency could impact on energy balance or appetite regulation.

Increased energy density of foodstuffs has also been proposed as a factor driving the increase in childhood obesity. Changes in family lifestyle, where the need for both parents to be out of the house in paid employment, have increased the consumption of preprepared convenience foods. These are generally rich in fats and sugars and have a higher energy density than meals prepared at home from fresh ingredients. Moreover, children are consuming increasing amounts of snack foods, in addition to meals, and these also increase the energy density of the overall diet. It is logical to assume that this change in food consumption has an impact upon overall energy intake in children, but once again methodological issues have made it difficult to demonstrate a relationship between energy density

and obesity risk. McCaffrey *et al.* (2008) investigated this potential association using a seven-year follow-up to a study initially conducted in primary school children (aged six to eight years). No relationship was noted between energy density of the children's diets and the gain in fat mass over this period. In contrast, Johnson *et al.* (2008) found that fat mass in nine-year-old children was related to energy density of the diet and dietary fat intake and inversely related to intakes of dietary fibre.

Regular consumption of 'fast food' is recognized as a behaviour that increases energy density of the diet and hence overall energy intake. Fast food can be defined as foodstuffs that are mass-produced convenience foods, generally purchased from self-service or takeaway outlets. The market for fast food is vast and reaches into all parts of the world. The McDonalds burger chain alone has a global turnover of around US$20 billion per year with over 38 600 outlets in 119 countries. Numerous studies show that children who are regular consumers of fast-food have higher habitual intakes of sugar and fat and lower intakes of fruits and vegetables, with an overall greater dietary density. In the United States consumption of ultra-processed foods accounts for 65% of dietary energy and 92% of energy from sugars in the diets of children (Neri *et al.*, 2019). A prospective study of three- to five-year-olds found that on average they consumed fast-food 2.1 times per week. Over the course of the two year cohort follow-up, the risk of transition from normal weight to overweight, or overweight to obese was increased by 38% for every instance of fast-food consumption per week. Among children who consumed fast-food more than three times per week the risk of becoming overweight or obese was increased by 2.17-fold (Emond *et al.*, 2020).

A growing body of research shows that the presence of fast-food outlets in children's everyday food environment is a risk factor for weight gain. Cheong *et al.*, (2019) reported that a high density of fast-food outlets around residential areas in Malaysia was associated with more overweight in children (OR 1.23, 95% CI 1.03–1.47). Similarly a six-year follow-up of a cohort of Swedish 0–14-year-olds showed greater odds of obesity among those living in neighbourhoods with more accessible fast-food outlets (Hamano *et al.*, 2017). A systematic review of studies from the UK concluded that fast-food shops and restaurants are more common in socially deprived neighbourhoods and that children who spend more time in such areas tend to consume more fast-food and have higher BMI (Turbutt *et al.*, 2019).

Sugar-sweetened beverages are an important element of the energy-dense diet that is associated with fast-food consumption. These drinks can contribute significantly to energy intake in children. Pure fruit juices are also considered in this category, even though parents widely perceive these to be a healthy alternative to other drinks, including water. A 100-ml serving of apple juice, for example, can deliver 11.8 g of sugar (a nearly identical quantity to a similar serving of cola), and consumption may displace less energy-dense, more nutrient-dense drinks such as milk (Table 6.5). Wang et al. (2008) reported that in the United States, energy intakes in children from sugar-sweetened beverages and fruit juices accounted for 10–15% of total energy intakes. The consumption of sugar-sweetened beverages appears to be a major culprit in weight gain associated with dietary patterns that include fast food. Although there was initial caution as to whether sugar-sweetened beverages caused weight gain (Ludwig et al., 2001), there is now clear evidence that they play a role in determining childhood body weight. Lim et al. (2009) followed a population of African-American preschool children over two years and found that there was a significant risk of obesity associated with high consumption of sugar-sweetened beverages. Odds of overweight increased by 4% for every 28 ml consumed per day.

Similarly, a case–control study of Spanish 5–18-year-olds noted a 3.46-fold (95% CI 1.24–9.62) increase in risk of obesity with greater than four servings per week (Martin-Calvo et al., 2015). The meta-analysis of Te Morenga et al. (2012) suggested that odds of overweight were higher (OR 1.55, 95% CI 1.32–1.82) in groups with the highest compared with the lowest intakes. These drinks may be particularly important in promoting weight gain, as the hypothalamic systems that regulate appetite and energy balance do not compensate for liquid food sources as efficiently as they do for solids.

6.4.2.3 Genetic disorders

There are several single-gene mutations that are known to promote early-onset obesity (Table 6.6). Until recently, it has always been assumed that these mutations are extremely rare and account for only a small proportion of childhood and adult obesity cases. The use of modern molecular techniques for population screening and the discovery of new gene targets are starting to change this perception, and it appears that up to 10% of all obese children may have an underlying genetic disorder. For example, confirmed deficiency of the leptin receptor had only been

Table 6.5 Energy and sugar content of beverages commonly consumed by children.

Beverage	Per 100-ml serving		
	Energy (kcal)	Energy (KJ)	Sugars (g)
Cow's milk (whole)	66	277	5.6
Apple juice (unsweetened)	49	205	11.8
Orange juice (unsweetened)	49	205	11.1
Fruit squash	55	230	12.8
Lemonade	63	264	15.9
Cola	43	180	11.9

Table 6.6 Genetic disorders associated with early-onset obesity.

Condition	Gene defect(s)	Contribution to obesity
Melanocortin receptor defects	MC1R, MC2R, MC3R, MC4R, MC5R	MC4R defects may explain 5% of all childhood obesity cases
FTO polymorphisms	FTO	Explains 1% of variation in population BMI. Sixteen per cent of population homozygous for obesity-related allele
Prader–Willi syndrome	Abnormalities of chromosome 15	One in 12 000–15 000 births
Leptin receptor defects	LepR	Up to 3% of cases of childhood obesity
Bardet–Biedl syndrome	Abnormalities of chromosomes 11 and 16	One in 125 000 births
MOMO	Unknown	Only 5 confirmed cases
Congenital leptin deficiency	Leptin	Only 12 confirmed cases

BMI, body mass index; MOMO, macrosomia, obesity, macrocephaly and ocular abnormalities.

observed in a single family, but a screen of 300 individuals with early-onset obesity revealed LepR defects in 3% of cases (Farooqi *et al.*, 2007). The *FTO* gene has been highlighted as a novel gene target for obesity research. Single nucleotide polymorphisms in *FTO* are common in the population (between 14 and 52%) and are associated with greater BMI. Individuals who are homozygous for the at-risk form of the FTO allele have 1.67-fold greater risk of obesity (Loos and Bouchard, 2008).

Many of the genetic disorders linked to obesity are associated with other abnormalities. In Bardet–Biedl syndrome, for example, obesity is just one outcome among a myriad abnormalities of growth and development, affecting the eyes, the gastrointestinal tract and the cardiovascular system. Other disorders induce obesity through effects upon the neuroendocrine control of appetite. Defects of MC4R (the melanocortin 4 receptor) are associated with binge eating disorders (Loos *et al.*, 2008). In Prader–Willi syndrome, there are defects of the chromosome 15q11–13 region that stem from either deletion of paternally derived alleles or epigenetic silencing (DNA methylation) of paternal alleles (Goldstone, 2004). Prader–Willi syndrome-affected children have a number of neurological defects and generally have learning difficulties. In infancy, they often fail to thrive, as they are unable to feed normally, but between one and six years gain weight at a prodigious rate due to extreme hyperphagia. Some adolescents with Prader–Willi syndrome will consume in excess of 5000 kcal/day if given free access to food. Management of the condition therefore requires strict control over portion sizes and the availability of food.

6.4.3 The consequences of childhood obesity
Soaring rates of childhood overweight and obesity have prompted fears about the impact of these trends upon the health of populations. Clearly, these concerns must focus upon the immediate health of the affected children, but it is also of importance to consider whether obesity in childhood increases risk of obesity and related disorders later in life.

6.4.3.1 Immediate health consequences
Obesity and overweight have important physical and psychological effects upon children and adolescents. Overweight children tend to grow and mature more rapidly and so attain a greater height than their leaner peers. In girls, the greater level of body fat drives earlier menarche (see Chapter 2). Overweight has important metabolic consequences and, as a result, disease states that were once extremely rare among children are increasing in prevalence. The metabolic syndrome, also referred

to as the insulin resistance syndrome, is defined as the combined presence of hyperinsulinaemia, hypertriglyceridaemia and cardiovascular disorders (hypertension). It is primarily a condition of adulthood, with a prevalence of just 4% in children. There are reports that in overweight children and adolescents, this may increase to 30–50% (Daniels *et al.*, 2005). Individual components of the syndrome are also noted in a high proportion of overweight children, who are more likely to have a profile of circulating lipids that is associated with greater risk of cardiovascular disease (elevated low-density lipoprotein-cholesterol and triglycerides, lower concentrations of high-density lipoprotein-cholesterol). Glucose intolerance is more likely in the obese child and so the increasing prevalence of overweight and obesity over the last few decades has seen a steady increase in the numbers of children with either pre-diabetes or frank type 2 diabetes (Mayer-Davis *et al.*, 2017). While type 1 diabetes has traditionally been known as 'early-onset' diabetes (incidence approximately 25 cases per 100 000 children), type 2 diabetes is increasingly common. In the United States, the estimated incidence is 12 per 100 000 children, while in the UK it is markedly lower at 0.72 per 100 000 (Reinehr, 2013; Candler *et al.*, 2018). Type 2 diabetes in children is strongly associated with obesity (>80% of cases) and is more common among children from ethnic minorities than in white populations (Candler *et al.*, 2018).

Overweight impacts upon liver function and obese children are more prone to hepatic steatosis and gallstones. High blood pressure is more likely among children who are obese. Cerebral hypertension can manifest as pseudotumour cerebri. Carrying excess weight puts strain upon the growing skeleton. Two thirds of patients diagnosed with Blount's disease, a bone-deformation condition of childhood, are obese. Thirty to fifty per cent of children with slipped capital femoral epiphysis, a defect of the growth plate in the thigh bone, are overweight or obese.

From a psychological perspective, overweight in the childhood years can be extremely destructive, lowering self-esteem, promoting depression and preventing happy social interactions. Children who are overweight are more likely to be bullied at school and are often discriminated against by their peers. Even very young children show a preference for thinner children as playmates and will equate obesity with laziness and other undesirable descriptions.

6.4.3.2 Tracking of obesity: consequences for the future
In the context of obesity, 'tracking' is the term used to describe the situation where body fatness at one stage of life correlates strongly with a later stage.

For example, if underweight children grow up to become underweight adults, their body fatness will be said to have tracked from one stage to another (Figure 6.17). Similarly, if overweight infants remain overweight in adolescence, their body fatness will be described as having tracked throughout childhood. Identification of tracking of overweight and obesity from childhood to adulthood and of risk factors for such tracking is important for two reasons. First, strong evidence of tracking would indicate that high levels of childhood obesity will exert effects upon adult body fatness and related health problems for many decades to come. In other words, if children who are obese grow up to be adults who are obese, the current generation of children may grow up with a major burden of type 2 diabetes and cardiovascular disease. Second, if overweight and obesity really do track to adulthood, then it may be possible to identify individuals at greatest risk of obesity and related disorders at an early phase of life and intervene at that stage.

In general, the literature in relation to obesity tracking shows only a moderate, weak association between BMI in childhood and adulthood but stronger associations between BMI in adolescence and later life. Studies that consider tracking are often limited by the span of time that can be reasonably covered by a follow-up study and by the confounding influences of parental BMI and genetic factors.

The Thousand Families cohort, a study of children born in the city of Newcastle between May and June 1947, provided a useful opportunity to consider tracking of body fatness from childhood to middle age. BMI at age nine years was weakly correlated with adult BMI, but this relationship was explained by lean, rather than fat, mass (Wright *et al.*, 2001). There was evidence of tracking from ages 13 to 50 years and children whose BMI was in the top quartile for the population were twice as likely to be in the top quartile for body fatness at age 50. However, as obesity was relatively uncommon in the 1950s and as the drivers of childhood obesity at that time may well be different to contemporary populations, the generalizability of these data may be questioned. Moreover, this study reported that most 50-year-olds with obesity had not been overweight as children. In contrast, Johannsson *et al.* (2006) suggested that tracking from infancy to adolescence meant that BMI in childhood was a strong predictor of overweight or obesity at age 15. Being overweight at age 6 or 9 was found to increase risk of overweight at 15 by 10.4- and 18.6-fold, respectively. Fifty-one per cent of overweight six-year-olds remained overweight after puberty. The Bogalusa Heart Study was a prospective cohort study from the United States, with adults who were initially studied at ages 9–11 followed to 19–35 years of age. Within this more contemporary study, overall tracking of overweight from childhood to adulthood was found to be around 22.5%, compared with 40% tracking of normal weight (Deshmukh-Taskar *et al.*, 2006).

The evidence to support the view that overweight in childhood predisposes the individual to overweight and obesity in adulthood is, therefore, rather modest. While it is clear that there is some influence of childhood body fatness on later weight classification, this is

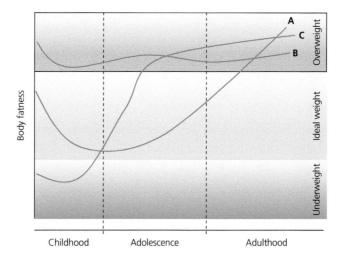

Figure 6.17 Tracking of overweight. An individual whose weight (body fatness) classification changes from childhood to adulthood is said not to be tracking (e.g. line A shows an adult onset of overweight). Where weight classification remains the same from childhood to adulthood (line B) or from adolescence to adulthood (line C), weight is tracking. The evidence of tracking of overweight is strongest from adolescence to adulthood.

just one component of a more complex aetiology for adult obesity. However, it is important to also consider whether childhood overweight and obesity might be an independent risk factor for adult disease states. Few studies have the power to consider this question in detail. The Thousand Families study surprisingly found that after adjusting for adult body fat, there was an inverse relationship between BMI at nine years and adult total cholesterol and triglyceride concentrations, but only for women. Other cardiovascular risk factors were unrelated to childhood BMI, and BMI at age 13 was completely unrelated to adult risk profile (Wright *et al.*, 2001). The greatest risk for adult disease appeared to be predicted by the combination of underweight during childhood and obesity in adulthood.

Juonala *et al.* (2005) found strong evidence of tracking of overweight from early childhood to adulthood. Individuals with BMI over the 80th centile between three and nine years had triple the risk of obesity between 24 and 39 years, and this risk increased to fourfold in those who were overweight in adolescence. Measurements of carotid intima-media thickness as a proxy for the early stages of atherosclerosis, however, showed no risk of cardiovascular disease associated with the childhood or adolescent obesity. All disease risk was related to adult obesity. Freedman *et al.* (2001) examined relationships between risk factors for cardiovascular disease and BMI in childhood. Although individuals who had been obese in childhood tended to have high circulating total cholesterol, low-density lipoprotein-cholesterol, insulin and triglyceride concentrations and higher blood pressure, these effects were all explained by their greater body fatness in adulthood (Figure 6.18). Systematic reviews of the relationship between childhood obesity and adult cardiovascular (Lloyd *et al.*, 2010) and metabolic (Lloyd *et al.*, 2012) disease found little evidence to suggest that childhood obesity is an independent risk factor. Risk appears entirely related to adult fatness and so tracking of obesity, particularly from adolescence, needs to be prevented. Although there is a lack of strong evidence to suggest that the obese child is at greater risk of disease in adulthood by virtue of their childhood adiposity, the balance of opinion appears to be that the obese child is more likely to be an obese adult and hence develop a high-risk metabolic profile. The treatment and prevention of paediatric obesity is therefore considered to be a very high priority for public health and clinical practice.

6.4.4 Treatment of childhood obesity

Once identified as being overweight or obese, children require rapid and well-thought-out intervention to limit the risk of health problems and of becoming an obese adult with related metabolic and cardiovascular disorders. However, the treatment of obese children poses special problems, as there is a need to maintain normal rates of growth, while simultaneously promoting loss of excess weight and reduction of fat mass. The strategy to be employed will depend upon the age of the child, partly because his/her capacity for autonomous decision making will change markedly between childhood and later adolescence but also because of the influence of normal growth. For very young children, for example, reducing rates of weight gain may be sufficient to correct overweight and obesity as the child will normalize body weight and fat mass through the growth process.

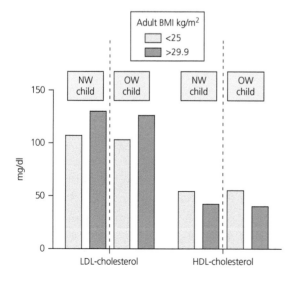

Figure 6.18 Risk factors for coronary heart disease in relation to childhood or adult overweight. Adult obesity is associated with raised circulating low-density lipoprotein (LDL)-cholesterol and lower high-density lipoprotein (HDL)-cholesterol concentrations. These are established risk factors for coronary heart disease. In adult individuals who were overweight during childhood, the risk profile associated with obesity is no different to that seen in adults who were of normal weight in childhood. These data suggest that adult risk of coronary heart disease is not directly influenced by childhood weight status. NW, normal weight; OW, overweight. *Source:* data drawn from Freedman *et al.* (2001).

The overriding aim in treating childhood obesity is to promote only slow and gradual reductions in fat mass and loss of excess weight. Slower rates of fat loss are easier to sustain and the gradual approach can be advantageous as children and their parents can be set simply achieved goals. With achievement of those goals comes the self-esteem and confidence that is necessary to achieve longer-term aims. However, the absence of an obvious and rapid change can also be disheartening. In some cases, fat loss may occur without any change or even an increase in body weight due to growth. Children who are obese and their parents therefore require close supervision and encouragement to sustain successful treatment.

Treating paediatric obesity requires a close integration of multiple approaches that include changes in nutrition, physical activity levels, sedentary time and wholesale lifestyle modifications that ideally impact upon whole families. The physical activity component can be particularly difficult to introduce as many overweight and obese children find exercise difficult and embarrassing. To promote fat loss, children need to engage in around 60 minutes per day of aerobic exercise, such as cycling, swimming, dancing or walking. To ensure compliance with any exercise programme, it is essential that the activities increase in intensity at a gradual rate and that the activities are tailored to the individual children. If the exercise is enjoyable, the children will maintain their involvement, whereas humiliating boot camp experiences will achieve no more than a short-term gain in energy expenditure. When children can be encouraged to take part in activities where they can succeed and show some mastery, self-esteem is increased, boosting motivation and the desire to stay active even at the end of treatment (Craig *et al.*, 1996). Alongside increased levels of exercise, parents should remove or limit access to elements of the environment that promote sedentary activity, such as televisions and computer games. Many of these changes are perhaps most effective if they are incorporated into whole lifestyle changes in which activity becomes a part of everyday life, (e.g. walking or cycling to school and other activities).

Dietary modifications to treat obesity must be introduced as long-term changes. It is obvious that any short-term dietary change that ceases as soon as an acceptable BMI is achieved will fail, as the individual will simply revert to their old eating habits and regain weight at the end of the treatment. With children, dietary changes should not be referred to as dieting and must be treated as a wholly positive experience. Rather than labelling certain foods as forbidden and to be wholly excluded, children should be encouraged to consume a pattern of diet that is

healthier overall but which still includes their preferred options such as sweets and chocolate (Grace, 2001). The child who is overweight requires a diet that delivers sufficient energy and nutrients to support growth that is based upon foods that are acceptable to children and that are easy to acquire and prepare. Epstein *et al.* (2008) compared the approaches of promoting healthy eating against restricting energy-dense foods in a group of children aged 8–12 years. All children and their parents were given the goal of keeping energy intake to 1000–1500 kcal per day and taught a traffic light classification of foodstuffs. One group was instructed to limit intakes of red light foods (high in sugar and fat), while the other was instructed to consume greater amounts of green light foods (mostly fruits and vegetables). At followup 12–24 months after the intervention, both groups of children had improved their BMI, but the healthy eating group had fared significantly better (Figure 6.16). This study highlights the importance of promoting a healthy lifestyle rather than simply dictating a restrictive diet. When given greater access to healthier foods, children find it easier to consume these as alternatives for energy-dense choices.

For most overweight and obese children, small gradual changes are sufficient to manage weight gain. For those with more severe or morbid obesity, the strategy is different as more rapid weight loss is necessary to avoid ill health. In these cases, low-calorie or very-low-calorie diets (800 kcal/day or less) may be merited but only under strict medical supervision (Caroli and Burniat, 2002).

Parents play a central role in the treatment of children with obesity. With younger children (under 11 years), at least, parents will generally have full control over food purchase and preparation, access to exercise opportunities and leisure activities and as such need to be the main targets for education and advice during periods of treatment (Golan *et al.*, 1998). Where at least one parent is actively participating in a weight loss programme alongside their children, the chances of success are increased (McLean *et al.*, 2003). Children enjoy monitoring the progress of their parents and setting their goals and rewards. This stimulates active engagement with treatment programmes. The influence of parents should ideally be applied to all children in a family. It is clearly unreasonable to expect a child who is obese to change their diet and increase activity levels if other family members do not.

With parents at the heart of treatment strategies, it is of concern to note that many parents of obese children do not recognize that their children have a problem. Carnell *et al.* (2005) surveyed parents of three- to five-year-old children through nursery and primary schools in London and found that only 1.9% of parents with children who were overweight and 17.1% of parents with children who were obese described their children as overweight. None of the parents described their children as 'very overweight', even though the prevalence of obesity among the children was actually 7.3%. However, although they were unable to correctly classify their children's body weights, the parents of infants who were overweight and obese were more than twice as likely than other parents to express concerns that their children may become obese later in life. Successful treatment of paediatric obesity can only begin once parents are ready to recognize the issue and engage with the relevant professionals. Parents are more likely to do this if their child is older, if the parents are themselves overweight or obese and if there is a belief that the health of the child may be at risk (Rhee *et al.*, 2005).

6.4.5 Prevention of childhood obesity

In the UK, the government's chief scientist published *Tackling Obesities: Future Choices – Project Report* (Butland *et al.*, 2007). This report highlighted obesity as a major public health problem, which by 2050 would be expected to cost the country £45 billion per year. Within this report, obesity was regarded as the normal passive physiological response to the modern obesogenic environment. To tackle the problem, there has to be massive societal change that changes the environment, as the epidemic cannot be prevented through individual action alone. These conclusions echo the statement made by the WHO to highlight the challenge, 'Obesity cannot be prevented or managed solely at the individual level. Committees, governments, the media and the food industry need to work together to modify the environment so that it is less conducive to weight gain' (Branca *et al.*, 2007).

Prevention of obesity is a far more effective public health strategy than treatment at any stage of life. Targeting prevention strategies at children is considered to be of primary importance, partly because the evidence suggests that obesity may track from childhood to adulthood, but primarily because sweeping lifestyle changes at this stage of life are more likely to be sustained by individuals over the longer term. While prevention strategies require a multi-agency approach which involves families, schools, the food industry and governments (Figure 6.19), they may be more effective if

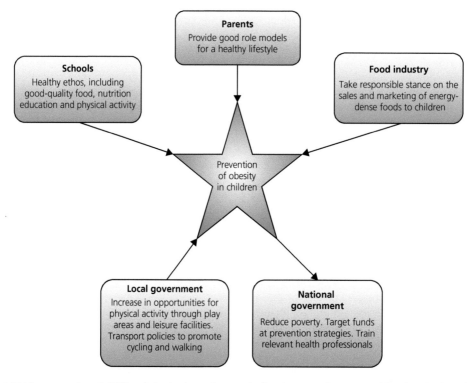

Figure 6.19 The prevention of childhood obesity depends upon the involvement of parents and families, food producers, schools and government agencies. None of these stakeholders has sufficient influence to be able to tackle the obesity problem in isolation.

tailored to suit the specific targets in the population. For example, interventions that promote breast-feeding may be an effective way of prevention obesity in infants, while targeting schools to increase physical activity, include more health-related subjects in the curriculum and limit access to energy-dense snacks would be an effective strategy for older school-age children (Daniels *et al.*, 2005).

The influence of parents and family upon the food choices and lifestyle behaviours of children is immense. Implementation of population-wide strategies for prevention of childhood obesity requires all members of the community to recognize the benefits of a healthy diet and greater level of physical activity. The food choices, attitudes and levels of activity adopted by parents will tend to be copied by their children. Parents undoubtedly shape the food choices of young children and even their ability to regulate their own intake and appetite (Birch and Davison, 2001; Cooke *et al.*, 2004). Campaigns to promote awareness of key issues are essential, and the constant coverage of the obesity epidemic and its causes through the printed and broadcast media should play a positive role.

Aside from parents and siblings, schools are the most important influence upon the health behaviours and knowledge of children. Schools are therefore seen as an ideal environment to set obesity prevention strategies and interventions. Schools can change behaviour in a number of different ways:

- Inclusion of healthy eating messages in the curriculum.
- Promotion of healthy living to both children and their parents.
- Inclusion of physical activity sessions across the whole curriculum on all days of the school week.
- Provision of open spaces and active play equipment.
- Limiting access to energy-dense snack foods through appropriate policies and removal of vending machines.
- Provision of healthy school meals.

There have been many published reports of school-based interventions, which have yielded rather patchy results. These reports generally show that interventions can be effective in promoting physical activity and/or dietary choices, but often without long-term effects, or observable impact upon risk of overweight. The 'SMART' lunch box intervention in the UK (Evans *et al.*, 2010) showed that materials targeting eight- to nine-year-olds and their parents could improve the quality of packed lunches taken into school, with greater adherence to government standards on school meals. Ribeiro and Alves (2014) showed the efficacy of two school-based

programmes in increasing physical activity, reducing sedentary time, improving intakes of fruits and vegetables and reducing fat consumption. The 'Eat Well and Keep Moving' intervention in the United States (Gortmaker *et al.*, 1999) was based on taught sessions from teachers in all curriculum areas. It achieved improvements in physical activity and dietary quality over a period of two years. Kipping *et al.* (2008, 2010) showed that the same programme could be imported into the UK, again with improvements in activity and intakes of fruits and vegetables over unhealthy snacks. None of these studies, however, reported any benefits in terms of obesity.

More recent interventions which have recognized that school-based interventions cannot succeed without parental engagement have also proven to be ineffectual in addressing the problem of overweight. The 'Healthy Lifestyles Programme' (HELP) operated in southwest England targeting 9–10-year-olds with one year of physical activity workshops, education sessions and behaviour-change goal setting with children and their parents. Two years from the start of HELP there was no effect on BMI of the children (Lloyd *et al.*, 2018). The 'West Midlands Active Lifestyle and Healthy Eating in School Children' (WAVES) study targeted five- to six-year-olds. A 12-month multi-arm trial of additional (30 minutes) physical activity, healthy lifestyle lessons, healthy eating and cooking sessions for children and parents and information about physical activity opportunities sent to parents, had no significant impact on BMI at 3 or 18 months after the intervention finished (Adab *et al.*, 2018). The systematic review of Calvert *et al.*, (2019) suggested that school-based interventions could be successful in promoting changes to dietary behaviours of children. The most effective interventions used increases in availability of healthy foods in schools, television and radio media to promote healthy lifestyles and active involvement of peers. However, efficacy in increasing physical activity is poor. Love *et al.* (2019) performed a meta-analysis of 25 trials which used robust accelerometer methods to monitor outcomes of school-based interventions that aimed to increase children's physical activity. There was no evidence that schools could significantly increase activity in children and adolescents.

The food industry, supermarkets and all elements of the food distribution network have a powerful influence upon the eating habits of the population and must therefore play a critical role in any obesity prevention strategy. To achieve societal change, the industry needs to be persuaded or forced by government to make changes to the formulation, pricing, availability and marketing of energy-dense, high-fat and high-sugar foodstuffs to discourage their consumption (Dehghan *et al.*, 2005; James, 2008b). Increasingly, national governments are implementing policies that attempt to force such behaviours from manufacturers and retailers. In 2014, the Mexican government introduced a tax of 1 peso per litre (equivalent to £0.04 per litre) on all non-alcoholic beverages containing added sugar. The UK followed suit in 2018 with a two-tier tariff called the Soft Drinks Industry Levy (SDIL), which imposed a tax of £0.24 per litre on drinks containing more than 8g per 100 ml sugar and £0.18 per litre on drinks with a sugar content of 5–8g per 100ml. Pure fruit juices and drinks with a high milk or calcium content were excluded from the SDIL. Sugar and soda taxes have also been implemented in France, Portugal and Ireland.

Sugar taxes undoubtedly have some impact on the purchase of sugar-sweetened beverages, although the impact is extremely limited when considered at the whole population level. Pedraza *et al.* (2019) reported that three years after the introduction of the Mexican tax, the energy consumption associated with sugar-sweetened beverages had reduced from 74 kcal per capita per day to 66 kcal per capita per day. In the UK, the implementation of the SDIL was accompanied by an increase in costs to consumers and some reformulation by manufacturers (Scarborough *et al.*, 2020). Between 2015 and 2018, the amount of sugar consumed in beverages fell from 15.5 g per capita per day to 10.8 g per capita per day (Bandy *et al.*, 2020), with the majority of that decrease preceding the introduction of SDIL and more reflecting the highly visible public health campaigns targeting reduction of sugar intake, particularly aimed at children. Public Health England (2019) found that while sugar intake from beverages may have declined in the UK following introduction of SDIL, intakes from some sources (puddings, cakes, ice cream) had increased slightly.

While taxation can clearly be shown to reduce sales of sugar-sweetened beverages and can therefore contribute to a healthier food environment for children, their capacity to influence overweight and obesity at the population level will be limited. Given that obesity has a complex, multifactorial basis (gene–environment interactions), a focus on a single component of the diet (sugar) is unlikely to have a major effect. The levels of taxation are quite low and the costs largely absorbed by manufacturers and retailers, so they do not have a major effect on consumers' shopping behaviours. To be truly effective, the taxes incurred need to be greater, but this risks having an undue impact on families of lower socioeconomic status.

Governments at national and local levels can have a major impact upon the fight against childhood obesity through the influence that they have upon all of the other agencies and individuals described earlier. Introducing policies, taxes or incentives that can influence food purchasing and consumer choices is one tool that could be applied. Similarly, governments can shape education policy and the priorities within school curricula. Changes to the built environment to encourage more leisure facilities, safe open spaces and the introduction of walking and cycling networks can help to promote physical activity.

SUMMARY

- Compared with adults, the energy and nutrient requirements of children are high. Increased demands are a product of growth and maturation. A nutrient- and energy-dense diet is essential to meet these demands as the small size of children means that they are unable to process a bulky diet.
- Children are vulnerable to micronutrient deficiencies and protein–energy malnutrition. Growth faltering is a common sign of these problems. Poverty, infectious disease or restrictive dietary practices are the major factors that drive undernutrition.
- Weaning is the introduction of complementary foods to the infant diet. The overall transition from a milk-based diet to a diet comprising an adult pattern of eating is an opportunity to teach children to follow a healthy lifestyle and comply with guidelines for healthy eating. The range of preferred foods that is actually consumed by children is rather narrow but strongly influenced by parental choices.
- Dental caries are a significant health issue in children and can be prevented through reducing intake of sugar and fluoridation of water.
- Schools provide suitable environments for the promotion of health in children. This can be achieved through placing health and nutrition in a prominent position in the curriculum, by encouraging daily physical activity and through introduction of high-quality school meals, breakfast clubs and other food-based initiatives.
- The prevalence of overweight and obesity in children has more than doubled in the first decade of the twenty-first century. This increase is primarily driven by increased consumption of energy-dense foodstuffs and declining energy expenditure associated with sedentary leisure activities.
- Successful strategies for the prevention of childhood obesity at the population level are dependent upon integrated activities of all stakeholders, including parents and children, schools, the food industry and local and national governments.

References

Adab, P., Barrett, T., Bhopal, R. *et al.* (2018). The West Midlands Active Lifestyle and Healthy Eating in School Children (WAVES) study: a cluster randomized controlled trial testing the clinical effectiveness and cost-effectiveness of a multifaceted obesity prevention intervention programme targeted at children aged 6–7 years. *Health Technology Assessment* **22**: 1–608.

Adair, L.S., Gordon-Larsen, P., Du, S.F. *et al.* (2014). The emergence of cardiometabolic disease risk in Chinese children and adults: consequences of changes in diet, physical activity and obesity. *Obestiy Reviews* **15**(Suppl 1): 49–59.

Ambroszkiewicz, J., Chełchowska, M., Szamotulska, K. *et al.* (2019). Bone status and adipokine levels in children on vegetarian and omnivorous diets. *Clinical Nutrition* **38**: 730–737.

Anderson, P.M., Butcher, K.F. and Schanzenbach, D.W. (2019). Understanding recent trends in childhood obesity in the United States. *Economics and Human Biology* **34**: 16–25.

Bailey, R.L., Catellier, D.J., Jun, S. *et al.* (2018). Total usual nutrient intakes of us children (under 48 months): findings from the Feeding Infants and Toddlers Study (FITS) 2016. *Journal of Nutrition* **148**: 1557S–1566S.

Bandy, L.K., Scarborough, P., Harrington, R.A. *et al.* (2020). Reductions in sugar sales from soft drinks in the UK from 2015 to 2018. *BMC Medicine* **18**: 20.

Barrera, C.M., Hamner, H.C., Perrine, C.G. and Scanlon, K.S. (2018). Timing of introduction of complementary foods to US infants, national health and nutrition examination survey 2009–2014. *Journal of the Academy of Nutrition and Dietetics* **118**: 464–470.

Bates, B., Lennox, A., Prentice, A. *et al.* (2014). *National Diet and Nutrition Survey: Results from Years 1–4 (combined) of the Rolling Programme (2008/2009 – 2011/12)*. London: Public Health England.

Bates, B., Lennox, A., Prentice, A. *et al.* (2011). *National Diet and Nutrition Survey Headline Results from Years 1, 2 and 3 (Combined) of the Rolling Programme (2008/2009–2010/11)*. London: Public Health England.

Bernabé, E., Ballantyne, H., Longbottom, C. and Pitts, N.B. (2020). Early introduction of sugar-sweetened beverages and caries trajectories from age 12 to 48 months. *Journal of Dental Research* **99**: 898–906.

Birch, L.L. and Davison, K.K. (2001). Family environmental factors influencing the developing behavioral controls of food intake and childhood overweight. *Pediatric Clinics of North America*, **48**: 893–907.

Black, M.M. (2003). The evidence linking zinc deficiency with children's cognitive and motor functioning. *Journal of Nutrition*, **133**: 1473S–1476S.

Borzekowski, D.L. and Robinson, T.N. (2001). The 30-second effect: an experiment revealing the impact of television commercials on food preferences of preschoolers. *Journal of the American Dietetic Association*, **101**: 42–46.

Boyland, E., Thivel, D., Mazur, A. *et al.* (2020). Digital food marketing to young people: a substantial public health challenge. *Annals of Nutrition and Metabolism* **76**: 6–9.

Boyland, E.J., Harrold, J.A., Kirkham, T.C. *et al.* (2011). Food commercials increase preference for energy-dense foods, particularly in children who watch more television. *Pediatrics* **128**: e93–100.

Branca, F., Nikogosian, H. and Lobstein, T. (eds). (2007). *The Challenge of Obesity in the WHO European Region and the Strategies for Response.* Copenhagen: World Health Organization.

Briefel, R., Hanson, C., Fox, M.K. *et al.* (2006). Feeding infants and toddlers study: do vitamin and mineral supplements contribute to nutrient adequacy or excess among US infants and toddlers? *Journal of the American Dietetic Association* **106**: S52–S65.

Brindal, E., Baird, D., Danthiir, V. *et al.* (2012). Ingesting breakfast meals of different glycaemic load does not alter cognition and satiety in children. *European Journal of Clinical Nutrition* **66**: 1166–1171.

Brophy, S., Cooksey, R., Gravenor, M.B. *et al.* (2009). Risk factors for childhood obesity at age 5: analysis of the millennium cohort study. *BMC Public Health* **9**: 467.

Brown, A. (2018). No difference in self-reported frequency of choking between infants introduced to solid foods using a baby-led weaning or traditional spoon-feeding approach. *Journal of Human Nutrition and Dietetics* **31**: 496–504.

Brown, A. and Lee, M. (2011). A descriptive study investigating the use and nature of baby-led weaning in a UK sample of mothers. *Maternal and Child Nutrition* **7**: 34–47.

Brown, C.L., Perrin, E.M., Peterson, K.E. *et al.* (2018). Association of picky eating with weight status and dietary quality among low-income preschoolers. *Academy of Pediatrics* **18**: 334–341.

Bundred, P., Kitchiner, D. and Buchan, I. (2001). Prevalence of overweight and obese children between 1989 and 1998: population based series of cross sectional studies. *BMJ* **322**: 326–328.

Burgess, J.A., Dharmage, S.C., Allen, K. *et al.* (2019). Age at introduction to complementary solid food and food allergy and sensitization: a systematic review and meta-analysis. *Clinical and Experimental Allergy* **49**: 754–769.

Butland, B., Jebb, S., Kopelman, P. *et al.* (2007). *Tackling Obesities: Future Choices – Project Report.* 2nd ed. London: Government Office for Statistics.

Butte, N.F. (2005). Energy requirements of infants and children. *Nestle Nutrition Workshop Series: Pediatric Programme* **58**: 19–32.

Calvert, S., Dempsey, R.C. and Povey, R. (2019). Delivering in-school interventions to improve dietary behaviours amongst 11- to 16-year-olds: a systematic review. *Obesity Reviews* **20**: 543–553.

Cameron, S.L., Taylor, R.W. and Heath, A.L. (2013). Parent-led or baby-led? Associations between complementary feeding practices and health-related behaviours in a survey of New Zealand families. *BMJ Open* **3**; e003946.

Candler, T.P., Mahmoud, O., Lynn, R.M. *et al.* (2018). Continuing rise of Type 2 diabetes incidence in children and young people in the UK. *Diabetic Medicine* **35**: 737–744.

Carnell, S., Edwards, C., Croker, H. *et al.* (2005). Parental perceptions of overweight in 3–5 y olds. *International Journal of Obesity* **29**: 353–355.

Caroli, M. and Burniat, W. (2002). Dietary management. In: *Child and Adolescent Obesity. Causes, Consequences and Management* (ed. W. Burniat, T. Cole, I. Lissau and E. Poskitt), 282–306. Cambridge: Cambridge University Press.

Carson, V., Hunter, S., Kuzik, N. *et al.* (2016). Systematic review of sedentary behaviour and health indicators in school-aged children and youth: an update. *Applied Physiology, Nutrition and Metabolism* **41**: S240–265.

Cheong, K., Yoon Ling, C., Kuang Hock, L. *et al.* (2019). Association between availability of neighborhood fast food outlets and overweight among 5–18 year-old children in peninsular Malaysia: a cross-sectional study. *International Journal of Environmental Research and Public Health* **16**: 593.

Child Poverty Action Group (2020). Child poverty facts and figures. https://cpag.org.uk/child-poverty/child-poverty-facts-and-figures (accessed 7 April 2021).

Chinn, S. and Rona, R.J. (2001). Prevalence and trends in overweight and obesity in three cross sectional studies of British children, 1974–94. *BMJ* **322**: 24–26.

Cofnas, N. (2019). Is vegetarianism healthy for children? *Critical Reviews of Food Science and Nutrition* **59**: 2052–2060

Cole, N.C., Musaad, S.M., Lee, S.Y., Donovan, S.M. (2018). Home feeding environment and picky eating behavior in preschool-aged children: A prospective analysis. *Eating Behaviour* **30**: 76–82.

Cole, T.J., Freeman, J.V. and Preece, M.A. (1995). Body mass index reference curves for the UK, 1990. *Archives of Disease in Childhood* **73**: 25–29.

Congdon, E.L., Westerlund, A., Algarin, C.R. *et al.* (2012). Iron deficiency in infancy is associated with altered neural correlates of recognition memory at 10 years. *Journal of Pediatrics* **160**: 1027–1033.

Connor, S.M. (2006). Food-related advertising on pre-school television: building brand recognition in young viewers. *Pediatrics* **118**: 1478–1485.

Cooke, L.J., Wardle, J., Gibson, E.L. *et al.* (2004). Demographic, familial and trait predictors of fruit and vegetable consumption by pre-school children. *Public Health Nutrition* **7**: 295–302.

Cowin, I. and Emmett, P. (2007). ALSPAC Study Team. Diet in a group of 18-month-old children in South West England, and comparison with the results of a national survey. *Journal of Human Nutrition and Dietetics* **20**: 254–267.

Craig, S., Goldberg, J. and Dietz, W.H. (1996). Psychosocial correlates of physical activity among fifth and eighth graders. *Preventive Medicine* **25**: 506–513.

Daniels, S.R., Arnett, D.K., Eckel, R.H. *et al.* (2005). Overweight in children and adolescents: pathophysiology, consequences, prevention, and treatment. *Circulation* **111**: 1999–2012.

Dehghan, M., Akhtar-Danesh, N. and Merchant, A.T. (2005). Childhood obesity, prevalence and prevention. *Nutrition Journal* **2**: 4–24.

Del-Ponte, B., Anselmi, L., Assunção, M.C.F. *et al.* (2019a). Sugar consumption and attention-deficit/hyperactivity disorder (ADHD): a birth cohort study. *Journal of Affective Disorders* **243**: 290–296.

Del-Ponte, B., Quinte, G.C., Cruz, S. *et al.* (2019b). Dietary patterns and attention deficit/hyperactivity disorder (ADHD): A systematic review and meta-analysis. *Journal of Affective Disorders* **252**: 160–173.

Department for Education. (2015). Standards for school food in England. https://www.gov.uk/government/publications/standards-for-school-food-in-england (accessed 7 April 2021).

Department of Health. (1998). *Dietary Reference Values for Energy and Nutrients for the United Kingdom*. London: Stationery Office.

Deshmukh-Taskar, P.R., Nicklas, T.A., O'Neil, C.E. *et al.* (2010). The relationship of breakfast skipping and type of breakfast consumption with nutrient intake and weight status in children and adolescents: the National Health and Nutrition Examination Survey 1999–2006. *Journal of the American Dietetic Association*, **110**: 869–878.

Deshmukh-Taskar, P., Nicklas, T.A., Morales, M. *et al.* (2006). Tracking of overweight status from childhood to young adulthood: the Bogalusa Heart Study. *European Journal of Clinical Nutrition* **60**: 48–57.

Dhar, T. and Baylis, K. (2011). Fast-food consumption and the ban on advertising targeting children: the Quebec experience. *Journal of Marketing Research* **48**: 799–813.

Djennane, M., Lebbah, S., Roux, C. *et al.* (2014). Vitamin D status of schoolchildren in Northern Algeria, seasonal variations and determinants of vitamin D deficiency. *Osteoporosis International* **25**: 1493–1502.

Dovey, T.M., Staples, P.A., Gibson, E.L. *et al.* (2008). Food neophobia and 'picky/fussy' eating in children: a review. *Appetite* **50**: 181–193.

Dubois, L., Farmer, A., Girard, M. *et al.* (2008). Social factors and television use during meals and snacks is associated with higher BMI among pre-school children. *Public Health Nutrition* 12: 1–13.

Dyson, A., Pizzutto, S.J., MacLennan, C. *et al.* (2014). The prevalence of vitamin D deficiency in children in the Northern Territory. *Journal of Paediatrics and Child Health* **50**: 47–50.

East, P., Delker, E., Blanco, E. *et al.* (2019). Effect of infant iron deficiency on children's verbal abilities: the roles of child affect and parent unresponsiveness. *Maternal and Child Health Journal* **23**: 1240–1250.

Eaton, S.B., Konner, M. and Shostak, M. (1988). Stone agers in the fast lane: chronic degenerative diseases in evolutionary perspective. *American Journal of Medicine* **84**: 739–749.

Ells, L.J., Hillier, F.C., Shucksmith, J. *et al.* (2008). A systematic review of the effect of dietary exposure that could be achieved through normal dietary intake on learning and performance of school-aged children of relevance to UK schools. *British Journal of Nutrition* **100**: 927–936.

Emond, J.A., Longacre, M.R., Titus, L.J. *et al.* (2020). Fast food intake and excess weight gain over a 1-year period among preschool-age children. *Pediatric Obesity* **15**: e12602.

Emond, J.A., Longacre, M.R., Drake, K.M. *et al.* (2019). Influence of child-targeted fast food TV advertising exposure on fast food intake: a longitudinal study of pre-school-age children. *Appetite* **140**: 134–141.

Epstein, L.H., Paluch, R.A., Beecher, M.D. *et al.* (2008). Increasing healthy eating compared with reducing high energy-dense foods to treat pediatric obesity. *Obesity* **16**: 318–326.

Eurostat. (2020) Children at risk of poverty or social exclusion. https://ec.europa.eu/eurostat/web/products-datasets/-/tespm040 (accessed 7 April 2021).

Evans, C.E., Greenwood, D.C., Thomas, J.D. *et al.* (2010). SMART lunch box intervention to improve the food and nutrient content of children's packed lunches: UK wide cluster randomised controlled trial. *Journal of Epidemiology and Community Health* **64**: 970–976.

Fagerberg, P., Langlet, B., Oravsky, A. *et al.* (2019). Ultra-processed food advertisements dominate the food advertising landscape in two Stockholm areas with low vs high socio-economic status. Is it time for regulatory action? *BMC Public Health* **19**: 1717.

Fangupo, L.J., Heath, A.M., Williams, S.M. *et al.* (2016). A baby-led approach to eating solids and risk of choking. *Pediatrics* **138**: e20160772.

Farooqi, I.S., Wangensteen, T., Collins, S. *et al.* (2007). Clinical and molecular genetic spectrum of congenital deficiency of the leptin receptor. *New England Journal of Medicine* **356**: 237–247.

Fernandez, C., McCaffery, H., Miller, A.L. *et al.* (2020). Trajectories of picky eating in low-income US children. *Pediatrics* **145**: e20192018.

Fewtrell, M.S. (2011). The evidence for public health recommendations on infant feeding. *Early Human Development* **87**: 715–721.

Fischer Walker, C.L., Ezzati, M., Black, R.E. (2009). Global and regional child mortality and burden of disease attributable to zinc deficiency. *European Journal of Clinical Nutrition* **63**: 591–597.

Food Foundation (2018). Millions of UK children are impacted by food poverty. https://foodfoundation.org.uk/millions-of-uk-children-are-impacted-by-food-poverty (accessed 7 April 2021).

Fox, M.K, Gearan, E., Cannon, J. *et al.* (2016). Usual food intakes of 2- and 3-year old U.S. children are not consistent with dietary guidelines. *BMC Nutrition* **2**: 67.

Freedman, D.S., Khan, L.K., Dietz, W.H. *et al.* (2001). Relationship of childhood obesity to coronary heart disease risk factors in adulthood: the Bogalusa Heart Study. *Pediatrics* **108**: 712–718.

Freeman, J.V., Cole, T.J., Chinn, S. *et al.* (1995). Cross sectional stature and weight reference curves for the UK, 1990. *Archives of Disease in Childhood* **73**: 17–24.

Furness, J., Oddie, S.J., Hearnshaw, S. (2020). Water fluoridation: current challenges. *Archives of Disease in Childhood* doi: 10.1136/archdischild-2019-318545.

Gahche, J.J., Herrick, K.A., Potischman, N., Bailey, R.L., Ahluwalia, N., Dwyer, J.T. (2019). Dietary supplement use among infants and toddlers aged <24 months in the United States, NHANES 2007–2014. *Journal of Nutrition* **149**: 314–322.

Garlick, P.J. (2006). Protein requirements of infants and children. *Nestle Nutrition Workshop Series: Pediatric Programme* **58**: 39–47.

Gibson, R.S., Heath, A.L., Szymlek-Gay, E.A. (2014). Is iron and zinc nutrition a concern for vegetarian infants and young children in industrialized countries? *American Journal of Clinical Nutrition* **100**(Suppl 1): 459S–68S.

Golan, M., Weizman, A., Apter, A. *et al.* (1998). Parents as the exclusive agents of change in the treatment of childhood obesity. *American Journal of Clinical Nutrition* **67**: 1130–1135.

Goldstone, A.P. (2004). Prader–Willi syndrome: advances in genetics, pathophysiology and treatment. *Trends in Endocrinology and Metabolism* **15**: 12–20.

Gomez, M.S., Novaes, A.P.T., Silva, J.P.D. *et al.* (2020). Baby-led weaning, an overview of the new approach to food introduction: integrative literature review. *Revista Paulista de Pediatria* **38**: e2018084.

Gorczyca, D., Paściak, M., Szponar, B. *et al.* (2011). An impact of the diet on serum fatty acid and lipid profiles in Polish vegetarian children and children with allergy. *European Journal of Clinical Nutrition* **65**: 191–195.

Gorczyca, D., Prescha, A., Szeremeta, K. and Jankowski, A. (2013). Iron status and dietary iron intake of vegetarian children from Poland. *Annals of Nutrition and Metabolism* **62**: 291–297.

Goris, J.M., Petersen, S., Stamatakis, E. *et al.* (2010). Television food advertising and the prevalence of childhood overweight and obesity: a multicountry comparison. *Public Health Nutrition* **13**: 1003–1012.

Gortmaker, S.L., Cheung, L.W., Peterson, K.E. *et al.* (1999). Impact of a school-based interdisciplinary intervention on diet and physical activity among urban primary school children: eat well and keep moving. *Archives of Pediatrics and Adolescent Medicine* **153**: 975–983.

Grace, C.M. (2001). Dietary management of obesity. In: *Management of Obesity and Related Disorders* (ed. P.G. Kopelman), 129–164. London: Martin Dunitz.

Griffith, R., von Hinke, S., Smith, S. (2018). Getting a healthy start: the effectiveness of targeted benefits for improving dietary choices. *Journal of Health Economics* **58**: 176–187.

Griffiths, C., Gately, P., Marchant, P.R. *et al.* (2013). A five year longitudinal study investigating the prevalence of childhood obesity: comparison of BMI and waist circumference. *Public Health* **127**: 1090–1096.

Guillaume, M., Lapidus, L. and Lambert, A. (1998). Obesity and nutrition in children: the Belgian Luxembourg Child Study IV. *European Journal of Clinical Nutrition* **52**: 323–328.

Gupta, P., Shah, D., Kumar, P. *et al.* (2019). Indian Academy of Pediatrics Guidelines on the Fast and Junk Foods, Sugar Sweetened Beverages, Fruit Juices, and Energy Drinks. *Indian Pediatrics* **56**: 849–863.

Gupta, S., Brazier, A.K.M. and Lowe, N.M. (2020). Zinc deficiency in low- and middle-income countries: prevalence and approaches for mitigation. *Journal of Human Nutrition and Dietetics* **33**: 624–643.

Gwamaka, M., Kurtis, J.D., Sorensen, B.E. *et al.* (2012). Iron deficiency protects against severe Plasmodium falciparum malaria and death in young children. *Clinical Infectious Disease* **54**: 1137–1144.

Hackett, A., Nathan, I. and Burgess, L. (1998). Is a vegetarian diet adequate for children. *Nutrition and Health* **12**: 189–195.

Halford, J.C., Boyland, E.J., Hughes, G. *et al.* (2007). Beyond-brand effect of television (TV) food advertisements/commercials on caloric intake and food choice of 5–7-year-old children. *Appetite* **49**: 263–267.

Hamano, T., Li, X., Sundquist, J. and Sundquist, K. (2017). Association between childhood obesity and neighbourhood accessibility to fast-food outlets: a nationwide 6-year follow-up study of 944,487 children. *Obesity Facts* **10**: 559–568.

Hamel, M.J., Otieno, P., Bayoh, N. *et al.*, (2011). The combination of indoor residual spraying and insecticide-treated nets provides added protection against malaria compared with insecticide-treated nets alone. *American Journal of Tropical Medicine and Hygiene* **85**: 1080–1086.

Hamlyn, B., Brooker, S., Oleinikova, K. *et al.* (2002). *Infant Feeding 2000*. London: Stationery Office.

Hardcastle, S.J. and Blake, N. (2016). Influences underlying family food choices in mothers from an economically disadvantaged community. *Eating Behaviours* 20: 1–8.

Health and Social Care Information Centre. (2012). *National Statistics Infant Feeding Survey – UK, 2010*. Leeds: Health and Social Care Information Centre.

Hearst, M.O., Jimbo-Llapa, F., Grannon, K. *et al.* (2019). Breakfast is brain food? The effect on grade point average of a rural group randomized program to promote school breakfast. *Journal of School Health* **89**: 715–721.

Hediger, M.L., Overpeck, M.D., Kuczmarski, R.J. *et al.* (2001). Association between infant breastfeeding and overweight in young children. *JAMA* **285**: 2453–2460.

Herrick, K.A., Storandt, R.J., Afful, J. *et al.* (2019). Vitamin D status in the United States, 2011–2014. *American Journal of Clinical Nutrition* **110**: 150–157.

Hill, J.O. and Peters, J.C. (1998). Environmental contributions to the obesity epidemic. *Science* **280**: 1371–1374.

Hobbs, M., Wade, A., Jones, P. *et al.* (2020). Area-level deprivation, childhood dental ambulatory sensitive hospitalizations and community water fluoridation: evidence from New Zealand. *International Journal of Epidemiology* **49**: 908–916.

Hovdenak, I.M., Stea, T.H., Magnus, P. *et al.* (2019). How to evaluate the effect of seven years of the Norwegian School Fruit Scheme (2007–2014) on fruit, vegetable and snack consumption and weight status: a natural experiment. *Scandinavian Journal of Public Health* 1403494819875923. doi: 10.1177/1403494819875923.

Howard Wilsher, S., Harrison, F., Yamoah, F. *et al.* (2016). The relationship between unhealthy food sales, socioeconomic deprivation and childhood weight status: results of a cross-sectional study in England. *International Journal of Behaviour, Nutrition and Physical Activity* **13**: 21.

Hughes, R.J., Edwards, K.L., Clarke, G.P. *et al.* (2012). Childhood consumption of fruit and vegetables across England: a study of 2306 6–7-year-olds in 2007. *British Journal of Nutrition* **108**: 733–742.

Huybrechts, I., Maes, L., Vereecken, C. *et al.* (2010). High dietary supplement intakes among Flemish preschoolers. *Appetite* **54**: 340–345.

Independent Food Aid Network. (2020). Mapping the UK's independent food banks. https://www.foodaidnetwork. org.uk/independent-food-banks-map (accessed 6 April 2021).

James, W.P. (2008a). The fundamental drivers of the obesity epidemic. *Obesity Reviews* **9**: 6–13.

James, W.P. (2008b). The epidemiology of obesity: the size of the problem. *Journal of Internal Medicine* **263**: 336–352.

Jenkins, K.T., Benton, D., Tapper, K. *et al.* (2015). A cross-sectional observational study of the nutritional intake of UK primary school children from deprived and non-deprived backgrounds: implications for school breakfast schemes. *International Journal of Behaviour, Nutrition and Physical Activity* **12**: 86.

Johannsson, E., Arngrimsson, S.A., Thorsdottir, I. *et al.* (2006). Tracking of overweight from early childhood to adolescence in cohorts born 1988 and 1994: overweight in a high birth weight population. *International Journal of Obesity* **30**: 1265–1271.

Johnson, L., Mander, A.P., Jones, L.R. *et al.* (2008). Energydense, low-fiber, high-fat dietary pattern is associated with increased fatness in childhood. *American Journal of Clinical Nutrition* **87**: 846–854.

Juonala, M., Raitakari, M.S.A., Viikari, J. *et al.* (2005). Obesity in youth is not an independent predictor of carotid IMT in adulthood: the cardiovascular risk in Young Finns Study. *Atherosclerosis* **185**: 388–393.

Keller, K.L., Kuilema, L.G., Lee, N. *et al.* (2012). The impact of food branding on children's eating behavior and obesity. *Physiology and Behaviour* **106**: 379–386.

Kemp, A. (2008) Food additives and hyperactivity. *BMJ* **336**: 1144.

Kennedy, E. and Davis, C. (1998). US department of agriculture school breakfast program. *American Journal of Clinical Nutrition* **67**: 798S–803S.

Kenney, E.L., Barrett, J.L., Bleich, S.N. *et al.* (2020). Impact of the healthy, hunger-free kids act on obesity trends. *Health Affairs* **39**: 1122–1129.

Kim, H.N., Kong, W.S., Lee, J.H. and Kim, J.B. (2019). Reduction of dental caries among children and adolescents from a 15-year community water fluoridation program in a township area, Korea. *International Journal of Environment Research and Public Health* **16**: 1306.

Kinderknecht, K., Harris, C. and Jones-Smith, J. (2020). Association of the healthy, hunger-free kids act with dietary quality among children in the US National School Lunch Program. *Journal of the American Medical Association* **324**: 359–368.

Kipping, R.R., Payne, C. and Lawlor, D.A. (2008). Randomised controlled trial adapting US school obesity prevention to England. *Archives of Disease in Childhood*, **93**, : 469–473.

Kipping, R.R., Jago, R. and Lawlor, D.A. (2010). Diet outcomes of a pilot school-based randomised controlled obesity prevention study with 9--10 year olds in England. *Preventive Medicine*, **51**, : 56–62.

Küpers, L.K., de Pijper, J.J., Sauer, P.J. *et al.* (2014). Skipping breakfast and overweight in 2- and 5-year-old Dutch children-the GECKO Drenthe cohort. *International Journal of Obesity* **38**: 569–571.

Laskowska-Klita, T., Chełchowska, M., Ambroszkiewicz, J. *et al.* (2011). The effect of vegetarian diet on selected essential nutrients in children. *Medycyna Wieku Rozwojowego* **15**: 318–325.

Leaf, A.A. (2007). RCPCH Standing Committee on Nutrition. Vitamins for babies and young children. *Archives of Disease in Childhood* **92**: 160–164.

León-Flández, K., Rico-Gómez, A., Moya-Geromin, M.Á. *et al.* (2017). Evaluation of compliance with the Spanish Code of self-regulation of food and drinks advertising directed at children under the age of 12 years in Spain, 2012. *Public Health* **150**: 121–129.

Lim, S., Zoellner, J.M., Lee, J.M. *et al.* (2009). Obesity and sugar-sweetened beverages in African-American preschool children: a longitudinal study. *Obesity* **17**: 1262–1268.

Liu, J., Hwang, W.T., Dickerman, B. *et al.* (2013). Regular breakfast consumption is associated with increased IQ in kindergarten children. *Early Human Development* **89**: 257–262.

Liu, D., Zhao, L.Y., Yu, D.M. *et al.* (2018). Dietary patterns and association with obesity of children aged 6–17 years in medium and small cities in China: findings from the CNHS 2010–2012. *Nutrients* **11**: 3.

Lloyd, J., Creanor, S., Logan, S. *et al.* (2018). Effectiveness of the Healthy Lifestyles Programme (HeLP) to prevent obesity in UK primary-school children: a cluster randomised controlled trial. *Lancet Child and Adolescent Health* **2**, : 35–45.

Lloyd, L.J., Langley-Evans, S.C. and McMullen, S. (2010). Childhood obesity and adult cardiovascular disease risk: a systematic review. *International Journal of Obesity* **34**: 18–28.

Lloyd, L.J., Langley-Evans, S.C. and McMullen, S. (2012). Childhood obesity and risk of the adult metabolic syndrome: a systematic review. *International Journal of Obesity* 36: 1–11.

Lok, K.Y., Chan, R.S., Lee, V.W. *et al.* (2013). Food additives and behavior in 8- to 9-year-old children in Hong Kong: a randomized, double-blind, placebo-controlled trial. *Journal of Developmental and Behavioral Pediatrics* 34: 642–650.

Loos, R.J. and Bouchard, C. (2008). FTO: the first gene contributing to common forms of human obesity. *Obesity Reviews* 9: 246–250.

Loos, R.J., Lindgren, C.M., Li, S. *et al.* (2008). Common variants near MC4R are associated with fat mass, weight and risk of obesity. *Nature Genetics* 40: 768–775.

Love, R., Adams, J., van Sluijs, E.M.F. (2019). Are school-based physical activity interventions effective and equitable? A meta-analysis of cluster randomized controlled trials with accelerometer-assessed activity. *Obesity Reviews* 20: 859–870.

Lozoff, B., Beard, J., Connor, J. *et al.* (2006). Long-lasting neural and behavioral effects of iron deficiency in infancy. *Nutrition Reviews* 64: S34–S43.

Lozoff, B., Smith, J.B., Kaciroti, N. *et al.* (2013). Functional significance of early-life iron deficiency: outcomes at 25 years. *Journal of Pediatrics* 163: 1260–1266.

Ludwig, D.S., Peterson, K.E. and Gortmaker, S.L. (2001). Relation between consumption of sugar-sweetened drinks and childhood obesity: a prospective, observational analysis. *Lancet* 357: 505–508.

Lutter, C.K. and Dewey, K.G. (2003). Proposed nutrient composition for fortified complementary foods. *Journal of Nutrition* 133: 3011S–3020S.

Lutter, C.K. and Rivera, J.A. (2003). Nutritional status of infants and young children and characteristics of their diets. *Journal of Nutrition* 133: 2941S–2949S.

Maffeis, C., Talamini, G. and Tatò, L. (1998). Influence of diet, physical activity and parents' obesity on children's adiposity: a four-year longitudinal study. *International Journal of Obesity* 22: 758–764.

Magarey, A.M., Daniels, L.A., Boulton, T.J. *et al.* (2001). Does fat intake predict adiposity in healthy children and adolescents aged 2–15 y? A longitudinal analysis. *European Journal of Clinical Nutrition* 55: 471–481.

Mangels, A.R. and Messina, V. (2001). Considerations in planning vegan diets: infants. *Journal of the American Dietetic Association* 101: 670–677.

Martin-Calvo, N., Martínez-González, M.A., Bes-Rastrollo, M. *et al.* (2015). Sugar-sweetened carbonated beverage consumption and childhood/adolescent obesity: a case-control study. *Public Health Nutrition* 17: 2185–2193.

Masood, M., Mnatzaganian, G., Baker, S.R. (2019). Inequalities in dental caries in children within the UK: Have there been changes over time? *Community Dentistry and Oral Epidemiology* 47: 71–77.

Matangila, J.R., Mitashi, P., Inocêncio da Luz, R.A. *et al.* (2015). Efficacy and safety of intermittent preventive treatment for malaria in schoolchildren: a systematic review. *Malaria Journal* 14: 450.

Mayer-Davis, E.J., Dabelea, D. and Lawrence, J.M. (2017). Incidence trends of type 1 and type 2 diabetes among youths, 2002–2012. *New England Journal of Medicine* 377: 301.

Mazzoleni, S., Magni, G. and Toderini, D. (2019). Effect of vitamin D3 seasonal supplementation with 1500 IU/day in north Italian children (DINOS study). *Italian Journal of Pediatrics* 45: 18.

Mbogori, T., Kimmel, K., Zhang, M. *et al.* (2020). Nutrition transition and double burden of malnutrition in Africa: A case study of four selected countries with different social economic development. *AIMS Public Health* 7: 425–439.

McCaffrey, T.A., Rennie, K.L., Kerr, M.A. *et al.* (2008). Energy density of the diet and change in body fatness from childhood to adolescence; is there a relation? *American Journal of Clinical Nutrition* 87: 1230–1237.

McCann, D., Barrett, A., Cooper, A. *et al.* (2007). Food additives and hyperactive behaviour in 3-year-old and 8/9-year-old children in the community: a randomised, double-blinded, placebo controlled trial. *Lancet*, **370**, : 1560–1567.

McLean, N., Griffin, S., Toney, K. *et al.* (2003). Family involvement in weight control, weight maintenance and weight-loss interventions: a systematic review of randomised trials. *International Journal of Obesity* 27: 987–1005.

McLennan, J.D. (2017). Changes over time in early complementary feeding of breastfed infants on the island of Hispaniola. *Pan American Journal of Public Health* 41: e39.

Methner, S., Maschkowski, G., Hartmann, M. (2017). The European School Fruit Scheme: impact on children's fruit and vegetable consumption in North Rhine-Westphalia, Germany. *Public Health Nutrition* 20: 542–548.

Menon, S., Peñalvo, J.L. (2019). Actions targeting the double burden of malnutrition: a scoping review. *Nutrients* 12: 81.

Moore, G.F., Tapper, K., Murphy, S. *et al.* (2007). Associations between deprivation, attitudes towards eating breakfast and breakfast eating behaviours in 9–11-year-olds. *Public Health Nutrition* 10: 582–589.

Moore, A.P., Milligan, P., Rivas, C. *et al.* (2012). Sources of weaning advice, comparisons between formal and informal advice, and associations with weaning timing in a survey of UK first-time mothers. *Public Health Nutrition* 15: 1661–1669.

Morison, B.J., Taylor, R.W., Haszard, J.J. *et al.* (2016). How different are baby-led weaning and conventional complementary feeding? A cross-sectional study of infants aged 6–8 months. *BMJ Open* 6: e010665.

Moya-Alvarez, V., Bodeau-Livinec, F. and Cot, M. (2016). Iron and malaria: a dangerous liaison? *Nutrition Reviews* 74: 612–623.

Mullan, B., Wong, C., Kothe, E. *et al.* (2014). An examination of the demographic predictors of adolescent breakfast consumption, content, and context. *BMC Public Health* 14: 264.

Muñoz, E.C., Rosado, J.L., López, P. *et al.* (2000). Iron and zinc supplementation improves indicators of vitamin A status of Mexican preschoolers. *American Journal of Clinical Nutrition* 71: 789–794.

Must, A. and Tybor, D.J. (2005). Physical activity and sedentary behavior: a review of longitudinal studies of weight and adiposity in youth. *International Journal of Obesity* 29: S84–S96.

Nathan, I., Hackett, A.F. and Kirby, S. (1997). A longitudinal study of the growth of matched pairs of vegetarian and omnivorous children, aged 7–11 years, in the north-west of England. *European Journal of Clinical Nutrition* 51: 20–25.

Neri, D., Martinez-Steele, E., Monteiro, C.A. and Levy, R.B. (2019). Consumption of ultra-processed foods and its association with added sugar content in the diets of US children, NHANES 2009–2014. *Pediatric Obesity* 14: e12563.

Neuberger, A., Okebe, J., Yahav, D. and Paul, M. (2016). Oral iron supplements for children in malaria-endemic areas. Cochrane Database of Systematic Reviews (2): CD006589.

Neville, L., Thomas, M. and Bauman, A. (2005). Food advertising on Australian television: the extent of children's exposure. *Health Promotion International* **20**: 105–112.

NHS England (2019). The Eatwell guide. https://www.nhs.uk/live-well/eat-well/the-eatwell-guide (accessed 6 April 2021).

Nigg, J.T., Lewis, K., Edinger, T. *et al.* (2012). Meta-analysis of attention-deficit/hyperactivity disorder or attention-deficit/ hyperactivity disorder symptoms, restriction diet, and synthetic food color additives. *Journal of the American Academy of Child and Adolescent Psychiatry* **51**: 86–97.

Noimark, L. and Cox, H.E. (2008). Nutritional problems related to food allergy in childhood. *Pediatric Allergy and Immunology* **19**: 188–195.

Norman, J., Kelly, B., McMahon, A.T. *et al.* (2020). Remember Me? Exposure to unfamiliar food brands in television advertising and online advergames drives children's brand recognition, attitudes, and desire to eat foods: a secondary analysis from a crossover experimental-control study with randomization at the group level. *Journal of the Academy of Nutrition and Dietetics* **120**: 120–129.

Nyakeriga, A.M., Troye-Blomberg, M., Dorfman, J.R. *et al.* (2004). Iron deficiency and malaria among children living on the coast of Kenya. *Journal of Infectious Disease* **190**: 439–447.

Ó Cathaoir K. (2017). Food marketing to children in Sweden and Denmark: a missed opportunity for Nordic leadership. *European Journal of Risk Regulation* **8**: 283–297.

O'Dowd, A. (2017). Spending on junk food advertising is nearly 30 times what government spends on promoting healthy eating. *BMJ* **359**: j4677.

Organisation for Economic Co-operation and Development. (2020). Poverty rate. https://data.oecd.org/inequality/poverty-rate.htm (accessed 7 April 2021).

Ohly, H., Crossland, N., Dykes, F. *et al.* (2019). A realist qualitative study to explore how low-income pregnant women use Healthy Start food vouchers. *Maternal and Child Nutrition* **15**: e12632.

Okada, C., Tabuchi, T. and Iso, H. (2018). Association between skipping breakfast in parents and children and childhood overweight/obesity among children: a nationwide 10.5-year prospective study in Japan. *International Journal of Obesity* **42**: 1724–1732.

Øvrum, A. and Bere, E. (2014). Evaluating free school fruit: results from a natural experiment in Norway with representative data. *Public Health Nutrition* **17**: 1224–1231.

Parkin, P.C., Koroshegyi, C., Mamak, E. *et al.* (2020). Association between Serum Ferritin and Cognitive Function in Early Childhood. *Journal of Pediatrics* **217**: 189–191.

Pedraza, L.S., Popkin, B.M., Batis, C. *et al.*,(2019). The caloric and sugar content of beverages purchased at different store-types changed after the sugary drinks taxation in Mexico. *International Journal of Behavioural Nutrition and Physical Activity* **16**: 103.

Pearce, J., Taylor, M.A. and Langley-Evans, S.C. (2013). Timing of the introduction of complementary feeding and risk of childhood obesity: a systematic review. *International Journal of Obesity* **37**: 1295–1306.

Perignon, M., Fiorentino, M., Kuong, K. *et al.* (2014). Stunting, poor iron status and parasite infection are significant risk factors for lower cognitive performance in Cambodian school-aged children. *PLoS One* **9**: e112605.

Pitchika, V., Standl, M., Harris, C. *et al.* (2020). Association of sugar-sweetened drinks with caries in 10- and 15-year-olds. *BMC Oral Health* **20**: 81.

Pollick, H. (2019). Children who live in mainly fluoridated us counties have less tooth decay. *Journal of Evidence Based Dental Practice* **19**: 217–219.

Popkin, B.M., Corvalan, C. and Grummer-Strawn, L.M. (2020). Dynamics of the double burden of malnutrition and the changing nutrition reality. *Lancet* **395**: 65–74.

Prentice, A.M. and Paul, A.A. (2000). Fat and energy needs of children in developing countries. *American Journal of Clinical Nutrition* **72**: 1253S–1265S.

Public Health England. (2020). National Diet and Nutrition Survey. https://www.gov.uk/government/collections/national-diet-and-nutrition-survey#history (accessed 6 April 2021).

Public Health England. (2019). National child measurement programme (NCMP): trends in child BMI. https://www.gov.uk/government/statistics/national-child-measurement-programme-ncmp-trends-in-child-bmi (accessed 7 April 2021).

Radesky, J., Chassiakos, Y.L.R., Ameenuddin, N. and Navsaria, D. (2020). Digital advertising to children. *Pediatrics* **146**: e20201681.

Rampersaud, G.C., Pereira, M.A., Girard, B.L. *et al.* (2005). Breakfast habits, nutritional status, body weight, and academic performance in children and adolescents. *Journal of the American Dietetic Association* **105**: 743–760.

Ranjani, H., Mehreen, T.S., Pradeepa, R. *et al.* (2016). Epidemiology of childhood overweight & obesity in India: A systematic review. *Indian Journal of Medical Research* **143**: 160–174.

Reilly, J.J., Armstrong, J., Dorosty, A.R. *et al.* (2005). Avon Longitudinal Study of Parents and Children Study Team. Early life risk factors for obesity in childhood: cohort study. *BMJ* **330**: 1357.

Reinehr, T. (2013). Type 2 diabetes mellitus in children and adolescents. *World Journal of Diabetes* **4**: 270–281.

Rennie, K.L., Wells, J.C., McCaffrey, T.A. *et al.* (2006). The effect of physical activity on body fatness in children and adolescents. *Proceedings of the Nutrition Society* **65**: 393–402.

Renninger, M., Hansen, B.H., Steene-Johannessen, J. *et al.* (2020). Associations between accelerometry measured physical activity and sedentary time and the metabolic syndrome: a meta-analysis of more than 6000 children and adolescents. *Pediatric Obesity* **15**: e12578.

Rhee, K.E., De Lago, C.W., Arscott-Mills, T. *et al.* (2005). Factors associated with parental readiness to make changes for overweight children. *Pediatrics* **116**,: e94–e101.

Ribeiro, R.Q. and Alves, L. (2014). Comparison of two school-based programmes for health behaviour change: the Belo Horizonte Heart Study randomized trial. *Public Health Nutrition* **17**: 1195–1204.

Roberts, C. Steer, T., Maplethorpe, N. *et al.* (2018). *National Diet and Nutrition Survey. Results from years 7 and 8 (combined) of the Rolling Programme*. London: Public Health England.

Robertson, S.M., Cullen, K.W., Baranowski, J. *et al.* (1999). Factors related to adiposity among children aged 3 to 7 years. *Journal of the American Dietetic Association* **99**: 938–943.

Robinson, S.M., Marriott, L.D., Crozier, S.R. *et al.* (2009). Variations in infant feeding practice are associated with body composition in childhood: a prospective cohort study. *Journal of Clinical Endocrinology and Metabolism* **94**: 2799–2805.

Robinson, T.N., Borzekowski, D.L., Matheson, D.M. *et al.* (2007). Effects of fast food branding on young children's taste preferences. *Archives of Pediatrics and Adolescent Medicine* **161**: 792–797.

Rudolf, M.C., Sahota, P., Barth, J.H. *et al.* (2001). Increasing prevalence of obesity in primary school children: cohort study. *BMJ* **322**: 1094–1095.

Russell, S.J., Croker, H., Viner, R.M. (2019). The effect of screen advertising on children's dietary intake: A systematic review and meta-analysis. *Obesity Reviews* **20**: 554–568.

SACN (2003) *Salt and Health*. London: Stationery Office.

Samman, M., Kaye, E., Cabral, H. *et al.* (2020). The effect of diet drinks on caries among US children: cluster analysis. *Journal of the American Dental Association* **151**: 502–509.

Sazawal, S., Black, R.E., Ramsan, M. *et al.* (2006). Effects of routine prophylactic supplementation with iron and folic acid on admission to hospital and mortality in pre-school children in a high malaria transmission setting: community-based, randomised, placebo-controlled trial. *Lancet* **367**: 133–143.

Scantlebury, R.J., Moody, A., Oyebode, O. and Mindell, J.S. (2018). Has the UK Healthy Start voucher scheme been associated with an increased fruit and vegetable intake among target families? Analysis of Health Survey for England data, 2001–2014. *Journal of Epidemiology and Community Health* **72**: 623–629.

Scarborough, P., Adhikari, V., Harrington, R.A. *et al.* (2020). Impact of the announcement and implementation of the UK Soft Drinks Industry Levy on sugar content, price, product size and number of available soft drinks in the UK, 2015–19: A controlled interrupted time series analysis. *PLoS Medicine* **17**: e1003025.

Schab, D.W. and Trinh, N.H. (2004). Do artificial food colors promote hyperactivity in children with hyperactive syndromes? A meta-analysis of double-blind placebo-controlled trials. *Journal of Developmental and Behavioral Pediatrics* **25**: 423–434.

Shamah, T. and Villalpando, S. (2006). The role of enriched foods in infant and child nutrition. *British Journal of Nutrition* **96**: S73–S77.

Sisson, S.B., Kiger, A.C., Anundson, K.C. *et al.* (2017). Differences in preschool-age children's dietary intake between meals consumed at childcare and at home. *Preventive Medicine Reports* **6**: 33–37.

Skinner, J.D., Bounds, W., Carruth, B.R. *et al.* (2004). Predictors of children's body mass index: a longitudinal study of diet and growth in children aged 2–8 y. *International Journal of Obesity* **28**: 476–482.

Smith, R., Kelly, B., Yeatman, H. *et al.* (2020. Advertising placement in digital game design influences children's choices of advertised snacks: a randomized trial. *Journal of the Academy of Nutrition and Dietetics* **120**: 404–413.

Stevens, L.J., Burgess, J.R., Stochelski, M.A.and Kuczek, T. (2015). Amounts of artificial food dyes and added sugars in foods and sweets commonly consumed by children. *Clinical Pediatrics* **54**: 309–321.

Stevens, L.J., Burgess, J.R., Stochelski, M.A. and Kuczek, T. (2014). Amounts of artificial food colors in commonly consumed beverages and potential behavioral implications for consumption in children. *Clinical Pediatrics* **53**: 133–140.

Tan, L., Ng, S.H., Omar, A. and Karupaiah, T. (2018). What's on YouTube? A case study on food and beverage advertising in videos targeted at children on social media. *Childhood Obesity* **14**: 280–290.

Taylor, A., Redworth, E.W. and Morgan, J.B. (2004). Influence of diet on iron, copper, and zinc status in children under 24 months of age. *Biology of Trace Elements Research* **97**: 197–214.

Taylor, R.W., Williams, S.M., Fangupo, L.J. *et al.* (2017). Effect of a baby-led approach to complementary feeding on infant growth and overweight: a randomized clinical trial. *Journal of the American Medical Association Pediatrics* **171**: 838–846.

Taylor, C.M., Hays, N.P. and Emmett, P.M. (2019). Diet at age 10 and 13 years in children identified as picky eaters at age 3 years and in children who are persistent picky eaters in a longitudinal birth cohort study. *Nutrients* **11**: 807.

Te Morenga, L., Mallard, S. and Mann, J. (2012). Dietary sugars and body weight: systematic review and meta-analyses of randomised controlled trials and cohort studies. *BMJ* **346**: e7492.

Torun, B. (2005). Energy requirements of children and adolescents. *Public Health Nutrition*: **8**, 968–993.

Townsend, E. and Pitchford, N.J. (2012). Baby knows best? The impact of weaning style on food preferences and body mass index in early childhood in a case-controlled sample. *BMJ Open* **2**: e000298.

Trussell Trust. (2020). What we do: our vision is for a UK without the need for food banks. https://www.trusselltrust.org/what-we-do (accessed 7 April 2021).

Turbutt, C., Richardson, J. and Pettinger, C. (2019). The impact of hot food takeaways near schools in the UK on childhood obesity: a systematic review of the evidence. *Journal of Public Health* **41**: 231–239.

Unicef. (2020). Child poverty. https://www.unicef.org/social-policy/child-poverty (accessed 7 April 2021).

United Nations. (2015) Sustainable Development Goals. https://www.un.org/sustainabledevelopment/sustainable-development-goals (accessed 7 April 2021).

Ustjanauskas, A.E., Harris, J.L. and Schwartz, M.B. (2014). Food and beverage advertising on children's web sites. *Pediatrric Obesity* **9**: 362–372.

Utter, J., Scragg, R., Mhurchu, C.N. *et al.* (2007). At-home breakfast consumption among New Zealand children: associations with body mass index and related nutrition behaviors. *Journal of the American Dietetic Association* **107**: 570–576.

Verhage, C.L., Gillebaart, M., van der Veek, S.M.C. and Vereijken, C.M.J.L. (2018). The relation between family meals and health of infants and toddlers: a review. *Appetite* **127**: 97–109.

Wang, Y.C., Bleich, S.N. and Gortmaker, S.L. (2008). Increasing caloric contribution from sugar-sweetened beverages and 100% fruit juices among US children and adolescents, 1988–2004. *Pediatrics* **121**: e1604–e1614.

Ward, D. and Ainsworth, P. (1998). The development of a nutritious low cost weaning food for Kenya infants. *African Journal of Health Science* **5**: 89–95.

Wardle, J., Carnell, S., Haworth, C.M. *et al.* (2008). Evidence for a strong genetic influence on childhood adiposity despite the force of the obesogenic environment. *American Journal of Clinical Nutrition* **87**: 398–404.

Weder, S., Hoffmann, M., Becker, K. *et al.* (2019). Energy, macronutrient intake, and anthropometrics of vegetarian, vegan, and omnivorous children (1–3 years) in Germany (VeChi Diet Study). *Nutrients* **11**: 832.

Wesnes, K.A., Pincock, C. and Scholey, A. (2012). Breakfast is associated with enhanced cognitive function in schoolchildren. An internet based study. *Appetite* **59**: 646–649.

Wessells, K.R. and Brown, K.H. (2012). Estimating the global prevalence of zinc deficiency: results based on zinc availability in national food supplies and the prevalence of stunting. *PLoS One* **7**: e50568.

Wijtzes, A.I., Jansen, W., Jaddoe, V.W. *et al.* (2015). Social inequalities in young children's meal skipping behaviors: the generation R study. *PLoS One* **10**(7): e0134487.

Wolstenholme, H., Heary, C., Kelly, C. (2019). Fussy eating behaviours: response patterns in families of school-aged children. *Appetite* **136**: 93–102.

World Health Organization. (2021). Malaria. https://www.who.int/news-room/fact-sheets/detail/malaria (accessed 7 April 2021).

World Health Organization. (2013). *Global Action Plan for the Prevention and Control of Non-Communicable Diseases 2013–2020.* Geneva: WHO.

World Obesity Federation. (2019). *Atlas of Childhood Obesity.* London: World Obesity Federation.

Wright, C.M., Parker, L., Lamont, D. *et al.* (2001). Implications of childhood obesity for adult health: findings from thousand families cohort study. *BMJ* **323**: 1280–1284.

Wright, C.M., Parkinson, K.N., Shipton, D. *et al.* (2007). How do toddler eating problems relate to their eating behavior, food preferences, and growth? *Pediatrics* **120**: e1069–e1075.

Wu, L., Sun, S., He, Y., Jiang, B. (2016). The effect of interventions targeting screen time reduction: A systematic review and meta-analysis. *Medicine* **95**: e4029.

Yen, C.E., Yen, C.H., Huang, M.C. *et al.* (2008). Dietary intake and nutritional status of vegetarian and omnivorous preschool children and their parents in Taiwan. *Nutrition Research* **28**: 430–436.

Yu, C.J., Du, J.C., Chiou, H.C. *et al.* (2016). Sugar-sweetened beverage consumption is adversely associated with childhood attention deficit/hyperactivity disorder. *International Journal of Environmental Research and Public Health* **13**: 678.

Zlotkin, S., Newton, S., Aimone, A.M. *et al.* (2013). Effect of iron fortification on malaria incidence in infants and young children in Ghana: a randomized trial. *Journal of the American Medical Association* **310**: 938–947.

Additional reading

If you would like to find out more about the material discussed in this chapter, the following sources may be of interest.

Michaelsen, K.F., Neufeld, L.M., Prentice A.M. (2020). *Global Landscape of Nutrition Challenges in Infants and Children.* Basel: Karger.

More, J. (2013). *Infant, Child and Adolescent Nutrition: A practical handbook.* Boca Raton, CA: CRC Press.

CHAPTER 7

Nutrition and adolescence

LEARNING OBJECTIVES

This chapter will enable the reader to:
- Describe the patterns of growth seen during the adolescent period.
- Discuss the changes in body composition associated with the pubertal phase of growth.
- Show an appreciation of the relationship between endocrine factors and nutritional status as determinants of bone growth and sexual maturation.
- Describe the processes that allow the growth of bone and how they are sensitive to micronutrient intake, physical activity and overweight.
- Discuss the physiological processes that determine requirements for energy, macronutrients and micronutrients during adolescence.
- Describe how the increasing independence associated with adolescence is a major factor in determining food choices during this life stage.
- Discuss the nutritional and physiological challenges of pubertal blockade during gender transition.
- Identify behaviours that may promote problems with nutritional status among adolescents, including restrictive dietary practices, excessive physical activity, disordered eating and the use of alcohol and tobacco products.
- Discuss the main features of anorexia nervosa and bulimia nervosa and identify key risk factors for the development of these eating disorders in adolescence.
- Describe the particular nutritional concerns that are associated with pregnancy during adolescence.

7.1 Introduction

Adolescence is the transitional stage that lies between childhood and adulthood. This stage of life is dominated by the physiological processes that surround puberty, which are accompanied by rapid growth and maturation. Alongside these biological processes, there are psychological changes as the child attains an adult capacity for cognitive processes and acquires the ability to take on adult responsibilities. The impact that the adolescent period has upon nutritional status is not only influenced by these biological and psychological changes but also strongly modulated by the sociocultural aspects of adolescence. In many developing countries, the transition from child to adult is mostly a physiological issue and, culturally, the child becomes an adult by passing through a coming-of-age ceremony. Thereafter, the boys take on the roles of adult men, and the girls marry and have children. In industrialized countries, the social construct of the 'teenager' is the dominant cultural pattern. This serves to extend the transition from child to adult and, in effect, the young adult lives for a longer period under the guidance of their parents. The teenager is culturally expected to undergo emotional trauma and erratic and occasionally rebellious behaviour. This chapter considers how these issues and behaviours, coupled with the biological demands of adolescence, impact nutritional requirements and status.

7.2 Physical development

7.2.1 Growth rate

During childhood, growth occurs at a rate of 5–6 cm per year, with a steady decline in growth velocity from infancy through to the onset of puberty. With puberty, both girls and boys go through a 'growth spurt' that lasts for approximately two to three years. In terms of height, the gain associated with the growth spurt is a significant proportion of final adult stature (15–20%). During this growth phase, girls gain approximately 20 cm (range 5–25 cm), while in boys, the gain is slightly greater at 23 cm

Nutrition, Health and Disease: A Lifespan Approach, Third Edition. Simon Langley-Evans.
© 2021 John Wiley & Sons Ltd. Published 2021 by John Wiley & Sons Ltd.
Companion website: www.wiley.com/go/langleyevans/lifespan3e

(10–30 cm). Peak height velocities achieved during the growth spurt are 9 and 10.5 cm per year for girls and boys, respectively (Tanner, 1989). Timing of the growth spurt is earlier in girls than in boys, occurring at around the time the breasts begin to grow (thelarche, one of the earliest indicators of female puberty). In boys, sexual maturation has generally advanced to a relatively late stage before the onset of the growth spurt. The increase in rates of height gain is matched by increases in weight. In boys, height and weight gains occur together, but in girls, weight gain lags behind height gain by three to six months. In both sexes, weight gain is proportionally greater than height gain (e.g. girls gain 20% of adult height and 50% of adult weight during the growth spurt), leading to an increased body mass index.

Although the pubertal growth spurt is a phase of major height and weight gain, it is not the main determinant of final adult height. Indeed, it is estimated that only 30% of the variation in adult height is explained by the rate of growth during its maximal phase during puberty (Tanner, 1989). Growth before puberty is in fact the main determinant of adult stature, and the height and weight gained during the growth spurt are simply superimposed upon the prepubertal growth rate. Boys tend to grow taller than girls because they enter puberty at a later age. Indeed, prior to puberty, boys and girls tend to be of similar stature (average height of Europeans at age nine for boys is 132 cm and for girls 131 cm), but by adulthood, males are typically 12–13 cm taller. Similarly, girls who are 'late developers' and enter puberty at an older age will generally attain a greater than average height due to their extended prepubertal growth phase.

The growth spurt impacts upon all parts of the body, but the timing of regional growth is uneven. Limb growth precedes the growth of the trunk by six to nine months, for example. Thickening of the skull and remodelling of tissues of the scalp, widening of the jaws and growth of the facial musculature are all events associated with the growth spurt and are more pronounced in boys than in girls, particularly later in puberty. Growth ceases in males between the ages of 18 and 20, which is usually two to three years after the end of the growth spurt. In females, growth usually ceases within two to three years of menarche, and on average, girls attain final adult height by the age of 16.5 years. In some cases, later sexual maturation allows growth to continue until 19 years.

Growth is sexually dimorphic, in terms of the timing and final achieved heights and the distribution of increasing mass. Males exhibit characteristic increases in size across the shoulders during puberty,

while in females, there is greater growth at the hips. These differences in skeletal growth occur due to hormone sensitivity of cartilage cells at these sites. At the hip, cells respond to oestrogen and this leads to greater pelvic girth to accommodate reproductive functions. Androgen sensitivity at the shoulders produces the characteristic male body shape and upper body strength.

7.2.2 Body composition

The rapid growth of adolescence is accompanied by remodelling of body composition in both sexes. In boys and girls, the larger body mass associated with greater stature is associated with an increase in muscle mass and hence the fat-free mass of the body (Figure 7.1). The growth spurt for muscle lags slightly behind the peak in linear growth, and as it is triggered by the events of puberty, it tends to occur earlier in females than in males. In fact, for a period between 12 and 14 years of age, girls will tend to be

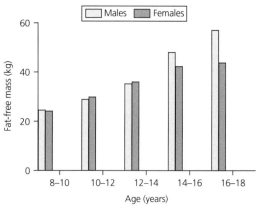

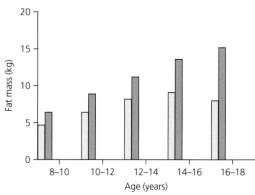

Figure 7.1 Accrual of lean and fat mass during the prepubertal and pubertal periods. During adolescence, there is a rapid increase in the lean body mass of males and females, coinciding with the pubertal growth spurt. Fat mass also increases but to a greater extent in females. *Source:* data from Guo *et al.* (1997).

more muscular than boys (Tanner, 1989). However, there are significant differences between the sexes in terms of fat deposition, which is greater in girls than in boys. As a result, while fat-free mass as a proportion of body weight increases from 80% to 90% in boys across the period of adolescence, this declines from 80% to 75% in girls.

The absolute mass of body fat in boys increases slightly between the ages of eight and the onset of the pubertal growth spurt and then declines (Figure 7.1). As a proportion of body mass, body fat increases from 15% at age eight to 17.5% at 12–14 years, but by the end of puberty, it is only 11% (Guo et al., 1997). In girls, puberty is associated with a steady increase in the amount of adipose tissue, as fat is deposited in the pelvic region, breasts, upper back, arms and subcutaneously. As a proportion of body mass, fat increases from 20% to 25% in females over the adolescent years.

7.2.3 Puberty and sexual maturation

It should be clear from the preceding sections that sexual maturation and the events surrounding puberty are the principal processes that determine many of the requirements for nutrients and changes in body composition that are associated with the adolescent period. Puberty has its onset earlier in girls (8–13 years of age) than in boys (9.5–13.5 years of age) and is typically of three to four years in duration. There are wide variations in timing and speed of maturation between individuals. In boys, the growth of the penis, for example, on average begins at the age of 12.5 years. However, in some boys, this will occur much earlier (10.5 years) and in others as late as 14.5 years. Thus, among a population of boys aged 13–15 years, the level of sexual maturation will show huge variation. Although the timings are variable, in boys, the sequence of maturational events is well conserved. Testicular enlargement is always the first event and the ensuing increase in hormone secretion drives penile growth, the appearance of pubic hair and the pubertal growth spurt.

As a result of the variability in timing of pubertal growth and maturation, it is more practical to consider adolescents in terms of their pubertal milestones than in terms of chronological age when reviewing influences of nutrition upon physiology. For this purpose, it is common to consider either skeletal age (see Section 7.2.4) or the sexual maturation rating (Tanner stage of development; Table 7.1). In girls, there is variability in terms of timing and sequencing of these stages. Breast stage 2 is often the first indicator of puberty and occurs on average at 10.8 years (range 8.8–12.8 years). In two

Table 7.1 Sexual maturation ratings (Tanner stages).

Stage	Both sexes
Pubic hair:	
1	None
2	Small amounts of long downy hair with little pigment
3	Coarse and curly extending across pubis
4	Adult-like features but not yet spreading to thighs
5	Adult pattern and features
Male genitals*	
1	Prepubertal appearance
2	Testes enlarging and scrotum reddening and thinning
3	Further enlargement of scrotum and testes; penis lengthening
4	Penis increasing in length and scrotum darkening further
5	Adult characteristics
Female breasts	
1	Prepubertal appearance
2	Breast bud formation and growth of areola
3	Areola continuing expansion. Breast elevating and extending beyond areola
4	Breast size and elevation increasing; nipple and areola extending as a secondary mound
5	Adult characteristics

* In males, staging based upon genital growth may be referred to as stages G1–G5.

thirds of girls, this will precede other events, but a significant proportion of girls will develop pubic hair ahead of breast budding (Tanner, 1989). Timing of menarche also varies and, while most girls have their first menstrual period at breast stage 4, around 25% will do so at stage 3. The sexual maturation ratings generally map well against growth rates. In girls, the pubertal growth spurt begins at around stage 2. In boys, the growth spurt is delayed and coincides with stage 4 (Figure 7.2).

The major changes in body composition described in Section 7.2.2 are partly features of growth during adolescence. They are also driven by the actions of sex steroids that are secreted as the hypothalamic–pituitary–gonadal and hypothalamic–pituitary–adrenal axes mature. The independent and parallel processes of puberty and adrenarche result in the development of the secondary sexual characteristics and produce endocrine changes that remodel body composition in a sex-specific manner (Figure 7.3).

Adrenarche usually occurs between the ages of 6 and 10 years. In boys, it is therefore a forerunner of puberty, but in girls it may occur alongside pubertal changes. During adrenarche, the adrenal cortex expands and completes differentiation into three

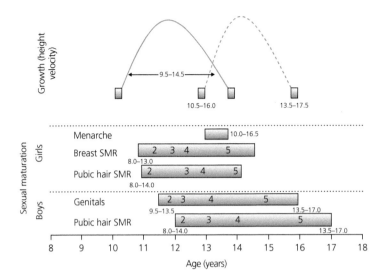

Figure 7.2 The relationship of growth velocity to pubertal staging in boys and girls. Average timings of pubertal (Tanner) staging are shown in the lower half of the figure. Age ranges beneath the pubertal staging boxes indicate the spread of values over which sexual maturation begins and ends. Height velocity curves at the top of the figure show the timings of the pubertal growth spurt in girls (—) and boys (- - -) and the average age of maximal growth velocity. It is clear from the figure that in girls, acceleration of growth precedes pubertal development, while in boys, this acceleration occurs at a more advanced stage. *Source:* adapted from Tanner (1989). Reproduced with permission from Castlemead Publications. SMR, sexual maturation rate.

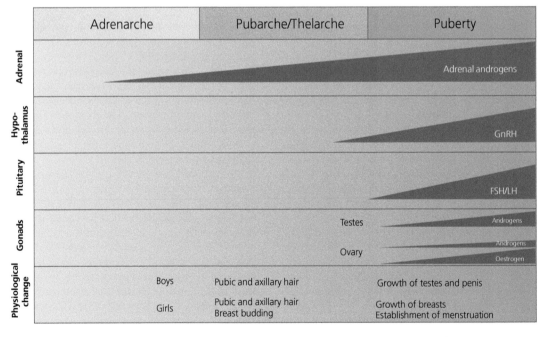

Figure 7.3 The key endocrine events of adolescence. Adrenarche and puberty are separate processes that promote endocrine maturation. Development of the adrenal gland increases secretion of androgens in both males and females (adrenarche). The adrenal androgens stimulate development of secondary sexual characteristics. Puberty begins with the maturation of the hypothalamus and the stable rhythm of production of gonadotrophin-releasing hormone (GnRH). FSH, follicle-stimulating hormone; LH, luteinizing hormone.

separate zones, the zona glomerulosa, the zona fasciculata and the zona reticularis. The zona reticularis synthesizes androgens, including androstenedione and dehydroepiandrosterone sulphate. These androgens initiate the appearance of the secondary sexual characteristics and symptoms associated with puberty, including acne, body odour, changes to the vocal cords and deepening of the voice and appearance of pubic and axillary hair.

The appearance of pubic hair is termed pubarche and is also driven by the endocrine signals that develop with the onset of puberty (Figure 7.3). True puberty begins with the hypothalamus achieving a regular pulsatile pattern of gonadotrophin-releasing hormone (GnRH) release. This is partly achieved as a response to leptin signalling of body fatness in both girls and boys (see Chapter 2) and is also driven by the maturation of glutaminergic neurones within the hypothalamus. Stimulation of the gonads by luteinizing hormone and follicle-stimulating hormone has characteristic effects in boys and girls. In boys, the testes enlarge and produce testosterone and androstenedione. These further stimulate the appearance of the secondary sexual characteristics and the growth of the penis and testes. Production of androgens promotes both linear growth and the growth of muscular tissue. The greater activity of these hormones in males results in the development of a larger body with a greater proportion of lean body mass. In girls, ovarian synthesis of oestrogen and progesterone also contributes to the secondary sexual characteristics but more importantly leads to the establishment of reproductive cycling and thelarche. Oestrogens stimulate the deposition of body fat, and hence, with advancing pubertal stages, the female body contains a greater proportion of fat than that of the male. Menarche is an indicator that the uterus and ovaries are fully mature, but this does not mark the end of the events of puberty. In girls, growth will continue for a short period, allowing a further increase in height of approximately 6 cm beyond menarche.

7.2.4 Bone growth

The mature skeleton is a complex tissue that comprises two main forms of bone, spongy trabecular bone and more dense cortical bone. Bones in different sites around the body differ in the relative amounts of the two forms that are present and within bones, there are different layers of cortical and trabecular bone, with the latter being more prominent in and around joints (see also Section 9.6.1.1). During adolescent growth, all the bones within the skeleton are increasing in size, but for the purposes of this text, the process will be described for the long bones (e.g. the femur or humerus).

Bones initially form from cartilaginous structures during the fetal period. The process of endochondral ossification converts these structures into mineralized (ossified) bone structures that are innervated and invaded by the cardiovascular system. Endochondral ossification ends in the first few years of life, and bone is then able to increase in size by virtue of the distribution of different zones of bone. The long bones in childhood comprise three regions (Figure 7.4). The shaft of the bone is called the diaphysis. This is mostly cortical bone surrounded by an external layer of connective tissue (the periosteum). This tissue is important in the growth process, as it allows an increase in bone girth. In mature bone, it is the point of connection for tendons and ligaments. There is also an internal layer of connective tissue (the endosteum), which surrounds the central medullary cavity, where the bone marrow is located. The end of the bone is called the epiphysis, which is mostly trabecular bone, with thin layers of cortical bone. In the growing bone, there is a layer between these two zones called the epiphyseal plate, which is composed of cartilage and partially calcified cartilage. It is this that allows linear growth to take place.

Within the epiphyseal plate, there are four layers of cells. Closest to the epiphysis lies a layer of resting chondrocytes (cartilage cells). The function of these cells is to anchor the epiphyseal bone to the growth zone. Beneath this layer, the chondrocytes are in a state of active multiplication by mitosis. Moving closer to the diaphysis, the cartilage of the plate begins to calcify. Within this zone are chondrocytes that are maturing and enlarging, and along the border of the epiphyseal plate and the diaphysis lies the fourth cell layer, which comprises chondrocytes that are dying and becoming calcified. In effect, the process pushes the epiphysis out from the diaphysis by depositing strips of bone over the top of the diaphysis and new cartilage cells just below the epiphysis, thus elongating the bone. The newly formed bone may be remodelled through the action of osteoblasts and other cells, and will be invaded by blood vessels. At the point of skeletal maturation, the cartilage is fully calcified and the epiphysis and diaphysis fuse together.

The same process occurs in all growing bones. While in the long bones the process relies on growth plates at the ends of the shaft, in other bones the growth plates exist as concentric rings, with growth progressing from the outside, in towards the centre. Bone maturity can be assessed by x-ray and is often used as a marker of pubertal development to

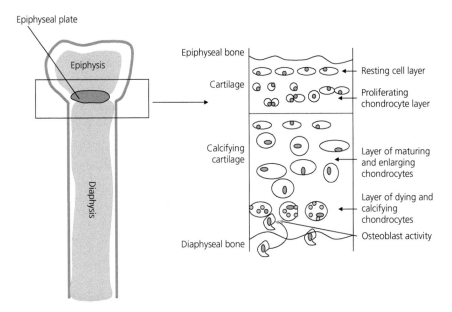

Figure 7.4 The growth of long bones. Long bones expand through activity within the epiphyseal growth plate, which lies at the interface of the bone shaft (diaphysis) and end (epiphysis). New cartilage cells (chondrocytes) are formed at the epiphyseal end of the growth plate, while mature cells on the diaphyseal end die and become calcified. The bone extends by virtue of this zone pushing the epiphysis away from the diaphysis.

supplement Tanner staging based on breast or genital maturation. In bones that are still growing, the epiphyses are imaged as less radiographically dense than the ossified bone, while in mature bones the fused epiphyses show as clear epiphyseal lines. Staging of maturity through skeletal ageing usually employs x-rays of the wrist or hand. These are then compared with atlases of images that consider the size and shape of bones, along with the degree of ossification (Tanner, 1989).

Bone growth occurs throughout childhood but is most rapid during adolescence, when approximately half of the eventual mass of the skeleton is laid down. There is a short continuation of the accrual of bone mass beyond the attainment of final height (Figure 7.5). In girls, the most rapid period of bone mineralization is between 12 and 15 years, while in boys, the peak lies between 14 and 17 years. During these brief periods, approximately 25% of adult bone mass is deposited, which is equivalent to the amount of bone mass which will be ultimately lost during late adulthood (Boreham and McKay, 2011). Peak bone mass, the point where bone mineral content and density are at its greatest, occurs between 25 and 35 years of age (Davies *et al.*, 2004).

Bone growth is strongly under the influence of genetic factors, which are believed to determine around 80% of the variation in adult bone mass.

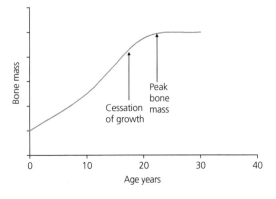

Figure 7.5 The accrual of bone mass. Much of the mass of the adult skeleton is deposited during the adolescent growth phase. The most rapid rate of bone mineralization coincides with the pubertal growth spurt. Deposition of bone continues beyond the cessation of growth, and peak bone mass is achieved in the third decade of life.

Many genes are important in formation, growth and maintenance of the skeleton, but those that appear to be of greatest importance during childhood and adolescent growth include the vitamin D receptor, type 1 collagen, oestrogen receptor beta (ERβ), leptin, insulin-like growth factor-1 (IGF-1), interleukin-6, low-density lipoprotein receptor-related protein-5 and osteocalcin (Davies *et al.*, 2004). Endocrine signals are also the major factors that drive bone growth. Growth hormone and IGF-1, for example, stimulate accrual of bone mass by promoting the proliferation of osteoblasts. The secretion of these hormones is increased during puberty through the actions of the sex steroids. The sex steroids exert direct effects on bone also. Adrenal-derived androgens increase the overall strength of bone, while estradiol increases bone thickness.

While genetics determine most of the variation in rates of bone growth and accrual of mineral, diet and lifestyle factors are also of importance. Physical activity stimulates bone mineralization, particularly high-impact sports (e.g. basketball, volleyball, rugby and gymnastics) or weight-bearing activities. Optimal bone mineralization is driven by activities of short and intense nature with frequent rest periods (Boreham and McKay, 2011). Activity-induced bone growth is greatest at the skeletal sites that bear the greatest load (Daly, 2007). In other words, bone tends to accrue at the greatest rate along lines of stress. This structural response to exercise is seen in both boys and girls, but once puberty is initiated it differs slightly. In boys, exercise stimulates bone thickening by expansion of the periosteum, while in girls, there is a contraction of the endosteum layer. Interventions of more than six-month duration that involve three or more periods of activity can increase bone mass by up to 6% (Boreham and McKay, 2011), and the benefits of activity in terms of bone mineral accrual are greatest in children who are active in the prepubertal and early pubertal stages (Davies *et al.*, 2004). A study of elite Finnish tennis female players showed that those who started their careers before puberty achieved two- to four-fold greater benefits from exercise-induced bone mineralization than those who started post-menarche (Kannus *et al.*, 1995). Welten *et al.* (1994) performed a longitudinal study of 13-year-old boys and girls with a follow-up to 27 years of age. Levels of physical activity in adolescence explained 17% of the variation in adult bone mineral density and were the main predictor of adult bone mass. Excessive exercise in adolescent girls can, however, be detrimental to bone health if it impacts upon menstrual cycle function (see Section 7.6.3).

Nutrition-related factors are known to be of importance in determining adolescent bone growth. Girls who have suffered from anorexia nervosa generally have reduced bone mineral density (BMD) into adulthood and are therefore at risk of bone disorders such as osteoporosis later in life. Eating disorders or excessive underweight is associated with reduced production of sex steroids and expression of IGF-1, hence limiting bone growth. Interestingly, overweight may also limit bone growth due to the inhibitory actions of leptin. Ducy *et al.* (2000) used mutant mouse strains to demonstrate that leptin is a negative regulator of skeletal growth. The *ob/ob* mouse, which lacks a functional leptin gene, and the *db/db* mouse, which does not express leptin receptors, have almost threefold greater bone volume than wild-type mice. Skeletal development can be normalized by administration of exogenous leptin. Children who are overweight will secrete more leptin and this may therefore reduce bone mineralization. As individuals with obesity tend to be leptin resistant, it might be argued that obesity in adolescence could provide some benefits for skeletal growth. However, as discussed in Chapter 6, excessive obesity in childhood can lead to deformation of the skeleton or damage to the epiphyses of the hip, associated with the need to bear a heavier load. Excess adiposity is generally associated with lower bone mineralization and impaired growth of the skeleton.

The main predictor of bone mass before puberty is lean mass, but beyond puberty, fat mass becomes more strongly associated with bone growth (Mosca *et al.*, 2013). El Hage *et al.* (2013) reported a lower whole-body bone mineral content in boys who were obese compared with those of healthy weight. Distribution of body fat may also play a key role, with central adiposity being associated with impaired bone growth at weight-bearing sites (Laddu *et al.*, 2013). Kondiboyina *et al.* (2020) followed a cohort of eight- to nine-year-olds and noted that not only did children who were overweight and obese have lower BMD (expressed per body weight), but they also gained less density than lean children over a nine-month period. Adolescents with obesity are sometimes noted to have higher BMD measures than healthy weight controls, but more detailed assessments of bone porosity and thickness and estimates of strength suggest that obesity is associated with changes in bone microarchitecture that increase risk of fractures (Singhal *et al.*, 2019). Children who are obese and overweight therefore appear to have a slowed rate of bone mass accrual and growth of the weight-bearing long bones fails to compensate for the excess weight carried.

The mechanisms that link obesity to bone growth are still not fully understood and may be complex. Adiposity may disrupt the endocrine signals that drive bone growth and maturation and is known to impact upon production of growth hormone (Perotti *et al.*, 2013) and sex hormones (Vandewalle *et al.*, 2014). Bone is also responsive to adipokines (including leptin and adiponectin) and pro-inflammatory cytokines (tumour necrosis factor α) that are produced by adipose tissue, and these agents may impact upon activity of osteoblasts and osteoclasts, resulting in altered rates of bone deposition (Campos *et al.*, 2013; Mosca *et al.*, 2013).

The major nutrient associated with skeletal growth is calcium, with increased intakes promoting accrual of bone mass, provided that vitamin D status is adequate. A randomized controlled trial in identical twins aged 9–13 showed that calcium 800 mg per day with vitamin D 400 ui per day produced significant gains in bone mass and strength over a six-month period (Greene and Naughton, 2011). However, not all studies report the same benefits. A randomized controlled trial providing 900 mg per day calcium to girls and boys whose habitual intake was below 800 mg per day resulted in no major impact on bone mineralization (Vogel *et al.*, 2017). In contrast, Ma *et al.* (2014) showed that providing supplements in the form of milk powders (calcium 300 or 600 mg/day with vitamin D 200 iu/day) resulted in greater accrual of bone mineral at the femoral neck among girls aged 12–14 years). The same protocol run over two years produced gains in BMD at the hip in boys and girls (Zhang *et al.*, 2014). Poor calcium intake is frequently reported in adolescents and is a major concern in the context of skeletal growth. The UK National Diet and Nutrition Survey (Roberts *et al.*, 2018) found that, among 11–18 year-olds, 11% of boys and 22% of girls consumed calcium at a level below the lower reference nutrient intake (LRNI). Similarly, the 2011–2014 US National Health and Nutrition Examination Survey found that 49% of boys and 68% of girls in the 12–19 years age group had calcium intakes below the estimated average requirement.

It seems unlikely that any benefits of calcium supplementation on bone mineralization in adolescence will have a lasting impact on bone health, unless supplements are continued beyond attainment of peak bone mass. Lambert *et al.* (2008) reported that 18 months of calcium supplements (792 mg/day) to 12-year-old girls with low habitual calcium intakes boosted whole-body BMD in the short term, but had no lasting effect when followed-up two years beyond the end of the supplementation period. A 12-year follow-up of a 1 g per day calcium supplement given to 8–12-year-olds in the Gambia for one year found that while supplementation boosted whole-body bone mineral accrual and bone areas in the middle of adolescence, there was no lasting effect on the skeleton (Ward *et al.*, 2014). Thus, while it is desirable to attain a higher peak bone mass through improvements to calcium nutrition during adolescence, short-term interventions are unlikely to achieve this aim.

7.3 Psychosocial development

Adolescence is a period of intense cognitive, emotional and social development. Over the period from 11 to 21 years of age, the individual undergoes a transition from a childlike way of thinking and interacting with others to a mature, adult level of functioning (Story *et al.*, 2002). These changes can impact significantly upon nutrition, as the transition process generates attitudes, beliefs and ways of thinking that can strongly influence food choices.

In the earliest stages of adolescence, children find it difficult to think in abstract terms. The average 11–14-year-old is able to focus only on present realities and thinks in concrete terms. The ability to process abstract concepts and make associations between current actions and later consequences is poorly developed. This can make health promotion at this stage very challenging, as these adolescents are unable to perceive that their current eating behaviours might impact upon their health three or more decades into the future. On a social and emotional level, the young adolescent increasingly strives to establish independence from parents and family. The peer group becomes overwhelmingly important and influential, and this can be a cause of conflict in the home as acceptance by peers often dictates a degree of rebellion against authority.

Between 15 and 17 years, the adolescent acquires a more advanced range of cognitive skills and begins to be able to think about abstract scenarios and consider the possibilities and intangible consequences that may stem from their actions. At this age, the individual can begin to grasp multiple viewpoints of a given situation or argument, and as a result, conflicts within families will reduce. The peer group remains hugely important, and the desire to be accepted by peers and to conform with the expectations of the social network can lead to the adolescent being very self-conscious about their appearance, behaviours and how they might be perceived by others. By the age of 18–21, the individual is capable of all advanced cognitive processes and will have established a firm view of their personal identity and their overall place within society and local culture. These young adults may still show immature behaviour and decision making, particularly under pressure, and will retain strong links with a wide social group of likeminded individuals of similar age.

7.4 Nutritional requirements in adolescence

The high rates of growth during adolescence carry significant increments in nutritional requirements over and above those seen in earlier childhood. Indeed, this stage of life has requirements for energy and nutrients that are greater than seen in adulthood, both in absolute terms and when expressed per body weight (Table 7.2). It is recognized that adolescence increases nutrient requirements, mostly due to growth. The remodelling of body shape and body composition and the maturation of organ systems also contribute to adolescence being a peak time in terms of nutrient requirements. Precise guidelines and recommendations for nutrient intakes in adolescence are, however, largely undefined. This is due to a lack of relevant research and due to the difficulties of reconciling chronological age and physiological stage of development. For some nutrients, it is more useful to set dietary reference values based upon height, body weight or energy intake, rather than age.

7.4.1 Macronutrients and energy

Estimating the energy requirements of adolescents represents a particular challenge, as the true energy requirement is more closely related to body size and the growth velocity than to age. The pubertal period sees an increase in height of 15–20% and a gain in weight that corresponds to approximately 50% of the final attained adult weight. The bulk of the

height gain and weight gain is through accrual of skeletal mass and lean body mass and therefore requires an anabolic state and hence a high demand for energy (Giovannini et al., 2000). The energy requirements of boys are greater than for girls at any given body weight, by virtue of their larger bulk of metabolically active tissue (lean body mass; Table 7.3). With the onset of puberty, therefore, the difference in energy requirements of males and females begins to diverge sharply. Adolescents often have higher levels of physical activity than seen in adults, and these also contribute significantly to energy requirements.

To deliver the energy needs of growth, the appetite of adolescents increases markedly. One of the challenges of this period is to manage intake such that optimal growth can be sustained, without excessive weight gain. As described in Chapter 6, the emergence of overweight and obesity during the adolescent years is an indicator of increased risk of obesity during adulthood. The major sources of energy within the diet are carbohydrate (which in adolescence should provide up to 55% of daily energy) and fat (no more than 35% of energy). There are no specific recommendations for these macronutrients in adolescence, but intakes need to be sufficient in order to spare protein for growth.

Protein demands reach their peak during the pubertal growth spurt (11–14 years in girls, 15–18 years in boys). In addition to growth, protein is required for the maintenance of existing tissues and the deposition of new lean mass. To maintain

Table 7.2 A comparison of nutrient requirements* between adults and children aged 11–18 years.

Nutrient	Age					
	11–14		15–18		19–50	
	Male	Female	Male	Female	Male	Female
Energy (kcal/day)	2500	2000	2500	2000	2500	2000
Protein (g/day)	42.1	41.2	55.2	45.0	55.5	45.0
Riboflavin (mg/day)	1.2	1.1	1.3	1.1	1.3	1.1
Vitamin A (retinol equiv./day)	600	600	700	600	700	600
Folate (µg/day)	200	200	200	200	200	200
Ascorbate (mg/day)	35	35	40	40	40	40
Cobalamin (µg/day)	1.2	1.2	1.5	1.5	1.5	1.5
Iron (mg/day)	11.3	14.8	11.3	14.8	8.7	14.8
Zinc (mg/day)	9.0	9.0	9.5	7.0	9.5	7.0
Calcium (mg/day)	1000	800	1000	800	700	700
Selenium (µg/day)	45	45	70	60	75	60
Magnesium (mg/day)	280	280	300	300	300	270

Data shown are UK estimated average requirements for energy, and reference nutrient intakes for protein and micronutrients (Public Health England, 2016).
* Selected nutrients.

Table 7.3 Energy requirements of adolescents are dependent upon physiological development and physical activity level.

Body weight (kg)	Basal metabolic rate (kcal/day)	Estimated average requirement (kcal/day)				
		Physical activity level				
		1.4	1.5	1.6	1.8	2.0
Boys:						
30	1186	1670	1789	1909	2148	2363
40	1362	1909	2052	2172	2458	2720
50	1539	2148	2315	2458	2768	3078
60	1715	2410	2578	2744	3078	3437
Girls:						
30	1093	1527	1646	1742	1957	2195
40	1227	1718	1837	1957	2195	2458
50	1360	1909	2028	2172	2458	2720
60	1494	2100	2243	2386	2697	2983

Data from Department of Health (1998). Physical activity level (PAL) of 1.0 corresponds to sleeping (basal rate); 1.2–1.4, lying or sitting at rest, reading, eating or watching television; 1.5–1.8, moderately active seated, for example, driving, playing piano or operating computer, and moderate standing activities; 1.9–2.4, walking 3–4 km/h and low-intensity sports. High-intensity sports and exercise will have PAL of 4.5–7.9. Average PAL for boys aged 10–18 years is 1.56 and for girls is 1.48 calculated from estimates of time spent sleeping, at school and engaged in light, moderate or high-intensity activities.

nitrogen balance in the face of growth and deposition of lean body mass, protein intake should be at a level corresponding to 12–14% of energy intake (Table 7.2). Most adolescents in the developed countries consume protein at a level beyond requirements. The UK National Diet and Nutrition Survey (Years 7 and 8; Roberts *et al.*, 2018) estimated mean protein intakes of 11–18-year-old boys to be 73.3 g/day, and girls 57g/day). Analysis of the US National Health and Nutrition Examination Surveys (2001–2015) suggested that 14–18-year-old boys consume 97 g per day and girls 63.9 g per day (Berryman *et al.*, 2018). Excessive intakes have been suggested as potentially detrimental to calcium homeostasis and bone growth.

7.4.2 Micronutrients

Micronutrients are essential during adolescence to ensure that the major physiological processes and functions can be maintained during the period of maximal growth (Olmedilla and Granado, 2000). Generally speaking, the demands for vitamins and minerals increase in proportion to energy requirements. For vitamins, there are few available data on which to base specific recommendations for adolescents. It is assumed that growth and the increased rates of energy use will increase requirements for riboflavin, thiamine and niacin. Protein metabolism and the synthesis of DNA and RNA will increase the demand for vitamin B6 and cobalamin. Folate is also required for these important synthetic processes, and it is a key nutrient in the synthesis of red

blood cells. The pubertal growth spurt sees a major (25%) increase in blood volume.

Most minerals and trace elements accumulate within the body in large amounts during adolescence due to increasing body mass and stature. For most of these minerals and elements, there are physiological adaptations in place to maximize absorption and bioavailability. Among the minerals, those of particular significance during the adolescent years are calcium, iron and zinc. Zinc is an essential nutrient for protein and nucleic acid synthesis and is a cofactor for many metabolically important enzymes. In adults, most zinc within the body is locked into muscle and bone. As these tissues gain in mass during adolescence, the accrual of zinc is at a maximal rate, and the biochemical measurements of zinc status in body fluids or hair often show declines as it is redistributed to bone and muscle. Poor zinc status can have important consequences, as zinc deficiency is associated with impaired growth, reduced appetite and delayed skeletal and sexual maturation.

The absorption of calcium from the diet (around 35–40%) during adolescence does not appear to be markedly greater than that at other stages of life. As described earlier in this chapter, bone mineralization is at a maximal rate during puberty, and hence, this is a peak period in terms of calcium requirements. The high reference nutrient intake set for the adolescent years (Table 7.2) reflects this accrual of bone mineral. Optimal use of calcium obtained within the diet is dependent on the supply of other nutrients, including vitamin D, phosphorus, protein, magnesium and ascorbate. Magnesium and phosphorus are also important skeletal minerals. The ratio of calcium to phosphorus in the diet becomes important at low intakes of calcium, when excessive intake of phosphorus leads to oversecretion of parathyroid hormone. This promotes release of calcium from bone. Ascorbate is an essential cofactor for the action of prolyl hydroxylase, which converts proline to hydroxyproline. This uncommon amino acid is incorporated into collagen, which is the major protein within bone, providing the basic fibrous structure into which calcium and other minerals are deposited.

Adolescence sees an increase in requirements for iron. This increase is driven partly by the increase in blood volume but mainly by the increase in lean body mass and the synthesis of the muscle protein myoglobin. The increase in lean mass is greater in boys than in girls, but the iron requirements of girls increase to a greater extent (Table 7.2) to compensate for blood losses associated with the onset of menstruation. Poor iron status is associated with iron deficiency anaemia, reduced ability to exercise and impaired cognitive abilities. Iron status is influenced by a variety of other nutrients and components of food (Figure 7.6). Phenolic compounds and phytates reduce absorption of non-haem iron, while ascorbate enhances absorption. It is desirable for adolescents to maintain high intakes of dairy products as a rich source of calcium, but as calcium inhibits uptake of iron, this can have a negative impact upon iron status. Individuals with poor vitamin A intakes will tend to develop problems with iron status. Vitamin A deficiency increases the occurrence of infectious disease, and the acute-phase response results in the sequestration of iron within the liver, reducing availability for the physiological processes associated with puberty.

7.5 Nutritional intakes in adolescence

Adolescents are frequently identified as being at risk of undernutrition, largely because their very high nutrient demands often appear incompatible with their range of preferred foods and patterns of eating. Surveys from all over the developed world identify high levels of potential nutrient deficiency. Interpretation of such surveys should, however, be very cautious. Nutritional surveys carried out at a national level often use estimates of intakes carried out over just a 24- or 48-hour period. These will rarely provide an accurate picture of nutritional status in the population and will be particularly

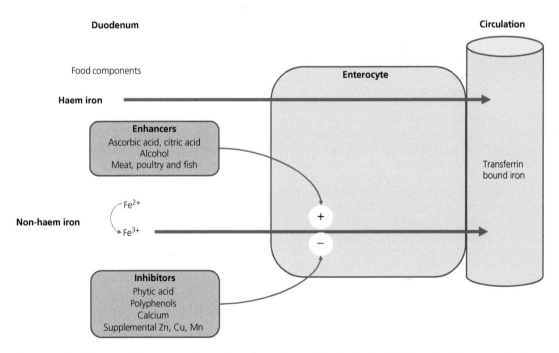

Figure 7.6 The absorption of iron. Haem iron and non-haem iron are absorbed in the duodenum by different mechanisms, and transported across enterocytes for binding to transferrin in circulation. Absorption of non-haem iron is sensitive to inhibitors and enhancers present in food.

misleading if the intention is to estimate the prevalence of low micronutrient intakes (Mackerras and Rutishauser, 2005). Even the well-designed National Diet and Nutrition Surveys (NDNS) carried out periodically in the UK (collecting data over a four-day period) may have problems with the validity and reliability of the data that are generated, due to issues of under-reporting. The disparity between estimates of intake and actual prevalence of nutrient deficiency disease perhaps best illustrates the perils and pitfalls of such survey data. In years 1 to 4 of the NDNS, for example, 46% of British girls aged 11–14 and 50% of girls aged 15–18 years were found to consume iron at a level below the LRNI (Bates *et al.*, 2014). However, assessment of iron status from blood samples showed the prevalence of iron deficiency anaemia (based on low haemoglobin and plasma ferritin) to be only 4.9%. Accurate estimation of the intakes of some micronutrients requires food records gathered over several weeks, with estimate ranging from around seven days for minerals and up to one month for some of the vitamins. Biochemical markers of micronutrient status are far more useful, but are challenging to obtain from children and adolescents.

In most developed countries, surveys indicate that adolescents consume adequate amounts of energy but that this energy is generally delivered through excessive consumption of fat and sugar. Years 1–4 of the UK NDNS (Bates *et al.*, 2014) reported that mean energy intake of adolescents was below the estimated average requirement but this age group had the lowest consumption of fruit and the highest consumption of chocolate, sweets, pasta, rice and pizza. Seventy-eight percent of the adolescents reported having consumed soft drinks within the four-day period and sweetened beverages provided 40% of non-milk extrinsic sugars. In Years 7 and 8 of NDNS (Roberts *et al.*, 2018), only 5% of adolescents were found to be consuming free sugars at or below the newly recommended maximum of 5% total energy. Only 10% of boys and 15% of girls consumed recommended amounts of dietary fibre (Roberts *et al.*, 2018). The HELENA study, which considered the diets of over 3000 adolescents in 10 European cities, also reported that energy intakes were in line with recommendations but that energy requirements were not met through fruit and vegetables, milk or dairy products (Diethelm *et al.*, 2012). While these foods were consumed well below population recommendations, intakes of saturated fats were high and polyunsaturated fatty acid intakes were considerably below age-specific references (Diethelm *et al.*, 2014).

Micronutrient intakes of adolescents are frequently identified as being below dietary reference values or population guidelines. This concern is illustrated by the UK NDNS, which showed high prevalence of intake below the LRNI for vitamin A, riboflavin, calcium, magnesium, potassium, zinc, selenium and iodine among both boys and girls (Roberts *et al.*, 2018). Low iodine status was verified biochemically (urinary iodine <50 µg/l). The diets of 11–18-year-old girls appeared particularly poor with more than a quarter being at risk of deficiency of magnesium (50% consumed below LRNI), selenium (45% consumed below LRNI) and zinc (27% consumed below LRNI); 9% of girls had haemoglobin concentration below the threshold of 12 g/dl and 24% had low serum ferritin. Similar concerns have been raised by surveys in Australia (Gallagher *et al.*, 2014) and the United States (Division of Laboratory Sciences, 2012) and HELENA (Diethelm *et al.*, 2014), with low intakes of iron, vitamin A, folate, iodine, calcium and magnesium emerging as a consistent theme.

7.5.1 Factors that influence food choice

Although reliable estimates of the prevalence of undernutrition with respect to specific micronutrients may be difficult to establish, it is clear that the diet of the typical adolescent does not comply with guidelines for healthy eating and may not deliver the full profile of nutrient requirements. This is of concern at a life stage when optimal nutrition is necessary for rapid growth and development. The reasons contributing to poor nutrition need to be explored. Suboptimal nutrition partly stems from the preferred range of foods that are consumed by adolescents and by the sometimes erratic meal patterns that are followed by this increasingly independent group of young people.

The range of influences upon adolescents' food choices is broad and varied (Figure 7.7). While current health status and other health behaviours are influential, food choices and eating behaviours are also determined by environmental factors and personal factors. Environmental factors include the influences of parents and family, socioeconomic factors, the influence of peers and exposure to media and sociocultural expectations. Personal factors include the values and beliefs of the individual (e.g. religious or ethical viewpoints), emotional and physiological needs and perceptions of body image. Several of these factors may interact with each other to influence behaviour. For example, dissatisfaction with appearance and body weight is common among adolescents (50% of girls and 20% of boys; Hill, 2002). Part of this dissatisfaction comes from

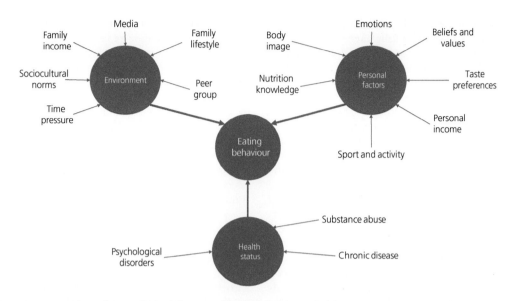

Figure 7.7 Factors that influence the food choices and eating behaviours of adolescents.

the exposure of adolescents to images in magazines and television programmes that depict thinness as the epitome of beauty and a state to aspire to. Girls in their mid-teens are particularly influenced by reported material depicting celebrities who are praised for weight loss and thinness and ridiculed for overweight or physical flaws. Thus, society shapes adolescents views of their own body size and shape and may prompt engagement in restrictive dietary practices (Hill, 2006).

Adolescence is in all ways a period of transition, both physically and emotionally. Food becomes an element of the developing autonomy of adolescents, and young people increasingly take control over the purchasing and preparation of meals. This can become embroiled in the general rebellion associated with the adolescent years, and poor food choices (fast convenience foods) may be particularly pleasurable because of their labelling as 'bad' foods by parents and other authorities (Hill, 2002). The main influences on the food choices of adolescents are, however, obvious ones. With appetite drives high to meet physiological demands, adolescents are strongly influenced by feelings of hunger and select foods that taste good, have favourable aroma and appearance and are familiar to them from earlier childhood exposures (Neumark-Sztainer et al., 1999).

Adolescents tend to feel constrained in terms of time, as they have to integrate their strong desire to sleep in late in the mornings with heavy workloads at school, busy social programmes, part-time jobs and sporting activities. This promotes preferences for foods that are readily available and that are easy and fast to prepare (Neumark-Sztainer et al., 1999). Adolescents who are taking responsibility for finding their own food for at least part of the day often find it hard to access more healthful alternatives (O'Dea, 2003). Outlets that sell high-fat, high-sugar fast foods can act as focal points for adolescents to meet with friends. There are some claims that poor food selections may be an element of achieving integration with the peer group and fulfilling social expectations, but the evidence to support this is not strong. Correlations of adolescents' food choices with parental preferences are considerably stronger than correlations with preferences of best friends (Hill, 2002).

While convenience and hedonic factors are strong factors that determine food choices, there are other factors that are of low importance to adolescents as a population group, but those may be major influences for some individuals with the population. These include the desire to enhance health or sporting performance, compliance with religious or family rules pertaining to food and issues relating to body image and influences of the media (Neumark-Sztainer et al., 1999).

7.5.2 Food consumed out of the home

While younger children will predominantly consume food in a supervised environment such as home or school, where food is purchased and prepared by adults, adolescents increasingly take responsibility for this themselves. Generally speaking, adolescents have some income that they can spend on food, and they begin to consume a considerable proportion of their daily energy and nutrient intakes in school or college, from vending machines, in snack bars, in fast-food restaurants, in sandwich shops or in the homes of their friends. Although school meals are increasingly being formulated to comply with nationally set standards (see Section 6.3.2), foods purchased from other sources tend to be of lower nutritional quality and of higher energy density. The HELENA study found that 7% of adolescents in their European sample bought their lunches out of school, in shops and fast-food restaurants. These children had higher intakes of sweets and bread (Müller *et al.*, 2013). The autonomy of adolescents in selection and preparation of foods may therefore be a determining factor leading to low micronutrient intakes.

Fast-food restaurants aim much of their marketing at adolescents and, indeed, a high proportion of their workforces have tended to be within this age group. Sometimes, these workers receive some of their remuneration in the form of free food (French *et al.*, 2001). Intakes of foods from fast-food restaurants increased rapidly over the last decades of the twentieth century and remain high in the early twenty-first century despite growing awareness of the importance of nutrition for health. Estimates of access to such establishments by adolescents vary considerably. The UK NDNS rolling programme years 1–6 found that 28.8% of adolescents consumed fast food once or twice per week (Taher *et al.*, 2019). A sample of 3030 US adolescents found that 35% of white, 54% of Black and 50% of Hispanic adolescents consumed fast food more than twice a week. This was partly driven by a lifestyle in which sleep quality was poor and fast food displaced breakfast (Mathew *et al.*, 2020). Winpenny *et al.*, (2020) followed a cohort of US adolescents into their early 30s and found that their mean fast-food consumption was 1.88 times per week, falling away when subjects found full-time jobs or became parents. A survey of 54 low and middle-income countries found that consumption of fast food is high among adolescents there too, with on average 55% of adolescents consuming fast food at least one day a week and 10.3% four to seven times a week. In South East Asia, consumption was particularly high, with Thailand having the greatest proportion of adolescents consuming fast food four to seven times a week (43.3%; Li *et al.*, 2020).

Consumption of food from takeaway outlets greatly increases the energy density of the diet and intakes of fat, sugar and sodium. Good sources of micronutrients such as grains, fruit, vegetables, legumes, seeds, milk and dairy products are displaced

from the diet by fast foods (Paeratakul *et al.*, 2003). The quality of the diet of adolescents is significantly reduced by regular consumption of takeaway foods (Taher *et al.*, 2019). The amount and type of foods consumed outside the home is dependent on socioeconomic status. While the main foods consumed by UK adolescents out of home and school are soft drinks, chocolate, chips and meat pies (Palla *et al.*, 2020), those of higher socioeconomic status are more likely to buy hot beverages in cafes and restaurants, while those of lower to mid-socioeconomic status buy more soft drinks and fast food (Cornelsen *et al.*, 2019). Adolescents will be more likely to buy food outside the home if they have an independent income, for example associated with a part-time job.

The convenience and time-saving attributes of snack foods and items from fast-food restaurants are a major attraction to busy adolescents, but the drivers of a fast-food-rich diet are more complex. The ease of access to fast-food restaurants is an important factor with several studies showing greater consumption by children who live in areas with a high density of outlets (Laxer and Janssen, 2014). Lower socioeconomic status and personal food preferences increase the likelihood of regular consumption, as does an unhealthy home eating environment (Bauer *et al.*, 2009). Strong maternal support for healthy eating and concerns about health and weight reduce consumption.

7.5.3 Meal skipping and snacking

In keeping with their increasing income and access to food outside the home, adolescents are the population group who are most likely to have erratic eating habits, with missed meals and high intakes of snack foods. Adolescents have strong appetites and tend to eat outside meal times in order to fulfil feelings of hunger and cravings for specific snack items (Neumark-Sztainer *et al.*, 1999). Skipping meals can impact significantly upon nutrient intakes, particularly as the meal that is most frequently missed is breakfast. Where the normal breakfast foods are fortified cereals with milk, this can produce marked reductions in micronutrient intakes. Some studies have estimated that up to one third of adolescents regularly miss breakfast. The major reason underpinning this behaviour appears to be a lack of time and low levels of hunger on rising in the morning (Shaw, 1998).

Breakfast is not the only meal that may be missed. In some families, adolescents either opt out of family meals or, if in the position of providing their own meals for at least some part of the day, will choose to adopt a 'grazing' pattern of snacking throughout the day. Breakfast is the most frequently missed meal of the day, followed by lunch and an evening meal (Prendergast *et al.*, 2016). Girls are more likely to miss the evening meal or lunch, while boys more frequently skip breakfast. The impact of missing main meals is to displace food intake towards snacks and sugar-sweetened beverages, generally purchased outside the home. Medin *et al.* (2019) found that skipping lunch tended to slightly reduce the total energy intake of Norwegian adolescents, but increased their intakes of fat and free sugars. The drivers of meal skipping have been attributed to cost of food, weight control and engagement with media (Custers and Van den Bulck, 2010; Prendergast *et al.*, 2016). A study of 12–16-year olds found that 11.8% skipped meals to watch television, 10.5% to play computer games and 8.2% to read books. All these activities are sedentary, reducing energy expenditure and, if accompanied by an increase in high-energy density snacks and drinks, would present a risk factor for becoming overweight.

The literature suggests that not all aspects of adolescent snacking are negative. Sebastian *et al.* (2008) reported that among US adolescents, snacking contributed around 25% of the daily energy intake and 43% of added sugar intake and was associated with greater total energy intake and higher intakes of carbohydrate. The contribution of snack foods to energy intake had increased markedly between 1978 and 2006 (Figure 7.8). However, high snack consumers also consumed more ascorbate and less protein and fat than adolescents with lower snack consumption. Intakes of milk and fruit were actually

increased by snacking, suggesting that awareness of healthy eating messages may influence some aspects of snacking behaviour. Breakfast cereals are a popular in-home snack food item, improving nutrient density for frequent snack consumers.

7.6 Potential problems with nutrition

7.6.1 Dieting and weight control

Restriction of dietary intake or other actions that can promote weight loss are commonplace behaviours among some groups of adolescents. Most surveys show that girls are more likely to indulge in such behaviours than boys but that 20–50% of adolescents of either sex will attempt some sort of weight loss behaviour (Neumark-Sztainer and Hannan, 2000), although the World Health Organization Collaborative Health Behaviours in School-Aged Children Study (Quick *et al.*, 2014) of 40 countries suggested a lower prevalence (Figure 7.9). Adolescents are prone to adopting dieting behaviour as a response to the major changes in body size and shape associated with puberty. Other influences include exposure to media items about body weight and dieting, parental concerns about weight gain, teasing from other children about weight and aspiration to share the dieting experiences of peers.

Some restrictive practices may improve the quality of the diet; for example, increasing intakes of fruits and vegetables in place of energy-dense snacks. These behaviours are more the norm for

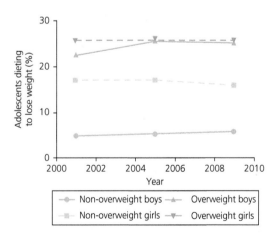

Figure 7.8 Dieting behaviours are commonplace among adolescents, including those who are not overweight. *Source:* reproduced with permission from Quick *et al.* (2014). © Nature Publishing Group.

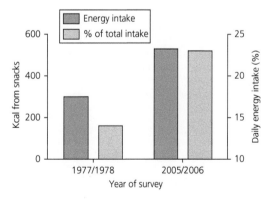

Figure 7.9 Snack foods comprise a significant proportion of daily intakes of energy, sugars and total and saturated fats among adolescents. This proportion increased between the 1977/1978 and 2005/2006 National Health and Nutrition Examination Surveys in the United States. *Source:* reproduced with permission from Sebastian *et al.* (2008). © Elsevier.

younger adolescents. Later in puberty, girls, in particular, develop increased concerns about their body image and become more likely to restrict weight gain in an unhealthy manner (Abraham, 2003). Unhealthy practices related to weight loss include meal skipping, use of dieting drugs, fasting, consumption of food substitutes (e.g. slimming shakes) and smoking. These can impact in a negative way upon nutritional status, particularly with respect to calcium and other micronutrients, and are associated with slower rates of growth, psychological disorders, and poor physical health (Neumark-Sztainer and Hannan, 2000). Longer-term health may also be compromised. Reduced bone mineralization and lower attained peak bone mass may, for example, increase risk of osteoporosis later in life. Interestingly, adolescents who dieted were shown by Neumark-Sztainer et al. (2006) to have threefold greater risk of overweight at a five-year follow-up. Adolescents who indulge in dieting behaviours may be eight times more likely to go on to develop eating disorders than those who do not diet (Neumark-Sztainer and Hannan, 2000).

Adolescents are immature in their thinking and understanding of the world. They are particularly sensitive to their need to fit in with their peers and conform to local cultural norms. These norms change over time and, as they shift, adolescent behaviours and their drivers shift with them. In contemporary western society, attitudes to what is a normal or desirable body shape for boys and girls are strongly driven by the media and so adolescents expectations of how they should look are shaped by what they see on internet and broadcast media. Dissatisfaction with their own body shape and size can lead to depression and behaviours that are believed to control body weight, including exercise, skipping meals, smoking and misuse of drugs (Weng et al., 2021; Sutin et al., 2020). As discussed in Research Highlight 7.1, weight stigma may be a factor that pressures adolescents to try to lose weight. Victimization by peers over appearance is a factor that prompts dieting behaviours (Sutin et al., 2020) and in some cases the victimization comes from the child's own family. Eisenberg et al. (2019) studied adolescents from immigrant families in Minnesota

Research Highlight 7.1 The impact of weight stigma on adolescent health and wellbeing.

The term 'weight stigma' is used to describe the discriminatory behaviours and stereotyping experienced by individuals in relation to their actual or perceived overweight. Weight stigma is built into the environment in contemporary western culture, where thinness is idealized and obesity is highlighted as a major public health concern. Weight stigma may be experienced by adolescents in the form of conscious teasing and bullying or as an unconscious bias exhibited by peers, family, health professionals and teachers. For example, Finn et al. (2020) provided teachers with a piece of assessment to grade accompanying the same piece of work with a picture of either an overweight or normal weight child. Teachers awarded lower grades when the work was believed to have been prepared by an overweight child, indicating an unconscious anti-fat bias. Unconscious anti-fat bias is also reported in adolescent groups (Cullin, 2020), a fact which threatens to undermine relationships between overweight children and their peers. Interestingly, this bias is greater in populations where overweight is more prevalent. Parents can also be a source of weight stigma, which is more prominent in households where parents express weight concerns to their children (Pudney et al., 2019). Weight stigma can be internalized by the person who experiences it, leading to a negative self-image and associated psychological disorders.

The consequences of weight stigma for adolescents are significant, shaping both psychological and physical development. Adolescents who experience high levels of weight stigma suffer low self-esteem, high levels of body dissatisfaction, more stress and depression, poor sleep patterns, worse academic performance and suicidal thoughts (Puhl and Lessard, 2020; Wang et al., 2021). When weight stigma is experienced by adolescents who are already sensitive to their own weight, it may result in a move towards unhealthy behaviours to control weight. Simone et al., (2019) followed a group of adolescents over 10 years and found that those who had been engaging with weight control measures at baseline and had experienced weight stigma were more likely to go on to use alcohol, cigarettes and cannabis.

While weight stigma experiences can prompt adolescents to adopt unhealthy weight control behaviours and lead to the development of eating disorders, it is also noted that it can prompt weight gain. Among Chinese adolescents, high exposure to weight stigma was associated with more emotional eating and uncontrolled eating (Wang et al., 2020). An 8.5-year follow-up of 11–12-year-olds found that high levels of weight stigma were associated with a 91% greater gain in fat mass and a 33% greater increase of body mass index than were observed in children who were not exposed to weight stigma (Schvey et al., 2019).

The unconscious and conscious bias against overweight that is present in society is a powerful force acting upon the immature minds of young people. Strategies that seek to tackle the rising prevalence of overweight and obesity in children require underpinning actions to limit stigmatization of overweight children in the environments that should provide a place of safety and support, namely home, school and in health services.

and found that depression and unhealthy weight control behaviours were in part driven by family members teasing them about their weight. An increased prevalence of dieting behaviours in the UK, rising from 6.8% of adolescents trying to lose weight in 1986, to 44% in 2015, was suggested to reflect an unintended consequence of the societal drive to combat the rising prevalence of childhood obesity (Solmi *et al.*, 2020).

7.6.2 The teenage vegetarian

Vegetarianism is a pattern of diet that has increased in popularity in most developed countries since the 1960s. There are many forms of vegetarian diet ranging from the semi-vegetarian to variations on the lacto-ovo vegetarian dietary pattern and to the more restrictive vegan patterns (Table 7.4). Adolescents are the population group most likely to make the switch from a mixed diet to a vegetarian diet. Girls are significantly more likely than boys to become vegetarians and estimates from the UK, Canada and Australia suggest that while veganism is extremely rare, around 8–10% of adolescent girls

Table 7.4 Vegetarian dietary practices.

Vegetarian diet	Practice defined as
Semi-vegetarian	Diet based on plant material but including some meat products
Pollotarian	A semi-vegetarian practice in which poultry but no mammalian meat is consumed
Pescetarian	A semi-vegetarian practice in which fish and shellfish are consumed
Pollo-pescetarian	A semi-vegetarian practice in which poultry, fish and shellfish are consumed; no mammalian meat is consumed
Ovo-vegetarian	All meat and dairy products are avoided but eggs are consumed
Lacto-vegetarian	All meat and eggs are avoided but dairy products are consumed
Ovo-lacto vegetarian	All meat is avoided but eggs and dairy products are consumed
Macrobiotic	Only whole grains and beans are consumed
Vegan	No animal products (including honey) or refined foods that might have been tested or processed with animal material are consumed
Fruitarian	Only fruit, nuts and seeds or material that can be obtained without harming plants are consumed
Raw vegan	Only fresh and uncooked fruit, nuts, seeds and vegetables are consumed
Jain vegetarian	No meat, eggs, honey or root vegetables are consumed but dairy products are acceptable

and 1–2% of boys (15–18 years) follow a lacto-ovo vegetarian diet. Pollo-vegetarianism and semi-vegetarianism may be considerably more common.

As expected, given the lower energy density of the diet, vegetarian adolescents typically have a lower body mass index and waist circumference and better metabolic profile. Segovia-Siapco *et al.* (2019b) reported that there was a strong correlation between intake of animal protein and both central adiposity and fat mass in vegetarian adolescents. Vegetarian adolescents in the cohort consumed less than half the animal protein intake of their omnivorous peers (Segova-Siapco *et al.*, 2019a). There are no long-term follow-up studies to confirm the future benefit of this, but being leaner during adolescence makes it less likely that the individual will be overweight in adult life (see Section 6.4.3.2). As with all forms of restrictive dietary practice in adolescence, there are concerns that vegetarianism could have a negative impact upon nutritional status and the capacity to maintain optimal rates of growth and development. Adolescents are likely to experiment with diets and to make unplanned and abrupt shifts from a diet including meat to some form of vegetarianism, or even veganism, without any informed guidance. This can increase the risk that the dietary pattern adopted will fail to deliver an adequate balance of nutrients.

The low digestibility of plant foods and the poor bioavailability of minerals from plant sources (particularly with high phytate intake) mean that intakes of protein, zinc and iron may be of concern in vegetarians (Amit, 2010). This is of major importance at a time of rapid growth. Plant foods are rich in phytic acid, which inhibits absorption of iron and calcium, and oxalates, which inhibit calcium uptake. The bioavailability of iron from a vegetarian diet is only 10% compared with 18% from a mixed diet (Hunt, 2003). An 80% increase in intake is therefore required to meet requirements (Amit, 2010), which is challenging without supplementation or careful dietary planning. Vegetarian girls were found to be six times more likely than omnivores to have low haemoglobin concentrations and were three times more likely to have reduced iron stores in the study of Thane *et al.* (2003). Krajcovicoca-Kuduckova *et al.* (1997) also reported low poor status in vegetarian adolescents compared with omnivores, and serum ferritin concentrations were lower in vegetarians studied by Gorczyca *et al.* (2013). Calcium uptake is poor from many plant sources, but some such as soya beans, broccoli and kale have relatively high bioavailability (Weaver *et al.*, 1999). Inclusion of dairy produce alongside such foods in the vegetarian diet should maintain healthy calcium status. In the absence of dairy produce, the vegan adolescent will need to take supplements of calcium and vitamin B12 (Amit, 2010).

Notwithstanding these concerns, the dietary intakes of vegetarian adolescents are generally considered healthier by virtue of their greater consumption of fruit and vegetables and complex carbohydrates. It is also reported that vegetarian adolescents are less likely to smoke, consume alcohol or use drugs (Robinson-O'Brien *et al.*, 2009). Vegetarians are less likely than omnivores to be overweight and obese. However, there is a greater prevalence of underweight, and vegetarian girls are more likely to suffer mental health disturbances and require medication for depression (Baines *et al.*, 2007). Forestell *et al.* (2012) reported that vegetarians have less food neophobia and experiment with a wider range of new food experiences than omnivores. However, their dietary choices were more motivated by weight control, and they were more likely to restrict their diet in an unhealthy manner. A vegetarian diet can be used as a cover to hide more serious restriction of the diet and disordered eating (Barrack *et al.*, 2019). A comparison of young women with eating disorders and unaffected controls found that those with eating disorders were almost five times more likely to have been vegetarian at some point, and four times more likely to currently follow a vegetarian diet (Barddone-Cone *et al.*, 2012). Controlling weight was the main reason why a vegetarian diet had been adopted. Vegetarian adolescents are also more likely to engage in binge eating with loss of control, supporting the idea that the vegetarian diet is a proxy for increased risk of disordered eating (Robinson-O'Brien *et al.*, 2009) and it may be a particular risk factor for orthorexia nervosa (Brytek-Matera, 2020; Section 7.6.4).

Vegetarian girls may exhibit problems with reproductive function. Vegetarianism is associated with longer cycle length, greater prevalence of amenorrhoea, anovulation and luteal phase defects. This may be partly explained by reduced body fatness and leptin secretion but may also relate to hypothalamic control over sex hormone secretion (Griffith and Omar, 2003). Vegetarians secrete lower levels of luteinizing hormone, even if cycles are regular. Diets rich in fibre and low in fat alter the profile of sex steroids that are synthesized within the ovary and increase cycle length (Goldin *et al.*, 1994).

7.6.3 Sport and physical activity

The impact of physical activity upon health and wellbeing is overwhelmingly positive at any stage of life. Adolescence is no exception to this, and

adolescents who are more active will be protected against overweight and obesity and will have enhanced skeletal growth. Exercise benefits bone mineralization, for example, with particularly strong effects in trabecular regions (Specker, 2006). Often, the diets of adolescents who are involved in sports are of higher quality than those of less active peers (D'Alessandro *et al.*, 2007). However, where levels of physical activity become more intense over longer and more frequent periods, such as in adolescents who become involved in organized sports or dance activities, this can impact upon energy balance, nutritional status, growth and development in an adverse manner.

Intense physical activity will, by definition, increase demands for energy, and the sporting teenager will need to consume more energy sources than a sedentary individual to maintain growth and sustain their performance. Requirements for protein may also be increased as physical activity will promote the deposition of muscle mass over and above that, which normally occurs in growth. This is most marked in adolescents who partake in events that are weight-class dependent, that is, where the optimal performance is associated with a highly muscular but lightweight body (e.g. martial arts and gymnastics) and endurance sports (swimming, long-distance running). Swimmers, for example, may increase their protein requirements from 0.73 g/kg (girls) to between 1.2 and 2.32 g/kg body weight per day (Petrie *et al.*, 2004). High-level physical activity also increases demands for micronutrients. Demand for most vitamins follows energy intake and use. Mineral requirements will increase as calcium, iron, magnesium, sodium, phosphorus and trace elements are incorporated into lean tissues and the skeleton as they grow under the influence of activity. Electrolyte and fluid status may also be perturbed by participation in sports.

Where physical activity is at a level that does not exert consistently high nutritional demands, there is unlikely to be any adverse impact upon physiological processes. Certain sports, however, particularly gymnastics, dance and the weight-class sports, can lead to delayed maturation. These activities often result in negative energy balance as individuals attempt to develop a lighter physique with greater muscular strength (Roemmich *et al.*, 2001). Energy deficit, poor nutritional status and reduced body fatness are particularly associated with amenorrhoea and menstrual cycle abnormalities in adolescent girls involved in intense sport. Menstrual cycle disorders were reported by 4.7% of Finnish athletes aged 14–16 and 38.7% of those aged 18–20 years (Ravi *et al.*, 2021). Fifty three percent of elite Chinese athletes (mean age 20 years) had amenorrhoea in the study of Meng *et al.* (2020), and Czajkowska *et al.* (2019) found that menarche was delayed and periods more severe (pain and heavy bleeding) in rhythmic gymnasts who participated in high-level sport before their first menstruation. The loss of the permissive effects of leptin on the hypothalamic–pituitary–ovarian axis as body fat declines may largely explain these problems. Hormones such as cortisol, which is secreted at higher levels during activity, may also suppress hypothalamic production of GnRH. Failure to produce oestrogen can impact upon growth, particularly of the skeleton, as oestrogen normally increases secretion of growth hormone and IGF-1. Only regular, intense activity will produce these effects. Lower levels of activity actually promote growth by stimulating growth hormone production.

The worst-case scenario associated with high-level sport in adolescence has become known as the 'female athlete triad' (Figure 7.10). This is noted where involvement in sport and exercise is at a high or elite level, particularly if the activity is associated with having a strictly controlled body weight that stems predominantly from a high proportion of lean body mass (Brunet, 2005). Aesthetic athletes (gymnasts, dancers, cheerleaders) are particularly at risk as their activity is in part judged on appearance. Long-distance runners are also at risk as an exceptionally lean body is advantageous for performance. A lean physique is generally achieved and maintained through the combination of activity itself and controlled eating. If the control over diet tips into disordered eating (see Section 7.6.4), the first

element of the triad is in place. This can also occur due to an individual's lack of awareness of energy requirements (Thein-Nissenbaum, 2013). The second element is amenorrhoea, which is a direct consequence of low body fat and loss of the stimulatory effect of leptin upon the hypothalamic–pituitary–ovarian axis. While amenorrhoea is seen in less than 5% of the general population during adolescence, 28% of aesthetic athletes and 65% of long-distance runners report menstrual irregularity (Thein-Nissenbaum, 2013). The third element is osteoporosis or osteopenia, which stems from inadequate bone mineralization. This will not only be mainly a result of the endocrine immaturity and suppressed reproductive cycling of the individual but can also be related to calcium intake. Avoidance of dairy products as a means of weight control is a common feature of this condition. While exercise is known to increase BMD in adolescents (see Section 7.4), young high-level female athletes have been reported to have low bone mineral and are prone to stress fractures. Emerging evidence suggests that this persists into adulthood as the lost bone mass cannot be replaced (Thein-Nissenbaum, 2013).

7.6.4 Eating disorders

Eating disorders are psychiatric conditions that manifest as extremely abnormal patterns of food intake and weight control. A number of such conditions have been identified, of which the best characterized are anorexia nervosa and bulimia nervosa. These conditions, together with binge eating disorder and the spectrum of conditions that fail to meet the diagnostic criteria for anorexia and bulimia

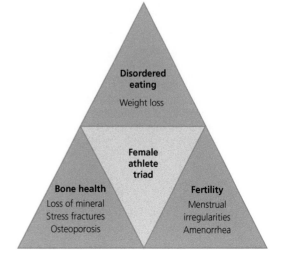

Figure 7.10 The female athlete triad is a syndrome of disordered eating resulting in reproductive and skeletal abnormalities. The syndrome is associated with high-level participation in sports that emphasize body size and appearance.

(partial eating disorders, eating disorders not otherwise specified and orthorexia nervosa; see Research Highlight 7.2), are believed to lie on a broad continuum of eating behaviours extending from normal eating to behaviours promoting underweight (including normal dieting) and to behaviours promoting severe overweight (Chamay-Weber *et al.*, 2005). All eating disorders are most common in young women and often first manifest during the adolescent years. Eating disorders, particularly anorexia, are among the major causes of death among adolescents in developed countries.

7.6.4.1 Anorexia nervosa

Anorexia nervosa is characterized by the adoption of a pattern of eating and physical activity that promotes severe weight loss. Individuals with anorexia generally have a highly distorted image of their own body size and shape and an intense fear of becoming fat or gaining weight. As a consequence, they impose a starvation regimen upon themselves. The full diagnostic criteria used for assessment of anorexia are shown in Table 7.5. Individuals with anorexia may adopt a purely restrictive dietary pattern, with minimal food intake, or may be of a bingeing–purging type whereby occasional episodes of excessive food intake are compensated through the use of

laxatives, diuretics, extreme exercise or techniques to induce vomiting. All of these behaviours surrounding food are often compounded by the presence of obsessions with food, ritualistic calorie counting, food hoarding and collection of food recipes (Abraham, 2003).

Individuals with anorexia undergo extreme weight loss and, if in adolescence, a failure of growth and delay of sexual maturation. Muscle wasting occurs, along with loss of subcutaneous fat. The body often grows a layer of downy hair (lanugo), and the individual develops gastrointestinal and renal disturbances. Electrolyte imbalances are common and result from dehydration and losses associated with purging behaviours. Treatment involves hospitalization and nutritional support to promote weight gain and metabolic stabilization. Psychotherapy is necessary to resolve the underlying condition. Getting individuals to treatment is challenging, as anorexia sufferers will often deny that they have a problem. As a result, mortality rates can be as high as 20%.

Anorexia is most common in women and is generally diagnosed between the ages of 15 and 23 years. The average age of onset is around 17 years. Anorexia is also seen in males, who account for around 10% of cases. Estimates of the prevalence of

Research Highlight 7.2 Orthorexia nervosa: a new eating disorder.

A number of eating disorders other than anorexia nervosa and bulimia nervosa are recognized by clinicians. These include binge-eating disorder, avoidant/restrictive food intake disorder and rumination syndrome. Orthorexia nervosa has been proposed as a new disorder under the eating disorders umbrella. While it is not formally recognized as a disorder covered by the *Diagnostic and Statistical Manual of Mental Disorders* (American Psychological Association, 2000), it is identified increasingly in clinical settings and there is a growing research literature on the subject. Orthorexia nervosa is characterized by an obsession with healthy eating. The sufferer becomes so fixated on healthy eating that they restrict their diet to an extreme, lose weight and develop associated medical complications. Orthorexia nervosa sufferers have a strong belief in nutrition as medicine and will compulsively check ingredients lists on foods and show and obsessive interest in the health qualities of what other people are eating (Cheshire *et al.*, 2020). They may be distressed if healthy foods are not available to them, be disgusted in the presence of unhealthy food and may exhibit body image concerns.

One of the key difficulties in studying orthorexia nervosa is the lack of strong diagnostic criteria. There are a number of scales to determine orthorexia nervosa, but none have robust psychometric properties (Opitz *et al.*, 2020). Many features of orthorexia nervosa are similar to anorexia nervosa, but with a stronger obsessive-compulsive element. Unlike anorexia the distribution of orthorexia nervosa appears to span all age groups, although one Polish study suggested a greater prevalence among 11–13-year olds (Lucka *et al.*, 2019). Estimates of prevalence range from 1% (Dunn *et al.*, 2017) to 8% (Koven and Abry, 2015). In contrast to anorexia nervosa, there is little difference in frequency between males and females (Strahler, 2019). Risk is increased in individuals who have a high level of nutrition knowledge and those involved in sporting activities. Young people with a strong sporting lifestyle may develop orthorexic characteristics because they are counting calories while in-training or because they feel guilt at missing training, or at underperformance (Kiss-Leizer *et al.*, 2019).

Whether orthorexia nervosa is classified as an independent eating disorder distinct from anorexia remains to be seen, but it is clear that growing knowledge about nutrition, access to information about the composition of food, availability of foods that are free from specific components (e.g. gluten or lactose) can fuel behaviours among young people. These may start as reasonable and appropriate lifestyle changes, which trip over into unhealthy actions in those with an already obsessive personality.

Table 7.5 Diagnostic criteria for eating disorders.

Disease	Criteria
Anorexia nervosa	Refusal to maintain body weight at or above minimally normal for age and height (<85% of expected weight) Intense fear of gaining weight or becoming fat, even though underweight Disturbance of the perception of body weight or shape; denial of seriousness of current underweight Amenorrhoea (absence of three consecutive menstrual periods)
Bulimia nervosa	Recurrent episodes of binge eating characterized by both of the following: • Eating an amount of food in a discrete period of time that is larger than most people would achieve in the same time, under similar circumstances • A sense of lack of control over eating during the bingeing episode Recurrent inappropriate behaviour to compensate for eating in order to control weight gain (e.g. use of laxatives, enemas or diuretics or excessive exercise) Binge eating and compensatory behaviour occurring at least twice a week for 3 months No undue influence of body shape and weight on behaviour The disturbance does not occur excessively during periods of anorexia nervosa

From *Diagnostic and Statistical Manual of Mental Disorders* (American Psychological Association, 2000).

the condition vary considerably, but 0.3–0.5% of the young female population are likely to be affected (Hoek and van Hoeken, 2003). The incidence of anorexia has not varied significantly since the 1930s in the United States, but in European countries, it appeared to increase between 1935 and the early 1980s. Risk may be higher among girls and young women who engage in particular activities. Arcelus *et al.* (2014) reported that anorexia occurs in 4% of ballet dancers.

The causes of anorexia are complex and not fully understood. The condition has always been more common in girls, particularly white girls from middle or high socioeconomic status. The key features of anorexia are very low self-esteem and a poor view of body image, and these psychological traits often stem from unhappiness in the home life of the individual. Common indicators of risk include having conflicts in the home (Felker and Stivers, 1994), a passive father and domineering mother, lack of independence for the adolescent or sexual or physical abuse. Anorexia may therefore be perceived as a failure of the individual to respond adequately to

the growing emotional challenges of adulthood (Baluch *et al.*, 1997). It is also argued that anorexia is a response to the pressures of a modern culture and society that idealizes a thin body shape and equates dieting and thinness with beauty and success. The marketing of this ideal to adolescent girls (and boys) is known to be highly effective (Hill, 2006). Field *et al.* (2008) reported that purging behaviour was associated with a desire to look like women in the media.

One important driver for anorexia may, in fact, be a genetic predisposition, which produces the eating disorder when coupled to sociocultural stimuli and/or emotional and psychological disturbance. Twin studies suggest a genetic component as anorexia may afflict both twins in a monozygotic (identical) pair, but this is not the case with dizygotic twins (Yilmaz *et al.*, 2015). Female relatives of anorexia sufferers are 11 times more likely to develop the disease than the rest of the population (Zipfel *et al.*, 2015) and the overall contribution of genetics to the anorexia risk profile is estimated to be 50–74% (Moskowitz and Weiselberg, 2017). The basis of the genetic association is not well understood, but single nucleotide polymorphisms in a number of genes have been found to associate with the condition (Paolacci *et al.*, 2020). A number of these are in genes that play a role in appetite regulation, including serotonin receptors and transporters, and dopamine receptors. Agouti-related peptide (AgRP) polymorphisms also associate with anorexia (Dardennes *et al.*, 2007) and animal models of anorexia suggest that regulation of mood and feeding behaviours may depend on interactions of AgRP neurons in the brain and the appetite regulatory hormone ghrelin (Méquinion *et al.*, 2020). Other genes implicated in the development of anorexia include epoxide hydroxylase-2, which plays a role in cholesterol metabolism and the oestrogen receptor β (Scott-van Zeeland *et al.*, 2014). A role for oestrogen is of interest as anorexia often first manifests during puberty.

7.6.4.2 Bulimia nervosa

Bulimia shares the same basic psychopathology as anorexia, namely, a distorted view of body size and shape, but despite this, it manifests in a different way and impacts upon a slightly different population (Fairburn and Harrison, 2003). While anorexia can begin to appear as early as eight years of age and reaches a peak of incidence in adolescence, development of bulimia before 13 years of age is unusual, and most sufferers are young adults (Gowers, 2008). Bulimia is estimated to affect approximately 1% of young women, although claims of prevalence rates of up to 3.2% in school girls have been reported and 4.4% in dancers (Arcelus *et al.*, 2014). The prevalence is 10 times higher in women than in men (Hoek and van Hoeken, 2003).

Bulimia is more challenging to identify than anorexia if one is working purely from physical symptoms. It is characterized by episodes of binge eating that occur on a frequent basis (Table 7.5). Usually, these binges involve the ingestion of between 1000 and 2000 kcal in a single two-hour session (Fairburn and Harrison, 2003), but there are reports that bulimics can take in 15 000 kcal during a binge. Sufferers sometimes report that during a binge, they lose all control and will eat raw food and food straight from tins and packets, stopping only when they are overcome by pain, fatigue or vomiting. The ability to take in larger binges is likely to develop over time as the normal signals from the gut that indicate satiety become suppressed.

Following binge sessions, the bulimia sufferer will take compensatory action to prevent weight gain. This can involve excessive exercising but more commonly uses techniques to purge the food from the body. Laxative substances or emetics are widely abused for this purpose. In between binges, there may be periods of intense food restriction to maintain control over body weight, but physically, the bulimia sufferer will often appear to be of normal or even slightly above average weight. Physiologically, however, there is an accrual of damage related to bingeing–purging cycles including loss of gut peristalsis and associated colonic problems, electrolyte imbalances and dehydration, damage to the salivary glands, malabsorption of fat soluble vitamins leading to deficiency of vitamin A and vitamin D, oesophagitis and erosion of dental enamel due to contact with stomach acid during vomiting.

As with anorexia, the development of bulimia is strongly linked to genetic factors and probably involves disturbances of the serotonergic system (Hinney and Volckmar, 2013). The profile of sufferers is similar to anorexia, with girls from home situations that create anxiety and depression being at greatest risk. Concerns about overweight that lead to dieting are also associated with greater risk and, in boys, negative paternal comments about weight are predictive of bingeing behaviours (Field *et al.*, 2008). Early menarche is also seen as a risk factor for bulimia in adolescent girls (Fairburn and Harrison, 2003). In the case of bulimia, the means of coping with emotional problems is to binge, which either provides a feeling of taking control over matters in an otherwise out of control life or a means of temporarily escaping from negative thoughts and feelings (Abraham, 2003). However, the bulimic individual falls into a negative cycle as the process of bingeing and purging creates feelings of shame, self-loathing and revulsion that exacerbate the initiating negative feelings (Figure 7.11).

Treatment for bulimia involves similar approaches to those used for anorexia. Hospitalization and the need for intense nutritional support are less likely as bulimia sufferers become malnourished less frequently. In adults, the prescribing of antidepressant medication can serve to reduce the frequency of bingeing and purging, but this benefit is often short lived and has not been reported in adolescents (Gowers, 2008).

7.6.5 The pregnant teenager
Each year around 12 million girls aged 15–19 years and a further 777 000 under 15 give birth (World Health Organization, 2020). The majority of these pregnancies occur in the impoverished and devel-

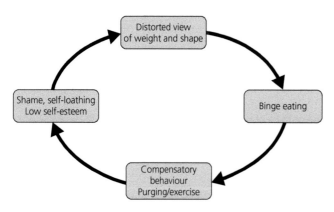

Figure 7.11 Bulimia nervosa as a cycle of behaviour driven by poor self-esteem. Individuals with bulimia go through frequent episodes of binge eating followed by use of laxatives and emetics or excessive exercise to compensate for ingested energy. The bingeing is seen as a way of dealing with anxiety and depression linked to poor self-esteem and feelings of low self-worth. Feelings of shame that follow the binge–purge episode actually serve to reinforce the initial problem and hence maintain the bulimic behaviour.

oping regions of the world. The highest adolescent pregnancy rates are observed in Sub-Saharan Africa (e.g. Central African Republic 229 adolescent pregnancies/1000 births; Mozambique 194/1000 births, Chad 179/1000 births, Mali 174/1000 births), with high rates in Asia and South America (Afghanistan 77/1000 births; Ecuador 111/1000 births, Mexico 71/1000 births; Brazil 59/1000 births). In contrast, developed countries typically have low adolescent birth rates (United States 19/1000 births, UK 14/1000 births, Australia 10/1000 births; Unicef, 2019). In addition to the live births, the developing regions of the world see up to 5.6 million adolescents have terminations of pregnancy, with the vast majority of these being carried out in unsafe conditions. Globally, complications associated with pregnancy and abortion are the main cause of death among adolescent girls (World Health Organization, 2020).

Adolescent pregnancy is a feature of poverty and low education. In developed countries, almost all such pregnancies are unplanned and result from either poor knowledge, or lack of access to contraception. Adolescent pregnancy rates are markedly greater in socially deprived settings. Among the developing countries, the highest adolescent pregnancy rates are seen in the poorest countries. In addition to poverty, cultures differ and early marriage and childbearing is socioculturally normalized. Globally, 12% of girls will marry before the age of 15 and 39% are married by 18 years. In cultures where education and employment opportunities for girls are limited but where marriage and childbearing are valued, adolescent girls may choose to become pregnant as their best option in life (World Health Organization, 2020). In developed countries, adolescent pregnancies are more likely among girls of lower socioeconomic status. In the UK, for example, more than half of adolescent pregnancies are seen in girls from socially deprived backgrounds, and pregnancy rates are six times more likely in socially deprived areas (Wallace et al., 2006).

The risks associated with pregnancy that were described in Chapter 3 (e.g. miscarriage, fetal death and maternal death) are considerably greater in adolescents than in older mothers. Adolescents have a fourfold greater risk of death during pregnancy than women over the age of 20 years. Postpartum haemorrhage (often related to iron deficiency anaemia) or obstructive labour due to the pelvis being too narrow for the passage of the baby is the major cause of maternal death among

15–19-year-old girls in developing countries. Adolescent pregnancies, particularly where the mother is under the age of 16 years, are significantly more likely to end in miscarriage, premature labour or low birth weight (Wallace et al., 2006). Risk of adverse outcomes of pregnancy for babies is also markedly higher (Figure 7.12). Stillbirth and neonatal death (infant death in the first 28 days postpartum) are significantly more common where mothers are below the age of 20 (Centre for Maternal and Child Enquiries, 2011). Girls aged 15–16 are significantly more likely (odds ratio, OR, 1.42, 95% confidence interval, CI, 1.06–1.89) to have low birth weight infants and to deliver prematurely (OR 1.87, 95% CI 1.51–2.31; Gibbs et al., 2012). Risks are higher in younger mothers. These observations were made in populations with good antenatal care, suggesting that factors related to biological immaturity drive many of the observed outcomes. Indeed, for adolescents in the developing world, antenatal care and medical supervision are likely to be poor. Teenagers in developed countries will often conceal their pregnancies until later in gestation because of the associated social stigma. This makes antenatal care, particularly strategies aimed at optimizing nutrition, extremely challenging. In addition to these immediate threats to health associated with pregnancy, the offspring of adolescent mothers are at risk in the long term. Low birth weight is associated with increased risk of cardiovascular disease and metabolic syndrome (Chapter 4). Children of adolescent mothers tend to remain

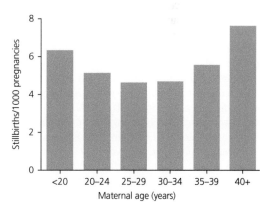

Figure 7.12 Adolescent pregnancy is associated with a number of adverse outcomes including stillbirth. Mothers under the age of 20 are 1.4 (95% CI 1.2–1.6) times more likely to have a stillbirth than 25–29-year-olds. *Source:* data from Centre for Maternal and Child Enquiries (2011).

socially disadvantaged, are less likely to succeed educationally and are more likely to have behavioural problems (Wallace *et al.*, 2006).

Nutritional status may be a critical element of the greater risk associated with adolescent pregnancy. The relationship between the nutritional status of adolescents and pregnancy outcomes is complex and poorly understood. It is clear, however, that there is major competition between maternal growth and the growth of the fetus and placenta. Growth generally continues during pregnancy and produces the apparently paradoxical situation of greater pregnancy weight gain than that seen in adult women but with lower eventual birth weights (Wallace *et al.*, 2006). Growth of adolescent girls continues for up to four years after menarche and is maximal between 13 and 15 years. The energy use needed to sustain growth appears to have priority over requirements for pregnancy and, as a result, adolescent mothers fail to deposit reserves of fat in early pregnancy and cannot sustain rapid rates of fetal growth in the second and third trimesters.

Adolescent mothers are more likely to consume alcohol, smoke tobacco and engage in other high-risk behaviours than older women. These factors may also contribute to the greater prevalence of adverse outcomes. These women are less likely to optimize nutritional status prior to conception, for example, they are unlikely to take folate supplements in the periconceptual period (Langley-Evans and Langley-Evans, 2002) and often enter pregnancy with low micronutrient reserves. A number of micronutrients are of particular concern. A study of 500 adolescent mothers-to-be in an inner city UK population found that the prevalence of anaemia was 11.9% in the first trimester and rose to 63.5% in the third trimester. Low intakes of iron and folate were noted (Baker *et al.*, 2009). Lee *et al.* (2014) reported low intakes (relative to the estimated average requirement) of vitamin D, vitamin E, iron, calcium and magnesium among 156 pregnant girls. Greater prevalence of vitamin D insufficiency was observed in pregnant adolescents (51% had 25-hydroxyvitamin D concentrations below 50 nmol/l) compared with older pregnant women (20% had low 25-hydroxyvitamin D concentrations; Ginde *et al.*, 2010). The systematic review of Marvin-Dowle *et al.* (2016) concluded that intakes of vitamin D, iron, calcium and selenium were the main concerns for pregnant girls.

The increased micronutrient demands of adolescence, coupled with sometimes chaotic eating habits on top of the demands of pregnancy mean that the nutritional status of the pregnant adolescent will be a cause for concern. Suboptimal nutrition will be more likely in girls who are in the rapid phase of pubertal growth during their pregnancy, and as discussed in Chapter 3, the risk of poor pregnancy outcomes will be greater. Competition for nutrients between the pregnancy and maternal growth and poorly understood issues related to how the placenta partitions nutrients between the mother and fetus are likely to play the major role in determining the relationship between maternal nutritional status and pregnancy outcomes.

7.6.6 The transgender teenager

It is increasingly recognized that individuals may develop a personal gender identity that is not consistent with their biological sex. Biological sex is binary (male or female) and is determined by chromosomes and characterized by the genitalia and sexual characteristics that develop during puberty. Gender identity is not binary and is represented as a spectrum with fully male or female sitting at the extremes (Figure 7.13). Some people will identify with a gender that is the same as their biological sex (cisgender), though with varying affinity for the other end of the spectrum, while others may be gender neutral, gender fluid, or may more strongly identify with the gender that is the opposite of their biological sex (transgender). Transgender people are generally diagnosed as having gender dysphoria, which is a psychological disorder that can lead to profound anxiety, depression and may end in suicide if unresolved.

Gender dysphoria is most likely to be identified during the adolescent years and the number of cases being referred to specialist gender identity services rose sharply between 2010 and 2020 in both the UK and United States (Handler *et al.*, 2019; Tavistock and Portman Trust 2020). Figure 7.13 shows the common treatment pathway for adolescents with gender dysphoria. Typically a period of two years psychological evaluation to confirm the condition will lead to administration of drugs to block the endocrine changes that drive puberty; typically a GnRH antagonist. A period of time on endocrine blockade, with continuing psychological evaluation, may lead to treatment with cross-sex hormones (testosterone to transboys, oestrogen to transgirls). From the age of 18, transgender individuals may elect to progress to full surgical gender reassignment.

Disrupting the normal endocrine changes associated with puberty may have significant implications for growth, impacting on demand for nutrients, establishment of mature body composition and bone deposition. There is not an extensive research

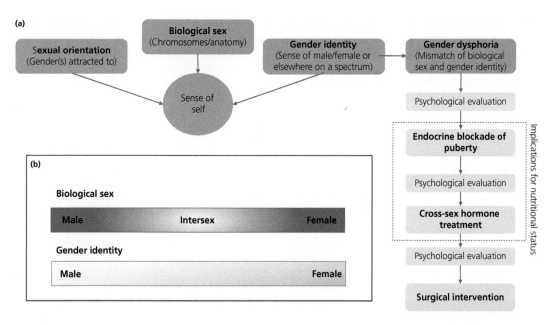

Figure 7.13 Gender identity and treatment of gender dysphoria in adolescents. a) Gender identity is a different concept to biologically determined sex and sexual orientation. A mismatch of biological sex and gender identity may result in treatment to enable a physiological transition from one gender to another. b) While biological sex is a binary concept, except in rare cases of intersex, gender identity covers a spectrum from fully female to fully male.

literature considering these issues and a complicating factor is that endocrine blockade may begin at a range of different ages due to delays in psychological presentation. Administration of GnRH antagonist would have markedly different consequences for a child at 13, before the pubertal growth spurt, compared with a 16-year-old, where the growth spurt may be near completion.

Gender dysphoria and the associated endocrine treatments can pose a number of nutrition-related challenges. First, gender dysphoria is closely associated with disordered eating. Body dissatisfaction is a key factor in gender dysphoria as the individual feels that they are in the wrong body, and so many adolescent sufferers will adopt eating strategies that attempt to block the physical changes associated with puberty. Gender dysphoria and anorexia nervosa are not uncommonly seen in the same individuals (Ristori *et al.*, 2019). Poor eating behaviours are more commonly observed in transboys (female to male transition) and transgirls (male to female transition) than in their cisgender classmates. Bishop *et al.* (2020) surveyed 80 794 US high school students and that found 2.7% identified as transgender or gender non-conforming. Among this group, meal skipping was more common, fast food and sugar-sweetened beverages were consumed more often, and consumption of fruit and milk was less common than in the cisgender population.

The metabolic impact of treatment with GnRH antagonist and cross-sex hormones appears to be low, according to one report of normal blood lipid concentrations and insulin sensitivity (Klaver *et al.*, 2020). Treatments shift body composition and shape towards the desired gender, so for transboys body fat decreases and lean body mass increases. In transgirls, the waist–hip ratio and fat mass increases (Schagen *et al.*, 2016; Klaver *et al.*, 2018). While this transition is a successful effect of treatment, transgender adolescents are significantly more likely to be obese than their cisgender counterparts (Klaver *et al.*, 2020). Some children with gender dysphoria receive different endocrine treatments, with GnRH antagonism replaced by antiandrogenic (cyproterone acetate) or pro-androgenic (lynestrol) progestins. This leads to the same shifts in body composition as treatment with GnRH antagonist and cross-sex hormones (Tack *et al.*, 2018).

The greatest concern in terms of growth and physical development associated with blockade of puberty relates to bone mineralization, since sex steroids are the main drivers of bone growth. Although normal sex hormone production is ablated during treatment there appear to be no lasting effects of treatments. Joseph *et al.* (2019) followed 12–14-year-olds who initiated GnRH antagonist treatment. After one year, their BMD z-scores had declined but overall bone mineral content had not changed. This reflected the fact that pubertal blockade had slowed bone accrual compared with age-matched untreated children. Vlot *et al.* (2017) reported the same effect, together with a reduction in bone turnover which was more pronounced in transboys than transgirls. However, when treatment with cross-sex hormones began accrual of bone caught up, such that by the age of 22 years there were no differences in bone mineralization. Delaying puberty therefore delays the deposition of bone mineral, but administration of sex hormones is sufficient to restore the expected level of bone mineralization. Children who are transitioning are advised to take vitamin D supplements during treatment, to maximize bone growth.

7.6.7 Alcohol

Adolescence is a time when individuals attempt to assert their individuality and independence from parents and family. This transition to adulthood can manifest in a variety of ways, but in many cultures, the rebellion of adolescence is heavily focused upon the misuse of alcohol and other substances. These behaviours are not of course unique to adolescents, but the adolescent years present the situation where the body first encounters such agents, often in an uncontrolled manner, at a time of maximum growth and maturation. In developed countries, there has been a trend for a reduction in prevalence of alcohol consumption among adolescents over the first two decades of the twenty-first century. In the UK the prevalence of drinking alcohol among 11–15-year-olds declined between 2003 and 2014, with only 6% consuming alcohol regularly in 2018 (NHS Digital, 2019a). An analysis of alcohol consumption in 25 European countries found that while there was a higher prevalence (18%) of heavy episodic (binge) drinking among adolescents in Germany, Finland, Denmark, Italy, Ireland, Belgium, Poland and the Netherlands than in other countries, the majority of adolescents in Iceland, Norway, Sweden, France, Portugal, Spain and Cyprus rarely drank alcohol on a frequent basis (Bräker and Soellner, 2016). Adolescents in Czechia, Estonia, Russia, Hungary and Lithuania were the populations most likely to consume alcohol on a regular basis (59% of adolescents compared with 0.7% regularly drinking in the Nordic, Iberian nations and France). These data suggest that there have been shifts away from unhealthy use of alcohol by the vast majority of adolescents, but alcohol still remains a significant risk to the health and nutritional status of significant numbers of children.

The metabolism of alcohol (Figure 7.14) occurs primarily within the liver, where it can be cleared by several pathways. Most metabolism is mediated by the cytosolic pathway in which alcohol dehydrogenase converts ethanol to acetaldehyde. This can then be cleared to acetate through the action of aldehyde dehydrogenases in the cytosol (ALDH1) or mitochondria (ALDH2). If alcohol consumption is excessive, these processes will have a number of effects upon nutritional status, primarily through increases in demand for thiamine, riboflavin and nicotinic acid. Alcohol dehydrogenase is also responsible for the conversion of retinol to retinaldehyde. Regular consumption of excessive alcohol will competitively inhibit retinol metabolism and hence impact upon vitamin A status.

If the capacity of the alcohol dehydrogenase pathway is exceeded, either due to the quantity of alcohol consumed or due to B vitamins being limiting nutrients, then detoxification follows the microsomal ethanol oxidation pathway. Cytochrome P450 enzymes catalyze the conversion of ethanol to acetaldehyde. As the expression of these enzymes is induced by ethanol, metabolism via this pathway has different consequences in individuals who consume frequently to those seen in irregular drinkers. Regular consumption increases the formation of free radical and carcinogenic intermediates. Clearance of xenobiotics, retinoids and steroids is more rapid and, as a consequence, hepatic vitamin D metabolism is disrupted. Damage to cells within the liver promotes cirrhosis. Specific damage to hepatic stellate cells further impacts on vitamin A status as these are the sites of liver storage. Acetaldehyde is itself a toxic intermediate and can cause injury to the liver and form adducts that promote cell death or carcinogenesis. Accumulation of lipid within the liver is commonly seen in alcohol abusers, and this stems from excess production of NADH from the alcohol dehydrogenase pathway and also from the actions of CYP4A1.

The effects of alcohol upon physiology and metabolism depend upon the nature and frequency of the exposure. In the short term, alcohol is associated with stimulation of the appetite and the consumption of energy-dense snacks. It is generally recognized that regular alcohol consumption contributes to excess weight gain in adolescents. Vågstrand *et al.* (2007) found that alcohol intake was positively correlated with body fat in 16–17-year-old girls, but not in boys. Croezen *et al.* (2009) reported that the risk of overweight was greater with alcohol consumption among 13–14-year-olds but not 15–16-year-olds (Figure 7.15). More frequent and excessive consumption has contrasting effects and may be extremely harmful to health and social development. While alcohol dependency

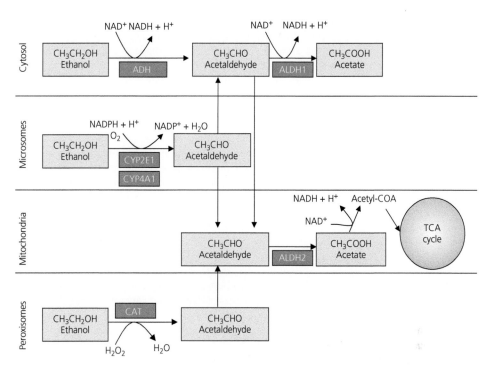

Figure 7.14 The metabolism of alcohol. Alcohol (ethanol) can be metabolized through cytosolic, microsomal or peroxisomal pathways. Cytosolic metabolism involves the enzymes alcohol dehydrogenase (ADH) and acetaldehyde dehydrogenase 1 (ALDH1). Where the cytosolic capacity is exceeded, microsomal metabolism uses the cytochrome P450 enzymes (CYP2E1 and CYP4A1). Acetaldehyde products of microsomal ethanol metabolism are cleared by acetaldehyde dehydrogenase 2 (ALDH2). Peroxisomal catalase (CAT) can also contribute to alcohol clearance.

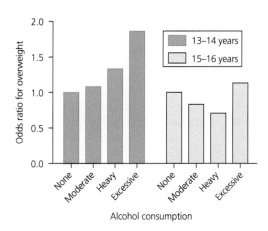

Figure 7.15 There is a weak association between alcohol consumption and body mass index in adolescents. In younger Dutch adolescents, heavy or excessive intake was associated with greater risk of overweight but the effect was absent in older adolescents. Intake: moderate, 1–3 glasses per occasion per week for girls and 1–5 for boys; heavy, 4–6 glasses for girls and 6–10 for boys; excessive >7 glasses for girls and >10 for boys. *Source:* reproduced with permission from Croezen *et al.* (2009). © Nature Publishing Group.

(alcoholism) may be rare among adolescents, alcohol abuse (a pattern of alcohol use in which the individual drinks in a manner that is hazardous to physical wellbeing and is likely to suffer problems with meeting obligations at home and at school) is increasingly a cause for concern. Alcoholics and alcohol abusers are often malnourished. This can stem from reduced nutrient intakes (alcoholic beverages displacing food intake), hyperexcretion of nutrients or reductions in bioavailability. Given the often marginal micronutrient intakes of adolescents, even moderate alcohol consumption may impact significantly upon nutritional status (Alonso-Aperte and Varela-Moreiras, 2000). Individuals who abuse alcohol are more likely to self-harm, suffer from attention deficit hyperactivity disorder, have learning difficulties and have problems with their behaviour and conduct. Adolescence is a critical period of development for the brain, during which regions in the hippocampus are rewired. These are centres that are responsible for memory. The adolescent brain appears more sensitive to alcohol than the adult, so excessive consumption during this stage may be particularly damaging (White and Swartzwelder, 2005).

Alcohol has known effects upon the skeleton, specifically the inhibition of osteoblast activity, which slows bone healing and turnover. However, there is evidence that in adults the relationship between alcohol and BMD is J-shaped, with low to moderate intakes actually stimulating accrual of greater bone mass (Wosje and Kalkwarf, 2007). The Tromso Fit Futures Study, which recruited 1038 boys and girls aged 15–19 years, found that bone mineralization was higher at the hip among those who reported consuming alcohol, but the study did not quantify alcohol intake (Winther *et al.*, 2014). However, with chronically excessive consumption or episodic binge drinking, is generally considered to limit peak bone mass (Zhu and Zheng, 2021). Adolescents who are regular consumers of alcohol have lower BMD at the hip and femoral neck (Dorn *et al.*, 2011).

7.6.8 Tobacco smoking

Among adult populations, the prevalence of smoking is in decline as awareness of the links between smoking and cancer, cardiovascular disease and pulmonary disease grows. The age group of 20–34-year-olds is the group in the population that is most likely to be smokers, but adolescence represents the life stage at which smoking is most likely to be initiated. Up to 75% of adolescents will experiment with cigarette smoking, and over 90% of adult smokers begin smoking in their teenage years. Although, cigarette smoking as a habit is in decline, it remains a significant issue among adolescents. In the UK, it is estimated that 3–6% of 11–15-year-olds smoke, with the highest prevalence in 14- and 15-year-olds (NHS, 2019a). In the United States, similar prevalence is reported, with 2–3% of middle school and 5.8% of high school students reporting smoking within 30 days of a national survey (Centers for Disease control and Prevention, 2019). Cigarette smoking is largely giving way to vaping e-cigarettes, as children find it easier to circumvent restrictions on purchasing these items and concealing their use than they do with tobacco products. Among 16–19-year-olds the use of e-cigarettes has been reported at 10.6% in the United States, 9.3% in Canada and 4.6% in England (Hammond *et al.*, 2019), although the US Centers for Disease Control and Prevention (2019) estimates that use is much higher.

As with alcohol consumption, cigarette smoking is often an act of rebellion among adolescents, and the habit is most commonly initiated to achieve social acceptance among peers. Other behaviours such as consuming caffeinated energy drinks are commonly associated with smoking (Larson *et al.*, 2014). The use of such drinks by adolescents is a cause for concern independently of smoking as their use may have serious health implications (see Research Highlight 7.3). There are suggestions that adolescents may also begin smoking as a means of addressing concerns about body weight or body image. Smoking is known to suppress weight gain. Typically, smoking males weigh 5 kg less than non-smokers (Hampl and Betts, 1999). Jensen *et al.* (1995) reported that hip circumference in young men was inversely correlated with excretion of cotinine (a breakdown product of nicotine). Awareness of the association between smoking and body weight appears to be greater among girls than boys, and there is evidence that this is an important influence on smoking behaviour in girls and young women (Potter *et al.*, 2004). Smokers are known to use the habit to control appetite and weight and, in particular, highlight the repression of sweet craving as a benefit of smoking (Coniglio *et al.*, 2020). Vaping of nicotine fluids is attractive for the same reason (Morean *et al.*, 2020). A survey by Jackson *et al.* (2019) found that among English adolescent smokers, 8% believed that vaping could control weight and 14% said they would use e-cigarettes if they were shown to restrict weight gain. Napolitano *et al.* (2020) found that adolescents who smoked cigarettes or vaped nicotine fluids had greater concerns about body shape and size and higher pathological eating scores.

The effects of smoking on the nutritional status of adults are well documented, but there have been few studies that have specifically addressed the issue in adolescents. As adolescent smokers are highly likely to have parents who smoke, it may be that their diets differ from non-smokers in the same respects as noted with adults. Indeed, Crawley and While (1996) reported that non-smoking teenagers' dietary intakes were similar to those of smokers if their parents were smokers. Typically, smokers have low circulating concentrations of folate, vitamin C, vitamin E and carotenoids, which may be explained by greater turnover due to oxidative stress (Tappia *et al.*, 1995). Dietary patterns also differ and smokers consume more meat, processed meat, eggs and fried foods. Adolescent boys who smoke tend to consume less fruit and fruit juices, while girls consume less fruit and vegetables (Hampl and Betts, 1999). Smoking among adolescents is associated with lower intakes of fibre, vitamin C, selenium, calcium and thiamine, and greater intakes of fat, sugar and alcohol (Crawley and While, 1996).

Smoking clearly impacts upon eating behaviours, and a number of explanations for this have been advanced. Primarily, the fact that an individual

Research Highlight 7.3 Safety of caffeinated energy drinks for adolescents.

Caffeinated energy drinks are sugar-sweetened beverages which contain added stimulants, typically caffeine and taurine or guarana. Often sold in 500 ml volumes they deliver around 150 mg caffeine per portion, which is a similar quantity to two servings of espresso coffee. They are marketed as an aid to maintain alertness and performance and the global sales market has grown considerably over the first two decades of the twenty-first century. Big brands such as Red Bull or Monster are highly visible and a popular among adolescents. Caffeinated energy drinks have no therapeutic value and as they contain non-regulated and some poorly understood ingredients, their safety for children and adolescence is strongly questioned.

Adolescents are known to be common consumers of energy drinks either as a means of staying awake at night to engage in social activities and online life (Calamaro et al., 2009), to engage with the experience and social acceptability of the products or to attempt to boost physical or mental performance. In the United States, consumption by adolescents increased sevenfold between 2000 and 2016 (Vercammen et al., 2019) and Miller et al. (2018) found that 41% of a sample of US adolescents reported consuming them at least once in the three months prior to survey. Among UK 11–15-year olds, 14% reported consuming energy drinks two to four times per week, with the beverages displacing breakfast (Brooks et al., 2018).

The major ingredient of energy drinks is caffeine. As adolescents are generally not regular consumers of tea and coffee, they have a lower pharmacological tolerance to caffeine than adults and this makes them more vulnerable to the acute toxic effects of caffeine when consumed as a high bolus dose. Adolescents are also likely to mix sweet energy drinks with alcohol and this will exacerbate the impact of the high caffeine dose. The reported adverse effects of excessive consumption of caffeinated beverages are severe. Kim et al. (2020) found that adolescents who consumed them more than three times a week were at greater risk of depression and suicidal ideation. Adolescent users have more mood disorders and exhibit low quality sleep (Seifert et al., 2011; Calamaro et al., 2012). Adverse physiological reactions include gastrointestinal, cardiovascular and neurological disturbances. The most severe reactions include heart palpitations, cardiac arrhythmias, low blood pressure associated with taurine, high blood pressure due to caffeine, seizures and even death (Wolk et al., 2012; Gunja and Brown, 2012; Ehlers et al., 2019; Moussa et al., 2021). Studies of adolescent rats and mice suggest that chronic exposure to caffeinated beverages has a deleterious effect on development of the brain and the skeleton (Serdar et al., 2019; Brown et al., 2020).

Although there are clear concerns about the safety of caffeinated energy drinks for adolescents they remain unregulated and available for sale to minors. The European Union introduced a requirement for all such products to be labelled as not suitable for adolescents and pregnant or breastfeeding women. In the UK and United States, there are voluntary codes of practice committing manufacturers to not advertise to children under 16 years of age. However, with reported cases of hospitalization and death of adolescents following excessive consumption of energy drinks, greater regulation by government and education of children and parents must be a high priority.

is a smoker indicates that they make less healthy choices in general. Poor dietary habits are therefore unsurprising. Indeed, individuals who cease smoking often also adopt very healthy dietary habits as an element of wholesale lifestyle changes. It is also proposed that food intake may be displaced by smoking and that cigarette smoking dulls the sense of taste, particularly for sweet foods (Hampl and Betts, 1999). The act of smoking may also determine meal frequency and duration. This might be particularly influential in adolescents, whose smoking habit is usually an illicit and furtive activity. The health consequences of cigarette smoking are well established, and clearly, the initiation of smoking in adolescence will be a risk factor for disease at later stages of life.

There is a well-established relationship between smoking and bone health in adults, with a 30% greater lifetime fracture risk in smokers compared with non-smokers. Reports of lower BMD are common, with the hip, spine and femoral neck all exhibiting lower BMD in smokers (Wong et al., 2007). The impact on the skeleton during adolescence is less well documented, but Jones et al. (2004) found that girls who smoked were significantly more likely to suffer fractures before age 18 if they smoked (OR 1.43, 95% CI 1.05–1.95). Regular smoking was associated with lower BMD at the hip and femoral neck in the study of Dorn et al. (2011) and also slowed the accrual of bone at the hip between the ages of 13 and 19 (Dorn et al., 2013). Välimäki et al. (1994) reported that men aged 20–29 had lower BMD if they had smoked in adolescence. Similar findings were noted in a comparison of 18–19-year-old men who smoked with non-smokers (Lorentzon et al., 2007). The mechanistic basis of these effects upon bone may lie in the metabolism of vitamin D and hence the availability of calcium for deposition of bone mineral. Serum 1,25 dihydroxycholecalciferol concentrations are lower in smokers compared with non-smokers, and this will inhibit intestinal uptake of calcium.

7.6.9 Drug abuse

While the majority of adolescents do not use illicit substances, this age group is the population subgroup that is most likely to experiment with abuse of hallucinogenic solvents, intravenous drugs, inhaled drugs and prescription drugs. Adolescents are experimental by nature and can be drawn to use of recreational drugs and abuse of toxic substances. Statistics from developed countries suggest that the numbers of adolescents using drugs increased significantly between the 1980s and the early part of the twenty-first century. In the UK, the 2019 survey of smoking, drinking and drug use among 11–15-year-olds found that 8% had used cannabis in the year of the survey, although among 15-year-olds this figure was 30%; 11% of boys and 8% of girls were possibly regular users. The report found that 4% used volatile intoxicants, 4% nitrous dioxide and 2% class A drugs (NHS Digital, 2019b). In the United States, around 50% of young people who vaped used cannabis products instead of nicotine fluids and 6.6% of 8th graders (13–14-year-olds) and 22% of 12th graders (17–18-year-olds) reported use of cannabis, with up to 6% doing so daily. Opioid misuse was reported by 2.7% and 2% abused other drugs including LSD, cocaine and amphetamines (National Institute on Drug Abuse, 2019). The Australian Institute of Health and Welfare (2020) reported that 8% if 12–17-year-olds used cannabis regularly and that ecstasy (3,4-methylenedioxymethamphetamine) was used by 2% of adolescents.

Abuse of drugs and other substances is often associated with undernutrition. This effect can be direct, by virtue of effects of drugs upon food intake, absorption of nutrients, urinary and faecal losses of nutrients and metabolic rate. The latter will often be elevated by substance abuse due to requirements to metabolize xenobiotics in the liver. In adolescents, there may be problems with micronutrient status that can potentiate the effects of drugs (both illicit and those administered for therapeutic purposes). The metabolism of xenobiotics in children and adolescents may differ from adults, particularly as the activities and expression of key enzymes and transporters are influenced by growth hormone and sex steroids during puberty (Akhlaghi et al., 2017). Indirect effects on nutritional status may be more important. For example, substance addiction will lead to crime and social exclusion, and this limits normal access to a healthy diet. The use of drugs is often associated with psychiatric disorders which can further impact on nutritional status. Piacentino et al. (2015) reported that among athletes who were users of anabolic steroids, eating disorders featured among the associated psychiatric disturbances. Adolescent girls in the UK Avon Longitudinal Study of Parents and Children cohort were more likely to use cannabis if they had high body dissatisfaction scores (Bornioli et al., 2019).

Drug use is also associated with other unhealthy behaviours and factors that can impact upon nutritional status. In a study of 3003 adolescents and young adults, the use of cannabis, amphetamines or LSD was associated with use of other drugs, tobacco smoking and alcohol consumption (Kotyuk et al., 2020). Consumption of snack foods tends to be greater, and drug users are more frequently from lower-income families or ethnic minority groups. Overall, drug use is therefore one manifestation of a wider spectrum of behaviours and influences that promote undernutrition. There are few studies that have been able to quantify the impact upon nutritional status, mainly because drug users are an unreliable group to survey accurately. Knight et al. (1994) were able to relate drug use to biochemical measures of nutritional status in a group of socially deprived, pregnant women. Use of cannabis, cocaine or phencyclidine was associated with reduced serum ferritin and poor ascorbate, folate and vitamin B12 status. This would be consistent with the imbalanced meals, erratic eating patterns and increased alcohol consumption that are associated with substance abuse.

Skeletal growth may be compromised by the abuse of solvents and drugs, although the negative influences have largely been demonstrated in animal models. Dündaröz et al. (2002) found that a group of young people who abused solvents had lower BMD than an age-matched control group, but could not dissect the possible confounding effects of cigarettes and alcohol. Animal studies are strongly indicative of a negative impact of inhalants upon skeletal growth and health (Crossin et al., 2019). There are several reports that abuse of opioids is also associated with loss of bone (Milos et al., 2011).

SUMMARY

- Adolescence is a life stage that is dominated by rapid rates of growth, remodelling of body shape and composition and sexual maturation. These physiological processes may be vulnerable if nutritional status is compromised.
- Puberty is associated with gains in lean body mass, rising fat mass in girls and rapid increases in bone mineralization.
- Requirements for energy and nutrients are higher during adolescence than at any other stage of life.

- Intakes of nutrients may be compromised by poor food choices that are related to the growing emotional and social independence of adolescents. Low iron, zinc, calcium and folate status is a concern in this sub-population.
- Nutrient status in adolescents may be impaired by experimentation with restrictive dietary practices such as vegetarianism or weight loss diets.
- Adolescents are a high-risk group for eating disorders. These conditions have a strong genetic component, but risk is increased by emotional disturbance, anxiety and depression.
- Adolescent pregnancy is a major challenge from a nutritional perspective. The competition for nutrients between fetal and continuing maternal growth increases the risk of poor pregnancy outcomes.
- Use of tobacco, alcohol and drugs can negatively impact upon nutritional status and normal growth and development in adolescents.

References

Abraham, S.F. (2003). Dieting, body weight, body image and self-esteem in young women: doctors' dilemmas. *Medical Journal of Australia* **178**: 607–611.

Akhlaghi, F., Matson, K.L., Mohammadpour, A.H. *et al.* (2017). Clinical pharmacokinetics and pharmacodynamics of antihyperglycemic medications in children and adolescents with type 2 diabetes mellitus. *Clinical Pharmacokinetics* **56**: 561–571.

Alonso-Aperte, E. and Varela-Moreiras, G. (2000). Drugsnutrient interactions: a potential problem during adolescence. *European Journal of Clinical Nutrition* **54**(Suppl): S69–S74.

American Psychiatric Association. (2000). *Diagnostic and Statistical Manual of Mental Disorders*, 4th ed. Washington DC: APA.

Amit, M. (2010). Vegetarian diets in children and adolescents. *Paediatrics and Child Health* **15**: 303–314.

Arcelus, J., Witcomb, G.L. and Mitchell, A. (2014). Prevalence of eating disorders amongst dancers: a systemic review and meta-analysis. *European Eating Disorders Review* **22**: 92–101.

Australian Institute of Health and Welfare (2020). Alcohol, tobacco and other drugs in Australia. https://www.aihw.gov.au/reports/alcohol/alcohol-tobacco-other-drugs-australia/contents/priority-populations/young-people (accessed 10 April 2021).

Baines, S., Powers, J. and Brown, W.J. (2007). How does the health and well-being of young Australian vegetarian and semi-vegetarian women compare with non-vegetarians? *Public Health Nutrition* **10**: 436–442.

Baker, P.N., Wheeler, S.J., Sanders, T.A. *et al.* (2009). A prospective study of micronutrient status in adolescent pregnancy. *American Journal of Clinical Nutrition* **89**: 1114–1124.

Baluch, B., Furnham, A. and Huszcza, A. (1997). Perception of body shapes by anorexics and mature and teenage females. *Journal of Clinical Psychology* **53**: 167–175.

Bardone-Cone, A.M., Fitzsimmons-Craft, E.E., Harney, M.B. *et al.* (2012). The inter-relationships between vegetarianism and eating disorders among females. *Journal of the Academy of Nutrition and Dietetics.* **112**, 1247–1252.

Barrack, M.T., West, J., Christopher, M. and Pham-Vera, A.M. (2019). Disordered eating among a diverse sample of first-year college students. *Journal of the American College of Nutrition* **38**: 141–148.

Bates, B., Lennox, A., Prentice, A. *et al.* (2014). *National Diet and Nutrition Survey: Results from years 1–4 (combined) of the rolling programme (2008/2009 – 2011/12)*. London: Public Health England.

Bauer, K.W., Larson, N.I., Nelson, M.C. *et al.* (2009). Fast food intake among adolescents: secular and longitudinal trends from 1999 to 2004. *Preventive Medicine* **48**: 284–287.

Berryman, C.E., Lieberman, H.R., Fulgoni, V.L. and Pasiakos, S.M. (2018). Protein intake trends and conformity with the dietary reference intakes in the United States: analysis of the National Health and Nutrition Examination Survey, 2001–2014. *American Journal of Clinical Nutrition* **108**: 405–413.

Bishop, A., Overcash, F., McGuire, J. and Reicks, M. (2020). Diet and physical activity behaviors among adolescent transgender students: school survey results. *Journal of Adolescent Health* **66**: 484–490.

Boreham, C.A. and McKay, H.A. (2011). Physical activity in childhood and bone health. *British Journal of Sports Medicine* **45**: 877–879.

Bornioli, A., Lewis-Smith, H., Smith, A. *et al.* (2019). Adolescent body dissatisfaction and disordered eating: Predictors of later risky health behaviours. *Social Science and Medicine* **238**: 12458.

Bräker, A.B. and Soellner, R. (2016). Alcohol drinking cultures of European adolescents. *European Journal of Public Health* **26**: 581–586.

Brooks, F.M., Klemera, E., Magnusson, J. and Chester, K. (2018). *Young People and Energy Drink Consumption in England: Findings from the WHO Health Behaviour in School aged Children (HBSC) Survey 2015. Detailed analysis on findings relating to consumption of energy drinks by young people.* Hatfield: University of Hertfordshire; 2018.

Brown, J., Villalona, Y., Weimer, J. *et al.* (2020). Supplemental taurine during adolescence and early adulthood has sex-specific effects on cognition, behavior and neurotransmitter levels in C57BL/6J mice dependent on exposure window. *Neurotoxicology and Teratology* **79**: 106883.

Brunet, M. (2005). Female athlete triad. *Clinical Sports Medicine* **24**: 623–636.

Brytek-Matera, A. (2020). Restrained eating and vegan, vegetarian and omnivore dietary intakes. *Nutrients* **12**: 2133.

Calamaro, C.J., Mason, T.B. and Ratcliffe, S.J. (2009). Adolescents living the 24/7 lifestyle: effects of caffeine and technology on sleep duration and daytime functioning. *Pediatrics* **123**: 1005–1010.

Calamaro, C.J., Yang, K., Ratcliffe, S., Chasens, E.R. (2012). Wired at a young age: the effect of caffeine and technology on sleep duration and body mass index in school-aged children. *Journal of Pediatric Health Care* **26**: 276–282.

Campos, R.M., de Mello, M.T., Tock, L. *et al.* (2013). Interaction of bone mineral density, adipokines and hormones in obese adolescents girls submitted in an interdisciplinary therapy. *Journal of Pediatric Endocrinology and Metabolism* **26**: 663–668.

Centers for Disease Control and Prevention. (2019). *Youth Risk Behavior Surveillance System*. https://www.cdc.gov/healthyyouth/data/yrbs/results.htm (accessed 10 April 2021).

Centre for Maternal and Child Enquiries. (2011). *Perinatal Mortality 2009*. London: CMACE.

Chamay-Weber, C., Narring, F. and Michaud, P.A. (2005). Partial eating disorders among adolescents: a review. *Journal of Adolescent Health* **37**: 417–427.

Cheshire, A., Berry, M. and Fixsen, A. (2020). What are the key features of orthorexia nervosa and influences on its development? A qualitative investigation. *Appetite* **155**: 104798.

Coniglio, K.A., Rosen, R., Burr, E.K. and Farris, S.G. (2020). Adherence to low-calorie and low-sugar diets is uniquely associated with distinct facets of appearance/weight-related smoking motivations. *Journal of Behavioural Medicine* **43**: 487–492.

Cornelsen, L., Berger, N., Cummins, S. and Smith, R.D. (2019). Socio-economic patterning of expenditures on 'out-of-home' food and non-alcoholic beverages by product and place of purchase in Britain. *Social Science and Medicine* **235**: 112361.

Crawley, H.F. and While, D. (1996). Parental smoking and the nutrient intake and food choice of British teenagers aged 16–17 years. *Journal of Epidemiology and Community Health* **50**: 306–312.

Croezen, S., Visscher, T.L., Ter Bogt, N.C. *et al.* (2009). Skipping breakfast, alcohol consumption and physical inactivity as risk factors for overweight and obesity in adolescents: results of the E-MOVO project. *European Journal of Clinical Nutrition* **63**: 405–412.

Crossin, R., Qama, A., Andrews, Z.B. *et al.* (2019). The effect of adolescent inhalant abuse on energy balance and growth. *Pharmacological Research Perspectives* **7**: e00498.

Cullin, J.M. (2020). Implicit and explicit fat bias among adolescents from two US populations varying by obesity prevalence. *Pediatric Obesity* **15**: e12747.

Custers, K. and Van den Bulck, J. (2010). Television viewing, computer game play and book reading during meals are predictors of meal skipping in a cross-sectional sample of 12-, 14- and 16-year olds. *Public Health Nutrition* **13**: 537–543

Czajkowska, M., Plinta, R., Rutkowska, M. *et al.* (2019). Menstrual cycle disorders in professional female rhythmic gymnasts. *International Journal of Environmental Research Public Health* **16**: 1470.

D'Alessandro, C., Morelli, E., Evangelisti, I. *et al.* (2007). Profiling the diet and body composition of subelite adolescent rhythmic gymnasts. *Pediatric Exercise Science* **19**: 215–227.

Daly, R.M. (2007). The effect of exercise on bone mass and structural geometry during growth. *Medicine and Sport Science* **51**: 33–49.

Dardennes, R.M., Zizzari, P., Tolle, V. *et al.* (2007). Family trios analysis of common polymorphisms in the obestatin/ghrelin, BDNF and AGRP genes in patients with anorexia nervosa: association with subtype, body-mass index, severity and age of onset. *Psychoneuroendocrinology* **32**: 106–113.

Davies, J.H., Evans, B.A. and Gregory, J.W. (2004). Bone mass acquisition in healthy children. *Archives of Disease in Childhood* **90**: 373–378.

Department of Health. (1998). *Dietary Reference Values for Energy and Nutrients for the United Kingdom*. London: Stationery Office.

Diethelm, K., Huybrechts, I., Moreno, L. *et al.* (2014). Nutrient intake of European adolescents: results of the HELENA (Healthy Lifestyle in Europe by Nutrition in Adolescence) Study. *Public Health Nutrition* **17**: 486–497.

Diethelm, K., Jankovic, N., Moreno, L.A. *et al.* (2012). Food intake of European adolescents in the light of different foodbased dietary guidelines: results of the HELENA (Healthy Lifestyle in Europe by Nutrition in Adolescence) Study. *Public Health Nutrition* **15**: 386–398.

Division of Laboratory Sciences. (2012). *Second National Report on Biochemical Indicators of Diet and Nutrition in the U.S. Population*. Atlanta, GA: Centers for Disease Control and Prevention.

Dorn, L.D., Beal, S.J., Kalkwarf, H.J. *et al.* (2013). Longitudinal impact of substance use and depressive symptoms on bone accrual among girls aged 11–19 years. *Journal of Adolescent Health* **52**: 393–399.

Dorn, L.D., Pabst, S., Sontag, L.M. *et al.* (2011). Bone mass, depressive, and anxiety symptoms in adolescent girls: variation by smoking and alcohol use. *Journal of Adolescent Health* **49**: 498–504.

Ducy, P., Amling, M., Takeda, S. *et al.* (2000). Leptin inhibits bone formation through a hypothalamic relay: a central control of bone mass. *Cell* **100**: 197–207.

Dündaröz, M.R., Sarici, S.U., Türkbay, T. *et al.* (2002). Evaluation of bone mineral density in chronic glue sniffers. *Turkish Journal of Pediatrics* **44**: 326–329.

Dunn, T.M., Gibbs, J., Whitney, N. and Starosta, A. (2017). Prevalence of orthorexia nervosa is less than 1 %: data from a US sample. *Eating and Weight Disorders* **22**: 185–192.

Ehlers, A., Marakis, G., Lampen, A. and Hirsch-Ernst, K.I. (2019). Risk assessment of energy drinks with focus on cardiovascular parameters and energy drink consumption in Europe. *Food Chemistry and Toxicology* **130**: 109–121.

Eisenberg, M.E., Puhl, R., Areba, E.M. and Neumark-Sztainer, D. (2019). Family weight teasing, ethnicity and acculturation: Associations with well-being among Latinx, Hmong, and Somali Adolescents. *Journal of Psychosomatic Research* **122**: 88–93.

El Hage, Z., Theunynck, D., Jacob, C. *et al* (2013). Bone mineral content and density in obese, overweight and normal weight adolescent boys. *Lebanese Medical Journal* **61**: 148–154.

Fairburn, C.G. and Harrison, P.J. (2003). Eating disorders. *Lancet* **361**: 407–416.

Felker, K.R. and Stivers, C. (1994). The relationship of gender and family environment to eating disorder risk in adolescents. *Adolescence* **29**: 821–834.

Field, A.E., Javaras, K.M., Aneja, P. *et al.* (2008). Family, peer, and media predictors of becoming eating disordered. *Archives of Pediatric and Adolescent Medicine* **162**: 574–579.

Finn, K.E., Seymour, C.M. and Phillips, A.E. (2020). Weight bias and grading among middle and high school teachers. *British Journal of Educational Psychology* **90**: 635–647.

Forestell, C.A., Spaeth, A.M. and Kane, S.A. (2012). To eat or not to eat red meat. A closer look at the relationship between restrained eating and vegetarianism in college females. *Appetite* **58**: 319–325.

French, S.A., Story, M., Neumark-Sztainer, D. *et al* (2001). Fast food restaurant use among adolescents: associations with nutrient intake, food choices and behavioral and psychosocial variables. *International Journal of Obesity* **25**: 1823–1833.

Gallagher, C.M., Black, L.J. and Oddy, W.H. (2014). Micronutrient intakes from food and supplements in Australian adolescents. *Nutrients* **6**: 342–354.

Gibbs, C.M., Wendt, A., Peters, S. *et al.* (2012). The impact of early age at first childbirth on maternal and infant health. *Paediatric Perinatology and Epidemiology* **26**(S1): 259–284.

Ginde, A.A., Sullivan, A.F., Mansbach, J.M. and Camargo, C.A. (2010). Vitamin D insufficiency in pregnant and nonpregnant women of childbearing age in the United States. *American Journal of Obstetrics and Gynecology* **202**: 436.e1–8.

Giovannini, M., Agostoni, C., Gianní, M. *et al.* (2000). Adolescence: macronutrient needs. *European Journal of Clinical Nutrition* **54**(Suppl 1): S7–S10.

Goldin, B.R., Woods, M.N., Spiegelman, D.L. *et al.* (1994). The effect of dietary fat and fiber on serum estrogen concentrations in premenopausal women under controlled dietary conditions. *Cancer* **74**: 1125–1131.

Gorczyca, D., Prescha, A., Szeremeta, K. and Jankowski, A. (2013). Iron status and dietary iron intake of vegetarian children from Poland. *Annals of Nutrition and Metabolism* **62**: 291–297.

Gowers, S.G. (2008). Management of eating disorders in children and adolescents. *Archives of Disease in Childhood* **93**: 331–334.

Greene, D.A. and Naughton, G.A. (2011). Calcium and vitamin- D supplementation on bone structural properties in peripubertal female identical twins: a randomised controlled trial. *Osteoporosis International* **22**: 489–498.

Griffith, J. and Omar, H. (2003). Association between vegetarian diet and menstrual problems in young women: a case presentation and brief review. *Journal of Pediatric and Adolescent Gynecology* **16**: 319–323.

Gunja, N. and Brown, J.A. (2012). Energy drinks: health risks and toxicity. *Medical Journal of Australia* **196**: 46–49.

Guo, S.S., Chumlea, W.C., Roche, A.F. *et al.* (1997). Age- and maturity-related changes in body composition during adolescence into adulthood: the Fels Longitudinal Study. *International Journal of Obesity* **21**: 1167–1175.

Hammond, D., Reid, J.L., Rynard, V.L. *et al.* (2019). Prevalence of vaping and smoking among adolescents in Canada, England, and the United States: repeat national cross sectional surveys. *BMJ* **365**: l2219.

Hampl, J.S. and Betts, N.M. (1999). Cigarette use during adolescence: effects on nutritional status. *Nutrition Reviews* **57**: 215–221.

Handler, T., Hojilla, J.C., Varghese, R. *et al.* (2019). Trends in referrals to a pediatric transgender clinic. *Pediatrics* **144**: e20191368.

Hill, A.J. (2006). Motivation for eating behaviour in adolescent girls: the body beautiful. *Proceedings of the Nutrition Society* **65**: 376–384.

Hill, A.J. (2002). Developmental issues in attitudes to food and diet. *Proceedings of the Nutrition Society* **61**: 259–266.

Hinney, A. and Volckmar, A.L. (2013). Genetics of eating disorders. *Current Psychiatry Reports* **15**: 423.

Hoek, H.W. and van Hoeken, D. (2003). Review of the prevalence and incidence of eating disorders. *International Journal of Eating Disorders* **34**: 383–396.

Hunt (2003).

Jackson, S.E., Brown, J., Aveyard, P. *et al.* (2019). Vaping for weight control: A cross-sectional population study in England. *Addictive Behaviours* **95**: 211–219.

Jensen, E.X., Fusch, C., Jaeger, P. *et al.* (1995). Impact of chronic cigarette smoking on body composition and fuel metabolism. *Journal of Clinical Endocrinology and Metabolism* **80**: 2181–2185.

Jones, I.E., Williams, S.M. and Goulding, A. (2004). Associations of birth weight and length, childhood size, and smoking withbone fractures during growth: evidence from a birth cohort study. *American Journal of Epidemiology* **159**: 343–350.

Joseph, T., Ting, J. and Butler, G. (2019). The effect of GnRH analogue treatment on bone mineral density in young adolescents with gender dysphoria: findings from a large national cohort. *Journal of Pediatric Endocrinology and Metabolism* **32**: 1077–1081.

Kannus, P., Haapasalo, H., Sankelo, M. *et al.* (1995). Effect of starting age of physical activity on bone mass in the dominant arm of tennis and squash players. *Annals of Internal Medicine* **123**: 27–31.

Kim, H., Park, J., Lee, S. *et al.* (2020). Association between energy drink consumption, depression and suicide ideation in Korean adolescents. *International Journal of Social Psychiatry* **66**: 335–343.

Kiss-Leizer, M., Tóth-Király, I. and Rigó, A. (2019). How the obsession to eat healthy food meets with the willingness to do sports: the motivational background of orthorexia nervosa. *Eating and Weight Disorders* **24**: 465–472.

Klaver, M., de Mutsert, R., Wiepjes, C.M. *et al.* (2018). Early Hormonal Treatment Affects Body Composition and Body Shape in Young Transgender Adolescents. *Journal of Sexual Medicine* **15**: 251–260.

Klaver, M., de Mutsert, R., van der Loos, M.A.T.C. *et al.* (2020). Hormonal treatment and cardiovascular risk profile in transgender adolescents. *Pediatrics* **145**: e20190741.

Knight, E.M., James, H., Edwards, C.H. *et al.* (1994). Relationships of serum illicit drug concentrations during pregnancy to maternal nutritional status. *Journal of Nutrition* **124**: 973S–980S.

Kondiboyina, V., Raine, L.B., Kramer, A.F. *et al.* (2020). Skeletal effects of nine months of physical activity in obese and healthy weight children. *Medicine and Science of Sports and Exercise* **52**: 434–440.

Kotyuk, E., Magi, A., Eisinger, A. *et al.* (2020). Co-occurrences of substance use and other potentially addictive behaviors: epidemiological results from the Psychological and Genetic Factors of the Addictive Behaviors (PGA) Study. *Journal of Behaviour and Addiction* **9**: 272–288.

Koven, N.S. and Abry, A.W. (2015). The clinical basis of orthorexia nervosa: emerging perspectives. *Neuropsychiatric Disorders and Treatment* **11**: 385–394.

Krajcovicová-Kudláčková, M., Simoncic, R., Béderová, A. *et al.* (1997). Influence of vegetarian and mixed nutrition on selected haematological and biochemical parameters in children. *Nahrung* **41**: 311–314.

Laddu, D.R., Farr, J.N., Laudermilk, M.J. *et al.* (2013). Longitudinal relationships between whole body and central adiposity on weight-bearing bone geometry, density, and bone strength: a pQCT study in young girls. *Archives of Osteoporosis* **8**: 156.

Lambert, H.L., Eastell, R., Karnik, K. *et al.* (2008). Calcium supplementation and bone mineral accretion in adolescent girls: an 18-mo randomized controlled trial with 2-y follow-up. *American Journal Clinical Nutrition* **87**: 455–462.

Langley-Evans, S.C. and Langley-Evans, A.J. (2002). Use of folic acid supplements in the first trimester of pregnancy. *Journal of the Royal Society of Health* **122**: 181–186.

Larson, N., DeWolfe, J., Story, M. and Neumark-Sztainer, D (2014). Adolescent consumption of sports and energy drinks: linkages to higher physical activity, unhealthy beverage patterns, cigarette smoking, and screen media use. *Journal of Nutrition Education and Behaviour* **46**: 181–187.

Laxer, R.E. and Janssen, I. (2014). The proportion of excessive fast-food consumption attributable to the neighbourhood food environment among youth living within 1 km of their school. *Applied Physiology Nutrition and Metabolism*, **39**: 480–486.

Lee, S., Young, B. E., Cooper, E. M. *et.al.* (2014). Nutrient inadequacy is prevalent in pregnant adolescents, and prenatal supplement use may not fully compensate for dietary deficiencies. *Childhood Obesity and Nutrition* **6**: 152–159.

Li, L., Sun, N., Zhang, L. *et al.* (2020). Fast food consumption among young adolescents aged 12–15 years in 54 low- and middle-income countries. *Global Health Action* **13**: 795438.

Lorentzon, M., Mellström, D., Haug, E. *et al.* (2007). Smoking is associated with lower bone mineral density and reduced cortical thickness in young men. *Journal of Clinical Endocrinology and Metabolism* **92**: 497–503.

Łucka, I., Domarecki, P. and Janikowska-Hołoweńko, D. (2019). The prevalence and risk factors of orthorexia nervosa among school-age youth of Pomeranian and Warmian-Masurian voivodeships. *Psychiatria Polska* **53**: 383–398.

Ma, X.M., Huang, Z.W., Yang, X.G. and Su, Y.X. (2014). Calcium supplementation and bone mineral accretion in Chinese adolescents aged 12–14 years: a 12-month, dose-response, randomised intervention trial. *British Journal of Nutrition* **112**: 1510–1520.

Mackerras, D. and Rutishauser, I. (2005). 24-Hour national dietary survey data: how do we interpret them most effectively? *Public Health Nutrition* **8**: 657–665.

Marvin-Dowle, K., Burley, V.J. and Soltani, H. (2016). Nutrient intakes and nutritional biomarkers in pregnant adolescents: a systematic review of studies in developed countries. *BMC Pregnancy and Childbirth* **16**: 268.

Mathew *et al.* (2020).

Medin, A.C., Myhre, J.B., Diep, L.M. and Andersen, L.F. (2019). Diet quality on days without breakfast or lunch – Identifying targets to improve adolescents' diet. *Appetite* **135**: 123–130.

Meng, K., Qiu, J., Benardot, D. *et al.* (2020). The risk of low energy availability in Chinese elite and recreational

female aesthetic sports athletes. *Journal of the International Society of Sports Nutrition* **17**: 13.

Méquinion, M., Foldi, C.J. and Andrews, Z.B. (2020). The Ghrelin-AgRP neuron nexus in anorexia nervosa: implications for metabolic and behavioral adaptations. *Frontiers in Nutrition* **6**: 190.

Miller, K.E., Dermen, K.H. and Lucke, J.F. (2018). Caffeinated energy drink use by U.S. adolescents aged 13–17: a national profile. *Psychology of Addictive Behaviour* **32**: 647–659.

Milos, G., Gallo, L.M., Sosic, B. *et al.* (2011). Bone mineral density in young women on methadone substitution. *Calcified Tissue International* **89**: 228–233.

Morean, M.E., Bold, K.W., Kong, G. *et al.* (2020). High school students' use of flavored e-cigarette e-liquids for appetite control and weight loss. *Addictive Behaviours* **102**: 106139.

Mosca, L.N., da Silva, V.N. and Goldberg, T.B. (2013). Does excess weight interfere with bone mass accumulation during adolescence? *Nutrients* **5**: 2047–2061.

Moskowitz, L. and Weiselberg, E. (2017). Anorexia Nervosa/Atypical Anorexia Nervosa. *Current Problems in Pediatric and Adolescent Health Care* **47**: 70–84.

Moussa, M., Hansz, K., Rasmussen, M. *et al.* (2021). Cardiovascular Effects of Energy Drinks in the Pediatric Population. *Pediatric Emergency Care* doi: 10.1097/PEC.0000000000002165.

Müller, K., Libuda, L., Diethelm, K. *et al.* (2013). Lunch at school, at home or elsewhere. Where do adolescents usually get it and what do they eat? Results of the HELENA Study. *Appetite* **71**: 332–339.

Napolitano, M.A., Lynch, S.B. and Stanton, C.A. (2020). Young adult e-cigarette users: perceptions of stress, body image, and weight control. *Eating and Weight Disorders* **25**: 487–495.

National Institute on Drug Abuse. (2019). Trends and statistics. https://www.drugabuse.gov/drug-topics/trends-statistics (accessed 9 April 2021).

Neumark-Sztainer, D. and Hannan, P.J. (2000). Weight-related behaviors among adolescent girls and boys: results from a national survey. *Archives of Pediatric and Adolescent Medicine* **154**: 569–577.

Neumark-Sztainer, D., Story, M., Perry, C. *et al.* (1999). Factors influencing food choices of adolescents: findings from focus-group discussions with adolescents. *Journal of the American Dietetic Association* **99**: 929–937.

Neumark-Sztainer, D., Wall, M., Guo, J. *et al.* (2006). Obesity, disordered eating, and eating disorders in a longitudinal study of adolescents: how do dieters fare 5 years later? *Journal of the American Dietetic Association* **106**: 559–568.

NHS Digital. (2019a). Smoking, drinking and drug use among young people in England 2018. https://digital.nhs.uk/data-and-information/publications/statistical/smoking-drinking-and-drug-use-among-young-people-in-england/2018/part-5-alcohol-drinking-prevalence-and-consumption (accessed 9 April 2021).

NHS Digital. (2019b). Statistics on Drug Misuse, England 2019. Part 4: Drug use among young people. https://digital.nhs.uk/data-and-information/publications/statistical/statistics-on-drug-misuse/2019/part-4-drug-use-among-young-people (accessed 9 April 2021).

O'Dea, J.A. (2003). Why do kids eat healthful food? Perceived benefits of and barriers to healthful eating and physical activity among children and adolescents. *Journal of the American Dietetic Association* **103**: 497–501.

Olmedilla, B. and Granado, F. (2000). Growth and micronutrient needs of adolescents. *European Journal of Clinical Nutrition* **54**(Suppl 1): S11–S15.

Opitz, M.C., Newman, E., Alvarado Vázquez Mellado, A.S. et al. (2020). The psychometric properties of Orthorexia Nervosa assessment scales: A systematic review and reliability generalization. *Appetite* 2020 **155**: 104797.

Paeratakul, S., Ferdinand, D.P., Champagne, C.M. et al. (2003). Fast-food consumption among US adults and children: dietary and nutrient intake profile. *Journal of the American Dietetic Association* **103**: 1332–1338.

Palla, L., Chapman, A., Beh, E. et al. (2020). Where do adolescents eat less-healthy foods? Correspondence analysis and logistic regression results from the UK National Diet and Nutrition Survey. *Nutrients* **12**: 2235.

Paolacci, S., Kiani, A.K., Manara, E. et al. (2020). Genetic contributions to the etiology of anorexia nervosa: New perspectives in molecular diagnosis and treatment. *Molecular Genetics and Genomic Medicine* **8**: e1244.

Perotti, M., Perra, S., Saluzzi, A. et al. (2013). Body fat mass is a strong and negative predictor of peak stimulated growth hormone and bone mineral density in healthy adolescents during transition period. *Hormone and Metabolic Research*, **45**, 748–753.

Petrie, H.J., Stover, E.A. and Horswill, C.A. (2004). Nutritional concerns for the child and adolescent competitor. *Nutrition* **20**: 620–631.

Piacentino, D., Kotzalidis, G.D., Del Casale, A. et al. (2020). Anabolic-androgenic steroid use and psychopathology in athletes: a systematic review. *Current Neuropharmacology* **13**: 101–121.

Potter, B.K., Pederson, L.L., Chan, S.S. et al. (2004). Does a relationship exist between body weight, concerns about weight, and smoking among adolescents? An integration of the literature with an emphasis on gender. *Nicotine and Tobacco Research* **6**: 397–425.

Prendergast, F.J., Livingstone, K.M., Worsley, A. and McNaughton, S.A. (2016). Correlates of meal skipping in young adults: a systematic review. *International Journal of Nutrition and Physical Activity* **13**: 125.

Public Health England. (2016). *Government Dietary Recommendations Government recommendations for energy and nutrients for males and females aged 1 –18 years and 19+ year*. London: PHE.

Pudney, E.V., Himmelstein, M.S. and Puhl, R.M. (2019). The role of weight stigma in parental weight talk. *Pediatric Obesity* **14**: e12534.

Puhl, R.M. and Lessard, LM. (2020). Weight Stigma in Youth: Prevalence, Consequences, and Considerations for Clinical Practice. *Current Obesity Reports* **9**: 402–411.

Quick, V., Nansel, T.R., Liu, D. et al. (2014). Body size perception and weight control in youth: 9-year international trends from 24 countries. *International Journal of Obesity* **38**: 988–994.

Ravi, S., Waller, B., Valtonen, M. et al. (2021). Menstrual dysfunction and body weight dissatisfaction among Finnish young athletes and non-athletes. *Scandinavian Journal of Medicine and Science in Sports* **31**: 405–417.

Ristori, J., Fisher, A.D., Castellini, G., et al., (2019). Gender Dysphoria and Anorexia Nervosa Symptoms in Two Adolescents. *Archives of Sexual Behaviour* **48**: 1625–1631.

Roberts, C. Steer, T., Maplethorpe, N. et al. (2018). *National Diet and Nutrition Survey. Results from years 7 and 8 (combined) of the Rolling Programme*. London: Public Health England.

Robinson-O'Brien, R., Perry, C.L., Wall, M.M. et al. (2009). Adolescent and young adult vegetarianism: better dietary intake and weight outcomes but increased risk of disordered eating behaviors. *Journal of the American Dietetic Association* **109**: 648–655.

Roemmich, J.N., Richmond, R.J. and Rogol, A.D. (2001). Consequences of sport training during puberty. *Journal of Endocrinological Investigation* **24**: 708–715.

Schagen, S.E, Cohen-Kettenis, P.T., Delemarre-van de Waal, H.A. and Hannema, S.E. (2016). Efficacy and safety of gonadotropin-releasing hormone agonist treatment to suppress puberty in gender dysphoric adolescents. *Journal of Sexual Medicine* **13**: 1125–1132.

Schvey, N.A., Marwitz, S.E., Mi, S.J. et al. (2019). Weight-based teasing is associated with gain in BMI and fat mass among children and adolescents at-risk for obesity: a longitudinal study. *Pediatric Obesity* **14**: e12538.

Scott-Van Zeeland, A.A., Bloss, C.S., Tewhey, R. et al. (2014). Evidence for the role of EPHX2 gene variants in anorexia nervosa. Molecular Psychiatry **19**: 724–732.

Sebastian, R.S., Cleveland, L.E. and Goldman, J.D. (2008). Effect of snacking frequency on adolescents' dietary intakes and meeting national recommendations. *Journal of Adolescent Health* **42**: 503–511.

Segovia-Siapco, G., Burkholder-Cooley, N., Haddad Tabrizi, S. and Sabaté, J. (2019b). Beyond meat: a comparison of the dietary intakes of vegetarian and non-vegetarian adolescents. *Frontiers in Nutrition* **6**: 86.

Segovia-Siapco, G., Khayef, G., Pribis, P. et al. (2019a). Animal Protein Intake Is Associated with General Adiposity in Adolescents: The Teen Food and Development Study. *Nutrients* **12**: 110.

Seifert, S.M., Schaechter, J.L., Hershorin, E.R. and Lipshultz, S.E. (2011). Health effects of energy drinks on children, adolescents, and young adults. *Pediatrics* **127**: 511–528.

Serdar, M., Mordelt, A., Müser, K. et al. (2019). Detrimental impact of energy drink compounds on developing oligodendrocytes and neurons. *Cells* **8**: 1381.

Shaw, M.E. (1998). Adolescent breakfast skipping: an Australian study. *Adolescence* **33**: 851–861.

Simone, M., Hooper, L., Eisenberg, M.E. and Neumark-Sztainer, D. (2019). Unhealthy weight control behaviors and substance use among adolescent girls: The harms of weight stigma. *Social Science and Medicine* **233**: 64–70.

Singhal, V., Sanchita, S., Malhotra, S. et al. (2019). Suboptimal bone microarchitecure in adolescent girls with obesity compared to normal-weight controls and girls with anorexia nervosa. *Bone* **122**: 246–253.

Solmi, F., Sharpe, H., Gage, S.H. et al. (2020). Changes in the prevalence and correlates of weight-control behaviors and weight perception in adolescents in the UK, 1986–2015. *JAMA Pediatrics* **175**: 267–275.

Specker, B.L. (2006). Influence of rapid growth on skeletal adaptation to exercise. *Journal of Musculoskeletal and Neuronal Interactions* **6**: 147–153.

Story, M., Holt, K. and Softka, A. (2002). *Bright Futures in Practice: Nutrition.* Arlington, VA: National Center for Education in Maternal and Child Health.

Strahler, J. (2019). Sex differences in orthorexic eating behaviors: A systematic review and meta-analytical integration. *Nutrition* **67–68**: 110534.

Sutin, A.R., Stephan, Y., Robinson, E. *et al.* (2020). Body-related discrimination and dieting and substance use behaviors in adolescence. *Appetite* **151**: 104689.

Tack, L.J.W., Craen, M., Lapauw, B. *et al.* (2018). Proandrogenic and antiandrogenic progestins in transgender youth: differential effects on body composition and bone metabolism. *Journal of Clinical Endocrinology and Metabolism* **103**: 2147–2156.

Taher, A.K., Evans, N. and Evans, C.E. (2019). The cross-sectional relationships between consumption of takeaway food, eating meals outside the home and diet quality in British adolescents. *Public Health Nutrition* **22**: 63–73.

Tanner, J.M. (1989). *Foetus into Man*, Ware: Castlemead Publications.

Tappia, P.S., Troughton, K.L., Langley-Evans, S.C. *et al.* (1995). Cigarette smoking influences cytokine production and antioxidant defences. *Clinical Science* **88**: 485–489.

Tavistock and Portman Trust (2020). *Gender Identity Development Service in 2019–20 same as 2018–19.* https://tavistockandportman.nhs.uk/about-us/news/stories/gender-identity-development-service-referrals-2019-20-same-2018-19 (accessed 10 April 2021).

Thane, C.W., Bates, C.J. and Prentice, A. (2003). Risk factors for low iron intake and poor iron status in a national sample of British young people aged 4–18 years. *Public Health Nutrition* **6**: 485–496.

Thein-Nissenbaum, J. (2013). Long-term consequences of the female athlete triad. *Maturitas* **75**: 107–112.

Unicef. (2019). *Early childbearing.* https://data.unicef.org/topic/child-health/adolescent-health (accessed 10 April 2021).

Vågstrand, K., Barkeling, B., Forslund, H.B. *et al.* (2007). Eating habits in relation to body fatness and gender in adolescents: results from the 'SWEDES' study. *European Journal of Clinical Nutrition* **61**: 517–525.

Välimäki, M.J., Kärkkäinen, M., Lamberg-Allardt, C. *et al.* (1994). Exercise, smoking, and calcium intake during adolescence and early adulthood as determinants of peak bone mass. Cardiovascular Risk in Young Finns Study Group. *BMJ* **309**: 230–235.

Vandewalle, S., Taes, Y., Fiers, T. *et al.* (2014). Sex steroids in relation to sexual and skeletal maturation in obese male adolescents. *Journal of Clinical Endocrinology and Metabolism* **99**: 2977–2985.

Vercammen, K.A., Koma, J.W., Bleich, S.N. (2019). Trends in energy drink consumption among U.S. adolescents and adults, 2003–2016. *American Journal of Preventive Medicine* **56**: 827–833.

Vlot, M.C., Klink, D.T., den Heijer, M. *et al.* (2017). Effect of pubertal suppression and cross-sex hormone therapy on bone turnover markers and bone mineral apparent density (BMAD) in transgender adolescents. *Bone* **95**: 11–19.

Vogel, K.A., Martin, B.R., McCabe, L.D. *et al.* (2017). The effect of dairy intake on bone mass and body composition in early pubertal girls and boys: a randomized controlled trial. *American Journal of Clinical Nutrition* **105**: 1214–1229.

Wallace, J.M., Luther, J.S., Milne, J.S. *et al.* (2006). Nutritional modulation of adolescent pregnancy outcome – a review. *Placenta* **27**: S61–S68.

Wang, Z., Dang, J., Zhang, X. *et al.* (2021). Assessing the relationship between weight stigma, stress, depression, and sleep in Chinese adolescents. *Quality of Life Research* **30**: 229–238.

Wang, Z., Wang, B., Hu, Y. *et al.* (2020). Relationships among weight stigma, eating behaviors and stress in adolescents in Wuhan, China. *Global Health Research Policy* **5**: 8.

Ward, K.A., Cole, T.J. and Laskey, M.A. (2014). The effect of prepubertal calcium carbonate supplementation on skeletal development in Gambian boys-a 12-year follow-up study. *Journal of Clinical Endocrinology and Metabolism* **99**: 3169–3176.

Weaver, C.M., Proulx, W.R. and Heaney, R. (1999). Choices for achieving adequate dietary calcium with a vegetarian diet. *American Journal of Clinical Nutrition* **70**: 543S–548S.

Welten, D.C., Kemper, H.C., Post, G.B. *et al.* (1994). Weight-bearing activity during youth is a more important factor for peak bone mass than calcium intake. *Journal of Bone and Mineral Research* **9**: 1089–1096.

Weng, C.B., Sheu, J.J. and Chen, H.S. (2021). Factors associated with unhealthy weight control behaviors among a representative sample of U.S. high school students. *Journal of School Nursing* doi:10.1177/1059840520965497.

White, A.M. and Swartzwelder, H.S. (2005). Age-related effects of alcohol on memory and memory-related brain function in adolescents and adults. *Recent Developments in Alcohol* **17**: 161–176.

Winpenny, E.M., Winkler, M.R., Stochl, J. *et al.* (2020). Associations of early adulthood life transitions with changes in fast food intake: a latent trajectory analysis. *International Journal of Behavioural Nutrition and Physical Activity* **17**: 130.

Winther, A., Jørgensen, L., Ahmed, L.A. *et al.* (2018). Bone mineral density at the hip and its relation to fat mass and lean mass in adolescents: the Tromsø Study, Fit Futures. *BMC Musculoskeletal Disorders* **19**: 21.

Wolk, B.J., Ganetsky, M., Babu, K.M. (2012). Toxicity of energy drinks. *Current Opinions in Pediatrics.* **24**, 243–251.

Wong, P.K., Christie, J.J. and Wark, J.D. (2007). The effects of smoking on bone health. *Clinical Science* **113**: 233–241.

World Health Organization. (2020). Adolescent pregnancy. https://www.who.int/news-room/fact-sheets/detail/adolescent-pregnancy (accessed 10 April 2021).

Wosje, K.S. and Kalkwarf, H.J. (2007). Bone density in relation to alcohol intake among men and women in the United States. *Osteoporosis International* **18**: 391–400.

Yilmaz, Z., Hardaway, J.A. and Bulik, C.M. (2015). Genetics and epigenetics of eating disorders. *Advances in Genomics and Genetics* **5**: 131–150.

Zhang, Z.Q., Ma, X.M., Huang, Z.W. *et al.* (2014). Effects of milk salt supplementation on bone mineral gain in pubertal Chinese adolescents: a 2-year randomized, double-blind, controlled, dose-response trial. *Bone* **65**: 69–76.

Zhu, X. and Zheng, H. (2021). Factors influencing peak bone mass gain. *Frontiers in Medicine* **15**: 53–69.

Zipfel, S., Giel, K.E., Bulik, C.M. *et al.* (2015). Anorexia nervosa: aetiology, assessment, and treatment. Lancet Psychiatry **2**: 1099–1111.

Additional reading

If you would like to find out more about the material discussed in this chapter, the following sources may be of interest:

Cameron, N., Bogin, B. (eds). (2012). *Human Growth and Development*. London: Academic Press.

Evans, J., Docter, A.D. (eds). (2020). *Adolescent Nutrition: Assuring the needs of emerging adults*. Cham: Springer Nature.

More, J. (ed.). (2013). *Infant, Child and Adolescent Nutrition. A practical handbook*. Boca Raton, CA: Taylor and Francis.

CHAPTER 8

The adult years

LEARNING OBJECTIVES

This chapter will enable the reader to:
- Show an awareness of the need to adjust diet and lifestyle during the adult years to promote maintenance of a healthy weight and avoid major disease states including cardiovascular disease, cancer and type 2 diabetes.
- Describe some of the different approaches taken by governments to promote healthy diet and lifestyle in populations.
- Describe the global trends in the prevalence of overweight and obesity.
- Demonstrate an understanding of the relationship between obesity, insulin resistance and risk of cardiovascular disease and diabetes.
- Describe optimal strategies for the management and treatment of obesity and related disorders.
- Discuss the diet-related risk factors for cardiovascular disease and show understanding of the extent to which dietary change can alter population level disease profiles.
- Critically review different approaches to nutritional epidemiology, showing an understanding of the limitations of observational and intervention studies.
- Describe the relationship between diet and cancer, showing an awareness of the elements of human diet and activity that may drive the processes of carcinogenesis and metastasis, and the factors that may play a role in cancer prevention.

8.1 Introduction

The preceding chapters in this book have considered the relationships between diet and health during periods of major physiological change. Demanding life stages and processes, such as development, growth, maturation and reproduction, all increase requirements for nutrients. Failure to deliver those nutrient demands can result in rapid onset of potentially disastrous outcomes for the individual or may set in place an increased risk of disease later in life. In contrast, the adult years from 19 to 65 are relatively 'quiet' from a nutritional perspective, but they do represent the stage of life at which most of the adverse consequences of poor nutrition and acquisition of unhealthy lifestyle behaviours in earlier life stages begin to manifest as major disease states. As discussed earlier in this book, the way in which the body responds to physiological challenges and variation in nutrition is determined by the cumulative effects of genetics, early life programming, lifestyle factors and the actions of the microbiome (see Research Highlight 8.1). The adult years are the life stage where these factors begin to impact heavily on lifestyle-related disease states. The main focus of this chapter is on nutrition-related diseases of adulthood and how diet and lifestyle change might offset risk of ill health and mortality.

8.2 Changing needs for nutrients

With the completion of growth at the end of the adolescent years, adult physiology becomes stable, with no further changes of a major nature until the degenerative processes associated with ageing begin to impact on organ functions (see Chapter 9). The peak of performance for most systems is achieved at around the age of 30 years but, with demand for most nutrients simply meeting the need for maintenance of function and repair processes, there is little variation in the need for nutrients across the earlier adult years. As there is no longer a demand associated with growth and maturation, requirements for most nutrients are lower in adulthood than were seen in adolescence. In most women, the menopause

Nutrition, Health and Disease: A Lifespan Approach, Third Edition. Simon Langley-Evans.
© 2021 John Wiley & Sons Ltd. Published 2021 by John Wiley & Sons Ltd.
Companion website: www.wiley.com/go/langleyevans/lifespan3e

Research Highlight 8.1 The microbiome, nutrition and health

The human body comprises a diverse community of human cells and microbial colonists, with microbial cells outnumbering human cells by at least tenfold. The presence of bacteria, fungi, viruses and protozoa in the body has major implications for human health as, in addition to potentially causing infectious disease, they produce a range of metabolic products and proteins which may either be harmful or beneficial to their human host (Ursell *et al.*, 2012; Calder *et al.*, 2018). The majority of organisms that exist in a commensal relationship with human cells are found in the gut, but local microbial communities exist in all parts of the body which are at the interface between the interior organs and the environment, such as the skin, mouth and vagina. The composition of the microbial community at each site will have specific characteristics. The core communities are established soon after birth and are relatively stable thereafter. However, rapid changes in composition can be achieved by using antibiotics or faecal transplant (Grehan *et al.*, 2010). Changes in the relative abundance of different groups of bacteria may occur with ageing or can be brought about through dietary change. As the presence of a vast microbial community puts a range of non-human enzymes and signalling molecules into the gut, the microbiome plays an important role in modifying the individual response to food, representing another reason why a one-size-fits-all approach to diet-health interventions is problematic (see Chapter 1).

The action of microbes, particularly bacteria, in the gut plays a role in human nutrition. The generation of vitamin K, for example, is bacterial dependent and humans also absorb vitamin B12 and riboflavin of bacterial origin (LeBlanc *et al.*, 2013). Other bacterial products may reflect the composition of the diet and some bacterial species may increase in abundance to exploit dietary changes. For example comparing the gut microbiome of American, Spanish and Japanese populations enabled Hehemann *et al.* (2012) to demonstrate that, in Japanese individuals, gut bacteria had capacity to degrade algal carbohydrates associated with consumption of sushi; a direct response to the presence of specific polysaccharides in the diet.

Bacterial products may be both beneficial and harmful to human health. For example, short chain fatty acids such as butyrate, generated by gut bacteria, are known to have anti-cancer properties. Dietary change to promote their generation may reduce risk of colon cancer. In contrast, the passage of bacterial cell wall material across the gut barrier leads to inflammation which is associated with autoimmune disease, type-2 diabetes and atherosclerosis (Rodriguez *et al.*, 2021).

Dietary patterns can alter the balance of species present in the core microbiome. A high-fat diet generates a profile of gut bacteria which promotes inflammation and even weight gain (Cani *et al.*, 2007). Obesity has a distinct microbiological 'signature' in the gut, which is reflected in the balance of *Bacteroides* and *Firmicutes* species (Ley *et al.*, 2005; Okubo *et al.*, 2018). When people who are obese lose weight through dietary change, the abundance of *Bacteroides* increases (Ley *et al.*, 2005). Other bacterial species are signatures for other conditions. In type-2 diabetes, *Betaproteobacteria* abundance is enriched, while *Firmicutes* and *Clostridia* are reduced in the gut. In addition to influencing inflammation this variation in the balance of species can determine fatty acid metabolism, dietary energy availability and even endocrine regulation of physiological processes (Ejtahed *et al.*, 2016).

will occur between the ages of 45 and 55 years. Although it has major endocrine effects that impact on physiological processes, menopause is of limited significance in terms of nutrition and health.

Beyond the change in demands associated with attainment of mature physique, protein and micronutrient requirements are unchanging across the earlier adult years. The requirements for protein are stable at 0.8 g/kg per day, and the requirements for vitamins and minerals are essentially similar at age 19 and age 60. However, this lack of change in demands masks the major change that is required in terms of the quality of diet across this time span. With ageing comes a need for the diet to become more nutrient dense (i.e. for the concentration of protein and micronutrients per unit of energy to increase). This reflects a downward shift in energy requirements with ageing.

Energy requirements of adults are lower than those of adolescents partly due to the loss of requirement for growth, but mainly due to typically lower levels of expenditure through physical activity.

Actual energy requirements of individual adults will vary widely, with sex, activity level, state of health and body size all contributing to this variation. For most adults engaged in sedentary occupations, energy requirements will fall not only relative to the adolescent years, but across the middle years of adulthood also. This is due to a decline in the resting metabolic rate (Figure 8.1).

Making adjustments to this protracted change in nutrient requirements can often be problematic, and overnutrition leading to overweight and obesity is commonplace among adults in westernized and, increasingly, the developing countries. Most of the major disease states – diabetes, cardiovascular disease (CVD) and cancer – which are reviewed later in this chapter are the consequence of this overnutrition. However, it is important to bear in mind that the undernutrition described earlier in this book in relation to children remains a significant problem among adult populations. Adult undernutrition will be observed in developing countries and in the developed countries of the world among particular

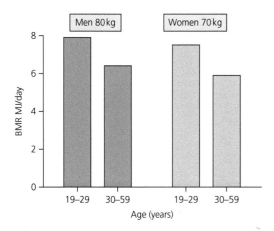

Figure 8.1 Basal metabolic rate (BMR) declines with age in men and women. Data show BMR estimates for men and women of average weight, derived from the Schofield equations:
Males aged 18–29 years: BMR = 0.063 × body weight + 2.869.
Males aged 30–59 years: BMR = 0.048 × body weight + 3.653.
Females aged 18–29 years: BMR = 0.062 × body weight + 2.036.
Females aged 30–59 years: BMR = 0.034 × body weight + 3.538.

subgroups in the population. Those at risk of malnutrition include the homeless, alcohol abusers, intravenous drug users, institutionalized individuals, the chronically ill, older people (see Chapter 9) and those infected with HIV. Whereas in children malnutrition rapidly becomes a life-threatening factor, among adults, undernutrition in these circumstances will generally be present over a longer term. Malnutrition in adults reduces the capacity to do physical work, which in many countries will impact on the ability to provide food and care for whole families. Undernutrition will also reduce the capacity of individuals to respond to metabolic trauma, triggered by infection, injury or surgery. Ultimately, the undernourished adult is as much at risk of premature death as the overweight or obese adult.

8.3 Guidelines for healthy nutrition

Decades of research that has considered the relationships between diet and disease have left no doubt that defining the optimal diet for a population is a complex process and that communicating dietary advice clearly to the population is a major challenge. Individuals respond metabolically to variation in the composition of the diet in different ways, and this variation will depend upon often poorly understood genetic factors, early life programming influences, the microbiome and lifestyle factors. However, it is clear that in general terms a healthier diet should be a varied diet in which carbohydrate provides the basic staple, with energy intakes from fat and protein providing lesser components of intake (Table 8.1). In most circumstances, healthy adults are advised to base meals on starchy foods, to consume five portions of fruit and vegetables per day, to consume two portions of fish per week (including one of oily fish) and to have low intakes of fats and sugars. Food intakes should be well spaced throughout the day, and breakfast remains an essential meal of the day, as in childhood.

Engagement of the public with healthy eating messages is variable and understanding is often poor. To a large extent, this results from the way in which the media portrays nutritional science. The reporting of studies of nutrition, health and disease is often overly simplistic and selective and fails to cover the limitations of studies. Reporting rarely describes an overview of a large body of evidence and instead represents single, isolated studies. Mixed messages and inappropriate reporting can induce scepticism and resentment, leading to rejection of established healthy eating guidelines by the public. For example, a report by Oyebode *et al.* (2014) demonstrating that consumption of seven or more portions of fruit and vegetables per day reduced all-cause mortality in the Health Survey for England prompted media reporting that existing guidelines should change and tabloid pronouncements about 'food police' and unreasonable demands for dietary change. However, the original paper had done no more than confirm well-established observations. Similarly, reporting of a meta-analysis on fats and CVD (Chowdhury *et al.*, 2014) concluded that there was little evidence

Table 8.1 General guidelines for intake of sugars, fats and salt by adults.

Nutrient	Maximum recommended intake (% of daily energy)*
Fats	
Saturated fatty acids	10
Polyunsaturated fatty acids	10
Monounsaturated fatty acids	12
Total fats	35
Sugars	
Milk sugars and starch	39
Free sugars	5[†]
Total carbohydrate	50
Salt	6 g/day

Source: Department of Health (1999). Crown copyright.
* Also referred to as population averages.
† Also referred to as free sugars.

to back up current advice to replace saturated fats with polyunsaturated fats prompted a media outcry about the merits of butter and further public misunderstanding of science. The media highlights and thrives upon disagreement and controversy, and as a result, the public struggle to understand how scientific evidence accumulates slowly, how the nature of our understanding tends to be provisional, and that the overall balance of data are more important than single studies. UK reporting of a call from Action on Sugar (2014) for aggressive action to reduce sugar consumption suggested to the public that single nutrients or classes of nutrients were drivers of disease, which, as described later in this chapter, is a viewpoint that most nutritional scientists would now reject and recognize as a mistake in early research into diet and cancer. This view was reinforced by changes to population guidelines to state that intakes of free sugars should be no more than 5% of energy intake (Scientific Advisory Committee on Nutrition, 2015). The growth of social media as an influencer of beliefs and behaviour is increasingly problematic. Prominent social media figures can promote dietary extremes to suit a particular agenda (usually a new diet book and personal profit), deride expert advice and condemn nutrition professionals as 'shills' for the food industry, without the need to fact check. Observing unqualified, self-styled nutrition gurus declaring that low-carbohydrate, high-fat diets are an ideal and that the dietary advice that has stood in place for more than 40 years is 'genocide' (Alliance for Natural Health, 2019), is difficult and hurtful for the dedicated professionals who have made public health and dietetic care their careers.

Despite these contradictions in the media and associated confusion among consumers, highly successful health promotion campaigns across westernized countries, such as the five-a-day campaign (NHS England, 2018), mean that many general messages about healthy nutrition are now widely recognized, but are not necessarily fully understood or adhered to. Communicating information such as that shown in Table 8.1 to the population presents a sizeable problem. Concepts such as percentage of daily energy intake are complex and mean nothing within the context of individuals' daily dietary choices. Even with successful campaigns such as five-a-day, understanding of the detail behind the generalized message is often weak. The need to consume five portions of fruit and vegetables per day is simple to remember, but defining a 'portion' (actually 80 g of fresh, frozen, canned or dried fruit, vegetables, salad, fruit juice) is beyond most people. As a result, most governments in westernized nations have sought to develop simple pictorial models to

act as a guide to healthy adults, showing what comprises a healthy and well-balanced diet. In the UK, the Balance of Good Health plate model was introduced in the mid-1990s for this purpose (Health Education Authority, 1995). The Food Standards Agency redesigned this model in 2007 and Public Health England refined it again in 2016, producing the new Eatwell Guide (Figure 8.2).

The Eatwell Guide works on a principle that is common to similar models that are used in other countries, for example, the US Food Pyramid (US Department of Agriculture, 2005). Foods are divided into food groups. Within the Eatwell model, there are fruits and vegetables, breads, cereals and potatoes, milk and dairy, meat, fish and alternatives and foods containing fat and sugar. The sectors on the plate (Figure 8.2) are supposed to reflect the relative amount of food intake that should come from each group; hence, breads, cereals and potatoes, fruits and vegetables should provide approximately two thirds of intake. The most recent iteration of the Eatwell Guide removed foods rich in free sugars completely and confined oils and spreads to a very small component, to emphasise the message that fats and sugars should be consumed at a minimal level. There are variations on this model (e.g. Japanese Spinning Top Food Guide, Swedish Food Circle), and within the US Food Pyramid, for example, fruits and vegetables are in their own separate food groups, and it is suggested that intakes of foods from the breads, cereals, pasta and rice group outweigh intakes of the fruit and vegetable groups. The Swedish Food Circle is similar in design to the Eatwell plate but crucially lacks the foods containing fat and sugar food group (hence discouraging their intake altogether) and separates vegetables into 'root vegetables' (starchy roots such as carrots and potatoes) and 'essential vegetables' (green leafy vegetables that are important micronutrient sources). The US Food Pyramid was first introduced in 1992 and was widely taken up by other countries in Europe, Australasia, Africa and Asia. An updated version of the pyramid model, MyPyramid, was introduced in the United States in 2005 to reflect some of the factors, including age, weight and ethnicity, that shape nutrient demands. In 2011, the US Department of Agriculture replaced the Food Pyramid with 'MyPlate', which recommends targets for food group consumption with detail on what and how much to eat within a daily energy allowance based on age, sex, body mass index (BMI) and level of physical activity. This provides a more personalized format for nutrition advice but required positive engagement with users who need to input their own health data. This latter point emphasizes

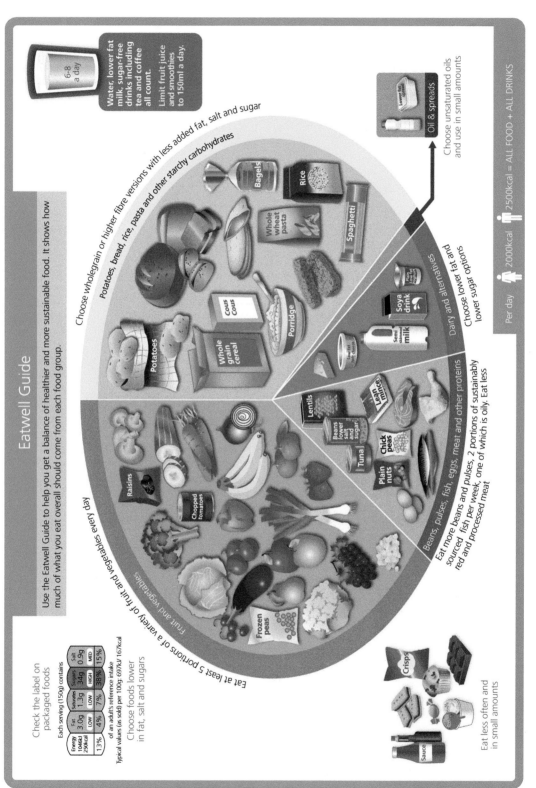

Figure 8.2 The Eatwell plate. This pictorial representation of the relative proportions of foods from each of five groups that should be included in a healthy diet is used as one of the key aids in health education in the United Kingdom. *Source*: Public Health England (2016).

the major problem with all such pictorial guidance schemes, as they can educate, but are of little practical use to individuals in daily life.

When confronted with the infinite variety of food products in supermarkets, individuals either forget or become confused by healthy eating messages. This has prompted many countries to promote improved food labelling schemes that provide clear and simple nutritional messages at the point of sale. In the UK, attempts to introduce a food 'traffic light' scheme in which foodstuffs would bear a label showing content of fat, saturated fat, sugar and salt highlighted as red for high, amber for medium and green for low has largely failed due to lack of commitment from supermarkets. It is now common practice for foods to be labelled with the less informative 'guideline daily amounts' (Figure 8.3). Consumers in Norway, Sweden, Iceland and Denmark have a simplified guide to healthy options when buying food in shops or eating out. The Livsmedelsverket Keyhole (Figure 8.3) symbol is a voluntary label, and food producers take responsibility for ensuring that foods bearing the symbol conform to regulations and are low in fat, sugar and salt and high in dietary fibre.

8.4 Disease states associated with unhealthy nutrition and lifestyle

8.4.1 Obesity
8.4.1.1 Classification of overweight and obesity

Obesity is normally defined on the basis of BMI (Table 8.2). This anthropometric measurement based on height and weight is actually a poor indicator of body fatness, so its usefulness in studying or managing obesity (which is essentially the presence of excess body fat) has been questioned. BMI cannot discriminate between lean tissue mass and fat mass and so will often misclassify individuals who are particularly muscular. However, for most clinical purposes and for epidemiological studies at the population level, BMI is a measurement that is fit for purpose. The BMI classifications shown in Table 8.2 are a generalization, and many obesity researchers argue that specific cut-offs should be used for different ethnic groups and should be age specific. South Asians, for example, have more body fat than white populations at any given level of BMI, when this is measured using robust methods such as computed tomography. A BMI of 27.0 may

Table 8.2 Classifying obesity using body mass index or waist circumference.

	Body mass index (kg/m2)
Underweight	<18.5
Desirable weight	18.5–24.9
Overweight	25.0–29.9
Obese	>30.0

	Waist circumference (cm)	
	Men	**Women**
Action level* 1	94	80
Action level 2	102	88

Source: data from Lean *et al.* (1995).
* Action levels 1 and 2 correspond to overweight and obese classifications and indicate the waist circumferences at which action to reduce weight would be beneficial to health.

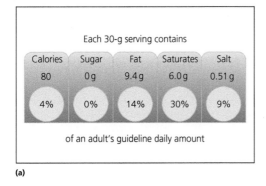

(a)

(b)

Figure 8.3 Symbols used in food labelling. a) A guideline daily amount-based food label. Guideline daily amounts on food labels represent the average requirements of an adult woman. Presenting front-of-pack information on energy, sugar, fats and salt is intended to enable consumers to make healthy choices. b) The Swedish National Food Administration Keyhole symbol. Only foods that are low in fat, sugar and salt can carry this logo, which allows consumers to identify the foods that comprise a healthy diet, both in shops and when eating out.

therefore be a more appropriate cut-off to define obesity in this ethnic group (Weisell, 2002).

Fat is distributed in different regions of the body and will be found in a subcutaneous layer, in depots with the abdomen and in depots around organs such as the heart and kidneys and present within tissues such as the liver and skeletal muscle. The fat stored in locations other than subcutaneously is termed visceral fat. The patterns of fat deposition within an individual may be critical determinants of their disease risk (see Sections 8.4.4.3.1 and 8.4.5.4.1) and will vary between the sexes. Males typically store fat in an android pattern, where most visceral fat accumulates in the abdomen. Women store fat in a gynoid pattern, with the buttocks and hips providing the main depots. In obesity, however, women will tend to adopt an android shape, as fat is stored centrally.

BMI cannot determine the patterns of fat distribution within the body, so other anthropometric tools are necessary. Historically, the waist–hip ratio, which simply required measurements of the circumference of the body around the waist and the hips, was viewed as a measure of abdominal fat deposition. Lean *et al.* (1995), however, suggested that waist circumference alone serves as a robust marker of central obesity, and this measure is now widely accepted (Table 8.2).

8.4.1.2 Prevalence and trends in obesity

The rise in the prevalence of obesity across the globe is well documented and widely reported. In most countries of the world, the proportion of obese adults increased by 40–50% between the mid-1990s and the first few years of the twenty-first century. In westernized countries, this increase in prevalence coincided with a decrease in overall energy intake, which strongly suggests that the rising trend was related to sedentary lifestyle.

The World Health Organization (2020) estimated that in 2016, globally, there were 1.9 billion adults who were overweight and 650 million who were obese over the age of 20, representing 39% and 13% of world population, respectively. Levels of obesity worldwide tripled between 1975 and 2016. As increasing economic prosperity brings about changes in diet and lifestyle in the developing countries, overweight and obesity have become a greater driver of disease and mortality than underweight. Among the countries of the European Union, it is estimated that 61% of adults are overweight or obese, with the highest rates seen in Malta and Latvia. 31% of Australian adults were obese in 2018 (Australian Institute of Health and Welfare, 2020). Table 8.3 shows data from the World Obesity Federation (2021), which highlight the countries with the greatest adult obesity problems, in different regions of the world.

Table 8.3 Global distribution of obesity in adults; countries within each region with the highest prevalence of obesity, 2001–2006.

Region	Men		Women	
	Country	(%)	Country	(%)
Europe	Malta	36.9	Georgia	36
	Greece	30.5	Turkey	35.9
	Georgia	30.2	Romania	34.1
Eastern Mediterranean	Qatar	39.5	Kuwait	49.1
	Kuwait	37.6	Egypt	48.8
	Bahrain	33	Qatar	43.2
North America and Caribbean	United States	42.2	Antigua and Barbuda	60
	Saint Kitts and Nevis	37.9	Bahamas	54.8
	Bahamas	31.8	Saint Kitts and Nevis	52.5
South and Central America	Argentina	31.4	Chile	38.4
	Chile	30.3	Argentina	33.4
	Venezuela	22.2	Ecuador	30.9
Africa	Seychelles	22	South Africa	41
	Mauritius	11.1	Seychelles	39
	South Africa	11	Mauritania	31.5
Southeast Asia	Maldives	7.9	Maldives	19.3
	Thailand	7	Sri Lanka	13.3
	Bhutan	4.5	Myanmar	13.1
Western Pacific	Cook Islands	68.7	Tonga	82.8
	Tonga	66.8	Cook Islands	70.7
	Niue	59.2	Samoa	68.6

Source: data from World Obesity Federation (2021).

The UK and the United States are among the most closely studied countries with regard to increasing obesity prevalence in both adults and children. The prevalence of obesity almost doubled in the UK between 1995 and 2015, and in fact prevalence quadrupled from 1980–2015 (Figure 8.4). Across the four UK nations, approximately 28% of adults are obese and a further 36% are overweight (England 28.7% obese, 35.6% overweight; Scotland 28% obese, 37% overweight; Wales 24% obese, 36% overweight; Northern Ireland 25% obese, 37% overweight). In the United States, the prevalence of obesity increased from 30.5% to 42.4% between 1999 and 2018 and the prevalence of severe obesity almost doubled from 4.7% to 9.2% over the same period. While US men are more likely to be obese than US women, 56.9% of non-Hispanic Black women were obese in 2018 (Centers for Disease Control and Prevention, 2021).

8.4.1.3 Causes of obesity in adulthood

While some associations between body fatness in childhood and early life experience may explain the development of obesity in adulthood (see earlier chapters), the adult lifestyle is the primary driver of weight gain and body fatness.

The combination of an excessive nutrient intake and a sedentary lifestyle promotes positive energy balance and adiposity. Positive energy balance will also be driven by genetic factors, and polymorphisms in genes that contribute to the regulation of appetite, energy metabolism and adipokine release may well predispose individuals to obesity. However, single-locus mutations that contribute to obesity are extremely rare, and most obesity-promoting genotypes are dependent on lifestyle factors to be fully expressed.

The rising prevalence of obesity across the globe over the last decades of the twentieth and first decade of the twenty-first centuries is almost wholly explained by changes in lifestyle over the same period. The availability and consumption of energy increased hugely relative to the 1970s and 1980s, and while intakes of sugars tended to decrease, fat consumption increased markedly (Prentice and Jebb, 1995). Food processing technology generated an infinite variety of inexpensive and attractive products. The low cost of this food contributed to increased portion sizes and with changing patterns of family life, more people chose to consume pre-packaged foods that were energy dense and nutrient poor. The increased use of cars in preference to walking and cycling, even over relatively short distances, contributed to a slump in physical activity and associated energy expenditure. Occupations that involved manual labour and heavy industry were replaced with desk-based jobs and leisure activities reinforced the sedentary way of living by becoming focused on television and the internet.

8.4.1.4 Treatment of obesity

Obesity is associated with significantly greater risk of major illness and premature death due to a variety of causes. Greenberg *et al.* (2007) estimated that a BMI greater than 30 kg/m^2 increased risk of death from any cause by 170% in a US population aged between 51 and 70 years. Banegas *et al.* (2003) estimated that in European countries 7.7% of all deaths were related to obesity, of which 70% were from CVD and 20% were cancer related. The association of obesity with diabetes, CVD and certain cancers is discussed in greater depth later in this chapter.

Given the importance of obesity and overweight as risk factors for life-threatening disease, the treatment and management of obesity is a major priority. Weight loss can be achieved through a wide variety of different approaches that use dietary change, increases in physical activity, pharmacological agents and bariatric surgery. Short-term weight loss carries no real health benefits, and there are some suggestions that weight cycling, in which individuals continually lose and then regain body weight, may actually increase risk of major disease. If the goal for obese individuals in the population is to lose weight for a sustained period, none of the approaches indicated above will be successful in isolation. Sustained weight loss depends upon wholesale lifestyle and behavioural changes that incorporate strategies for reducing energy intake while increasing expenditure through activity.

Dietary approaches to losing weight are legion, and a massive multibillion-pound industry has grown up around the global obesity pandemic. Most, if not all, of the restrictive diet practices that

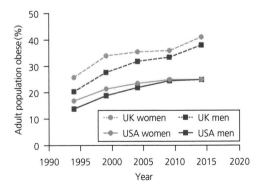

Figure 8.4 Trends in adult obesity 1993–2015 in the USA and UK.

are advocated will be effective in the short term but are unlikely to produce sustained weight loss (Figure 8.5). The more bizarre and difficult it is to follow the commercial/fad diet programmes, the harder the users will find the process, reducing the likelihood that the new eating pattern will be successfully incorporated into a permanent lifestyle change. The most effective strategies for reducing energy intake will be those that require less will-power to follow. In this respect, reducing energy intake by limiting snacking (which may contribute in excess of 300 kcal/day to the typical diet) or reducing portion sizes may be a helpful strategy (Jebb, 2005). Reductions of energy intake of approximately 500 kcal per day would be expected to produce weight loss of around 0.25 kg per week. This slow gradual weight loss is more likely to be successful in the longer term. Intermittent fasting is one approach to reducing energy intake without the problem of sustaining a continual restraint on food intake (Varady, 2011). Typically, this involves two days per week of severe caloric restriction (<200 kcal/day) and five days of ad libitum intake. In the short term, this brings about weight loss that is equivalent to continuous restriction (Klempel *et al.*, 2012, Kroeger *et al.* 2012), and this loss may be sustained to one year (Arguin *et al.*, 2012).

Many weight-loss diets have been designed to reduce fat intake, working on the assumption that if obesity is increased body fatness, then consuming less fat will promote weight loss. This is of course overly simplistic, and most studies show that decreasing fat intake has only short-term effects on body weight and that these are almost certainly the result of reducing the energy density of the diet (Jebb, 2005).

There is major interest in diets that limit carbo-hydrate intake. These have been shown to be as effective as low-fat diets in terms of weight loss but confer more metabolic benefits (Frigolet *et al.*, 2011). The Atkins diet, for example, reduces intake of carbohy-drates to just 10–30% of daily energy intake and allows unlimited consumption of protein and fat. Weight loss is supposed to occur as the lower blood sugar resulting from carbohydrate restriction pro-motes ketosis and lowers insulin concentrations. This is proposed to stimulate lipolysis and inhibit lipogen-esis. However, it is far more likely that the greater pro-tein intakes associated with such diets promote satiety and simply reduce overall energy intake. Consumption of high-protein, low-carbohydrate diets results in the body entering a ketogenic state, and the resulting increase in β-hydroxybutyrate concentrations will suppress appetite and increase gluconeogenesis. The latter is proposed to increase energy expenditure (Veldhorst *et al.*, 2009). A high-protein diet will also favour the deposition of fat-free mass over fat mass, where weight regain occurs (Westerterp-Plantenga *et al.*, 2012). Low-carbohydrate, high-fat diets (ketogenic diets) are discussed in more detail in Research Highlight 8.2, but essentially are appropriate only for short-term treatment of pre-existing obesity-related conditions, rather than as diets to prevent weight gain and disease.

Another approach to modifying the diet is to restrict intake of carbohydrates to those with a lower glycaemic index (GI). GI is a ranking system that rates different carbohydrate sources according to their impact upon blood glucose and insulin con-centrations. Simple sugars that are rapidly absorbed, producing a large spike in blood glucose, have high GI, while complex carbohydrates that require greater digestion and release glucose into the blood in a slow sustained fashion have low GI. True GI will vary between individuals due to variation in the response to different foodstuffs. Low-GI diets appear to promote weight loss in animal studies, but data from human trials remain controversial. Miller *et al.* (2011) reported that an intervention to increase consumption of low-GI foods resulted in weight loss and a reduction in waist circumference, but this study only considered short-term weight loss and did not have a control group. In contrast, Papadaki *et al.* (2014) found no significant benefits of a low-GI diet upon weight or symptoms of the metabolic syndrome, and Ajala *et al.* (2013) concluded from a meta-analysis that low-GI diets had no significant benefits over other dietary approaches for weight loss in subjects with type 2 diabetes. Although some studies suggest that low-GI diets promote weight loss of 5% or more over a 12-month period, this

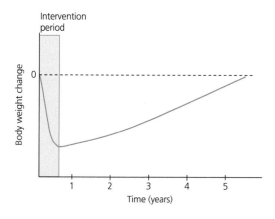

Figure 8.5 Weight loss is often followed by regain. Weight loss interventions generally result in weight loss for their duration in compliant individuals. Weight regain will begin once the intervention is complete, and full regain of lost weight will usually occur within a five-year period.

Research Highlight 8.2 Ketogenic diets, weight and metabolic health

For the past six decades the advice to increase intakes of complex carbohydrates and reduce fat consumption, while replacing saturated fats with plant-derived oils, has been at the heart of population level dietary guidelines. This has been driven by understanding of the relationships between diet, cholesterol metabolism and atherosclerosis. More recently, it has become clear that cardiovascular disease is also driven by inflammation and insulin resistance. Observations that a low-carbohydrate, high-fat (ketogenic) diet can be effective in promoting weight loss and improving insulin sensitivity in obese subjects have resulted in an interest in the use of ketogenic diets in prevention of obesity and related disorders. This interest has been stoked by controversial and highly biased articles that have questioned the central dogma of replacing animal fats with complex carbohydrates and plant oils (Malhotra *et al.*, 2017; Harcombe, 2017).

Ketogenic diets are marginally more effective than standard low-fat, energy-restricted diets in promoting weight loss. A systematic review of 17 randomized controlled trials found that ketogenic diets led to greater weight loss (–2 kg, 95% CI –3.1 to 0.9 kg) compared with low-fat diets and also reduced the number of cardiovascular events in people who were overweight and obese (Sackner-Bernstein *et al.*, 2015). However, most of these studies had a follow-up of less than 12 months. Bueno *et al.* (2013) showed that in studies of longer duration, the magnitude of difference in weight loss between ketogenic and low-fat diets was negligible in clinical terms (0.91 kg). In addition to a modest impact on weight loss, ketogenic diets are more effective than usual care in patients with type-2 diabetes, in terms of promoting weight loss, managing HbA1c and improving insulin sensitivity (Bhanpuri *et al.*, 2018).

Ketogenic diets may therefore be beneficial for some groups of individuals with specific medical conditions, if followed for short periods and supervised by an appropriate health professional. There is no robust evidence to show that long-term use of a ketogenic diet is of benefit in preventing weight gain or metabolic disease in otherwise healthy individuals. A ketogenic diet may be associated with gastrointestinal disturbance, halitosis and vitamin deficiencies. The metabolic benefits may also be overstated. Hall *et al.* (2016) compared weight and fat loss among a group of men who alternated between low-fat and ketogenic diets. There were no difference in either measure over four weeks on each diet. Imamura *et al.* (2016) examined insulin sensitivity across ketogenic, high saturated fat, high poly- and monounsaturated fatty acid diets. The biggest improvement in insulin sensitivity was seen with high polyunsaturated fatty acids, which is entirely consistent with current dietary guidelines for healthy adults. From a cardiometabolic perspective, a ketogenic diet may be detrimental. Randomized controlled trials in healthy (Retterstol *et al.*, 2018) and overweight (Bueno *et al.*, 2013) participants consistently show that ketogenic diets increase low-density lipoprotein-cholesterol concentrations.

may occur simply because subjects seeking lower-GI foods consume more fruits and vegetables and reduce consumption of processed, refined foods, which tend to be more energy dense (Jebb, 2005).

Individuals with higher-grade obesity (BMI over 35 kg/m²) may be advised to follow a very-low-calorie diet. This type of diet focuses on severely reducing energy intake to approximately 800–1200 kcal per day. This often promotes rapid weight loss of around 1 kg per week. However, such a diet is largely ineffective as a tool for achieving longer-term weight loss. Vogels and Westerterp-Plantenga (2007) reported that in a group which followed a very-low-calorie diet for six weeks, achieving an average weight loss of 7.2 kg, 87% of the individuals regained the lost weight within two years.

Mild to moderate exercise such as walking or housework is sufficient to increase energy expenditure, and even with no change in dietary intakes, sedentary individuals taking on such activities in addition to normal activity should experience some weight loss. However, weight loss associated with physical activity alone will be minor, and exercise is most effective when coupled to a change in diet (Shaw *et al.*, 2006). Higher-intensity exercise

produces greater improvements in weight profile than mild to moderate activity but, for any individual to succeed, it is important that exercise and weight loss goals are realistic and achievable.

Pharmacological agents are considered appropriate for patients who either cannot or do not lose weight using conventional approaches. They are a suitable adjunct to lifestyle advice and change but should only be used for the short term since all carry some form of undesirable adverse effects and several promising weight loss drugs have been withdrawn because of safety concerns (rimonabant, sibutramine, lorcaserin). Typically, anti-obesity drugs have their maximum effect over a period of seven to eight months, beyond which users will tend to start regaining weight unless adequate lifestyle changes have also been implemented.

Orlistat is a widely used anti-obesity drug that works by inhibiting lipase activities and hence reducing the absorption of fat across the gut. On a diet that provides 30% of energy in the form of fat, approximately one third of the fat will be lost in the faeces (Bray and Ryan, 2007). Orlistat has been shown to promote loss of approximately 7% of body weight in obese individuals over a two-year period.

Similar effects were noted with sibutramine, which is a central inhibitor of serotonin, noradrenaline and dopamine reuptake. This drug inhibits appetite and also promotes energy expenditure by activating thermogenesis. Apfelbaum *et al.* (1999) showed that sibutramine was highly effective alongside a very-low-calorie diet, allowing patients to maintain weight loss associated with their initial dietary change, for at least one year. However, sibutramine was linked to some negative cardiovascular events, prompting discontinuation of use on safety grounds. Phentermine/topiramate and naltrexone/bupropion are drugs licensed for use as appetite suppressants, but both carry significant safety concerns (e.g. phentermine may cause birth defects so cannot be used by women who may be planning a pregnancy and naltrexone can increase suicidal thoughts and actions). The glucagon-like peptide-1 mimetic, semaglutide, is a drug that has a long half-life and can be administered by injection once a week. Semaglutide increases insulin secretion and is also an appetite suppressant. When administered weekly in conjunction with lifestyle modification, semaglutide induced a 15% loss of body weight over 68 weeks in adults who were obese and overweight (Wilding *et al.*, 2021).

Bariatric surgery is an extreme approach to treating obesity and would normally be reserved only for the morbidly obese (BMI over 40 kg/m²). There are a number of different surgical approaches, which include gastric banding or stomach resection to limit the size of the stomach, or major surgery to limit the capacity of the gut to absorb nutrients (Figure 8.6) removed and the small remnant is joined directly to the ileum, bypassing the jejunum and duodenum. Roux-en-Y bypass surgery limits stomach capacity and induces malabsorption by creating a pouch within the stomach, which empties directly into the ileum.

Bariatric surgery is significantly more effective in affecting weight loss in people who are morbidly obese than non-surgical methods. The meta-analysis of Gloy *et al.* (2013) considered 11 randomized controlled trials of bariatric surgery and compared them with non-surgical approaches. The study found that the additional mean weight loss with surgery was 26 kg. However, surgery is not effective in all cases. Nedeljkovic-Arsenonvic *et al.* (2020) followed a group of 66 patients following Roux-en-Y bypass and found that 2 showed no weight loss at six months post-surgery and only 38 maintained lost weight to five years. Where successful, surgically induced weight loss reduces death rates associated with diabetes and the metabolic syndrome. Kwok *et al.* (2014) reported a marked reduction in deaths related to stroke (hazard ratio, HR, 0.49, 95% confidence interval, CI, 0.32–0.75) and myocardial infarction risk is similarly reduced (HR 0.46, 95% CI 0.30–0.69; Gloy *et al.*, 2013). Follow-up of a cohort of 17 998 women following bariatric surgery showed a significant reduction in risk of both premenopausal (HR 0.72, 95% CI 0.54–0.94) and postmenopausal (HR 0.55, 95% CI 0.42–0.72) breast cancer (Feigelson *et al.*, 2020).

8.4.2 Type 2 diabetes

Diabetes mellitus is a condition in which control over blood glucose homeostasis is lost through impairment of either the production of insulin by the pancreas or through impairment of the actions of insulin in the main target tissues (liver, skeletal muscle). Type 1 diabetes mellitus (formerly described as insulin-dependent diabetes) is the result of destruction of the β cells of the pancreas, leading to either an absence of or low production of insulin. Type 1 diabetes is generally of early onset,

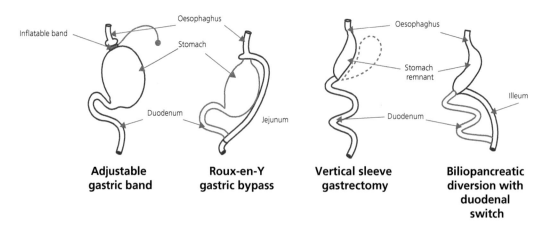

Adjustable gastric band   **Roux-en-Y gastric bypass**   **Vertical sleeve gastrectomy**   **Biliopancreatic diversion with duodenal switch**

Figure 8.6 Types of bariatric surgery.

and many sufferers will be diagnosed in childhood. Type 2 diabetes mellitus (non-insulin-dependent diabetes) is characterized by either blunted insulin production in response to ingestion of carbohydrates or, more commonly, extremely high plasma insulin concentrations with a blunted response to insulin (insulin resistance; see following text). Type 2 diabetes generally first appears in the middle years of adulthood.

The simplest diagnostic tools used to identify individuals with type 2 diabetes are the presence of symptoms such as thirst and polyuria or the observation of a raised fasting plasma glucose concentration (>126 mg/dl glucose in venous blood). However, the fasting plasma glucose method is less reliable and will tend to underdiagnose type 2 diabetes in the population. The oral glucose tolerance test is a more robust method, which should always be used to confirm any provisional diagnosis. In an oral glucose tolerance test, the patient is fasted overnight and then provided with a solution of glucose (usually a 75-g load) to drink. This promotes a rapid increase in blood glucose concentrations (Figure 8.7). In healthy individuals, this promotes a release of insulin, which drives the excess blood glucose into the liver and skeletal muscle and brings blood glucose back to the baseline concentration within two hours of loading. Among individuals with glucose intolerance (a prediabetic state), the peak in plasma glucose will tend to be greater than in healthy individuals, and concentrations will remain elevated (>140 mg/dl) after two hours. In

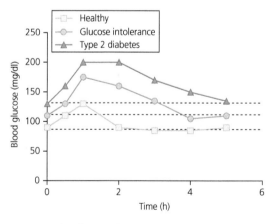

Figure 8.7 The glucose tolerance test. Patients consume an oral load of 75 g glucose. This promotes a rise in blood glucose concentrations. Blood samples at two hours into the test can discriminate between healthy people (glucose should have returned to the baseline, normal range of below 110 mg/dl), those who are glucose intolerant (glucose will remain above 140 mg/dl) and those with frank diabetes (glucose will remain above 200 mg/dl).

individuals with type 2 diabetes, the peak in blood glucose will be over 200 mg/dl and the return to baseline concentrations greatly delayed (Figure 8.7).

The risk of developing type 2 diabetes is strongly influenced by genetic factors. Individuals who have a sibling with type 2 diabetes are four times more likely to develop the disease than individuals with no family history. There are some rare forms of type 2 diabetes that are attributable to defects of specific genes. These maturity-onset diabetes of the young (MODY) variants of type 2 diabetes are associated with defects of hepatocyte nuclear factor 4α (MODY1), glucokinase (MODY2), hepatocyte nuclear factor 1α (MODY3), insulin promoter factor 1 (MODY4), hepatocyte nuclear factor 1β (MODY5) and neurogenic differentiation factor 1 (MODY6). It has proven difficult however to firmly identify genes that drive the risk of type 2 diabetes in the rest of the population, as it is clear that several genes or polymorphisms of genes are likely to play a role and, more importantly, that these genetic influences are modified by environmental factors (McIntyre and Walker, 2002). Candidate genes that may contribute to risk of type 2 diabetes include the insulin gene itself, sulfonylurea receptor-1, insulin receptor substrate-1, peroxisome proliferator-activated receptor gamma and glycogen synthase. All of these show polymorphisms in humans that have variants that appear to predispose to type 2 diabetes. Obesity is the main diet- and lifestyle-related risk factor for type 2 diabetes. Storage of fat in adipose tissue impairs insulin sensitivity in target tissues by promoting the delivery of fat in the form of triacylglycerides to peripheral tissues and by direct production of antagonists of insulin action by the adipocytes (Roche *et al.*, 2005).

The prevalence of type 2 diabetes is rapidly increasing all over the world, and it is estimated that it currently affects 462 million individuals worldwide and contributes to a million deaths per year (Khan *et al.*, 2020). It is the ninth most common cause of death. The highest prevalence is seen in Western Europe, but because of the close relationship between obesity and type 2 diabetes, high prevalence is noted in the Pacific Ocean states (e.g. Tonga, Nauru). The countries with the largest numbers of people with type 2 diabetes are China (88.5 million), India (66 million) and the United States (29 million).

The migration of certain ethnic minorities to westernized countries has resulted in greater prevalence of type 2 diabetes in those migrant populations. As reported by Patel *et al.* (2006), Asian Indians in the UK exhibit greater prevalence of obesity and type 2 diabetes than the white populations of the UK and considerably higher prevalence than non-migrant Indians. Similar observations are noted in migrant Indians living in South Africa, where the association between migrant status and type 2 diabetes is more marked if the migrants retain their traditional diet and lifestyle (Misra and Ganda, 2007). The finding that migration promotes an increase in prevalence rates adds weight to the argument that the risk of type 2 diabetes is strongly associated with a thrifty genotype (Neel, 1962) or thrifty phenotype (Hales and Barker, 2001). Generations of undernutrition and regular famine will either programme traits or select for genetic traits that promote the most efficient use of metabolic substrates. On encountering an environment where energy is widely available, this metabolic thrift will drive development of obesity and associated disorders.

The concept of thrift, whether acquired through programming or through genetic selection, is also supported by studies of the two populations with the highest global prevalence of type 2 diabetes. The Pima Indians of Arizona and the Nauruan islanders exhibit type 2 diabetes rates of 40–50%, and in both populations, the shift to endemic diabetes was associated with a rapid shift in availability of high-energy foods and adoption of sedentary patterns of work and physical activity. However, the situation with migrant populations may be less clear-cut, as migration brings social inequalities, stress and greater prevalence of unhealthy behaviours such as smoking and alcohol consumption in addition to a nutritional transition (Misra and Ganda, 2007).

Type 2 diabetes is a major risk factor for CVD (see following text) but is also associated with a range of other complications that arise due to the damaging effects of chronically high blood glucose concentrations upon the vasculature and nerves. Within the eye, glucose causes damage to the vessels that supply the retina (non-proliferative diabetic retinopathy), which causes leakage of plasma into the retina and blurs vision. In more severe diabetes, abnormal blood vessels develop on the face of the retina (proliferative diabetic retinopathy). This reduces normal blood flow to the tissue and can cause blindness. Within the kidneys, high glucose concentrations cause loss of nephrons, which can lead to chronic renal failure in people with diabetes. The legs and feet are vulnerable, as nerve damage (diabetic neuropathy) numbs sensation and leads to greater risk of physical injury. With lower blood flow to the limbs (a further consequence of diabetes), these injuries are prone to infection and ulceration. Amputation of feet and lower limbs can be a consequence of failure to heal these ulcers successfully.

The treatment and management of type 2 diabetes relies upon a mixture of dietary and lifestyle change and medication. Monitoring of blood glucose concentrations is an essential element of management of the condition, as this allows carbohydrate intakes to be tailored to fluctuations in blood glucose, which may be influenced by the time since the last food consumption or by levels of physical activity. Clinical monitoring is also recommended, with regular screening of the glycosylated haemoglobin (HbA1c) concentration providing a good indicator of the quality of glycaemic control (target HbA1c concentration is 6.5–7.5%; Figure 8.8).

Patients with type 2 diabetes who are of optimal body weight may be able to maintain good control over blood glucose concentrations through relatively simple management of the carbohydrate content of their diet. In individuals who are overweight or obese, the priorities will shift so as to couple weight loss to glycaemic control. There is no 'diabetic diet' as such, and the guidelines given to people with diabetes are broadly in line with the healthy eating guidelines for adults that were outlined earlier in this chapter (Dyson *et al.*, 2018). Patients with diabetes are advised to increase intakes of complex carbohydrates and reduce intakes of simple sugars, in effect taking on a low-GI diet. Intakes of dietary fibre should be high, and it is suggested that complex carbohydrates should be consumed with every meal or snack to delay absorption of glucose into the circulation. Meals should be regular and low-fat options should be the mainstay of intake. Special foods aimed at people with diabetes are not necessary and often have a

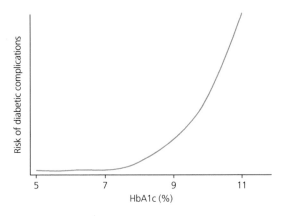

Figure 8.8 Glycosylated haemoglobin (HbA1c) percentage is a measure of the degree of glycation of haemoglobin and as such serves as a marker for longer-term blood glucose concentration. Relatively small increases in HbA1c are associated with significant increases in risk of cardiovascular disease and nephropathy. Risk of complications increases sharply with values of 7.5% or greater.

high-fat content to maintain palatability, so should be avoided. In 2018, Diabetes UK published new guidelines on the prevention and management of type 2 diabetes. At the core of those guidelines was an emphasis on a person-centred and culturally-sensitive approach (Dyson *et al.*, 2018). Patients require regularly updated diabetes education and nutritional advice delivered by dietitians. The focus of management of the disease is on achieving and sustaining a weight loss of at least 5% following diagnosis. This and enhanced glycaemic control is best delivered through the adoption of a Mediterranean or similar healthy dietary pattern built around increasing intakes of wholegrains, fruit, vegetables, nuts, pulses and oily fish, and reducing intakes of red meat, refined carbohydrates and alcohol (Dyson *et al.*, 2018).

Where patients are overweight or obese and have difficulties in maintaining satisfactory glycaemic control, pharmacological agents are widely used (Table 8.4). These agents are designed to either boost insulin secretion, inhibit glucagon release or inhibit gluconeogenesis. All these actions will reduce circulating glucose and enable the patient to maintain glucose homeostasis.

8.4.3 The metabolic syndrome

The metabolic syndrome, also called the insulin resistance syndrome or syndrome X, is a cluster of metabolic and physiological disturbances that all stem from the occurrence of insulin resistance in an individual. Insulin resistance is the state in which the response to insulin is blunted, and hence, individuals who are insulin resistant need to produce more insulin to regulate their blood glucose concentrations. Insulin is a powerful metabolic regulator and has effects in skeletal muscle, the liver, the brain, the kidney and vascular tissues. As a result, insulin resistance will impact upon multiple organ systems, producing a broad spectrum of effects (Figure 8.9). The metabolic syndrome is strongly linked to CVD as most of the functional defects that accompany insulin resistance are all independent risk factors for coronary heart disease (CHD) and stroke (see later sections in this chapter). Lakka *et al.* (2002) estimated that metabolic syndrome increases risk of CVD mortality threefold.

Insulin resistance can be measured in individuals using a variety of different techniques, but mostly, the homeostasis model assessment – insulin resistance scale is applied. This scale is determined using the calculation:

$$\left(\frac{\text{plasma insulin concentration} \times \text{plasma}}{\text{glucose concentration}} \right) / 22.5$$

An alternative is the quantitative insulin sensitivity check index (known as QUICKI), which is calculated as:

Table 8.4 Drug treatment for type-2 diabetes.

Drug class	Example	Mode of action
Metformin	Metformin	Inhibitor of gluconeogenesis; increases insulin sensitivity
Sulfonylureas	Glipizide	Increase insulin secretion by pancreatic β-cells
Meglitinides	Nateglinide	Increase insulin secretion by pancreatic β-cells
Thiazolidinediones	Rosiglitazone	Activate peroxisome proliferator activated receptor-γ, resulting in a decrease in circulating fatty acids and increase in glucose oxidation
DPP-4 inhibitors	Sitagliptin	Inhibition of dipeptidyl peptidase-4 prolongs the action of glucagon-like peptide-1. This inhibits glucagon release and increases insulin secretion
GLP-1 receptor agonists	Liraglutide	Activates the glucagon-like peptide-1 receptor to increase insulin secretion
SGLT-2 inhibitors	Canagliflozin	Inhibit the sodium-glucose transport protein 2, to limit glucose reabsorption by the kidneys

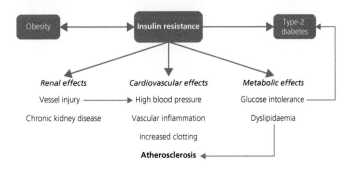

Figure 8.9 Schematic representation of the consequences of insulin resistance.

$$1 \Big/ \left(\frac{\log \text{fasting insulin concentration} + \log \text{fasting}}{\text{glucose concentration}} \right)$$

These results can be used alongside other diagnostic criteria to confirm the presence of the metabolic syndrome. A number of diagnostic definitions are in use, and that used by the World Health Organization is shown in Table 8.5.

The basic actions of insulin are to stimulate glucose uptake by the muscle and liver and to inhibit lipolysis. In individuals who are insulin resistant, these functions will be impaired, blood glucose clearance is reduced and circulating lipid concentrations rise. However, some other functions of insulin are not impaired, and the high circulating insulin concentrations that are associated with insulin resistance will increase these functions. For example, insulin promotes elevations of blood pressure, and this function is not lost in the individual who is insulin resistant.

The origins of metabolic syndrome may vary considerably between individuals. Certainly, obesity promotes insulin resistance, possibly because factors such as cytokines produced from adipose tissue act as antagonists of insulin action. Insulin resistance itself will promote deposition of lipid in adipose tissue, as adipocytes often retain greater sensitivity to insulin than other tissues. This promotes storage of energy in the adipose tissue in preference to the liver or muscle. Obesity should therefore be regarded as both a cause and a consequence of insulin resistance.

Table 8.5 World Health Organization diagnostic criteria for the metabolic syndrome.

Criteria*	Defined by
Insulin resistance	Measure of resistance in top 25% for population
Impaired glucose tolerance	Raised fasting glucose, impaired glucose tolerance Test or type 2 diabetes
Hypertension	Systolic pressure >159, diastolic pressure >89
Central obesity	BMI > 30 kg/m². Waist–hip ratio >0.9 in men or 0.8 in women
Raised triglycerides	Serum triglycerides >2.0 mmol/l
Reduced HDL-cholesterol	HDL-cholesterol <1.0 mmol/l
Microalbuminuria	Urinary albumin excretion >30 mg/day

Source: data from Alberti and Zimmet (1998). Reproduced with permission of Wiley.
* Individuals manifesting one of the first two criteria and two of the remaining criteria should receive a diagnosis of metabolic syndrome.

Concentrations of hormones such as cortisol also become elevated in obese individuals, and these may oppose the actions of insulin. There are a number of genetic defects that may also contribute to risk. Loss or impairment of insulin-responsive elements in a number of different pathways that control lipid or carbohydrate metabolism would be expected to promote the development of an insulin-resistant phenotype.

8.4.4 Cardiovascular disease

8.4.4.1 What is cardiovascular disease?
CVD is a term that collectively describes a number of different conditions, which include CHD, cerebrovascular disease and peripheral artery disease. All these conditions stem from the same basic pathology, which is the development of atherosclerosis within major arteries.

8.4.4.1.1 Atherosclerosis
Atherosclerosis is the process through which deposits of cholesterol, collagen and calcium accumulate within the intimal layer of arteries, resulting in the occlusion of the arterial lumen and a focus for the formation of clots (thrombosis). Atherosclerotic plaques can form in any of the arterial vessels of the body, and each individual may potentially have tens or hundreds of plaques. The main feature of plaques is the accumulated mass of cholesterol-bearing foam cells and vascular smooth muscle cells (Figure 8.10). Most plaques are stable as they are covered in a fibrous crust. Should this crust split, the resultant release of collagen and other material will provide the focus for thrombosis, which can trigger potentially fatal consequences.

There are two prerequisites for the initiation of plaque formation. The first requires the accumulation of oxidized low-density lipoprotein (LDL)-cholesterol within the arterial intima. LDL is responsible for the transport of cholesterol away from the liver to deliver it to sites that require it for metabolism, (e.g. the adrenal glands) where it is used to manufacture steroid hormones. Some of this circulating LDL-cholesterol can be deposited in the arterial wall. Cholesterol may be transferred from low- to high-density lipoprotein (HDL), which carries it back to the liver. However, the conditions within the intimal layer will also tend to favour the oxidation of LDL-cholesterol by reactive oxygen species (ROS). The LDL-cholesterol complex is vulnerable to ROS attack, despite having antioxidant defences, due to the high polyunsaturated fatty acid (PUFA) density present within the phospholipid shell. Oxidative damage will spread from the lipids

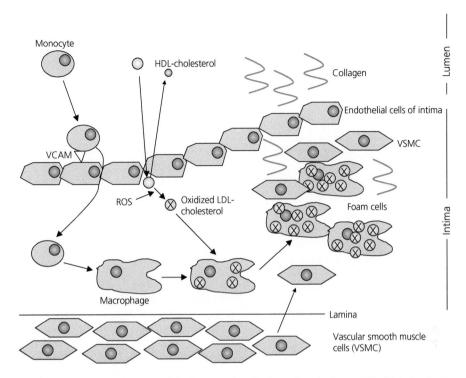

Figure 8.10 Events leading to the formation of the fatty streak and atherosclerotic plaque. HDL, high-density lipoprotein; LDL, low-density lipoprotein; ROS, reactive oxygen species; VCAM, vascular cell adhesion molecule.

to the key apolipoprotein B100, which is required to recognize the LDL receptor on target tissues.

The second key event in atherosclerosis is damage to the endothelial lining of the intima. This is generally due to inflammation, which can be triggered by local injury, infection or raised circulating concentrations of inflammatory cytokines, as is seen in individuals with obesity. Endothelial inflammation attracts monocytes, a class of undifferentiated white blood cell. Monocytes bind to vascular cell adhesion molecule on the endothelial surface, allowing movement through to the underlying intimal zone. Here, the presence of cytokines associated with endothelial inflammation drives differentiation of the monocytes to macrophages.

Macrophages bear a scavenger receptor that is able to recognize and bind oxidized LDL-cholesterol. Macrophages that have taken up oxidized LDL will remain in the intima and steadily accumulate this oxidized material, eventually becoming foam cells. The first sign of atherosclerosis in blood vessels is the appearance of a yellowish spot, termed a fatty streak. The accumulated foam cells promote the proliferation of vascular smooth muscle cells in the intima, and thus, the plaque becomes established. Vascular smooth muscle cells secrete collagen into the plaque, providing the associated protein accumulation. Established plaques will also accrue calcium and this causes stiffening of the arteries.

8.4.4.1.2 Coronary heart disease
CHD is also referred to as ischaemic heart disease. It is the result of atherosclerotic plaque formation within the coronary arteries, which supply the heart muscle with oxygen and nutrients. Formation of plaques will occlude these arteries causing chest pain, termed angina pectoris. The potentially life-threatening aspect of atherosclerosis in the coronary arteries results from thrombosis, causing full occlusion of the vessels. The heart muscle, starved of oxygen, will then begin to die, forming a damaged area called an infarct. In individuals surviving this injury (myocardial infarction), future heart function will be impaired, and they may suffer from arrhythmias and other cardiac problems.

Although deaths from CHD have generally been in decline in westernized countries throughout the 1990s and the early twenty-first century, CHD remains the leading cause of death in the western hemisphere. Alongside this, the disease has increased in prevalence in the developing countries, as they enter economic and nutritional transition. Figure 8.11 shows the prevalence rates for CHD in selected countries and highlights the fact that the

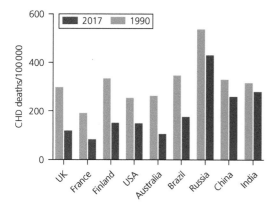

Figure 8.11 Coronary heart disease mortality in men and women in selected countries.

disease is most prevalent in countries of the former Soviet Union (e.g. Russia) and has the lowest prevalence in Southern Europe (e.g. France). There can be considerable variation within countries. For example, in the UK, the lowest rates of CHD are seen among men and women in the south and eastern parts of England. CHD rates among the male population of Scotland are at a level 60% above those in southern England. This variation largely reflects regional differences in diet and lifestyle.

8.4.4.1.3 Cerebrovascular disease

Cerebrovascular disease manifests itself when individuals suffer a cerebrovascular accident, or stroke. Strokes occur when the blood supply to the brain is interrupted, which can lead to reversible or irreversible damage. Strokes may be haemorrhagic, in which case blood leaks from vessels into the brain tissue. These strokes are unrelated to atherosclerosis and

are the product of raised blood pressure. Ischaemic strokes are caused by blockage of the arterial supply to the brain due to atherosclerosis and thrombosis. Strokes are the second most common cause of death in the UK and other European countries.

8.4.4.1.4 Peripheral artery disease

Peripheral artery disease stems from the formation of atherosclerotic plaques in arteries other than those supplying the heart or brain. Typically, these problems affect the legs. Often, peripheral artery disease will manifest as pain during exercise, which is termed claudication. In severe cases, these plaques will lead to ischaemic injury to the limbs, resulting in amputation.

8.4.4.1.5 Hypertension

Hypertension, or raised blood pressure, is often included as one of the CVDs. However, raised blood pressure is not truly a disease state and should instead be regarded as a risk factor or clinical indicator for other CVDs. High blood pressure is associated with increased risk of both CHD and stroke. In the case of CHD, it may be that atherosclerosis impairs the ability of the major vessels to contract or dilate to maintain normal pressure, but it is also the case that raised pressure causes a form of arterial damage, called shear stress, that can act as the focus for plaque formation. Higher blood pressures will also make atherosclerotic plaques less stable.

8.4.4.2 Risk factors for cardiovascular disease

The classical risk factors for CVD are generally defined as modifiable or non-modifiable characteristics (Figure 8.12). Non-modifiable risk factors include age, sex and ethnicity. The strong association

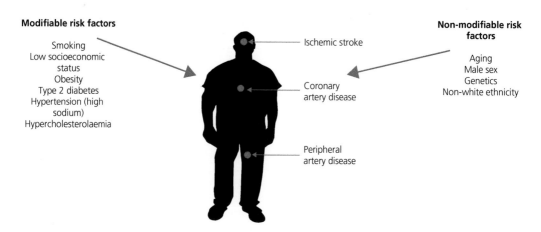

Figure 8.12 Risk factors for cardiovascular disease.

of risk with sex can be clearly seen in Figure 8.11, which shows death rates from CHD to be lower in women than men in all countries. Much of the protection associated with female sex disappears after the menopause, and it is suggested that this is due to postmenopausal women adopting an android pattern of abdominal fat deposition. Risks of CHD and stroke both increase with increasing age and this may, at least in part, be explained by rising blood pressure that typically occurs with ageing.

Certain ethnic groups exhibit increased risk of CVD within westernized nations. Individuals of South Asian descent (i.e. populations from India, Bangladesh and Pakistan) have increased risk of CHD, which appears to be related to a greater propensity to develop abdominal obesity. Patel *et al.* (2006) compared a population of Gujarati migrants in the UK with a non-migrant Gujarati population in India. The UK population had considerably greater BMI, raised circulating lipids and other CVD risk factors compared with the Indian group. Thus, the combination of a South Asian heritage with a westernized lifestyle appeared to increase CVD risk. African-Caribbean populations are at greater risk of stroke-related death than other ethnic groups, and this appears to be due to a genetic predisposition to hypertension.

Aspects of lifestyle that increase CVD risk are generally considered to be modifiable risk factors (Figure 8.12). Lower socioeconomic status can be included in this category. Lower socioeconomic status is an indicator of a number of different factors that include lower income, poor health behaviours, such as smoking, and a diet of lower quality. Ramsay *et al.* (2007) reported that lower socioeconomic status in adulthood was a risk factor for CHD in men aged 52–74. Men who had manual occupations were significantly more likely to suffer from fatal or nonfatal CHD and were more likely to be smokers, to be overweight and to be physically inactive, when compared with those in non-manual occupations.

Smoking increases risk of CVD through a number of mechanisms, including increasing concentrations of clotting factors and thereby increasing risk of thrombosis, by promoting endothelial dysfunction and by increasing oxidative stress. Obesity and related disorders, including type 2 diabetes, are major risk factors for CHD and other cardiovascular conditions. Abdominal obesity in particular will increase risk. Factors that contribute to development of obesity, such as physical inactivity, are independently associated with greater risk of CVD. The nutrition-related risk factors for CVD, including obesity, are described in more detail in the next section.

8.4.4.3 Nutrition-related factors and risk of cardiovascular disease

8.4.4.3.1 Obesity

The major lifestyle-related risk factors for CVD are cigarette smoking and obesity. At a time when the prevalence of smoking is declining in most westernized populations, the secular trend for increasing prevalence of obesity is reducing the beneficial impact of smoking reduction (Hu *et al.*, 2000) and is rapidly becoming the main contributor to CHD and stroke-related death. Bender *et al.* (2006) reported that obesity increased risk of CVD death by 2.2-fold in men and 1.6-fold in women (comparing BMI of over 30 kg/m^2 to BMI in the ideal range).

Determining the influence of obesity on CVD risk independent of all other risk factors is almost impossible. Individuals who are obese will also tend to be the individuals who are least physically active and who have raised blood pressure, type 2 diabetes, insulin resistance and dyslipidaemia, all of which are associated with greater risk of atherosclerosis. However, it is clear that all anthropometric measures of overweight and obesity, whether considering BMI, waist–hip ratio or total percentage body fat, determined by bioimpedance, are powerful indicators of increased CVD risk. Abdominal fat deposition is most strongly related to risk, presumably because fat stored centrally either triggers or is a marker of metabolic events that impact upon mechanisms that drive atherosclerotic plaque formation. Leander *et al.* (2007) reported that the presence of excess central fat was also strongly predictive of risk of a further nonfatal or fatal myocardial infarction in individuals who had undergone treatment for a first infarction.

Obesity clearly increases CVD risk via a number of different routes. Blood pressure becomes elevated in obesity, as the blood volume increases in proportion to the greater body size. Individuals with obesity also become hypertensive because the homeostatic regulation of blood pressure is abnormal. Factors produced from the adipose tissue, including leptin, will also contribute to elevated blood pressure. Obesity is associated with increased circulating concentrations of a number of clotting factors including fibrinogen, factor VII and factor VIII. This increases the likelihood of thrombosis in subjects with established atherosclerosis. Morbid obesity is a major risk factor for death from acute pulmonary thromboembolism (Blaszyk *et al.*, 1999).

Adipose tissue is a source of a wide range of adipokines, cytokines and other factors that can modulate the process of atherosclerosis. Adiponectin, for example, suppresses inflammation and tends to accumulate in the vascular wall following local trauma. Adiponectin will block atherosclerosis as it prevents the transformation of macrophages to foam cells at an early stage in the formation of the fatty streak. However, in obesity, concentrations of adiponectin tend to be low, and so this protective mechanism is less effective. The pro-inflammatory cytokines tumour necrosis factor-α and interleukin-6 (IL-6) are also produced by adipose tissue and with obesity, their secretion is increased. IL-6, in particular, appears to drive atherosclerosis and thrombosis as it induces the production of C-reactive protein and fibrinogen, increasing blood viscosity. IL-6 suppresses the activity of lipoprotein lipase in macrophages, and this promotes the uptake of lipids by the fatty streak. IL-6 has also been linked to development of hypertension and promotes endothelial cell dysfunction.

Interventions that promote weight loss and increase physical activity produce clear benefits in terms of CVD risk factors but not necessarily cardiovascular outcomes. In patients with hypertension, for example, weight loss is associated with a lowering of blood pressure (Siebenhofer *et al.*, 2011). The Look AHEAD Research Group (2007) reported that an intensive lifestyle intervention over a 12-month period in over 5000 adults who were obese or overweight with type 2 diabetes reduced body weight by an average of 8.9%. This weight loss was associated with lowered blood pressure, reduced use of diabetes and hypertension medication, increased physical fitness, raised HDL-cholesterol and lowered LDL-cholesterol concentrations. A meta-analysis of randomized controlled trials of glucose lowering drugs in people with or at risk of type 2 diabetes found that drug therapies were effective in managing diabetes and had modest effects in prevention of major adverse cardiovascular events (relative risk, RR, 0.92, 95% CI 0.89–0.95; Ghosh-Swaby *et al.*, 2020). Semlitsch *et al.* (2016) highlighted that while dietary change could reduce blood pressure alongside weight loss, the effects were small and it was unclear whether they would reduce cardiovascular morbidity and mortality. Similarly, a meta-analysis of 122 randomized controlled trials of behavioural and pharmacological interventions to promote weight loss and prevent obesity-related disorders, reported that weight loss strategies prevented type 2 diabetes but could find no strong evidence of cardiovascular benefit (LeBlanc *et al.*, 2018). Although the cardiovascular benefit of weight loss achieved through lifestyle modification is difficult to corroborate, it is clear that greater weight loss achieved through bariatric surgery does transform the cardiovascular risk profile of patients. A meta-analysis of 29 208 surgical patients compared with 166 200 non-surgical controls and concluded that bariatric surgery reduced risk of cardiovascular death, stroke and myocardial infarction by 50% (Kwok *et al.*, 2014).

8.4.4.3.2 Diabetes

People with type 2 diabetes are at significantly greater risk of CVD and of fatal outcomes associated with CVD events than the non-diabetic population. Men with type 2 diabetes have two- to threefold greater CVD mortality, and in women, the risk is even greater (three- to fourfold; Goff *et al.*, 2007). Twice as many people with type 2 diabetes than those without show clinical evidence of atherosclerosis, and death rates following myocardial infarction are two to three times higher where diabetes is present. Diabetes tends to be associated with other classical risk factors for CVD, including obesity, hypertension and dyslipidaemia, and this undoubtedly explains some of the increased risk. However, insulin resistance is the main driver of CVD risk in diabetes.

Insulin resistance impacts upon atherosclerosis and the associated disease outcomes (myocardial infarction and stroke) at several different levels (Bansilal *et al.*, 2007). The processes that drive endothelial cell dysfunction, the uptake of oxidized lipid by macrophages to form foam cells and the development of a chronic inflammatory state that favours plaque formation are all consequences of insulin resistance and the associated hyperglycaemia and dyslipidaemia. The cytokines and adipokines that are the products of adipocytes are major players in mediating these effects, as described earlier, in the context of obesity. Insulin resistance is associated with elevated leptin, IL-6 and tumour necrosis factor-α and lower concentrations of adiponectin, all of which will contribute to the development of atherosclerosis and a hypercoagulant state that promotes thrombosis. In addition to these factors, insulin resistance favours the production of angiotensinogen by the adipocytes. This is the precursor of angiotensin II, which promotes vasoconstriction and elevated blood pressure and also increases the vascular expression of monocyte chemoattractant protein-1, vascular cell adhesion molecule-1 and intracellular adhesion molecule-1, all of which drive the recruitment and binding of monocytes to the intima in the early stages of atherosclerosis. Plasminogen activation inhibitor-1 is also overexpressed by the adipocytes in insulin resistance, which promotes the formation of clots around existing, unstable atherosclerotic plaques.

Interventions that target type 2 diabetes, either through improved control over blood glucose or through improving other associated metabolic abnormalities (e.g. dyslipidaemia), generally show that cardiovascular risk declines with successful management. An intensive programme to manage glycaemia, blood pressure, microalbuminuria and dyslipidaemia in the Steno-2 Study (Gaede *et al.*, 2003) showed that over an eight-year period CVD risk was reduced by 53% in patients with type 2 diabetes. The UK Prospective Diabetes Study (1998) showed that intensive control of blood glucose using oral drugs or insulin reduced risk of myocardial infarction by 39%.

8.4.4.3.3 Dietary fat and cholesterol transport
Risk of CVD is strongly related to circulating concentrations of total cholesterol, lipoproteins and triglycerides. Reference ranges for these lipids are shown in Table 8.6. High total cholesterol, hypertriglyceridaemia, raised LDL-cholesterol and low HDL-cholesterol are all risk factors for atherosclerosis. The main basis for this risk stems from the fact that cholesterol uptake by macrophages as they become foam cells is an essential process in plaque formation. HDL-cholesterol reduces risk as it is responsible for carrying excess cholesterol away from the arterial wall to the liver. Concentrations of triglycerides tend to be inversely correlated with HDL-cholesterol. The strong association between dyslipidaemia (an abnormal lipid profile) and CVD risk has made manipulation of cholesterol and triglycerides a primary target for interventions designed to prevent disease, both in individuals and at the population level. Statins are a class of drug that are designed specifically to lower LDL-cholesterol concentrations. These agents, such as lovastatin, are inhibitors of 3-hydroxy-3-methylglutaryl-CoA reductase, which is the rate-limiting step in the pathway of cholesterol biosynthesis. Statins effectively lower cholesterol concentrations, and this in turn leads to up-regulation of LDL receptors in the liver, which causes LDL to be more rapidly cleared from circulation.

Table 8.6 Reference ranges for plasma lipids in adults.

	Reference range (mmol/l)*	Healthy range (mmol/l)
Triglycerides	0.70–1.80	0.70–1.70
Total cholesterol	3.50–7.80	<5.20
HDL-cholesterol	0.80–1.70	>1.15
LDL-cholesterol	2.30–6.10	<4.0

* The reference range is the range of values that would be within the normal distribution for the population. There are sex differences in these ranges, with triglyceride concentrations tending to be higher in men and HDL-cholesterol higher in women.

Statins are undoubtedly effective drugs and have potential in both the primary prevention (i.e. administration to high-risk individuals without disease) and secondary prevention (administration to individuals with disease) of cardiovascular disease. Gould *et al.* (2007) analyzed interventions using statins and found that they reduced total cholesterol concentrations by between 4% and 34% and LDL-cholesterol concentrations by up to 52%, with no effect on HDL-cholesterol; 1 mmol/l reductions in total cholesterol were shown to reduce prevalence of CHD events by 29.5% and CHD death rates by 24.5%. When used in the primary prevention of CVD, statins significantly reduce the risk of non-fatal myocardial infarctions and strokes and lower overall cardiovascular mortality (RR 0.80, 95% CI 0.71–0.91; Yebyo *et al.*, 2019). The meta-analysis of Singh *et al.* (2020) focused on 11 randomised controlled trials that recruited patients without established CVD and who had near optimal to borderline high serum LDL-cholesterol concentrations. Statins reduced risk of myocardial infarction (RR 0.56, 95% CI 0.47–0.67) and stroke (RR 0.78, 95% CI 0.63–0.96) but had no significant effect on cardiovascular mortality. In secondary prevention of CVD, statins are highly effective. Introducing statin therapy after myocardial infarction significantly reduced risk of further cardiovascular events in the study of Schubert *et al.* (2020). The greatest benefits were seen where LDL-cholesterol concentrations were reduced to the greatest extent. Comparing patients in the highest quartile of LDL-cholesterol reduction with the lowest quartile showed a 23% reduction in further myocardial infarction, stroke and cardiovascular death.

Dietary change provides the alternative strategy for minimizing the prevalence of dyslipidaemia and the associated burden of CVD. Strategies for preventing CVD have long been focused on controlling circulating cholesterol concentrations, which are overwhelmingly determined by de novo synthesis rather than dietary consumption. The major determinants of total cholesterol are intakes of saturated and polyunsaturated fatty acids, as demonstrated by the Keys equation:

$$\Delta \text{cholesterol concentration} = 0.026 \times$$
$$(2.16\Delta \text{ saturated fatty acid intake} - 1.65\Delta \text{PUFA}$$
$$\text{intake} - 6.66\Delta \text{cholesterol intake} - 0.53)$$

For several decades, the public health message has been to reduce total intakes of fat, to consume less saturated fat and to consume more starchy carbohydrates as an alternative energy source (see Section 8.3). This is a message familiar to most people in westernized countries, but it is now becoming clear that this may need more nuance, as there are also interactions between carbohydrates in the diet and the metabolism and transport of cholesterol.

Saturated fats (see Figure A2 in the Appendix) increase total cholesterol concentrations in circulation and elevate LDL-cholesterol. PUFA have the opposite effect. HDL-cholesterol concentrations are increased by greater consumption of all classes of fatty acids (saturates, PUFA and monounsaturated fatty acids, MUFA) if these fats replace carbohydrate in the diet. Interestingly, saturated fatty acids may be more effective than PUFA and MUFA in this respect. Replacing fats in the diet with carbohydrates actually increases serum triglyceride concentrations. This means that following advice to replace saturated fats in the diet with carbohydrate is likely to have little cardiovascular benefit, since this will effectively lower both LDL-cholesterol and HDL-cholesterol and increase triglyceride concentrations (Hu and Willett, 2002). The more effective strategy is to replace the saturated fats in the diet with alternative fats. MUFA and PUFA in place of saturates would lower LDL-cholesterol, and although there would be no increase in HDL-cholesterol, the HDL–LDL ratio would be improved. It is thought that substitution of saturated fatty acids with MUFA and PUFA would carry additional benefits as the unsaturated fatty acids improve insulin sensitivity and risk of diabetes, which effectively reduces CVD risk independently of direct effects on the process of atherosclerosis. The replacement of saturated fats with MUFA and PUFA is more impactful than low-carbohydrate, high-fat (ketogenic) diets, for example, and is more sustainable as a lifestyle modification to prevent disease (see Research Highlight 8.2).

Although changes to the profile of fatty acids in the diet appears to have beneficial effects in terms of the ratio of HDL to LDL-cholesterol in circulation, there are meta-analyses that suggest that replacing saturated fatty acids with mostly n-6 PUFA does not reduce cardiovascular mortality or CHD events (Chowdury et al., 2014, Hamley 2017). This may be attributed to a number of factors. First, the way in which the diet is altered in randomized controlled trials may impact on the outcome, given that carbohydrate may also determine cardiovascular outcomes. Second, recruitment of subjects to a randomized controlled trial is a critical step. If subjects already have advanced cardiovascular disease, this may limit the capacity of dietary change to alter outcomes. Furthermore, trials may be of insufficient duration. The systematic review and meta-analysis of Hooper et al. (2020) included trials with a minimum intervention time of 24 months and found that reducing

saturated fat intake significantly reduced the risk of coronary heart disease events (RR 0.79, 95% CI 0.66–0.93) and that the benefit was dose dependent. Greater reductions in fat intake led to greater reductions in serum cholesterol and greater reductions in disease risk.

There has been considerable concern over the high levels of trans-fatty acids present in the processed foods consumed in the westernized nations. Trans-fatty acids (see Figure A2 in the Appendix) are derived from both MUFA and PUFA and are formed during the processing of vegetable oils to convert them to solids. The majority of trans-fatty acids in the human food chain are associated with this industrial hydrogenation of vegetable oils, and they are primarily consumed in margarines and in deep-fried foods. Trans-fatty acids formed in food processing generally have similar effects to saturated fatty acids and will increase LDL-cholesterol concentrations (Hu and Willett, 2002). The trans-fatty acids inhibit the enzyme delta 6 desaturase and therefore disrupt the metabolism of essential fatty acids and the generation of prostaglandins and inflammatory mediators. This contributes to endothelial cell dysfunction. Chowdhury et al. (2014) found that risk of CHD events was increased by 16% when comparing the highest and lowest thirds of trans-fatty acid consumption. Naturally occurring trans-fatty acids are found in dairy products and include vaccenic acid and conjugated linoleic acid. Some isomers of these fatty acids have been shown to protect against atherosclerosis and even cause regression of existing atherosclerotic lesions in mice (Toomey et al., 2003), but beneficial effects in humans have not been convincingly demonstrated. Gayet-Boyer et al. (2014) found that ruminant trans-fatty acids consumed at up to 4.19% of daily energy intake were not associated with changes in LDL-cholesterol or HDL-cholesterol concentrations, suggesting that while not beneficial for health, these fatty acids do not increase CVD risk in the same way as those generated through industrial processing. Similarly, a randomized controlled trial of ruminant trans-fatty acids at 2% of dietary energy for a period of four weeks had no effect on arterial function, inflammation or clotting factors. These ruminant-derived trans-fatty acids normally make up less than 0.5% of total fatty acid intake from food in the western diet. Intake may be significant in individuals who consume conjugated linoleic acid supplements, but studies of such supplements suggest that the impact of conjugated linoleic acid upon LDL-cholesterol is essentially the same as industrially generated trans-fatty acids (Brouwer et al., 2013).

A number of intervention trials have suggested that greater intakes of n-3 fatty acids are protective against CVD. Bucher *et al.* (2002) noted that eicosapentaenoic acid and docosahexaenoic acid were associated with significantly lower mortality from CVD, whether consumed as part of the normal diet or if taken as supplements. The greatest benefits were noted in individuals with established CVD. Abdelhamid *et al.* (2020) performed a meta-analysis of 86 randomised controlled trials of n-3 PUFA and cardiovascular outcomes, which included 162796 participants. This analysis concluded that there was sufficient high quality evidence to support the hypothesis that n-3 PUFA reduce cardiovascular mortality (RR 0.92, 95% CI 0.86–0.99). This benefit was associated with consumption of n-3 supplements or foods enriched with n-3 PUFA or alphalinolenic acid. Consuming oily fish did not reduce CVD risk. An analysis comparing supplementation of n-3 PUFA at doses over 1 g per day with lower doses or placebo found that higher doses were associated with lower risk of myocardial infarction and CVD mortality compared with both lower doses and the control (Lombardi *et al.*, 2020).

A number of food products have been developed to reduce total cholesterol through the inclusion of plant stanols and stanol esters. There is a large global market for low-fat spreads containing these agents, which block the absorption of exogenous dietary cholesterol and endogenous biliary cholesterol in the small intestine. This has the effect of reducing circu-lating cholesterol and increasing expression of hepatic LDL receptors (Figure 8.13). It is well-established that plant stanols and stanol esters reduce serum LDL-cholesterol. Musa-Veloso *et al.* (2011) considered 113 randomised controlled trials and found that intakes of 2–3 g per day reduced LDL-cholesterol concentrations by up to 17%. There are no data available on whether these compounds can significantly impact on CVD outcomes since studies of sufficient size and duration have not been published. A theoretical calculation based on the known LDL-cholesterol lowering effect of plant stanols suggests that an intake of 3 g per day could reduce risk of atherosclerotic CVD events by approximately 8.8% (Gylling *et al.*, 2020).

8.4.4.3.4 Folic acid and plasma homocysteine

Homocysteine is a sulphur-containing amino acid, which is found in circulation bound to proteins (70%) and other sulphates (5%) or as homocysteine dimers (25%). Elevated plasma homocysteine is recognized as a risk factor for CVD. Risk associated with elevated concentrations of homocysteine is independent of all other CVD risk factors and appears to be graded and linear, that is, as plasma homocysteine concentration increases, the increase in CVD risk is directly proportional.

The normal range of homocysteine concentrations in human plasma is considered to be 5–15 µmol/l. The range 16–100 µmol/l represents mild-to-moderate hyperhomocysteinaemia, and concentrations over

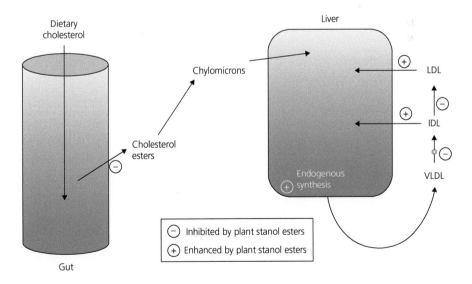

Figure 8.13 Plant stanol esters lower circulating low-density lipoprotein (LDL)-cholesterol concentrations. This is partially achieved through inhibition of cholesterol ester uptake from the gut. This increases endogenous synthesis, but production of LDL is inhibited and the reuptake from circulation is enhanced. As a result, circulating LDL falls. IDL, intermediate-density lipoprotein; VLDV, very low density lipoprotein.

100 μmol/l represent severe hyperhomocysteinae-mia. Hyperhomocysteinaemia is reported in up to half of patients with atherosclerosis. Concentrations of homocysteine are determined by the flux through two biochemical pathways, both of which are subject to regulation by micronutrients (Figure 8.14).

The methionine cycle involves reactions that either demethylate or remethylate methionine and homocysteine, respectively. This cycling is critical in determining the availability of methyl groups for a variety of processes, including synthesis of phos-phatidylcholine and the methylation of DNA in epi-genetic gene silencing. When methionine is in excess, concentrations of homocysteine will increase unless it can be converted to cysteine via the trans-sulphuration pathway. The rate-limiting step in this pathway, catalysed by cystathionine-β-synthase, requires vitamin B6 as a cofactor. If methionine is limiting, then homocysteine will be remethylated by methionine synthase. This step requires vitamin B12 and an adequate supply of methyltetrahydro-folate, which is derived from folate in the folate cycle. Thus, the metabolism and circulating concen-tration of homocysteine are controlled by the B vitamins, of which folic acid appears to be the most important.

There are well-described inborn errors of metab-olism that impact upon the three key enzyme steps in the methionine–homocysteine cycle identified in Figure 8.14. Individuals with these inherited disor-ders share the characteristics of having severe hyperhomocysteinaemia and premature atheroscle-rotic disease. This emphasizes the potential impor-tance of homocysteine as a risk factor for CVD. In addition to these inborn errors of metabolism, a relatively common polymorphism of methylenetet-rahydrofolate reductase (MTHFR C677T) is associ-ated with increased CVD risk. The TT variant of MTHFR C677T leads to enzyme activity being two thirds lower than in individuals with the CC variant. Individuals with TT are therefore predisposed to a higher circulating homocysteine concentration as their capacity to form MTHF for the methionine synthase step of the methionine cycle is impaired. Holmes *et al.* (2011) reported that homocysteine concentrations were up to 4 μmol/l higher in the TT population than in CC, but that the effect was only seen where folate intake was habitually low.

The Homocysteine Studies Collaboration (2002) reviewed evidence from 30 studies that had consid-ered homocysteine in relation to CVD, following on from some smaller meta-analyses that suggested hyperhomocysteinaemia increased CHD risk by 70%. The aim of the Homocysteine Studies Collaboration was to assess the likely impact of a 25% reduction in population plasma homocysteine concentrations. It was suggested that such a reduc-tion would reduce risk of both CHD (OR 0.73, 95% CI 0.64–0.83) and stroke (OR 0.77, 95% CI 0.66–0.90). For CHD, at least, this reduction in risk would be dependent on the MTHFR genotype of individu-als. Klerk *et al.* (2002) also noted that MTHFR

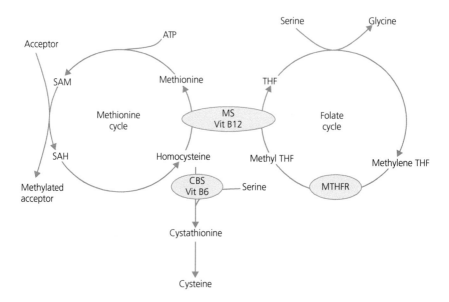

Figure 8.14 The methionine and folate cycles. CBS, cystathionine-β-synthase; MS, methionine synthase; MTHFR, methylenetetrahydrofolate reductase; SAH, S-adenosylhomocysteine; SAM, S-adenosylmethionine; THF, tetrahydrofolate; Vit, vitamin.

genotype modified CHD risk, but found that other factors could modify this risk. In European populations, carrying the TT genotype increased CHD risk (OR 1.16, 1.05–1.28), but in North America, where folate status is better due to fortification, there was no evidence that TT impacted significantly on CHD risk. In Asian countries with low folate status, the TT genotype was associated with 68% greater risk of stroke (Holmes *et al.* 2011).

A variety of mechanisms have been proposed to explain the association of hyperhomocysteinaemia with CVD risk. Homocysteine may initiate atherosclerosis through oxidative processes and by causing endothelial cell injury. In the presence of ferric or cupric ions, homocysteine will auto-oxidize, and the ensuing production of hydrogen peroxide could be an early step in LDL-cholesterol oxidation. In particular, this process inhibits the formation of nitric oxide, which normally serves to protect LDL-cholesterol from oxidation within the vessel wall. Animal studies indicate that experimentally induced hyperhomocysteinaemia promotes changes in the arterial wall that are early stages in the process of atherosclerosis, including endothelial cell dysfunction, activation of thrombosis and increased adhesion of monocytes.

Given the epidemiological findings that hyperhomocysteinaemia increases CVD risk and the presence of apparently robust biological mechanisms to explain the association, there is considerable interest in the use of B vitamins, and particularly folate, to modify this risk factor. A number of studies have shown that supplements of folate, vitamin B12 and vitamin B6 at doses up to 20 times normal intakes could reduce plasma homocysteine by up to 32%, with folate providing the strongest effect. Malinow *et al.* (1998) studied the impact of supplementing breakfast cereals with folate at doses ranging from 127 to 665 µg/day. All doses were effective in reducing plasma homocysteine, and the effect of folate was dose dependent. Since 1998, staple foods in the United States have been fortified with folic acid. In that time, there have been a 50% decrease in the prevalence of hyperhomocysteinaemia and a significant decrease in stroke-related death rates.

While there is good evidence that hyperhomocysteinaemia is a biomarker for CVD risk and that folic acid and other B vitamins can lower circulating homocysteine, the evidence exploring the potential for B vitamins to reduce CVD risk is inconsistent. Observational studies are supportive of a cardioprotective role for folate. For example, a case–control study of elderly Chinese coronary artery disease patients compared with age- and sex-matched controls suggested a dose-dependent relationship

between serum folate and disease risk, with a 25% lower risk in subjects in the highest compared with the lowest quartile of serum folate (RR 0.75, 95% CI 0.65–0.96; Long *et al.*, 2020). A systematic review of prospective cohort studies concluded that for every 250 µg increment of folate intake, CHD risk was reduced by 21% (Jayedi and Zargar, 2019). For vitamin B6, a 13% reduction of risk was associated with each 0.5 mg increment in intake.

Randomized controlled trials, however, do not wholly support the observational findings. The VITATOPS Trial Study Group (2010) found no cardiovascular benefit of 3.4 years of supplementation with 2 mg folic acid, 25 mg vitamin B6 and 0.5 mg vitamin B12 per day in men and women who had previously suffered a stroke. The B-PROOF trial administered placebo or a daily supplement of 400 µg folic acid and 0.5 mg vitamin B12 for two years (van Dijk *et al.*, 2015). At the two-year follow-up there was no impact on carotid intima-media thickness, a marker of arterial stiffness and atherosclerosis. Five to seven years after baseline there were no effects of supplement on cardiovascular outcomes (Araghi *et al.*, 2021). The HOPE 2 trial successfully lowered homocysteine concentrations using a mixed supplement of folic acid, vitamin B6 and vitamin B12 over five years (Lonn *et al.*, 2006). This was associated with reduced risk of stroke (OR 0.75, 95% CI 0.59–0.97), but the supplements did not impact on myocardial infarction or overall cardiovascular mortality. The HOPE 2 results are mirrored in meta-analyses of folic acid supplementation and CVD risk. Wang *et al.* (2019) reviewed studies of folic acid supplements given to patients with established CVD and found a 25% reduction in stroke risk but no other cardiovascular benefits. An analysis of the impact of homocysteine-lowering interventions reached the same conclusion (RR for stroke 0.90, 95% CI 0.82–0.99; Marti-Carvajal *et al.*, 2017).

The evidence is therefore consistent with folate status determining circulating homocysteine concentrations and risk of stroke. However, the homocysteine-lowering effect of folate may not be a mechanistic link and this could explain why trials designed to examine the impact of interventions targeting homocysteine are less effective than expected in lowering CVD risk. Folate could determine cardiovascular health by enhancing nitric oxide synthesis and hence improving vascular endothelial function; by dampening inflammatory processes; or by exerting effects on epigenetic regulation of gene expression. It should also be noted that responses to folic acid supplements would be heavily influenced by genotype. The analysis of

Long *et al.* (2020) suggest that Chinese populations may derive greater cardiovascular benefit from folic acid supplements than Europeans. Age could also be a key factor, with most randomized controlled trials recruiting older patients, with established disease risk. It is noteworthy that while folic acid had no impact on carotid intima-media thickness in the 65–70 year old patients in the B-PROOF trial (van Dijk *et al.*, 2015), folate status was associated with the same measure of arterial stiffness in a slightly younger cohort (Durga *et al.*, 2005).

8.4.4.3.5 Antioxidant nutrients

Given the importance of LDL oxidation and uptake of the oxidized complex by macrophages in the aetiology of atherosclerosis, it is suggested that antioxidant nutrients present within the diet may be protective against CVD. LDL is a rich target for ROS attack as each LDL complex comprises a spherical arrangement of approximately 2700 phospholipids around a hydrophobic core of cholesterol and cholesterol esters. Around 50% of the fatty acids in the phospholipid shell are polyunsaturated, and the presence of a high density of double bonds serves to increase the likelihood of reaction with free radicals. Oxidation of these fatty acids can establish chain reactions that will spread through the phospholipid shell, eventually leading to oxidation of apoprotein B100. Antioxidant protection within LDL is provided primarily by vitamin E (α-tocopherol), with between five and nine molecules inserted into the phospholipid shell of each LDL complex. In addition to vitamin E, the core of the LDL will contain other fat-soluble antioxidants, including β-carotene, lycopene, ubiquinone and polyphenolics.

Increased consumption of foods that are rich in antioxidants has been shown in epidemiological studies to provide protection against CVD. Law and Morris (1998) showed that higher levels of consumption of fruits and vegetables could significantly reduce CHD risk. Tea, the world's most commonly consumed beverage, may also deliver a range of antioxidant phytochemicals (flavonoids and catechins) that have a cardioprotective effect (Arab *et al.*, 2013).

In general, studies that have considered the impact of specific antioxidant nutrients upon risk provide results that are consistent with the hypothesis that consumption of antioxidants will oppose LDL oxidation and protect against atherosclerosis. Abbey (1995) performed a series of studies that showed that vitamin E could inhibit LDL oxidation in vitro and that LDL obtained from volunteers who had taken vitamin E supplements was also protected from copper-induced oxidation. The CHAOS

intervention study (Stephens *et al.*, 1996) evaluated the impact of supplementing patients with established atherosclerosis with vitamin E at doses of 400 or 800 iu per day over a period of over 500 days. The study found that supplements led to a 47% reduction in risk of nonfatal myocardial infarction. Nagao *et al.* (2012) found that stroke mortality was lower in patients with the highest circulating concentrations of α- and γ-tocopherol in a Japanese population. Similarly, the Finnish ATBC trial found lower cardiovascular mortality in subjects with higher α-tocopherol intake (Wright *et al.*, 2006). The EURAMIC study (Kardinaal *et al.*, 1993) compared fat-soluble antioxidant status in fat biopsies (a marker of long-term intake) from men who had suffered a myocardial infarction event and healthy controls. No difference in vitamin E status was reported, but there was evidence that the patients who had a myocardial infarction had consumed less β-carotene and fewer fat-soluble antioxidants in total. Other studies suggest a protective role for carotenoids, with β-cryptoxanthin and lutein emerging as cardioprotective in the study of Koh *et al.* (2011).

The overall effectiveness of vitamin E and other antioxidant nutrients in lowering CVD risk appears to depend upon their source. Knekt *et al.* (2004) performed a meta-analysis of nine major cohort studies, comprising more than 290 000 people that had considered the impact of dietary sources of vitamin E, vitamin C and the carotenoids and the impact of supplements of these nutrients on the risk of CHD. Within the normal diet, comparing the highest quintile of vitamin E intake, with the lowest quintile of intake, showed a reduced risk of CHD (OR 0.77, 95% CI 0.64–0.92). Carotenoids had a similar protective effect (OR 0.83, 95% CI 0.73–0.95), with α-carotene, β-carotene, β-cryptoxanthin and lutein, but not lycopene, all contributing to this effect. In contrast, vitamin C within the normal diet had no significant impact upon CHD risk. This evidence argues in favour of supplementation as a strategy for CVD prevention. To attain the doses of fat-soluble antioxidant vitamins required to obtain significant cardiovascular protection through diet alone would necessitate sizeable increases in consumption of fats and oils that would probably offset any benefit. However, the Knekt analysis also evaluated the impact of antioxidant supplements and concluded that while supplemental vitamin C produced a dose-dependent reduction in CHD risk (500 mg/day ascorbate reduced risk by 25%), vitamin E supplements were ineffective. It is likely therefore that the benefits associated with increased intakes of vitamin E and carotenoids may be, at least in part, explained by other components present in the foods that are their richest sources. The wider literature indicates little benefit of antioxidant supplements for cardiovascular health. The US Physicians Health Study II (Sesso *et al.*, 2008), for example, showed that after eight years of follow-up of men aged over 50 taking daily supplements of vitamin E 400 iu and vitamin C 500 mg per day, there was no significant difference in myocardial infarction, stroke or cardiovascular death. A meta-analysis of 43 randomized controlled trials of anti-oxidant supplements concluded that they had no impact on cardiovascular mortality, although combining supplement mixtures with selenium did have a beneficial effect (antioxidants without selenium RR CVD death 1.05, 95% CI 0.97–1.15; antioxidants with selenium RR 0.77, 95% CI 0.62–0.97; Jenkins *et al.*, 2020).

8.4.4.3.6 Sodium and blood pressure

Blood pressure is the pressure generated within the vascular tree when blood pushes against the arterial walls. In measurement of blood pressure, two components are determined. The systolic pressure is the pressure generated when blood is ejected from the left ventricle of the heart, while the diastolic pressure is the pressure between heartbeats. Table 8.7 shows the normal ranges of values for systolic and diastolic pressures and the different classifications of prehypertension and hypertension. From a clinical perspective, the cut-off points generally used in treatment of hypertension are systolic blood pressure (SBP) of 140 mmHg and diastolic blood pressure (DBP) of 90 mmHg.

In Westernized countries, blood pressure will generally increase with age in both men and women, and systolic pressure is 20–30 mmHg higher at age 75 than at age 24. Men have higher blood pressure than women. Rising blood pressure is associated with increased risk of stroke death in both sexes. In men, comparing the highest decile of the blood pressure distribution (SBP 151 mmHg,

DBP 98 mmHg) with the lowest decile (SBP <112 mmHg, DBP <71 mmHg) indicates an eight-fold greater risk of stroke death with the higher pressure. In women, a fourfold greater risk is noted. The association between stroke risk and blood pressure applies across the whole of the population distribution of blood pressures, so men who may not be considered for antihypertensive treatment (SBP 137–142 mmHg, DBP 89–92 mmHg) have fourfold greater risk of stroke death than those in the population who have the lowest blood pressures.

High blood pressure is driven by a number of non-modifiable risk factors, which, in addition to increasing age, includes male sex, ethnicity and a number of genetically determined disorders of renal and vascular function. For example, the syndrome of apparent mineralocorticoid excess is a genetic disorder of the renal form of 11β-hydroxysteroid dehydrogenase, which allows cortisol to bind to the aldosterone receptor. This leads to sodium retention and hypertension. Modifiable factors that increase blood pressure include lower socioeconomic status, physical inactivity, high intakes of alcohol and dietary factors.

Within diet, sodium intake is the major concern in relation to blood pressure. On a low-salt (sodium chloride) diet, homeostatic mechanisms ensure that the kidneys will excrete any excess sodium via the urine. Acute and modest changes in sodium intake will be comfortably accommodated by these mechanisms. In salt-sensitive individuals (Figure 8.15) and with age-related declines in renal function, the capacity of the kidneys to clear excess sodium may be exceeded with high intakes of salt. As a result, sodium will be retained necessitating a movement of water from the intracellular compartment to the extracellular compartment. Effectively, the required dilution of circulating sodium will produce an increase in blood volume. With more blood to be pumped by the heart, blood pressure increases. Over a relatively short period of time, these blood pressure changes can become fixed as the vessels accommodate to the raised pressure by reducing their elasticity. Greater resistance to flow will push blood pressure still higher.

Animal studies clearly show the relationship between sodium intake and blood pressure. Rats, for example, provided with a solution of 1.5% sodium chloride instead of water to drink, show increases of SBP of around 40 mmHg within three to five days of treatment. Experiments with chimpanzees showed that increasing salt intake from 5 to 15 g per day led to a rise in blood pressure of 30 mmHg SBP and 10 mmHg DBP over a

Table 8.7 Normal and hypertensive blood pressure references.

Category	Blood pressure (mmHg)	
	Systolic	Diastolic
Normotensive	<120	<80
Prehypertensive	120–139	80–89
Hypertensive:		
Stage 1	140–159	90–99
Stage 2	160+	100+

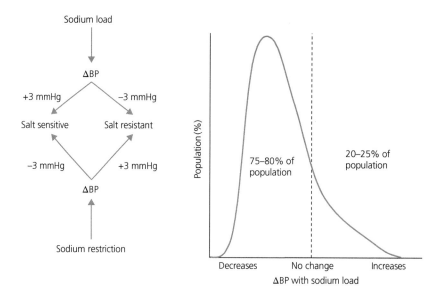

Figure 8.15 Salt sensitivity and resistance. Individuals are defined as salt sensitive if the ingestion of a sodium load induces an increase in blood pressure and if the adoption of sodium restriction leads to a corresponding decrease in blood pressure. Individuals with the opposite response are termed salt resistant. Salt resistance is seen in a minority of individuals (20–25% of the population), while most humans exhibit a degree of salt sensitivity. BP, blood pressure.

period of 16 months. As in the rodent studies, this effect was reversible.

Epidemiological studies of the association between sodium and blood pressure in humans have been rather controversial due to concerns regarding the analytic methods used and potential confounding factors. However, that such a relationship exists is irrefutable. One of the first major studies to consider this issue was INTERSALT (Elliott *et al.*, 1989), which considered 10 000 people in 52 populations across 32 different countries. The full analysis showed that blood pressure was related to sodium excretion, which provides the most robust marker of intake. Every 100 mmol sodium greater excretion predicted an 11.3 mmHg rise in SBP and 6.4 mmHg rise in DBP. Moreover, when considering four rural populations in INTERSALT, with the lowest salt intakes, blood pressure was lower than in westernized populations, and there was no age-related rise in blood pressure, unlike all other populations in the study.

The findings of INTERSALT were reproduced by the more recent European Prospective Investigation into Cancer and Nutrition Norfolk study (Khaw *et al.*, 2004), which studied 23 104 men and women aged 45–79. Comparing the lowest to the highest quintile of sodium excretion, there was a 7.2 mmHg SBP difference in men and a 3.0 mmHg difference in women. These differences appear to be very small in the context of Table 8.7, but at the whole population

level would be highly significant. In the UK, a 5-mmHg reduction of SBP for the whole population would halve the number of hypertensive individuals, reducing stroke-related deaths by 14% and CHD deaths by 9%.

Given this potentially very powerful impact of minor shifts in the population blood pressure profile, it is of major importance to develop and evaluate interventions that could reduce sodium intake. The Trials of Hypertension Prevention study (Cook *et al.*, 1998), which included 2382 participants, evaluated the effectiveness of counselling to reduce sodium intake and promote weight loss over a four-year period. At the end of the trial, sodium reduction alone had reduced the prevalence of hypertension by 18%. Similarly, the Dietary Approaches to Stop Hypertension (DASH) study showed that a diet low in fat, high in fibre, low in sodium and rich in magnesium and potassium could reduce SBP and DBP in hypertensive individuals by 11 mmHg and 5.5 mmHg, respectively, over just an eight-week period (Sacks *et al.*, 2001). The low sodium DASH diet is now recognized as a standard for the prevention and management of hypertension (Table 8.8).

Huang *et al.* (2020) conducted a systematic review and meta-analysis of 133 randomized controlled trials of sodium reduction interventions and blood pressure. The analysis found that interventions to reduce sodium intake were effective in reducing 24-hour

Table 8.8 The Dietary Approaches to Stop Hypertension (DASH) and Mediterranean diets

Diet	Food group	Recommendation
Mediterranean	Whole grains, vegetables, fruits, seeds, olive oil, nuts and legumes	Basis for every meal
	Poultry, eggs, yoghurt and cheese	Consume moderate portions daily to weekly
	Wine	Consume in moderation
DASH	Whole grains	7–8 servings per day
	Vegetables	4–5 servings per day
	Fruits	4–5 servings per day
	Lean meats or fish	2 or fewer servings per day
	Dairy (low fat)	2–3 servings per day
	Nuts, seeds and pulses	4–5 servings per week
	Fats and oils	2–3 servings per day
		5 servings or fewer per week
	Whole grains	7–8 servings per day
	Vegetables	4–5 servings per day

urinary sodium excretion by an average of 130 mmol/l, which is the equivalent of a 7.6 g per day reduction in salt intake. These interventions reduced blood pressure in a dose-dependent manner with participants in the highest quintile of sodium reduction exhibiting a decline of blood pressure of –5.74 mmHg (95% CI –7.67 to –3.81 mmHg) compared with –3.21 mmHg (95% CI –4.13 to –2.28 mmHg) in the lowest quintile (Huang *et al.*, 2020). The blood pressure lowering effect was greatest in subjects who were hypertensive, with the highest blood pressure at baseline being associated with the greatest blood pressure decrease at follow-up. Greater benefits were also noted in older adults and in subjects of non-white ethnicity. On average, a 50 mmol/l decrease in sodium excretion (equivalent to 2.9 g per day lower salt intake) was associated with a 4.26 mmHg decline in systolic and 2.07 mmHg decrease in diastolic pressure (Huang *et al.*, 2020). While in an individual sense, reductions in blood pressure of this magnitude are of limited significance, across a national population reductions in average pressure due to sodium reduction, would represent tens of thousands of cardiovascular events avoided.

The UK rolling programme of National Diet and Nutrition Surveys estimated that while the recommendation is for adults to consume no more than 7 g salt per day (men) or 5 g salt per day (women), the average intakes for men and women were 7.5 g and 6.8 g per day in 2018/19 (Ashford *et al.*, 2020). For men, this represented a reduction in intake of approximately one third since 2001. Progress in reducing the salt intake of the population represents a public health nutrition success in the UK, but new evidence from the GenSalt trial in China suggests that the response to salt reduction may not be beneficial in all individuals

(Chen, 2010). GenSalt considered the blood pressure response to seven days of low-salt (3 g/day) or high-salt (18 g/day) diets. On average, salt reduction decreased blood pressure by 7–8 mmHg (SBP), and high salt increased pressure by 5–6 mmHg. Responses were slightly greater in women than in men and were greatest in older subjects (Figure 8.16). Importantly, the blood pressure response to variation in salt intake followed a normal distribution around the mean changes, with approximately 23% of subjects increasing blood pressure in response to salt reduction and reducing blood pressure with a high-salt diet. GenSalt found that 32.4% of the Chinese population was salt sensitive (i.e. increased blood pressure with increasing sodium intake) and has been able to explore the mechanisms underlying salt sensitivity through genomic analyses. A clear role for genes involved in blood pressure regulatory pathways (the renin-angiotensin system, the sympathetic

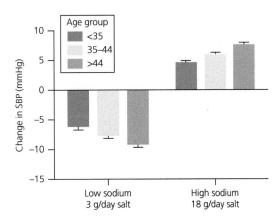

Figure 8.16 The effect of low- and high-salt diets on systolic blood pressure (SBP) in a Chinese population; the GenSalt study. *Source:* data from Chen (2010).

nervous system and the natriuretic hormone system) and ion and water channels has been identified (Liu *et al.*, 2020).

Other minerals may play a role in determining blood pressure. Calcium, for example, is believed to lower blood pressure, but studies with supplements show that even megadoses (twice normal daily intake) produce only minor changes. Similarly, magnesium is believed to be of importance as hypertensives often manifest low serum magnesium concentrations. However, supplemental magnesium has no significant effect upon blood pressure in humans. Increasing potassium intakes will lower blood pressure. INTERSALT suggested that a 50 mmol per day increase in potassium excretion would be associated with 3 mmHg lower SBP and 2 mmHg lower DBP.

8.4.5 Cancer
8.4.5.1 What is cancer?
Cancers, or tumours, can arise in any of the tissues of the body. They develop through a process termed carcinogenesis and are essentially the products of uncontrolled cell division. All mammalian cells have a limited capacity for cell division, termed the Hayflick limit. In humans, differentiated cells can divide only 52 times before undergoing apoptosis (programmed cell death), but in cancer, the processes that control cell division are lost through genetic mutation. Prevention of cell division beyond the Hayflick limit is achieved by action of the products of genes called proto-oncogenes and anti-oncogenes.

Proto-oncogenes are genes whose protein products participate in cell–cell signalling and signal transduction pathways. Under normal circumstances, these proteins are expressed at levels that do not allow cell division to occur and are represented as the c-forms of the gene, for example, c-ras or c-myc. Mutations of the proto-oncogenes render them oncogenes (cancer genes), which actively drive unregulated mitotic cell division. The oncogenic forms are given the 'v-' prefix, for example, v-ras. A large number of proto-oncogenes have now been identified, and all are known components of signal transduction pathways. Ras, for example, is a membrane-associated G protein and in the mutated form is frequently found in colorectal tumours. The *Trk* genes are tyrosine kinases and Raf is a threonine kinase.

Anti-oncogenes are also called tumour suppressor genes. Most of their protein products are factors that prevent cell division. For example, the p53 protein is a transcription factor that promotes the expression of other genes that suppress mitosis. Mutations of p53 will therefore allow unregulated cell division to occur. p53 mutations are among the most common found in human tumours. Some other tumour suppressors have roles in repairing DNA damage that might lead to mutations of anti-oncogenes or proto-oncogenes. For example, mutations of *BRCA1* are known to greatly increase risk of breast cancer. *BRCA1* and the related *BRCA2* gene encode enzymes that have a role in repairing double-stranded DNA breaks.

The process of developing cancer follows three defined stages (Figure 8.17). Carcinogenesis is initiated

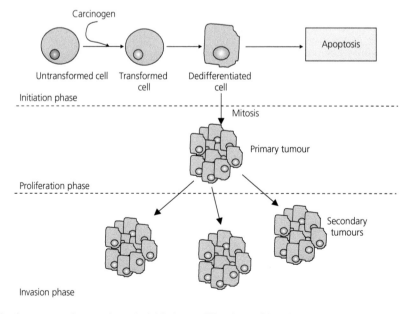

Figure 8.17 The three stages of tumourigenesis: initiation, proliferation and invasion.

with damage to either proto-oncogenes or anti-oncogenes, resulting in cells that are actively expressing oncogenes or have the inhibitory affectors of the cell cycle silenced. Such mutations are commonplace within cells and tissues and are generally repaired without any adverse consequences. However, should a mutated oncogene not undergo repair and should the cell be stable and able to survive in the mutated form, then it becomes transformed. A transformed cell dedifferentiates, essentially losing all of its specialized structures and functions. In many cases, the transformed cell will not be viable and will be eliminated through apoptosis. If this does not occur, the cell will proliferate through mitotic divisions to form a primary tumour. Many tumours are benign and grow only slowly, but others are more aggressive and will invade tissues rapidly. Often, these aggressive tumours will shed cells into the circulation, which then act as the focus for development of secondary tumours (metastases) in other organs.

The initiation phase of carcinogenesis depends upon contact between cells and carcinogenic agents. These include all factors that are capable of inducing genetic mutations through DNA damage. Thus, ionizing radiation, ultraviolet radiation, chemical agents and certain viruses (e.g. human papillomavirus) are all carcinogenic. Most carcinogen exposures are either lifestyle or occupation related. Occupations that involve exposure to hazardous chemicals, for example, asbestos or pesticides, are associated with elevated cancer risk. Carcinogenic exposures also occur due to tobacco smoking, exposure to environmental pollution, excessive sunlight exposure and the presence of carcinogenic chemicals in the food chain.

8.4.5.2 Diet is a modifiable determinant of cancer risk

While tobacco smoking and environmental or occupational exposures are most obviously viewed as risk factors for cancer, it is becoming clear that diet and lifestyle factors related to diet are major determinants of risk of cancer in all organs and tissues. Some estimates suggest that up to 70% of all cancer deaths may be attributable to diet-related factors (Doll and Peto, 1981), although it is more generally accepted that 30–40% of risk is diet related. The historic view that specific components of the diet (e.g. vitamin C, alcohol, fat, protein) are able to modify cancer risk is changing. It is now recognized that foods and their constituents influence cancer initiation and progression in many different ways. There is convincing evidence that some diet-related agents increase risk of cancer, while other dietary behaviours have a protective effect.

The most obvious way in which the diet can increase the risk of cancer is by directly delivering carcinogenic chemicals to the body. Later in this chapter, agents such as safrole are discussed as carcinogens that are normally present within certain foodstuffs. Intakes of such agents at levels that are hazardous are unusual, and so they are not generally considered as a major threat to human health. Most carcinogens that are ingested as components of food at levels that pose risk will be present either as contaminants or as products of cooking. Nitrosamines are a good example of the latter. The nitrosamines are derived from nitrites combined with secondary amino groups on certain amino acids or proteins. The most commonly occurring dietary nitrosamine is N-nitrosodimethylamine. Such compounds are present in high quantities in cooked, processed meats and in salted foods and pickles and are formed as by-products of food processing. Nitrosamines can also be inhaled as components of tobacco smoke. Nitrosamines are associated with a range of different cancers, particularly within the digestive tract. Larsson *et al.* (2006) reported that stomach cancer risk was elevated twofold in women consuming high levels of N-nitrosodimethylamine derived from salami, ham and sausages. Similarly, high intakes of nitrosamines and foods rich in nitrosamines are associated with risk of rectal and oesophageal cancers (Le Marchand *et al.*, 2002). A case–control study of bladder cancer found that cancer patients were more likely to have had high consumption of amine- and nitrosamine-rich foods (salami, pastrami, corned beef, liver) than controls in the two years prior to diagnosis (Catsburg *et al.* 2014).

Some foods may also deliver compounds to the body that themselves may be only weakly carcinogenic but which when processed through phase I metabolism in the liver generate potent carcinogenic forms (Figure 8.18). A good example of this is benzo(a)pyrene (B(a)P), which is a polycyclic aromatic hydrocarbon formed during combustion. B(a)P can be present on grains and cereals as an environmental pollutant but is more likely to enter the body during the cooking of meats, particularly if the meat is charred on the outside. B(a)P is metabolized by aryl hydrocarbon hydroxylase (cytochrome P450 1B1) to form a series of hydroxyl and diol intermediates. These products, and most notably the B(a)P diol epoxides, are able to form adducts with DNA, leading to damage and mutation.

The metabolism of nitrosamines may also determine their ultimate carcinogenicity. Nitrosamines are metabolized by the cytochrome P450, CYP2E1. This can exist in different forms as there is a

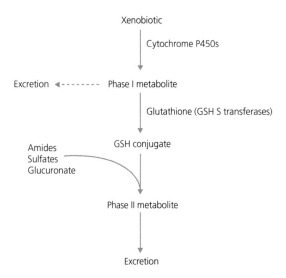

Figure 8.18 Xenobiotics (chemicals that are not components of normal mammalian biochemistry) are metabolized via phase I and phase II systems. Phase I metabolism generates metabolites that are conjugated with glutathione (GSH; phase II) and further compounds that enable urinary excretion.

polymorphism of the *CYP2E1* gene, with some individuals having a gene with 96 bp 5′ insert. In a study of a Hawaiian population, individuals with the 5′ insert had 60% greater risk of rectal cancer

(Le Marchand *et al.*, 2002). This increased risk may be further elevated by consumption of a nitrosamine-rich diet. Individuals carrying the gene with the 5′ insert were noted to have up to threefold greater risk of rectal cancer if consuming a diet rich in processed meats.

Components of the diet may also interact with each other or with other cancer risk factors to modify risk of cancer. Stomach cancer is generally preceded by inflammatory disorders of the stomach lining, which permit infection with bacteria that promote carcinogenesis (e.g. *Helicobacter pylori*) or which increase the likelihood of cell transformation occurring in the presence of carcinogens (Figure 8.19). A high-sodium diet is proposed to irritate the stomach mucosa and promote localized inflammation (gastritis). In addition to promoting infection, high salt concentrations appear to alter expression of certain *H. pylori* genes, and this may contribute to tumour initiation (Loh *et al.*, 2007). Nitrosamines may also promote development of gastric carcinomas once gastritis is established.

Once within the body, the ability of carcinogens to drive the formation of tumours, or for tumours to become established, may be modulated by other components of the diet. Antioxidant nutrients have an anticarcinogenic function as they have the capacity to neutralize free radicals such as the hydroxyl

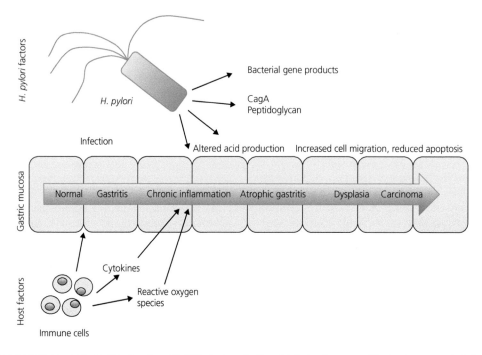

Figure 8.19 Infection of the gastric mucosa with *Helicobacter pylori* is a risk factor for cancer. The host response to infection promotes inflammation and cell damage. Bacterial products change the nature of the gastric mucosa and can prevent apoptosis and inhibit tumour suppressor functions.

radical, which unquenched can cause DNA strand scission or modify base sequences. It is also proposed that some components of the diet can modulate the access of carcinogens to their sites of action. For example, certain non-nutrient components of plant foodstuffs may bind carcinogenic compounds and prevent their absorption across the gut and therefore have anti-tumour properties (see Section 8.4.5.5). Other anti-tumour agents are active post-absorption and bind carcinogens to prevent their interaction with DNA. The actions of nutrients may differ according to stage of tumourigenesis, and while they may be protective against initiation, they may promote proliferation and invasion.

8.4.5.3 Nutritional epidemiology and cancer

The study of the relationship between diet and cancer has been one of the main areas of focus for nutritional epidemiologists over the last four decades. A wide range of different methodological approaches have been adopted, each yielding data suggestive of associations between particular components of the diet and either increased or decreased risk of cancers at different sites of the body.

8.4.5.3.1 Ecological studies

Ecological studies involve comparing prevalence rates for specific diseases between different regions of a country or between different countries. They can also look at changes in prevalence rates within a population over an extended period of time. To uncover the underlying reasons between temporal or geographical variation in disease rates, the ecological studies explore variation in putative exposures that might explain the patterns of disease. For example, it is widely reported that there is a strong correlation between risk of breast cancer in women and total fat intake. This assertion is based on the observation that on a global scale, the nations with the highest breast cancer death rates (e.g. the UK, Netherlands, New Zealand, Canada, Denmark and the United States) are those with the highest per capita fat intakes. The nations with the lowest death rates from breast cancer (Thailand, Japan, Taiwan, El Salvador) are those with the lowest fat intakes. This example typifies the limitations of ecological studies, which at best can only be suggestive of a diet–cancer relationship. In the example described earlier, it is not possible to establish whether the women dying of breast cancer are the same women who were exposed to high fat intake, nor is it possible to exclude important confounding factors that are known to impact on breast cancer risk and that vary between these nations (e.g. age at menarche

and menopause, age at first pregnancy, number of pregnancies, use of oral contraceptives). All ecological studies must be followed up with studies using more reliable methodologies. In the case of the putative relationship between fat and breast cancer, there is actually little reliable evidence to suggest a major risk (Mazhar and Waxman, 2006).

8.4.5.3.2 Migrant studies

Migrant populations, that is, groups of people who have moved from a country where they have been established for many generations to a new country, were widely used in early studies of diet and cancer. Migrant populations provide the ability to discriminate between influences of genetics and influences of the environment in the aetiology of disease. Genetic changes in migrant populations occur slowly as they often require three or more generations to mix significantly with the indigenous peoples of their new homeland. Environmental changes such as exposure to pollutants or background radiation will exert effects immediately. Dietary changes often occur within two generations as younger people, in particular, will take on the dietary patterns of the new country very readily.

Studies of Japanese migrants to the United States in the period following the Second World War provided some of the first clues to the dietary basis of cancers of the stomach and colon. Over three generations, the US Japanese developed colon cancer rates fivefold above those seen in Japan, while stomach cancer rates fell by 80%. These observations were taken as evidence that high salt intake was a risk factor for stomach cancer, while a high-red-meat, low-fibre diet could increase risk of colon cancer. Lee *et al.* (2007) reported on changes in prevalence of cancers among Korean migrants to the United States. In South Korea, rates of certain cancers are very high, and this has been attributed to high intakes of salted foods and foods rich in nitrosamines. Among the male population of US Koreans, migration decreased prevalence rates of stomach, liver and gall bladder cancers, while risk of cancers of the colon and prostate appeared to increase (Figure 8.20). This illustrates that the shift to a more westernized lifestyle produces profound changes in cancer risk and investigation of the nature of those lifestyle changes could inform understanding of the diet–cancer relationship.

8.4.5.3.3 Studies of populations with unique characteristics

There are some groups of individuals living among national or continental populations, whose beliefs and lifestyles set them apart. Through comparisons of

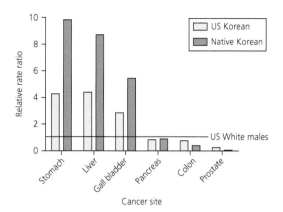

Figure 8.20 Cancer rates in male Korean migrants to the United States compared with the native South Korean population. Migration is associated with significantly decreased prevalence of cancers of the stomach, liver and gall bladder, but these cancers still remain more common than in the full US population. Migration increased risk of colon and prostate cancers. *Source:* data from Lee *et al.* (2007).

such groups with the broader population, it may be possible to elucidate nutritional factors that could explain variance in cancer risk. For example, some orders of English nuns who follow a vegetarian diet have been useful in exploring relationships between

meat consumption and breast cancer risk. The nuns are celibate and therefore not reproductively active, so they represent a high-risk group for these tumours. As they also abstain from alcohol and tobacco smoking, the influence of diet can be studied in the absence of these other risk factors (Willett, 1990). As described in Research Highlight 8.3, the Seventh Day Adventist population of the United States has also proved highly informative when examining the impact of a vegetarian diet and other lifestyle factors on risk of cancer.

8.4.5.3.4 Case–control studies

Case–control studies have been a valuable investigative tool for considering relationships between diet and cancer. Essentially, in a case–control study, researchers will recruit subjects who have been diagnosed with the disease of interest. These cases will then be compared with a suitably matched control group without the disease to ascertain the factors that could explain why the cases but not the controls developed the disease. For example, Hawrysz *et al.* (2020) recruited 187 patients with newly diagnosed lung cancer and analysed their adherence to a Polish adaptation of the Mediterranean diet (Table 8.8) using a food frequency questionnaire. Comparison with 252 controls showed that moderate smokers

Research Highlight 8.3 The US Seventh Day Adventist health studies and cancer

The Seventh Day Adventist church is a Protestant Christian domination founded in the 1860s. It has over 20 million members largely centred in Africa, Central and South America. Approximately 7% of Adventists live in the United States, where the church was founded. Adventist theology has a strong focus on staying healthy and Adventists largely abstain from alcohol (only 7% of US Adventists are drinkers) and tobacco smoking (1% of US Adventists smoke). The church encourages members to adhere to a diet that is either vegetarian or consistent with the kosher laws of Judaism. In the United States, the Adventist population is split roughly 50 : 50 between omnivores and vegetarians, with around 8% following a vegan diet.

The Adventist population in the United States have been a focus for large prospective cohort studies, particularly focused on cancer outcomes. The nature of the Adventist lifestyle enables such studies to analyse risk, either without the confounding effects of smoking and alcohol or with those variables very well adjusted for. Moreover, the population is large enough to be able to draw robust conclusions. Data considering the difference between diet and health outcomes in Adventists compared with non-Adventists have helped to establish how lifestyle determines cancer risk, while comparing vegetarian and omnivorous Adventists helps to provide more detail. There are three noteworthy Adventist cohort studies.

The Adventist Mortality Study began in 1958 and recruited 22 940 Californian Adventists. This group showed markedly reduced risk of cancer compared with non-Adventists (Le and Sabate, 2014). Adventists had 79% lower risk of lung cancer and colorectal cancer (30% lower), breast cancer (15% lower) and prostate cancer (8% lower) were significantly reduced by the Adventist lifestyle.

The Adventist Health Study 1 cohort was recruited in 1973, with the aim of examining which aspects of the Adventist diet offered protection against cancer. It found that vegetarians were at lower risk than omnivores for cancers of the breast, colon, bladder, prostate and stomach (Tantamango *et al.*, 2011); Le and Sabate, 2014; Fraser *et al.*, 2015). The beneficial features of a vegetarian diet were high fibre and low intakes of animal produce.

The Adventist Health Study 2 is still continuing at the time of writing. It completed baseline recruitment of 96 000 Adventists between 2001 and 2007. The early findings on cancer suggest that a vegan diet may be beneficial. Vegan Adventists exhibited a lower risk of prostate cancer (hazard ratio, HR, 0.65, 95% CI 0.49–0.85; Tantamango-Bartley *et al.*, 2016). A similar benefit was reported for breast cancer, although this was not statistically significant (HR 0.78, 95% CI 0.58–1.05, comparing vegans with omnivores; Penniecook-Sawyers *et al.*, 2016).

with greatest adherence to the Mediterranean diet had lower risk of lung cancer than those with lowest adherence (OR 0.34, 95% CI 0.15–0.76). Similarly, a case–control study to consider relationships between low-fat foods and colorectal cancer in New Zealand recruited 806 patients with colorectal cancer and 1025 controls and observed that a high preference for low-fat food alternatives, over the year before recruitment to the study, was associated with reduced cancer risk (Sneyd and Cox, 2020).

There are a number of important problems with this approach that can undermine confidence in any findings. First, the recruiting of suitable control populations is often fraught with difficulty, and case–control studies are highly vulnerable to influences of confounding factors. It is impossible to exclude the possibility that controls are undiagnosed cases or cases waiting to happen. Finally, all exposure data (i.e. data relating to diet) are either collected well after the period during which carcinogenesis was initiated or have to be collected retrospectively. Asking people to recall their typical diet from a decade previously is bound to introduce considerable bias to a study.

8.4.5.3.5 Cohort studies

Prospective cohort studies that are able to follow a population over an extended period of time provide a very powerful tool for examining relationships between diet and cancer. Prospective cohorts require very large populations (tens of thousands of people) to be recruited to allow for the fact that specific cancers are actually uncommon events. Baseline data on diet and other exposures can be collected at the start of the study and at intervals thereafter. These data can then be related to the occurrence of disease over the duration of the study. Although many prospective studies are plagued by inaccurate estimation of the exposure data in the initial stages, there are several major prospective cohorts that have informed much of what we know about diet–cancer relationships.

The US Nurses' Health Study (Colditz and Hankinson, 2005) began to collect data on diet and alcohol consumption among US women in 1980 and has included over 80 000 participants. By sustaining the follow-up of these women over three decades, it has proved possible to investigate the role of diet in the aetiology of many cancers and other disease states. The Nurses' Health Study is one of the key cohorts that have yielded evidence to show a proposed relationship between fat intake and risk of breast cancer to be fallacious. The EPIC cohort was established in 1992 and by 2006 had recruited 521 448 individuals across 23 centres in 10 European countries (Gonzalez, 2006). The chief advantage of such a large study is that the actual number of cancer cases will be high, which greatly increases the chances of observing diet–cancer relationships. EPIC used a range of dietary assessment methods to obtain baseline data from participants and was designed to follow-up for at least 20 years. The UK Biobank is a long-term prospective cohort of 500 000 participants aged 40–69 years at baseline. Participants were recruited between 2006 and 2010 and the cohort baseline data included sampling for biomarkers in blood, saliva and urine, information on their health and wellbeing, weight, blood pressure diet, cognitive function and mental health (Sudlow et al., 2015). The UK Biobank study focuses heavily on the role of lifestyle–genotype interactions as determinants of disease risk.

8.4.5.3.6 Intervention studies

As discussed in Chapter 1, intervention studies (particularly placebo-controlled randomized controlled trials) are generally seen as the gold standard in epidemiology. Intervention studies are arguably the most effective tool for studying the relationship between any dietary component and cancer risk. Typically, an intervention will seek to provide volunteers with a diet that is either supplemented with a putative protective factor or which has a reduced content of a suspected harmful agent. The volunteers can then be followed up over a period to assess the impact on cancer risk. Many of these very expensive intervention trials have been performed to assess efficacy of antioxidants, dietary fibre and other agents in cancer prevention, but despite their power, many of the trials examining associations with cancer have proven inconclusive or have yielded results of an unexpected nature. For example, the CARET trial was an intervention trial in which supplements of β-carotene were provided to smokers and other individuals at high risk of lung cancer. It was initiated because observational studies had indicated that higher serum carotenoid concentrations were associated with lower lung cancer mortality, particularly among smokers. The CARET trial was abandoned at an early stage when it was noted that the supplements actually increased rather than decreased cancer mortality (Omenn et al., 1996). It is thought that this increase occurred because although vitamin A may block carcinogenesis at the initiation stage, it may accelerate the progression of tumours at the proliferation and invasion stages. The meta-analysis of Druesne-Pecollo et al. (2014) estimated that β-carotene supplements increased risk of stomach and lung cancers by up to 34% in non-smokers and up to 54% in smokers and asbestos workers. The World Cancer Research Fund

(2018d) has now identified β-carotene supplements as a causative factor for lung cancer.

The CARET experience highlights some of the main drawbacks of almost all diet–cancer intervention trials. Most trials, for reasons of good scientific method, seek to only manipulate subjects' intakes of a single nutrient. This instantly renders them unrepresentative of a typical human diet. Moreover, selected doses are often based on too little information and may be insufficient to elicit an effect, or too high to be safe. CARET emphasizes the frequent disparity between evidence gathered from case–control studies and cohort studies and randomized controlled trials that have been developed to test the anti-cancer properties of specific micronutrients.

Much of the divergence between randomized controlled trials and observational studies may be explained by timing of supplementation in relation to the progression from a transformed cell to a cancerous lesion. Folic acid, for example, is well documented to prevent the early stages of cancer, and it does so by maintaining normal patterns of DNA methylation and gene silencing and by providing a precursor for nucleotides that are required for DNA repair following damage. However, folic acid will also promote the replication of established tumour cells through the same mechanisms as a plentiful supply of nucleotides is required for tumour growth. Similarly, β-carotene will prevent DNA damage

through antioxidant properties but may act as a mitogen that enhances replication of transformed cells through interference with retinoid metabolism and associated signalling pathways (Goralczyk, 2009). Randomized controlled trials have to recruit people at high risk of disease to observe benefits in a timely manner, so there is a strong risk that nutrients that may have differential effects on tumour initiation and proliferation may have markedly different effects to their effects when consumed as part of a long-term dietary pattern by low-risk healthy individuals. It is commonplace, for example, to recruit individuals who have previously been treated for a cancer and who are at high risk of recurrence. For example, Alberts *et al.* (2000) recruited patients who had undergone surgery to remove colorectal tumours for a study of the potential benefits of fibre supplementation. This is not representative of the population and their risk in relation to diet.

8.4.5.3.7 Cancer risk is a product of the whole diet

All of the approaches to the study of diet–cancer relationships outlined run the risk of producing erroneous results if they fail to take into account the ways in which nutrients interact with each other, with the genes carried by individuals, with the microbiome and with other risk factors in the environment (Figure 8.21). Much of the research into diet and

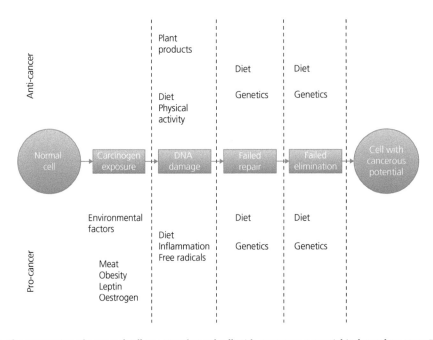

Figure 8.21 The progression of a normal cell to a transformed cell with cancerous potential is dependent upon DNA damage, a failure to repair that damage and the evasion of systems that eliminate damaged cells. Environmental factors, including diet, interact with genetic factors at all stages of the process.

cancer conducted in the latter part of the twentieth century is now recognized as being of limited value as the emphasis then was on specific nutrients and risk. Humans consume foods with mixed and variable components, not single nutrients in isolation. It was therefore overly simplistic to assume that intakes of a single nutrient are representative of the whole range of dietary and environmental exposures experienced by individuals. The CARET study described earlier typifies this and highlights the fact that nutritional factors impact on cancer risk at all stages of the development and progression of the disease. The progression from a damaged cell to a cell with cancerous potential during the initiation phase of cancer is influenced by interactions of genetics and lifestyle (Figure 8.21). These can be both pro-cancer and anti-cancer in nature.

The human diet comprises varied mixtures of foods, each providing different combinations of nutrients, prepared in a variety of different ways. This means that within each food and within each meal, there is considerable scope for interactions between nutrients and between nutrients and the non-nutrient components of foodstuffs. Having a varied diet is desirable as it increases the chances that a broad array of protective agents will be ingested and minimizes the risk of repetitive exposure to harmful factors. As such, it will be the combinations of factors in the habitual diet of any individual that confer cancer risk, rather than intakes of specific nutrients or foods. For example, in relation to colon cancer risk, a diet high in processed and red meats, which promotes excessive weight gain carries significantly greater risk than one high in fish, vegetables, fruits and rich sources of dietary fibre. Dietary patterns can be complex and, when considering the cancer reductions associated with a Mediterranean dietary pattern for example, it is challenging to ascertain where the benefits are derived from. Is the reduced risk associated with the latter diet due to the lower intake of meat or saturated fats, or could it be explained by greater intakes of antioxidants from plant materials? Almost certainly it is a combination of these factors that provides the observed benefit and then the level of benefit will be modified by stage of life, body fatness, genotype and the status of the microbiome. These are questions that invariably cannot be answered by randomized controlled trials and so systematic review and meta-analysis of decades of research is the strongly favoured methodology at present.

Studies of diet and cancer are of considerable importance as it is clear that lifestyle modifications have the potential to reduce population and individual level risk of cancers at a number of sites

(Table 8.9). Clear identification of factors or combinations of factors that may increase or decrease risk will help to refine dietary guidelines given to populations and will inform the design of future dietary interventions. The focus of contemporary studies of diet and cancer relationships, is very much on broader classes of foodstuffs, such as meats or wholegrains. The 2020 World Cancer Research Fund Third Expert Report on food, nutrition and cancer indicates that the main risk factors for cancer are alcohol and meat consumption, while a prudent diet based upon fruits, vegetables and foods rich in dietary fibre reduce risk (Table 8.9). Obesity also has a critical role in determining cancer risk, and increasing physical activity may be protective.

8.4.5.4 Dietary factors that may promote cancer
8.4.5.4.1 Obesity
Excessive weight gain and body fatness, whether attributable to poor diet, low physical activity levels or both, are firmly associated with cancers at all sites around the body. Large prospective cohort studies indicate that overweight and obesity are major risk factors. For example, an eight-year follow-up of over 3.6 million Spanish adults indicated that high BMI was associated with increased prevalence of cancers of the uterus, kidney, gall bladder, thyroid and colon, together with postmenopausal breast cancer, myelomas and lymphomas (Recalde et al., 2021). Weight gain in adulthood also increases risk. An eight-year follow-up of the EPIC cohort found that a weight gain of 0.4–5 kg per year was associated with greater risk of gall bladder, thyroid and postmenopausal breast cancers (Christakoudi et al., 2021). Weight loss reduced risk of uterine and colon cancers. Arnold et al. (2015) estimated that globally in 2012, 481 000 new cancers in adults over 30 years of age were attributable to overweight and obesity. The greatest burden of cancers related to excess weight was seen in the more highly developed countries, consistent with previous estimates that 6.4% of all female and 3.4 of all male cancers in European populations were related to overweight (Figure 8.22; Bergstrom et al., 2001). The third expert report of the World Cancer Research Fund (2018a) concluded that there was convincing evidence that being overweight or obese was associated with increased risk of postmenopausal breast cancer and cancers of the prostate, kidney, endometrium, liver, pancreas, oesophagus (adenocarcinoma), gall bladder, stomach, colon, mouth, pharynx and larynx (Table 8.10). Being overweight between the ages of 18 and 30 is associated with lower risk of premenopausal breast cancer.

Table 8.9 Diet and cancer risk.

Dietary factor	Cancer site									
	Breast	Colorectal	Prostate	Lung	Oesophageal	Kidney	Endometrial	Mouth, larynx and pharynx	Stomach	Liver
Processed meat		↑↑↑		↑					↑	
Red meat		↑↑		↑						
Fish		↓								↓
Grilled and barbecued meat/fish									↑	
Non-starchy vegetables				↓				↓		
Vegetables				↓	↓				↓	
Fruit		↓		↓						
Citrus fruits									↓	
Wholegrains		↓↓								
Fibre		↓↓								
Foods containing carotenoids	↓			↓						
Foods containing isoflavones										
Foods containing β-carotene				↓						
β-carotene supplements				↑↑↑						
Dairy products	↓	↓↓	↑							
Calcium in foods or supplements		↓↓	↑							
Salted foods									↑	
Coffee				↑		↓↓	↓↓		↑	↓↓
Alcohol	↑↑	↑↑↑			↑↑↑			↑↑↑	↑↑	↑↑↑

Data extracted from World Cancer Research Fund (2020). ↑ denotes increased risk of cancer; ↓ denotes decreased risk of cancer. ↑↑↑/↓↓↓ indicates convincing evidence; ↑↑/↓↓ indicates probable association ↑/↓ indicates limited evidence of association.

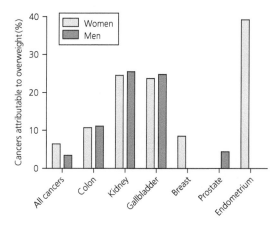

Figure 8.22 Contribution of obesity and overweight to cancer risk in European men and women. *Source:* data from Bergstrom *et al.* (2001).

The mechanisms through which obesity increases cancer risk are varied and largely unidentified and may be specific to each tumour site. Individuals who are obese produce greater background concentrations of pro-inflammatory cytokines, and in tissues such as the colon, the presence of a persistent, low-level inflammation will increase risk of tumour growth. Obesity is also associated with insulin resistance and raised concentrations of sex steroids and insulin-like growth factor-1. All these factors will promote the growth and metabolic activity of tumour cells and hence drive the proliferative and invasion phases of cancer.

Breast cancer risk is strongly related to the duration of production of oestrogens. As described in Chapter 2, obesity in childhood is associated with an earlier menarche and hence a longer phase of oestrogen production, while obesity beyond the menopause will allow for oestrogen production beyond the phase of normal ovarian function. The association between female BMI and breast cancer

risk is dependent on stage of life. Premenopausal women of greater BMI are apparently protected against breast cancer (World Cancer Research Fund, 2018a), with some studies suggesting that BMI of 30 or greater may halve risk. The underlying mechanism for this is unknown, but it has been suggested that it may a benefit associated with anovulation due to leptin resistance impacting on the endocrine regulation of the menstrual cycle. This results in low concentrations of progesterone which is known to stimulate cell proliferation in the breast (Dowsett and Folkerd, 2015).

In postmenopausal women, however, there is a significant increase in risk, particularly with central adiposity. Each 5-kg increment in BMI over 'normal' weight is associated with a 12% increase in risk (World Cancer Research Fund, 2018a). Oestrogens are produced beyond the menopause through the action of aromatases in adipose tissue that convert androgens to a range of oestrogen metabolites. Insulin resistance associated with obesity increases the production of androgens and hence drives this process. Oestrogens are mitogenic and will promote tumour growth. It is suggested that before the menopause, the actions of oestrogens are opposed by progesterone, but following the menopause, this protective action of progesterone will be lost. The association of obesity with breast cancer mortality may also be explained by delays in recognizing symptoms and detecting breast lumps at an early stage of cancer due to the accumulation of fatty tissue in the breasts.

Effects of body fatness on cancer risk may vary within a tissue. Organs and tissues are not homogenous and comprise varied cell types that may give rise to different types of tumour with differing origins and risk factors. Oesophageal cancers, for example, may be squamous cell carcinomas (derived from epithelial cells) or adenocarcinomas (derived from glandular cells). Both types of tumour are related to direct

Table 8.10 Estimates of risk of cancer associated with physical activity and obesity.

Cancer site	RR (95% CI) for each 5kg/m2 increase in BMI	RR (95% CI) comparing highest with lowest total physical activity level
Colorectal	1.05 (1.03–1.07)	0.80 (0.72–0.88)
Oesophageal (squamous cell)	0.64 (0.56–0.73)	
Oesophageal (adenocarcinoma)	1.48 (1.35–1.62)	
Breast (premenopause)	0.93 (0.90–0.97)	
Breast (postmenopause)	1.12 (1.09–1.15)	0.87 (0.79–0.96)
Prostate	1.08 (1.04–1.12)	
Kidney	1.30 (1.25–1.35)	
Gall bladder	1.25 (0.15–1.37)	

Data Source: World Cancer Research Fund (2020).

exposures to carcinogens entering the gastrointestinal tract (e.g. alcohol, tobacco smoke). While squamous carcinomas of the oesophagus are strongly related to infection by the human papillomavirus, adenocarcinomas are associated with obesity. This relationship may be driven through greater gastric reflux with greater abdominal fat deposition. Acid damage may promote chronic tissue inflammation and carcinogenesis. Evidence suggests that obesity is associated with lower risk of squamous cell carcinomas (World Cancer Research Fund, 2018a), but it may be an artefact of weight loss occurring in people with undiagnosed cancers (Abnet *et al.*, 2018). Figure 8.23 summarises the apparent disparities in evidence relating obesity to cancers of the breast and oesophagus.

8.4.5.4.2 Meat

The initial interest in meat consumption as a risk factor for cancer stemmed from now discounted observational studies that suggested that high intakes of animal protein and saturated fat increased risk. However, it is now believed that formation of nitrosamines and heterocyclic amines during the cooking and preservation of meats is the main vehicle through which meat products contribute to cancer risk. Although there is some limited evidence that meat intake is associated with risk of cancers of the lung and stomach, the main association is with colorectal cancer when there is convincing evidence that high intakes of red meat and processed meat play a causal role (World Cancer Research Fund, 2018b). Processed meats include all products that are preserved either by curing, salting, smoking or the addition of nitrates and nitrites.

Several cohort studies have shown an increased risk of colorectal cancer associated with meat consumption. A large study of male health professionals in the United States (Giovannucci *et al.*, 2004) found that regular consumption of meat increased risk (RR 3.6) compared with rare or infrequent consumption of meat. Processed meat and red meats are generally identified as the main contributor to risk, with white meat (poultry) apparently having little or no impact. The meta-analysis of the World Cancer Research Fund (2018b) found that the relative risk for colorectal cancer for every 100 g per day increment of red meat intake was 1.12 (95% CI 1.00–1.25) and for processed meat was 1.16 for every 50 g per day increment of intake (95% CI 1.08–1.26). Current advice is that intakes of red meat should be limited to 500 g/week (cooked weight) with avoidance of processed meats (World Cancer Research Fund, 2008). There is some limited evidence that consumption of chargrilled and barbecued meats are a risk factor for stomach cancer (World Cancer Research Fund, 2018c), which may be related to formation of heterocyclic amines and polyaromatic hydrocarbons during cooking. There is no convincing evidence that poultry or egg intake is related to cancer risk. High intakes of fish are associated (limited suggestive evidence) with lower risk of cancers of the liver (World Cancer Research Fund, 2015a) and colon (World Cancer Research Fund, 2018b) which may be related to anti-inflammatory activity of n-3 fatty acids.

As stated above, red and processed meat may directly deliver carcinogens formed during preservation and cooking to the body, and these are believed to play a major role in colorectal cancer. The high iron content of red meat may also play a role as iron has the potential to drive the generation of ROS (Figure 8.24). Meat is also an energy-dense food, so high consumption can lead to weight gain.

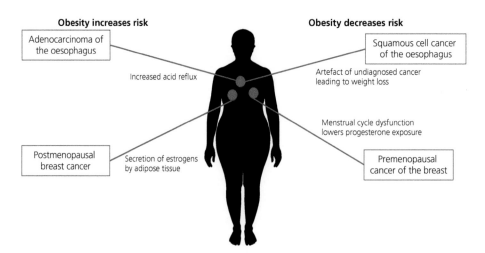

Figure 8.23 Obesity has differential effects on risk of tumour types at the same sites.

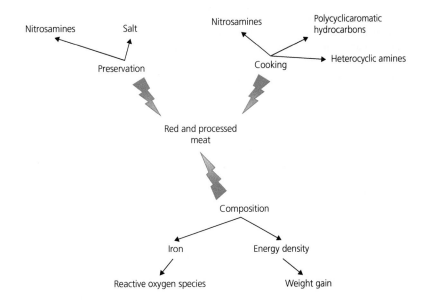

Figure 8.24 Possible routes from meat intake to colorectal cancer.

Heterocyclic amines are formed in the cooking of all meats, including poultry, so the lack of evidence linking consumption of white meats to cancer is perplexing. The explanation may be that peptides derived from red, but not white, meats undergo metabolism in the colon, greatly increasing their mutagenicity. N-nitrosation generates N-methyl-N-nitroso compounds that form adducts with DNA. Many of these adducts are excised during DNA repair processes and can be detected in the colon as a marker of carcinogenic processes. Lewin *et al.* (2007) studied healthy volunteers who were allocated to consume either a vegetarian diet or a diet rich in red meat. In a third element of the study, the high meat intake was supplemented with fibre. Shedding of cells containing the adduct O^6-carboxymethyl guanine was determined in faecal samples. The high-meat diet greatly increased this marker of carcinogenic processes, and high-fibre intake partially offset this effect (Figure 8.25). Thus, delivery of N-nitroso compounds to the colon may be an important means through which red meat increases risk of colorectal cancer.

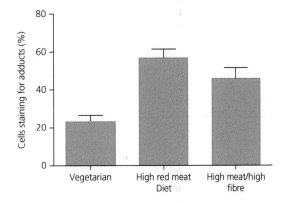

Figure 8.25 Healthy volunteers consumed vegetarian, high-meat or high-meat, high-fibre diets for periods of 10 days. Exfoliated colonic cells shed in faecal matter were stained for 0^6-carboxymethyl guanine. Meat increased appearance of these positive cells and fibre partially offset this effect. *Source:* data from Lewin *et al.* (2007).

8.4.5.4.3 Alcohol

The extent of alcohol consumption within groups is extremely varied both across and within global populations. While some groups never consume alcoholic beverages, there are others where around 10% of energy is consumed as alcohol. Globally, the average annual consumption of alcohol by adults is 6.4 litres of pure alcohol per capita. The highest consumption is seen in Europe where consumption varies between 7 and 15 litres per year per capita, with greatest consumption seen in Czechia, Lithuania and Moldova, followed by Germany, France, Portugal, Ireland and Belgium (Ritchie and Roser, 2019). The UK National Diet and Nutrition Survey years 1 and 2 analysis (Bates *et al.*, 2011) reported that consumption beyond recommendations (14 units per week) was commonplace, with 28% of men and 19% of women consuming double the recommended limits. Between 2005 and 2016, UK alcohol consumption declined slightly and a greater proportion of adults reported being teetotal

(Office for National Statistics, 2016). More British men than women consume alcohol and the occurrence of binge drinking and overall consumption is greater in people of higher socioeconomic status. These trends are a major concern as globally alcohol consumption is associated with 2.8 million deaths per annum (Ritchie and Roser, 2019) and alcohol has been positively identified as a carcinogen in humans.

There is high level evidence that alcohol consumption is a risk factor for cancers of the mouth, pharynx, larynx, stomach, liver, oesophagus (squamous cell), breast (pre- and postmenopause) and colon (World Cancer Research Fund, 2015a, 2016, 2018b, 2018e, 2018f; Table 8.11). The mechanisms of action proposed include direct DNA damage by ethanol and acetaldehyde, the main product of alcohol degradation in the liver; activation of microsomal phase I metabolism; and delivery of other carcinogens that may be present in alcoholic beverages, such as nitrosamines. It is also suggested that alcohol in drinks may increase the bioavailability of ethanol-soluble carcinogens across the digestive tract. Alcohol is also associated with generation of ROS.

Most epidemiological studies suggest that risk of breast cancer increases with alcohol consumption although care has to be taken in adjusting analysis for tobacco smoking as a confounder and consumption of alcoholic beverages is often under-reported. Meta-analysis of well-designed cohort studies (Smith-Warner *et al.*, 1998) showed that for every 10 g per day increase in alcohol consumption, risk of breast cancer rose by 9%. Risk of oesophageal and other head and neck cancers is increased by up to tenfold in heavy drinkers (over 80 g alcohol per day), a hazard that is further increased by cigarette smoking. The meta-analyses performed by the

World Cancer Research Fund demonstrate dose-dependent relationships between alcohol and cancers of the liver (2015a), stomach (2018c), colon (2018b), mouth, pharynx and larynx (2018e), oesophagus – squamous cell (2016) and breast (2018f). Moderate alcohol consumption is associated with lower risk of kidney cancer (World Cancer Research Fund, 2015b) but the mechanism underpinning this association is unknown.

Rehm *et al.* (2007) performed a systematic review of the literature examining whether alcohol-related cancer risk could be ameliorated through cessation of drinking. Alcohol consumption increased risk of oesophageal cancer by 2.7-fold in people who consumed alcohol compared with those who never consumed it (Figure 8.26). Cessation of drinking produced an initial increase in risk, which is also seen in relation to breast cancer (Willett, 2001), but by five years post-cessation of drinking significant health benefits became apparent.

8.4.5.4.4 Specific carcinogens in food
Foodstuffs deliver a huge range of chemical agents that are not normally regarded as nutrients to the body. Some of these are present as contaminants, entering the food chain during production and preparation; others are generated during the process of cooking. In addition, there is a vast array of agents that are the products of the complex secondary metabolism of plants. As described in the following paragraphs, some of the non-nutrient components of

Table 8.11 Estimates of risk of cancer associated with alcohol consumption.

Cancer site	RR (95%CI) for each 10g/day increase in alcohol consumption
Colorectal	1.07 (1.05–1.08)
Oesophageal (squamous cell)	1.25 (1.12–1.41)
Liver	1.04 (1.02–1.06)
Breast	1.05 (1.02–1.08)
Mouth, pharynx and larynx	1.15 (1.09–1.22)
Stomach	1.0 (1.00–1.04)
Kidney	0.92 (0.86–0.97)

Source: World Cancer Research Fund (2020).

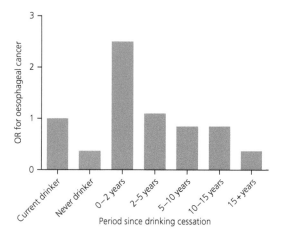

Figure 8.26 Risk of oesophageal cancer associated with alcohol consumption is significantly higher when comparing current drinkers with individuals who have never consumed alcohol. Cessation of alcohol drinking initially increases risk of cancer but over the longer term restores risk to the equivalent of never drinking. OR, odds ratio. *Source:* data from Rehm *et al.* (2007).

food may have anti-cancer properties. It is also the case that some of these factors are directly carcinogenic and if consumed in excess may directly promote the development of primary tumours.

A simple test was developed by Bruce Ames and his colleagues in the 1970s to screen potential carcinogenic agents from food or from other sources. The Ames test assesses the mutagenic capacity of compounds and works on the assumption that any agent capable of damaging DNA will have the potential to have carcinogenic effects. The test involves growing mutant strains of *Salmonella typhimurium* that lack genes for key enzymes involved in amino acid metabolism, on media lacking those amino acids (Figure 8.27). Any colonies that grow in the presence of a suspected carcinogen must have undergone mutation to be able to use the limiting medium and therefore signal that the test chemical is a mutagen. The number of colonies that grow will provide an index of how potent a mutagen, the agent, is. Many compounds that are not carcinogens could produce a positive Ames test result, and some carcinogens that only become active when metabolized within the human body, such as B(a)P, give a negative Ames test result. The main disadvantage of the Ames test is that the test organism is a prokaryote and thus, it is a poor model for studying potential

harm to humans. The test can be improved by using eukaryotic yeast cells instead of bacteria and by adding extracts of rodent liver to the test medium to introduce hepatic phase I and phase II xenobiotic metabolism (Figure 8.27).

There are some important Ames test-positive agents that can regularly appear in the human food chain and promote carcinogenesis. Several such agents are present in commonly consumed herbs. Basil and tarragon, for example, deliver estragole, while comfrey contains carcinogenic alkaloids. Generally speaking, however, these agents are not consumed in significantly large amounts and risk is negligible. The same is true of safrole, a compound found in cinnamon and nutmeg. Safrole is also present in peppercorns, which are used to produce the pepper used in cooking and as a condiment in most western cuisines. In Taiwan, the habit of chewing betel is associated with oesophageal cancer. Betel is essentially ground areca nut mixed with leaves and lime (calcium hydroxide) to form a chewable quid that has a high safrole content. Red peppers and chilli peppers have their characteristic flavour due to the presence of capsaicin. Capsaicin is mutagenic in the Ames test and has been shown to be carcinogenic in animal studies. Archer and Jones (2002) studied different ethnic groups in the United States,

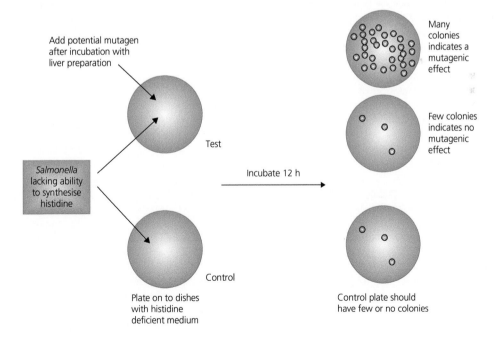

Figure 8.27 The Ames test is used to assess the potential mutagenicity of chemical agents. *Salmonella* lacking pathways to synthesize histidine are plated on to histidine-free medium. Bacterial growth can only occur if mutation reinstates the synthetic pathway. Refinements of the Ames test include a pre-incubation of suspected mutagens with mammalian liver to generate phase I metabolites, which may be mutagenic in their own right.

where capsaicin-containing peppers are widely used in Mexican, Creole and Cajun cooking. Evidence was found to relate high consumption of capsaicin to increased risk of gastric cancer. The meta-analysis of Du *et al.* (2021) concluded that moderate to high consumption of chilli was associated with a greater risk of stomach cancer (OR 1.96, 95% CI 1.59–2.42) that was dose dependent.

A variety of fungal toxins are known to be potent carcinogens, providing a concern over some foods grown in the tropics. Peanuts, for example, can be a source of aflatoxins, which are highly active liver carcinogens (World Cancer Research Fund, 2015a). Ochratoxins are also fungal contaminants, arising through development of mildews on cereal crops. A systematic review of nine studies found that risk of liver cancer was 4.75-fold greater for people with the highest level of exposure to Aflatoxin B1 compared with the lowest exposure (Liu *et al.*, 2012). While controls over the quality of imported peanuts and other foods from at-risk areas minimize aflatoxin and ochratoxin exposures of western populations, in the developing world contamination of staple foods is widespread. Most contamination occurs after harvest due to storage in unventilated, hot and humid conditions with poor hygiene. Maize and groundnut crops are particularly at risk, and consumption of these staples in West Africa is associated with high circulating concentrations of aflatoxin–albumin adducts in both children and adults (Egal *et al.*, 2005). Simple procedures to reduce contamination, such as sun-drying of crops and storage in natural-fibre bags, can reduce exposure in affected areas (Turner *et al.*, 2005). Contamination of crops also occurs outside Africa. A study of popcorn in Mexico found that almost half of samples tested were contaminated with aflatoxins and that theoretical exposure of the population was 16–20 times greater than recognised safe limits (Morales-Moo *et al.*, 2020). In two regions of Texas with liver cancer rates, exposure to aflatoxin contamination was shown to have increased between 2004 and 2014 (Xue *et al.*, 2021). Western populations may suffer increasing exposure to these carcinogens as climate change leads to wetter and warmer conditions that favour fungal growth on crops.

8.4.5.5 Dietary factors that may reduce cancer risk

8.4.5.5.1 Complex carbohydrates

Much of the literature that discusses the associations between complex carbohydrates and risk of cancer will refer to the influence of dietary fibre. Dietary fibre is a term that is perhaps better replaced, as it is more appropriate to discuss the influence of non-starch polysaccharides and insoluble starches. The complex carbohydrates within the human diet are a diverse group of materials that share the common property of resisting digestion and hence are able to pass through the digestive tract to the colon relatively unchanged. The complex carbohydrates include cellulose from plant materials, insoluble starches (largely of vegetable or cereal origin), lignans (of vegetable origin), phytoestrogens and chitin (from fungal cell walls and shellfish). 'Fibre' is therefore not a single substance, and the effects of fibre reported in the literature should be expected to vary according to the source of the material in the diet, as the composition of fruit, vegetable or cereal-derived fibre will differ considerably. There is an extensive literature that links higher consumption of complex carbohydrates to lower risk of cancer at several sites. It is difficult to isolate dietary fibre as a beneficial component of the diet, as individuals who have higher intakes of these complex carbohydrates from plant materials will also tend to have lower intakes of meat and the associated putative carcinogenic agents described earlier.

It is widely reported that complex carbohydrate consumption reduces the risk of cancers of the breast and ovary in women. These cancers are largely driven by hormonal factors, which implies that complex carbohydrates may somehow modify the production of oestrogens beyond the menopause, which is the major risk factor for these cancers. Certainly, feeding high-fibre diets to rodents protects the animals against development of chemically induced mammary tumours, and a meta-analyses of case–control studies in human populations suggested that a 20 g per day increase in fibre intake would reduce risk of breast cancer by approximately 15% (Howe *et al.*, 1990). However, large prospective cohort studies, including the US Nurses' Health Study, have suggested that there is little benefit associated with increased intakes of complex carbohydrates with respect to breast cancer (Willett, 2001). Interventions in which women have made lifestyle changes favouring a low-fat, high-fibre diet have produced small reductions in risk of breast cancer over follow-up periods of around 8–10 years, but these may be attributed more to the associated weight and body fat loss than to specific effects of complex carbohydrates (Forman, 2007).

Case–control studies spanning more than 40 years have suggested that higher intakes of complex carbohydrates, particularly those of vegetable rather than cereal origin, are associated with lower risk of colorectal cancer. However, these observations are not supported by all large prospective cohort studies performed in European and US settings. The Nurses' Health Study, for example, found that there was no difference in risk of colorectal cancer between groups with the highest compared with the lowest intakes of dietary fibre (Fuchs *et al.*, 1999) and, in fact, the highest intakes of vegetable fibre were actually associated with a 35% increase in colorectal cancer risk. Kato *et al.* (1997) reported no association between dietary fibre intake and colorectal cancer, a finding echoed by the Netherlands Cohort Study (Wark *et al.*, 2005). This prospective study of 120 852 people found that dietary fibre intake was not associated with risk of two types of colon tumour. A pooled analysis of 13 prospective cohorts concluded that an inverse association between fibre intake and colorectal cancer risk was present, but that this was explained by other dietary risk factors. In addition to this apparent indication that the case–control data were misleading, a number of intervention trials of dietary fibre supplementation found that administration of fibre to individuals with previous history of colorectal cancer failed to prevent either tumour recurrence or short- to medium-term survival (Alberts *et al.*, 2000).

Discrepancies in earlier literature may be attributable to small cohort sizes and a lack of sufficient cases of colorectal cancer to draw firm conclusions. Strong support for a protective effect of complex carbohydrates against colorectal cancer was provided by the EPIC study (Bingham, 2006). With over half a million participants across 10 different countries, EPIC had unprecedented power to consider any putative diet–cancer association. The heterogeneity of diets between European countries means that the range of nutrient intakes is extremely broad, which enhances the prospects of detecting significant influences. As reviewed by Bingham (2006), EPIC found that when comparing dietary fibre intakes in the highest quintile (mean 35 g/day) with the lowest quintile (15 g/day), the relative risk for colorectal cancer was 0.58 (95% CI 0.41–0.85), with beneficial effects of fibre becoming apparent at intakes of around 20 g per day. The main benefit in this study appeared to be associated with intakes of cereal fibre. Risk of colorectal cancer is obviously determined by complex interactions of nutrients and other factors. The EPIC study was able to assess some of these interactions and noted that the greatest colorectal cancer risk was associated with the highest intakes of meat and lowest intakes of fibre, when compared with the lowest intakes of meat and highest intakes of fibre (Bingham, 2006). The most recent meta-analyses from the Third Expert Report of the World Cancer Research Fund (2018b)

indicate that for each 10-g increment in fibre intake risk of colorectal cancer declines by 9% (RR 0.91, 95% CI 0.87–0.94). Similarly, increasing intakes of wholegrains reduces risk (RR 0.83, 95% CI 0.78–0.95 for each 90-g increment in wholegrain intake).

The mechanism through which complex carbohydrates are proposed to protect the colon from tumourigenesis is shown in Figure 8.28. Entry of complex carbohydrates into the large intestine provides substrates for the growth of the bacterial species that make up the colonic microflora. Fermentation of complex carbohydrates is associated with reproduction and metabolism of these organisms and has several beneficial effects for the human host. First, the presence of fibre itself within the faecal material has the effect of bulking up the stool, but this is further enhanced by accumulation of bacteria and retention of water. The larger and softer stool that results is more rapidly moved through the colon and this reduced transit time minimizes the length of time that potential carcinogens will be present within the colon. The larger stool also has a reduced surface area to volume ratio, which effectively means that any carcinogenic agents are more likely to be buried within the faecal material rather than on an exterior surface that might come into contact with the colonic mucosal cells. Wholegrains in the stool may also have the capacity to bind and neutralize carcinogens. The fermentation of the complex carbohydrates by the microflora will also generate short-chain fatty acids, which include butyrate, propionate and acetate. This reduces the pH of the colon, which reduces the likelihood of inflammation of the mucosa. More importantly, butyrate is an inducer of apoptosis and inhibits the transformation of cells in the colonic epithelium (Chai *et al.*, 2000). Thus, use of complex carbohydrate by bacteria generates potent antitumour agents within the human colon. The nature of the carbohydrates reaching the colon may determine the profile of bacterial species present, and some of the more soluble complex carbohydrates have been proposed to favour the growth of beneficial *Bifidobacteria* over other species such as *Escherichia coli* or *Bacteroides* (Slavin, 2003). Fibre and wholegrain material may also protect through reduction of insulin resistance and associated inflammation. Wholegrains also deliver material such as vitamin E, selenium and polyphenols, which could protect through an antioxidant mechanism.

The functional food industry exploits the fibre–colorectal cancer relationship and markets two classes of product on the basis of their potential protective properties. Probiotic foods supply bacterial species such as *Lactobacilli* directly to the gut with

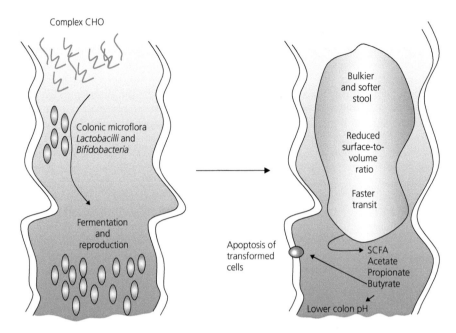

Figure 8.28 Proposed mechanism to explain the protective influence of complex carbohydrate in colorectal cancer. CHO, carbohydrate; SCFA, short-chain fatty acids.

the intention of boosting fermentation by species that generate short-chain fatty acids. Prebiotics are complex carbohydrates such as inulin or fructo-oligosaccharides that are intended to enter the colon and selectively stimulate the reproduction of *Lactobacilli* and *Bifidobacteria*.

Another explanation of the protective effects of complex carbohydrates in the colon is that foods that are rich in fibre will also deliver other cancer-preventive compounds. Folate, for example, will tend to be consumed in greater quantities with fibre-rich foods. There is also a wide range of non-nutrient compounds present in plants that have anti-tumour and tumour-suppressing properties, and these could confound the apparent relationship between colorectal cancer and fibre.

8.4.5.5.2 Milk and dairy produce

Milk and dairy produce represent the main sources of bioavailable calcium within the human diet and play an important role in maintaining bone health (see Chapter 9). There is some conflicting literature regarding milk, other dairy foods and calcium rich foodstuffs and cancer. These foods appear to be generally beneficial, but may increase risk of prostate cancer. Meta-analysis from the World Cancer Research Fund (2018b) concluded that for every 400 g per day increment in dairy product intake, the risk of colorectal cancer decreased by 13% (RR 0.87,

95% CI 0.83–0.90). Given that milk is the main dairy item consumed in such bulk, it is unsurprising that this effect was largely related to milk intake. Analysis also highlighted that there is a relationship between calcium and colorectal cancer, with a 6% reduction in risk for each 200 mg per day increase in consumption. Calcium may be protective as it binds free fatty acids and unconjugated bile acids in the gut, which reduces inflammation. Calcium has also been shown to inhibit cell proliferation and promote differentiation in vitro.

While calcium sources appear protective in the colon and rectum, there is inconclusive evidence in relation to breast cancer. No relationship exists between calcium or dairy foods and postmenopausal breast cancer (World Cancer Research Fund, 2018f), but for premenopausal cancers each 200 g per day increment in dairy intake is associated with a 5% reduction in risk.

A harmful impact of calcium rich foods in prostate cancer may stem from calcium down-regulation of the formation of 1,25-dihydroxyvitamin D. Experimental studies show that 1,25-dihydroxyvitamin D is a suppressor of cell proliferation in the prostate. Risk of non-advanced prostate cancer increases by an estimated 9% with every 400 g per day increment of dairy consumption (World Cancer Research Fund, 2014). This is primarily associated with higher intakes of low-fat milk and cheese.

8.4.5.5.3 Non-starchy vegetables, fruit and carotenoids

There is a very robust literature relating to the cancer-preventive properties of agents present in fruits and vegetables and, in fact, some of the most convincing evidence in cancer epidemiology relates to the strong inverse relationship between consuming diets rich in fruits and vegetables and risk of cancers at all sites. Ames and Wakimoto (2002) combined evidence from two major reviews of the evidence and concluded that 75% of all studies showed clear protective effects. Generally, a higher intake of fruits and vegetables had the potential to halve the risk of cancer, with most of the convincing data relating to squamous cell cancers of the digestive tract, lung and liver. Greatest benefits were noted for pancreatic and stomach cancers, while the only cancer showing little associated benefit was prostate cancer. The Third Expert Report of the World Cancer Research Fund reported probable anti-cancer effects of non-starchy vegetables for cancers of the mouth, pharynx and larynx, colon and rectum (World Cancer Research Fund, 2018b, 2018e). Fruit intake is associated with lower risk of colorectal, stomach and lung cancers (World Cancer Research Fund, 2018b, 2018c, 2018d). Foods that are rich in carotenoids reduce risk of breast cancer (World Cancer Research Fund, 2018f) and lung cancer (World Cancer Research Fund, 2018d).

Fruits and vegetables are foodstuffs that deliver a very broad range of putative cancer-preventing nutrients and agents, including dietary fibre and folic acid. Most attention has focused on the possible impact of the antioxidant nutrients they deliver, most notably the vitamins A, C and E and selenium. These are proposed to primarily act through protection of DNA from oxidative damage mediated by ROS but may also prevent tumour formation and proliferation by other mechanisms. Quenching of ROS action will prevent some conversion of inactive precursors to active carcinogens. There is also some evidence that vitamin C and retinol have the capacity to induce apoptosis in tumour cells.

Foods rich in antioxidant nutrients are clearly beneficial in protecting against cancer at many sites. For example, fruit and non-starchy vegetables reduce risk of CRC by 2% for every 100 g per day intake (RR 0.98, 0.96–0.99; World Cancer Research Fund, 2018b) and consumption of vegetables is weakly associated with lower risk of adenocarcinoma of the oesophagus (World Cancer Research Fund, 2016). Although it is now recognized that the benefits of these foods go beyond the delivery of the classical antioxidant nutrients (see Section 8.4.5.5.5), much of the literature has focused on these nutrients in an attempt to isolate factors that could be used as cancer-preventive supplements. In considering the associations between the antioxidant nutrients and cancer risk, it is necessary to dissociate the evidence from observational studies at the population level, based upon intake of food, and intervention trials using supplements, as these frequently yield widely contrasting results. Vitamin E, for example, was first identified as potentially beneficial when rodent studies showed that it could prevent mammary tumour formation. However, in humans, there is no evidence of protection against breast cancer associated with normal ranges of intake. The World Cancer Research Fund (2018c) reports that higher intakes of citrus fruits may have a protective role in stomach cancer (RR/100-g increment of intake 0.76, 95% CI 0.58–0.99), but only for cancers of the gastric cardia (the top portion of stomach where the stomach meets the oesophagus). This may be related to the antioxidant functions of vitamin C.

The most effective specific antioxidant nutrients (as opposed to antioxidant-rich foods) in relation to cancer risk are the carotenoids, notably those which are precursors of retinol (β-carotene, α-carotene and β-cryptoxanthin). Carotenoid-rich foods appear to provide protection against cancer of the breast (World Cancer Research Fund, 2018f). Circulating concentrations of β-carotene and lutein are associated with lower risk of all breast cancers, while dietary intakes of β-carotene and α-carotene may reduce risk of oestrogen receptor negative tumours. Foods containing β-carotene are associated with lower lung cancer risk, but the effect is modest (RR 0.99, 95% CI 0.98–1.00 per 700 µg increment of β-carotene, intake; World Cancer Research Fund, 2018d). However, supplemental β-carotene is recognized as having a causative role in lung cancer and should be avoided.

Following on from the wealth of studies suggesting that the antioxidant components of fruit and vegetables account for at least some of the protective effects that accompany consumption of these foods, there have been a multitude of cancer intervention trials designed around supplementation with vitamins A, C and E and with selenium. The CARET trial mentioned earlier in this chapter typifies the null or often negative outcomes of such trials, with unexpectedly increased cancer mortality associated with supplementation (Omenn et al., 1996). Almost all studies that have administered single antioxidant nutrients or combinations of antioxidant nutrients have failed to show the benefits predicted by case–control or other observational studies. Bjelakovic et al. (2004) performed a meta-analysis of intervention trials performed to prevent gastrointestinal and liver cancers using antioxidants. Fourteen large randomized trials including over 170 000 individuals were considered, and no benefits of vitamins A, C and E or selenium were noted, regardless of whether they were given alone or in combination. In fact, there was evidence of an increase in death rates associated with supplementation (RR of death 1.06, 95% CI 1.02–1.10). This latter finding was supported by the work of Lawson *et al.* (2007) who considered risk of prostate cancer in a population of almost 300 000 US men. Men consuming seven doses of multivitamin supplements per week were at greater risk of fatal cancers (RR 1.98, 95% CI 1.07–3.66) than men who did not take supplements. Clearly, the benefits of fruit and vegetable intake cannot be solely attributed to their antioxidant content, and the promise of antioxidant supplement therapy in cancer prevention strategies cannot be realistically delivered.

One of the main reasons why antioxidant supplements fail to prevent cancer is most likely to be an arbitrary dose selection that may be considerably higher than required. At high concentrations, some antioxidants may take on a prooxidant activity that would promote oxidative processes. Providing supplements of single nutrients shows a lack of consideration of the interactions between antioxidant nutrients and between the antioxidants and other components of the diet such as fibre, which may be critical in mediating the protective effects of plant-derived foodstuffs. It is also important to appreciate that ROS play a normal role in several processes, including the destruction of precancerous or cancerous cells. Inhibiting these processes may allow tumours to progress beyond the initiation stage of carcinogenesis (Bjelakovic and Gluud, 2007).

8.4.5.5.4 Folic acid

As with complex carbohydrates, a large proportion of the early cancer epidemiology literature identified that poor dietary intakes of folic acid were associated with increased risk of cancers at many sites. Closer scrutiny of the data has proven less convincing but some consensus is now emerging through meta-analysis of available data. In relation to pancreatic cancer, there is evidence of a protective influence of folate but this is only observed in case–control and not cohort studies. Fu *et al.* (2021) reported that comparing highest to the lowest intakes of folate there was an 18% reduction in risk. Analysis of data for colorectal cancer is similarly equivocal. There is no association between serum folate and cancer risk, and no evidence of benefit associated with folate supplementation, but across cohort studies the greatest intakes are associated with reduced risk compared with the lowest intakes of folate (RR 0.71, 95% CI -0.59–0.86; Moazzen *et al.*, 2018). Higher folate intakes are also associated with lower risk of squamous cell cancers of the oesophagus but not adenocarcinomas (Sun *et al.*, 2020). Folate may reduce risk of premenopausal breast cancer and is associated with lower risk of postmenopausal estrogen receptor-negative and estrogen receptor/progesterone receptor-negative tumours (Zeng *et al.*, 2019).

Folate status is extensively determined by genotype for a number of polymorphisms of genes in the folic acid cycle, such as the MTHFR C677T polymorphism described earlier in this chapter. The TT variant is associated with greater risk of thyroid cancer, oesophageal cancer and non-Hodgkin lymphoma, although the risk associated with this genotype may vary with other factors, including ethnicity (Tang *et al.*, 2014). Surprisingly, the TT variant of this polymorphism, which is associated with the lowest concentrations of folate in circulation, appears to be protective against colorectal cancer (Sharp and Little, 2004). The explanation for this paradox lies in the fact that two mechanisms may underlie the association between folate and cancer risk. Both of these putative mechanisms of protection involve folate increasing the stability of DNA. Folate is critical in the synthesis of nucleotides, and poor folate status is associated with limited synthesis of thymine, so instead, uracil is incorporated into DNA during cell replication or DNA repair processes. Uracil misincorporation promotes DNA strand breaks and is associated with cell transformation. The TT variant of MTHFR is associated with lower folate concentrations but individuals with this gene variant appear to be more effective at synthesizing nucleotides for DNA repair and therefore have lower levels of uracil misincorporation. This would explain why there are lower rates of colorectal cancer among the TT-carrying population (Duthie *et al.*, 2004).

The other protective mechanism depends upon the role of folate in determining levels of DNA methylation. Methylation of DNA at CpG islands in promoter regions effectively silences the expression of key genes. Low folate status results in hypomethylation and activation of gene expression and it is proposed that, in susceptible individuals, this will result in the expression of normally silenced proto-oncogenes. New methods for the early detection of colorectal cancer are making use of detection of differentially methylated genes in blood and faecal samples, but it is unclear whether this is due to tumour cells exhibiting altered methylation patterns or whether these genes play a causal role in cancer development (Cho *et al.*, 2020).

8.4.5.5.5 Non-nutrient components of plant foodstuffs

As described earlier, non-starchy vegetables and fruits are recognized as having a cancer-preventive role within the diet. It is becoming clear that these benefits are not associated with compounds that are traditionally classed as nutrients. A wide range of putative cancer-preventive bioactive compounds are present within foods of plant origin. There is evidence from in vitro studies and animal models that these may be protective either against specific cancers or possibly all cancers, but as yet, little evidence exists to firmly support claims made regarding human disease. The impact of such compounds is therefore encompassed by data considering plant-based foods in relation to cancer.

Allium vegetables have been widely reported as having anti-cancer benefits, although these were not singled out in the Third Expert Report of the World Cancer Research Fund. The principal allium vegetables in the human diet are onions, garlic and chives, which have a distinctive flavour due to the presence of allicin and allyl sulphides. Higher consumption of these foods has been widely reported to reduced risk of a number of cancers, particularly in the upper digestive tract. Observational studies comparing highest and lowest consumption of allium vegetables suggest protection against squamous cell carcinomas of the oesophagus, for example (Guercio *et al.*, 2016). A meta-analysis of 97 cohort studies considering diet in relation to ovarian cancer suggested that allium

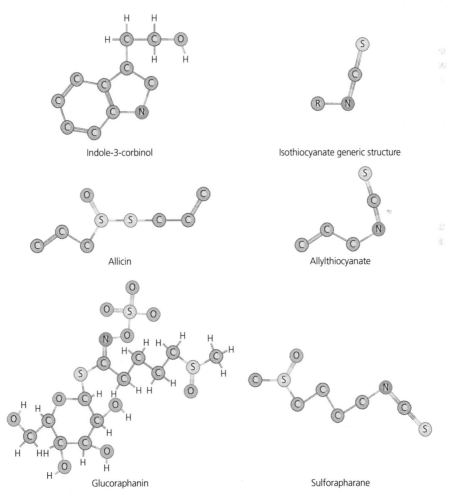

Figure 8.29 Plant-derived anti-cancer agents include a number of chemicals of the isothiocyanate and indole classes. Many of these are delivered in the diet as glucuronides (e.g. glucoraphanin) which are subsequently converted to isothiocyanates (sulforapharane).

vegetables may reduce risk (RR 0.79, 95% CI 0.64–0.96; Khodavandi *et al.*, 2021). As allicin has antimicrobial activity, it has been proposed that it protects against stomach cancer by limiting infection by *H. pylori*. There is, as yet, little evidence to support this assertion, and it has been noted that allicin also has direct antiproliferative activity in cell culture and can activate autophagic cell death in tumour cells (Xiang *et al.*, 2018).

Phytoestrogens such as the soy isoflavones are proposed to confer protection against breast cancer by modifying circulating oestrogen concentrations after the menopause. For example, a case–control study of breast cancer among Chinese patients found markedly lower cancer risk was associated with high intakes of the soy isoflavones and their precursors (Feng *et al.*, 2021). Foods rich in phytoestrogens may also contribute to the overall bulk of antioxidants that are delivered by plant foodstuffs. These antioxidants also include polyphenolic compounds, terpenoids (such as limonene) and the flavonoids (including quercetin and myricetin). These potent antioxidants may provide some protection against cancer by reducing oxidative damage to DNA (Shree *et al.*, 2021). There are other modes of action though, and many of these compounds are known to inhibit mutagenicity in the Ames test, although curiously some of the flavonoids such as quercetin appear to be mutagens according to this test. Quercetin can act as conjugator of carcinogens within the digestive tract and hence reduce the bioavailability of harmful agents. It also is an inducer of apoptosis (programmed cell death) in some tumour cells (Shi *et al.*, 2020). Some phenolics also have the capacity to inhibit angiogenesis, thereby restricting the formation of new blood vessels around primary tumours and limiting the capacity for metastasis (Fresco *et al.*, 2006). Polyphenols have not been specifically studied in relation to human cancer, so the actual efficacy of such agents in cancer prevention is largely unknown.

Cruciferous vegetables (broccoli, Brussels sprouts, cauliflower, cabbage, cress, bok choy) in the diet are strongly associated with lower risk of cancer. These foods are rich in glucosinolates, which are precursors of a range of compounds that have anti-cancer activity (Figure 8.29). Protective effects of cruciferous vegetables have been reported for a number of cancers, including stomach cancer (Wu *et al.*, 2013), colon and rectum (Tse and Eslick, 2014) and non-Hodgkin lymphoma (Sergentanis *et al.*, 2018). Two major classes of glucosinolate derivatives have been identified: the isothiocyanates (e.g. sulphopharane) and the indoles (e.g. indole-3-carbinol). Isothiocyanates and indoles are present in plants as their glucosinolate conjugates, but chopping or chewing releases myrosinase which cleaves off the bioactive compounds (Houghton *et al.*, 2013; Razis and Noor, 2013). Sulforaphane is the product of glucoraphanin, while glucobrassicin is the precursor for indole-3-carbinol. Once ingested, the indoles and isothiocyanates undergo further transformation in the acid environment of the stomach, yielding many derivatives. The principal anti-cancer activity of the indoles and isothiocyanates derives from their effects upon xenobiotic metabolism. Isothiocyanates are potent inducers of glutathione-S-transferases and therefore activate phase II metabolism, while the indoles activate both phase I and phase II pathways. These compounds therefore increase the potential for cells to detoxify and eliminate xenobiotics prior to tumour initiation. There is also evidence of anti-tumour activity post-initiation. The indole-3-carbinol derivative diindolylmethane and sulforaphane have both been shown to induce apoptosis and limit cancer cell proliferation in vitro.

SUMMARY

- The adult years (19–65) are associated with decreasing energy requirements and therefore adjustment to a more nutrient-dense pattern of dietary intake. Undernutrition remains a significant issue among sub-populations, but for the majority of adults, a healthy diet and lifestyle aimed at preventing obesity and related metabolic disorders are a high priority.
- Obesity and overweight are increasing in prevalence all over the world due to greater availability of food and declining physical activity levels.
- Risk of type 2 diabetes is the product of an interaction between genetic factors and environmental influences. Obesity-related insulin resistance is the main feature of this condition.
- The metabolic syndrome represents a complex cluster of disorders including hypertension, renal dysfunction and disordered lipid and glucose metabolism. All these disorders are driven by insulin resistance. The metabolic syndrome is a major risk factor for development of cardiovascular disease.
- Atherosclerosis is the process through which deposits of cholesterol and collagen in the arterial wall promote occlusion of blood flow and clot formation. This provides the fundamental basis of CHD, cerebrovascular disease and peripheral artery disease.
- The major dietary risk factors for CVD are high intakes of saturated fats, trans-fatty acids and sodium and obesity and related metabolic disorders. Increasing intakes of n-3 fatty acids, folic acid and plant-derived antioxidant nutrients may reduce risk.

- Cancer risk is strongly related to the overall quality of the diet. Risk is greatest with obesity and high intakes of red or processed meats and low intakes of fruits and vegetables.
- Attempts to identify specific dietary components that may be cancer preventive have been largely unsuccessful, and attention is now strongly focused upon the putative antitumour agents that are present in fruits and vegetables.

References

Abbey, M. (1995). The importance of vitamin E in reducing cardiovascular risk. *Nutrition Reviews* **53**: S28–S32.

Abdelhamid, A.S., Brown, T.J., Brainard, J.S. *et al.* (2020). Omega-3 fatty acids for the primary and secondary prevention of cardiovascular disease. *Cochrane Database of Systematic Reviews* (3): CD003177.

Abnet, C.C., Arnold, M. and Wei, W.Q. (2018). Epidemiology of esophageal squamous cell carcinoma. *Gastroenterology* **154**: 360–373.

Action on Sugar. (2014). Action on sugar www.actiononsugar.org (accessed 11 April 2021).

Australian Institute of Health and Welfare. (2020). Overweight and obesity. https://www.aihw.gov.au/reports/australias-health/overweight-and-obesity (accessed 11 April 2021).

Ajala, O., English, P. and Pinkney, J. (2013). Systematic review and meta-analysis of different dietary approaches to the management of type 2 diabetes. *American Journal of Clinical Nutrition* **97**: 505–516.

Alberti, K.G.M.M. and Zimmet, P.Z. (1998). Definition, diagnosis and classification of diabetes mellitus and its complications. Part 1: Diagnosis and classification of diabetes mellitus. Provisional report of a WHO consultation. *Diabetic Medicine* **15**: 539–553.

Alberts, D.S., Martinez, M.E., Roe, D.J. *et al.* (2000). Lack of effect of a high-fiber cereal supplement on the recurrence of colorectal adenomas. *New England Journal of Medicine* **342**: 1156–1162.

Alliance for Natural Health. (2019). UK Govt panel sticks to ancient, outdated low-fat guidelines. 7 August. https://www.anhinternational.org/news/uk-govt-panel-sticks-to-ancient-outdated-low-fat-guidelines (accessed 11 April 2021).

Ames, B.N. and Wakimoto, P. (2002). Are vitamin and mineral deficiencies a major cancer risk? *Nature Reviews Cancer* **2**: 694–704.

Apfelbaum, M., Vague, P., Ziegler, O. *et al.* (1999). Long-term maintenance of weight loss after a very-low-calorie diet: a randomized blinded trial of the efficacy and tolerability of sibutramine. *American Journal of Medicine* **106**: 179–184.

Arab, L., Khan, F. and Lam, H. (2013). Tea consumption and cardiovascular disease risk. *American Journal of Clinical Nutrition* **98**(6 Suppl): 1651S–1659S.

Araghi, S., Kiefte-de Jong, J.C., van Dijk, S.C. *et al.* (2021). Long-term effects of folic acid and vitamin-B12 supplementation on fracture risk and cardiovascular disease: extended follow-up of the B-PROOF trial. *Clinical Nutrition* **40**: 1199–1206.

Archer, V.E. and Jones, D.W. (2002). Capsaicin pepper, cancer and ethnicity. *Medical Hypotheses* **59**: 450–457.

Arguin, H., Dionne, I.J., Sénéchal, M. *et al.* (2012). Short- and long-term effects of continuous versus intermittent restrictive diet approaches on body composition and the metabolic profile in overweight and obese postmenopausal women: a pilot study. *Menopause* **19**: 870–876.

Arnold, M., Pandeya, N., Byrnes, G. *et al.* (2015). Global burden of cancer attributable to high body-mass index in 2012: a population-based study. *Lancet Oncology* **16**: 36–46.

Ashford, R., Jones, K., Collins, D. *et al.* (2020). *National Diet and Nutrition Survey: Assessment of salt intake from urinary sodium in adults (aged 19 to 64 years) in England, 2018 to 2019*. London: Public Health England.

Banegas, J.R., Lopez-Garcia, E., Gutierrez-Fisac, J.L. *et al.* (2003). A simple estimate of mortality attributable to excess weight in the European Union. *European Journal of Clinical Nutrition* **57**: 201–208.

Bansilal, S., Farkouh, M.E. and Fuster, V. (2007). Role of insulin resistance and hyperglycemia in the development of atherosclerosis. *American Journal of Cardiology* **99**: 6B–14B.

Bates, B., Lennox, A., Bates, C. and Swan, G. (2011). *National Diet and Nutrition Survey: Headline results from years 1 and 2 (combined) of the rolling programme (2008/2009 – 2009/10)*. London: Food Standards Agency.

Bender, R., Zeeb, H., Schwarz, M. *et al.* (2006). Causes of death in obesity: relevant increase in cardiovascular but not in all-cancer mortality. *Journal of Clinical Epidemiology* **59**: 1064–1071.

Bergstrom, A., Pisani, P., Tenet, V. *et al.* (2001). Overweight as an avoidable cause of cancer in Europe. *International Journal of Cancer* **91**: 421–430.

Bhanpuri, N.H., Hallberg, S.J., Williams, P.T. *et al.* (2018). Cardiovascular disease risk factor responses to a type 2 diabetes care model including nutritional ketosis induced by sustained carbohydrate restriction at 1 year: an open label, non-randomized, controlled study. *Cardiovascular Diabetology* **17**: 56.

Bingham, S. (2006). The fibre-folate debate in colo-rectal cancer. *Proceedings of the Nutrition Society* **65**: 19–23.

Bjelakovic, G. and Gluud, C. (2007). Surviving antioxidant supplements. *Journal of the National Cancer Institute* **99**: 742–743.

Bjelakovic, G., Nikolova, D., Simonetti, R.G. *et al.* (2004). Antioxidant supplements for prevention of gastrointestinal cancers: a systematic review and meta-analysis. *Lancet* **364**: 1219–1228.

Blaszyk, H., Wollan, P.C., Witkiewicz, A.K. *et al.* (1999). Death from pulmonary thromboembolism in severe obesity: lack of association with established genetic and clinical risk factors. *Virchows Archive* **434**: 529–532.

Bray, G.A. and Ryan, D.H. (2007). Drug treatment of the overweight patient. *Gastroenterology* **132**: 2239–2252.

Brouwer, I.A., Wanders, A.J. and Katan, M.B. (2013). Trans fatty acids and cardiovascular health: research completed? *European Journal of Clinical Nutrition* **67**: 541–547.

Bucher, H.C., Hengstler, P., Schindler, C. *et al.* (2002). N-3 polyunsaturated fatty acids in coronary heart disease: a meta-meta- analysis of randomized controlled trials. *American Journal of Medicine* **112**: 298–304.

Bueno, N.B., de Melo. I.S., de Oliveira, S.L. and da Rocha Ataide, T. (2013). Very-low-carbohydrate ketogenic diet v. low-fat diet for long-term weight loss: a meta-analysis of randomised controlled trials. *British Journal of Nutrition* **110**: 1178–1187.

Calder, P.C., Carding, S.R., Christopher, G. *et al.* (2018). A holistic approach to healthy ageing: how can people live longer, healthier lives? *Journal of Human Nutrition and Dietetics* **31**: 439–450.

Cani, P.D. and Delzenne, N.M. (2007). Gut microflora as a target for energy and metabolic homeostasis. *Current Opinions in Clinical Nutrition Metabolism and Care* **10**: 729–734.

Catsburg, C.E., Gago-Dominguez, M., Yuan, J.M. *et al.* (2014). Dietary sources of N-nitroso compounds and bladder cancer risk: findings from the Los Angeles bladder cancer study. *International Journal of Cancer* **134**: 125–135.

Centers for Disease Control and Prevention. (2021). Adult obesity facts. https://www.cdc.gov/obesity/data/adult. html (accessed 11 April 2021).

Chai, F., Evdokiou, A., Young, G.P. *et al.* (2000). Involvement of p21(Waf1/Cip1) and its cleavage by DEVD-caspase during apoptosis of colorectal cancer cells induced by butyrate. *Carcinogenesis* **21**: 7–14.

Chen, J. (2010). Sodium sensitivity of blood pressure in Chinese populations. *Current Hypertension Reports* **12**: 127–134.

Cho, N.Y., Park, J.W., Wen, X. *et al.*, (2020). Blood-based detection of colorectal cancer using cancer-specific DNA methylation markers. *Diagnostics* **11**: 51.

Chowdhury, R., Warnakula, S., Kunutsor, S. *et al.* (2014). Association of dietary, circulating, and supplement fatty acids with coronary risk: a systematic review and meta-analysis. *Annals of Internal Medicine* **160**: 398–406.

Christakoudi, S., Pagoni, P., Ferrari, P. *et al.* (2021). Weight change in middle adulthood and risk of cancer in the European Prospective Investigation into Cancer and Nutrition (EPIC) cohort. *International Journal of Cancer* **148**: 1637–1651.

Colditz, G.A. and Hankinson, S.E. (2005). The nurses' health study: lifestyle and health among women. *Nature Reviews Cancer* **5**: 388–396.

Cook, N.R., Kumanyika, S.K. and Cutler, J.A. (1998). Effect of change in sodium excretion on change in blood pressure corrected for measurement error: the trials of hypertension prevention, phase I. *American Journal of Epidemiology* **148**: 431–444.

Department of Health. (1999) *Dietary Reference Values for Energy and Nutrients for the United Kingdom.* London: Stationery Office.

Doll, R. and Peto, R. (1981). The causes of cancer: quantitative estimates of avoidable risks of cancer in the United States today. *Journal of the National Cancer Institute* **66**: 1191–1308.

Dowsett, M. and Folkerd, E. (2015). Reduced progesterone levels explain the reduced risk of breast cancer in obese premenopausal women: a new hypothesis. *Breast Cancer Research and Treatment* **149**: 1–4.

Druesne-Pecollo, N., Keita, Y., Touvier, M. *et al.* (2014). Alcohol drinking and second primary cancer risk in patients with upper aerodigestive tract cancers: a systematic review and meta-analysis of observational studies. *Cancer Epidemiology, Biomarkers and Prevention* **23**: 324–331.

Du, Y., Lv, Y., Zha, W. *et al.* (2021). Chili consumption and risk of gastric cancer: a meta-analysis. *Nutrition and Cancer* **73**: 45–54.

Durga, J., Bots, M.L., Schouten, E.G. *et al.* (2005). Low concentrations of folate, not hyperhomocysteinemia, are associated with carotid intima-media thickness. *Atherosclerosis* **179**: 285–292.

Duthie, S.J., Narayanan, S., Sharp, L. *et al.* (2004). Folate, DNA stability and colo-rectal neoplasia. *Proceedings of the Nutrition Society* **63**: 571–578.

Dyson, P.A., Twenefour, D., Breen, C. *et al.* (2018). Diabetes UK evidence-based nutrition guidelines for the prevention and management of diabetes. *Diabetic Medicine* **35**: 541–547.

Egal, S., Hounsa, A., Gong, Y.Y. *et al.* (2005). Dietary exposure to aflatoxin from maize and groundnut in young children from Benin and Togo, West Africa. *International Journal of Food Microbiology* **104**: 215–224.

Ejtahed, H.S., Soroush, A.R., Angoorani, P. *et al.* (2016). Gut microbiota as a target in the pathogenesis of metabolic disorders: a new approach to novel therapeutic agents. *Hormone and Metabolic Research* **48**: 349–358.

Elliott, P., Marmot, M., Dyer, A. *et al.* (1989). The INTERSALT study: main results, conclusions and some implications. *Clinical and Experimental Hypertension* **11**: 1025–1034.

Feigelson, H.S., Caan, B., Weinmann, S. *et al.* (2020). Bariatric surgery is associated with reduced risk of breast cancer in both premenopausal and postmenopausal women. *Annals of Surgery* **272**: 1053–1059.

Feng, X.L., Ho, S.C., Zhan, X.X. *et al.* (2021). Serum isoflavones and lignans and odds of breast cancer in pre- and postmenopausal Chinese women. *Menopause* **28**: 413–422.

Forman, M.R. (2007). Changes in dietary fat and fiber and serum hormone concentrations: nutritional strategies for breast cancer prevention over the life course. *Journal of Nutrition* **137**: 170S–174S.

Fraser, G.E., Orlich, M.J. and Jaceldo-Siegl, K. (2015). Studies of chronic disease in Seventh-day Adventists. *International Journal of Cardiology* **184**: 573.

Fresco, P., Borges, F., Diniz, C. *et al.* (2006). New insights on the anticancer properties of dietary polyphenols. *Medicinal Research Reviews* **26**: 747–766.

Frigolet, M.E., Ramos Barragán, V.E. and Tamez González, M. (2011). Low-carbohydrate diets: a matter of love or hate. *Annals of Nutrition and Metabolism* **58**: 320–334.

Fu, H., Zeng, J., Liu, C. *et al.* (2021). Folate intake and risk of pancreatic cancer: a systematic review and updated meta-analysis of epidemiological studies. *Digestive Disease Science* doi: 10.1007/s10620-020-06525-7.

Fuchs, C.S., Giovannucci, E.L., Colditz, G.A. *et al.* (1999). Dietary fiber and the risk of colorectal cancer and adenoma in women. *New England Journal of Medicine*, **340**: 169–176.

Gaede, P.H., Jepsen, P.V., Larsen, J.N. *et al.* (2003). The Steno-2 study: intensive multifactorial intervention reduces the occurrence of cardiovascular disease in patients with type 2 diabetes. *Ugeskrift for Laeger* **165**: 2658–2661.

Gayet-Boyer, C., Tenenhaus-Aziza, F., Prunet, C. *et al.* (2014). Is there a linear relationship between the dose of ruminant trans-fatty acids and cardiovascular risk markers in healthy subjects: results from a systematic review and meta-regression of randomised clinical trials. *British Journal of Nutrition* **112**: 1914–1922.

Ghosh-Swaby, O.R., Goodman, S.G., Leiter, L.A. *et al.* (2020). Glucose-lowering drugs or strategies, atherosclerotic cardiovascular events, and heart failure in people with or at risk of type 2 diabetes: an updated systematic review and meta-analysis of randomised cardiovascular outcome trials. *Lancet Diabetes and Endocrinology* **8**: 418–435.

Giovannucci, E., Rimm, E.B., Stampfer, M.J. *et al.* (2004). Intake of fat, meat, and fiber in relation to risk of colon cancer in men. *Cancer Research* **54**: 2390–2397.

Gloy, V.L., Briel, M., Bhatt, D.L. *et al.* (2013). Bariatric surgery versus non-surgical treatment for obesity: a systematic review and meta-analysis of randomised controlled trials. *BMJ* **347**: f5934.

Goff, D.C., Jr, Gerstein, H.C., Ginsberg, H.N. *et al.* (2007). Prevention of cardiovascular disease in persons with type 2 diabetes mellitus: current knowledge and rationale for the Action to Control Cardiovascular Risk in Diabetes (ACCORD) trial. *American Journal of Cardiology* **99**: 4i–20i.

Gonzalez, C.A. (2006). The European prospective investigation into cancer and nutrition (EPIC). *Public Health Nutrition* **9**: 124–126.

Goralczyk, R. (2009). Beta-carotene and lung cancer in smokers: review of hypotheses and status of research. *Nutrition and Cancer* **61**: 767–774.

Gould, A.L., Davies, G.M., Alemao, E. *et al.* (2007). Cholesterol reduction yields clinical benefits: meta-analysis including recent trials. *Clinical Therapeutics* **29**: 778–794.

Greenberg, J.A., Fontaine, K. and Allison, D.B. (2007). Putative biases in estimating mortality attributable to obesity in the US population. *International Journal of Obesity* **31**: 1449–1455.

Grehan, M.J., Borody, T.J., Leis, S.M. *et al.* (2010). Durable alteration of the colonic microbiota by the administration of donor fecal flora. *Journal of Clinical Gastroenterology* **44**: 551–561.

Guercio, V., Turati, F., La Vecchia, C., *et al.* (2016). Allium vegetables and upper aerodigestive tract cancers: a meta-analysis of observational studies. *Molecular Nutrition and Food Research* **60**: 212–222.

Gylling, H., Strandberg, T.E., Kovanen, P.T., Simonen, P. (2020). Lowering low-density lipoprotein cholesterol concentration with plant stanol esters to reduce the risk of atherosclerotic cardiovascular disease events at a population level: a critical discussion. *Nutrients* **12**: 2346.

Hales, C.N. and Barker, D.J. (2001). The thrifty phenotype hypothesis. *British Medical Bulletin* **60**: 5–20.

Hall, K.D., Chen, K.Y., Guo, J. *et al.* (2016). Energy expenditure and body composition changes after an isocaloric ketogenic diet in overweight and obese men. *American Journal of Clinical Nutrition* **104**: 324–333.

Hamley, S. (2017). The effect of replacing saturated fat with mostly n-6 polyunsaturated fat on coronary heart disease: a meta-analysis of randomised controlled trials. *Nutrition Journal* **16**: 30.

Harcombe, Z (2017). Dietary fat guidelines have no evidence base: where next for public health nutritional advice? *British Journal of Sports Medicine* **51**: 769–774

Hawrysz, I., Wadolowska, L., Slowinska, M.A. *et al.* (2020). Adherence to prudent and Mediterranean dietary patterns is inversely associated with lung cancer in moderate but not heavy male Polish smokers: a case–control study. *Nutrients* **12**: 3788.

Health Education Authority. (1995) *Enjoy Healthy Eating. The Balance of Good Health*. London: HEA.

Hehemann, J.H., Kelly, A.G., Pudlo, N.A. *et al.* (2012). Bacteria of the human gut microbiome catabolize red seaweed glycans with carbohydrate-active enzyme updates from extrinsic microbes. *Proceedings of the National Academy of Science of the United States of America* **109**: 19786–19791.

Holmes, M.V., Newcombe, P., Hubacek, J.A. *et al.* (2011). Effect modification by population dietary folate on the association between MTHFR genotype, homocysteine, and stroke risk: a meta-analysis of genetic studies and randomised trials. *Lancet* **378**: 584–594.

Homocysteine Studies Collaboration. (2002). Homocysteine and risk of ischemic heart disease and stroke: a meta-analysis. *JAMA* **288**: 2015–2022.

Hooper, L., Martin, N., Jimoh, O.F. *et al.* (2020). Reduction in saturated fat intake for cardiovascular disease. *Cochrane Database of Systematic Reviews* (5): CD011737.

Houghton, C.A., Fassett, R.G. and Coombes, J.S. (2013). Sulforaphane: translational research from laboratory bench to clinic. *Nutrition Reviews* **71**: 709–726.

Howe, G.R., Hirohata, T., Hislop, T.G. *et al.* (1990). Dietary factors and risk of breast cancer: combined analysis of 12 case-control studies. *Journal of the National Cancer Institute* **82**: 561–569.

Hu, F.B. and Willett, W.C. (2002). Optimal diets for prevention of coronary heart disease. *JAMA* **288**: 2569–2578.

Hu, F.B., Stampfer, M.J., Manson, J.E. *et al.* (2000). Trends in the incidence of coronary heart disease and changes in diet and lifestyle in women. *New England Journal of Medicine* **343**: 530–537.

Huang, L., Trieu, K., Yoshimura, S. *et al.* (2020). Effect of dose and duration of reduction in dietary sodium on blood pressure levels: systematic review and meta-analysis of randomised trials. *BMJ* **368**: 315.

Imamura, F., Micha, R., Wu, J.H. *et al.* (2016). Effects of saturated fat, polyunsaturated fat, monounsaturated fat, and carbohydrate on glucose-insulin homeostasis: a systematic review and meta-analysis of randomised controlled feeding trials. *PLoS Medicine* **13**: e1002087.

Jayedi, A. and Zargar, M.S. (2019). Intake of vitamin B6, folate, and vitamin B12 and risk of coronary heart disease: a systematic review and dose-response meta-analysis of prospective cohort studies. *Critical Reviews in Food Science and Nutrition* **59**: 2697–2707.

Jebb, S.A. (2005). Dietary strategies for the prevention of obesity. *Proceedings of the Nutrition Society* **64**: 217–227.

Jenkins, D.J.A., Kitts, D., Giovannucci, E.L. *et al.* (2020). Selenium, antioxidants, cardiovascular disease, and all-cause mortality: a systematic review and meta-analysis of randomized controlled trials. *American Journal of Clinical Nutrition* **112**: 1642–1652.

Kardinaal, A.F., Kok, F.J., Ringstad, J. *et al.* (1993). Antioxidants in adipose tissue and risk of myocardial infarction: the EURAMIC Study. *Lancet* **342**: 1379–1384.

Kato, I., Akhmedkhanov, A., Koenig, K. *et al.* (1997). Prospective study of diet and female colorectal cancer:

the New York University Women's Health Study. *Nutrition and Cancer* **28**: 276–281.

Khan, M.A.B., Hashim, M.J., King, J.K. *et al.* (2020). Epidemiology of type 2 diabetes – global burden of disease and forecasted trends. *Journal of Epidemiology and Global Health* **10**: 107–111.

Khaw, K.T., Bingham, S., Welch, A. *et al.* (2004). Blood pressure and urinary sodium in men and women: the Norfolk cohort of the European prospective investigation into cancer (EPIC- Norfolk). *American Journal of Clinical Nutrition* **80**: 1397–1403.

Khodavandi, A., Alizadeh, F., Razis, A.F.A. (2021). Association between dietary intake and risk of ovarian cancer: a systematic review and meta-analysis. *European Journal of Nutrition* doi: 10.1007/s00394-020-02332-y.

Klempel, M.C., Kroeger, C.M., Bhutani, S. *et al.* (2012). Intermittent fasting combined with calorie restriction is effective for weight loss and cardio-protection in obese women. *Nutrition Journal* **11**: 98.

Klerk, M., Verhoef, P., Clarke, R. *et al.* (2002). MTHFR 677C– > T polymorphism and risk of coronary heart disease: a meta-analysis. *JAMA* **288**: 2023–2031.

Knekt, P., Ritz, J., Pereira, M.A. *et al.* (2004). Antioxidant vitamins and coronary heart disease risk: a pooled analysis of 9 cohorts. *American Journal of Clinical Nutrition* **80**: 1508–1520.

Koh, W.P., Yuan, J.M., Wang, R. *et al.* (2011). Plasma carotenoids and risk of acute myocardial infarction in the Singapore Chinese Health Study. *Nutrition, Metabolism and Cardiovascular Disease* **21**: 685–690.

Kroeger, C.M., Klempel, M.C., Bhutani, S. *et al.* (2012). Improvement in coronary heart disease risk factors during an intermittent fasting/calorie restriction regimen: relationship to adipokine modulations. *Nutrition and Metabolism* **9**: 98.

Kwok, C.S., Pradhan, A., Khan, M.A. *et al.* (2014). Bariatric surgery and its impact on cardiovascular disease and mortality: a systematic review and meta-analysis. *International Journal of Cardiology* **173**: 20–28.

Lakka, H.M., Laaksonen, D.E., Lakka, T.A. *et al.* (2002). The metabolic syndrome and total and cardiovascular disease mortality in middle-aged men. *JAMA* **288**: 2709–2716.

Larsson, S.C., Bergkvist, L. and Wolk, A. (2006). Processed meat consumption, dietary nitrosamines and stomach cancer risk in a cohort of Swedish women. *International Journal of Cancer* **119**: 915–919.

Law, M.R. and Morris, J.K. (1998). By how much does fruit and vegetable consumption reduce the risk of ischaemic heart disease? *European Journal of Clinical Nutrition* **52**: 549–556.

Lawson, K.A., Wright, M.E., Subar, A. *et al.* (2007). Multivitamin use and risk of prostate cancer in the National Institutes of Health-AARP Diet and Health Study. *Journal of the National Cancer Institute* **99**: 754–764.

Le, L.T. and Sabaté, J. (2014). Beyond meatless, the health effects of vegan diets: findings from the Adventist cohorts. *Nutrients* **6**: 2131–2147.

Le Marchand, L., Donlon, T., Seifried, A. *et al.* (2002). Red meat intake, CYP2E1 genetic polymorphisms, and colorectal cancer risk. *Cancer Epidemiology, Biomarkers and Prevention* **11**: 1019–1024.

Lean, M.E., Han, T.S. and Morrison, C.E. (1995). Waist circumference as a measure for indicating need for weight management. *BMJ* **311**: 158–161.

Leander, K., Wiman, B., Hallqvist, J. *et al.* (2007). Primary risk factors influence risk of recurrent myocardial infarction/death from coronary heart disease: results from the Stockholm Heart Epidemiology Program (SHEEP). *European Journal Cardiovascular Preventive and Rehabilitation* **14**: 532–537.

LeBlanc, E.S., Patnode, C.D., Webber, E.M. *et al.* (2018). Behavioral and pharmacotherapy weight loss interventions to prevent obesity-related morbidity and mortality in adults: updated evidence report and systematic review for the US Preventive Services Task Force. *JAMA* **320**: 1172–1191.

LeBlanc, J.G., Milani, C. and de Giori, G.S. (2013). Bacteria as vitamin suppliers to their host: a gut microbiota perspective. *Current Opinions in Biotechnology* **24**: 160–168.

Lee, J., Demissie, K., Lu, S.E. *et al.* (2007). Cancer incidence among Korean-American immigrants in the United States and native Koreans in South Korea. *Cancer Control* **14**: 78–85.

Lewin, M.H., Bailey, N., Bandaletova, T. *et al.* (2007). Red meat enhances the colonic formation of the DNA adduct O6- carboxymethyl guanine: implications for colorectal cancer risk. *Cancer Research* **66**: 1859–1865.

Ley, R.E., Bäckhed, F., Turnbaugh, P. *et al.* (2005). Obesity alters gut microbial ecology. *Proceedings of the National Academy of Science of the United States of America* **102**: 11070–11075.

Liu, Y., Chang, C.C., Marsh, G.M. and Wu, F. (2012). Population attributable risk of aflatoxin-related liver cancer: systematic review and meta-analysis. *European Journal of Cancer* **48**: 2125–2136.

Liu, Y., Shi, M., Dolan, J., He, J. (2020). Sodium sensitivity of blood pressure in Chinese populations. *Journal of Human Hypertension* **34**: 94–107

Loh, J.T., Torres, V.J. and Cover, T.L. (2007). Regulation of *Helicobacter pylori* cagA expression in response to salt. *Cancer Research* **67**: 4709–4715.

Lombardi, M., Chiabrando, J.G., Vescovo, G.M. *et al.* (2020). Efficacy of different doses of omega-3 fatty acids on cardiovascular outcomes: rationale and design of a network meta-analysis. *Minerva Cardioangiology* **68**: 47–50.

Long, P., Liu, X., Li, J. *et al.* (2020). Circulating folate concentrations and risk of coronary artery disease: a prospective cohort study in Chinese adults and a Mendelian randomization analysis. *American Journal of Clinical Nutrition* **111**: 635–643.

Lonn, E., Yusuf, S., Arnold, M.J. *et al.* (2006). Homocysteine lowering with folic acid and B vitamins in vascular disease. *New England Journal of Medicine* **354**: 1567–1577.

Look AHEAD Research Group. (2007). Reduction in weight and cardiovascular disease risk factors in individuals with type 2 diabetes: one-year results of the look AHEAD trial. *Diabetes Care* **30**: 1374–1383.

Malhotra, A., Redberg, R.F. and Meier, P. (2017). Saturated fat does not clog the arteries: coronary heart disease is a chronic inflammatory condition, the risk of which can be effectively reduced from healthy lifestyle interventions. *British Journal of Sports Medicine* **51**: 1111–1112.

Malinow, M.R., Duell, P.B., Hess, D.L. *et al.* (1998). Reduction of plasma homocyst(e)ine levels by breakfast cereal fortified with folic acid in patients with coronary heart disease. *New England Journal of Medicine* **338**: 1009–1015.

Martí-Carvajal, A.J., Solà, I., Lathyris, D. and Dayer, M. (2017). Homocysteine-lowering interventions for preventing cardiovascular events. *Cochrane Database of Systematic Reviews* (17): CD006612.

Mazhar, D. and Waxman, J. (2006). Dietary fat and breast cancer. *Quarterly Journal of Medicine* **99**: 469–473.

McIntyre, E.A. and Walker, M. (2002). Genetics of type 2 diabetes and insulin resistance: knowledge from human studies. *Clinical Endocrinology* **57**: 303–311.

Miller, C.K., Headings, A., Peyrot, M. *et al.* (2011). A behavioural intervention incorporating specific glycaemic index goals improves dietary quality, weight control and glycaemic control in adults with type 2 diabetes. *Public Health Nutrition* **14**: 1303–1311.

Misra, A. and Ganda, O.P. (2007). Migration and its impact on adiposity and type 2 diabetes. *Nutrition* **23**: 696–708.

Moazzen, S., Dolatkhah, R., Tabrizi, J.S. *et al.* (2018). Folic acid intake and folate status and colorectal cancer risk: a systematic review and meta-analysis. *Clinical Nutrition* **37**: 1926–1934.

Morales-Moo, T., Hernández-Camarillo, E., Carvajal-Moreno, M. *et al.* (2020). Human health risk associated with the consumption of aflatoxins in popcorn. *Risk Management and Healthcare Policy* **13**: 2583–2591.

Musa-Veloso, K., Poon, T.H., Elliot, J.A. and Chung, C. (2011). A comparison of the LDL-cholesterol lowering efficacy of plant stanols and plant sterols over a continuous dose range: results of a meta-analysis of randomized, placebo-controlled trials. *Prostaglandins Leukotrienes and Essential Fatty Acids* **85**: 9–28.

Nagao, M., Moriyama, Y., Yamagishi, K. *et al.* (2012). Relation of serum α- and γ-tocopherol levels to cardiovascular disease-related mortality among Japanese men and women. *Journal of Epidemiology* **22**: 402–410.

Nedeljkovic-Arsenovic, O., Banovic, M., Radenkovic, D. *et al.* (2020). Five-year outcomes in bariatric surgery patients. *Medicina (Kaunas)* **56**: 669.

Neel, J.V. (1962). Diabetes mellitus: a 'thrifty' genotype rendered detrimental by 'progress'? *American Journal of Human Genetics* **14**: 353–362.

NHS England. (2018). 5 a day: what counts? Eat well. https://www.nhs.uk/live-well/eat-well/5-a-day-what-counts (accessed 11 April 2021).

Office for National Statistics. (2016). UK Opinions and Lifestyle Survey https://data.gov.uk/dataset/45f08b71-dcc4-4ce7-90b7-c9b393e95e8a/opinions-and-lifestyle-survey (accessed 11 April 2021).

Okubo, H., Nakatsu, Y., Kushiyama, A. *et al.* (2018). Gut microbiota as a therapeutic target for metabolic disorders. *Current Medicinal Chemistry* **25**: 984–1001.

Omenn, G.S., Goodman, G.E., Thornquist, M.D. *et al.* (1996). Risk factors for lung cancer and for intervention effects in CARET, the Beta-Carotene and Retinol Efficacy Trial. *Journal of the National Cancer Institute* **88**: 1550–1559.

Oyebode, O., Gordon-Dseagu, V., Walker, A. *et al.* (2014). Fruit and vegetable consumption and all-cause, cancer and CVD mortality: analysis of Health Survey for England data. *Journal of Epidemiology and Community Health* **68**: 856–862.

Papadaki, A., Linardakis, M., Plada, M. *et al.* (2014). Impact of weight loss and maintenance with ad libitum diets

varying in protein and glycemic index content on metabolic syndrome. *Nutrition* **30**: 410–417.

Patel, J.V., Vyas, A., Cruickshank, J.K. *et al.* (2006). Impact of migration on coronary heart disease risk factors: comparison of Gujaratis in Britain and their contemporaries in villages of origin in India. *Atherosclerosis* **185**: 297–306.

Penniecook-Sawyers, J.A., Jaceldo-Siegl, K., Fan, J. *et al.* (2016). Vegetarian dietary patterns and the risk of breast cancer in a low-risk population. *British Journal of Nutrition* **115**: 1790–1797.

Prentice, A.M. and Jebb, S.A. (1995). Obesity in Britain: gluttony or sloth? *BMJ* **311**: 437–439.

Public Health England (2016). The Eatwell Guide. https://www.gov.uk/government/publications/the-eatwell-guide (accessed 11 April 2021).

Ramsay, S.E., Whincup, P.H., Morris, R.W. *et al.* (2007). Are childhood socio-economic circumstances related to coronary heart disease risk? Findings from a population-based study of older men. *International Journal of Epidemiology* **36**: 560–566.

Razis, A.F. and Noor, N.M. (2013). Cruciferous vegetables: dietary phytochemicals for cancer prevention. *Asian Pacific Journal of Cancer Prevention* **14**: 1565–1570.

Recalde, M., Davila-Batista, V., Díaz, Y. *et al.* (2021). Body mass index and waist circumference in relation to the risk of 26 types of cancer: a prospective cohort study of 3.5 million adults in Spain. *BMC Medicine* **19**: 10.

Rehm, J., Patra, J. and Popova, S. (2007). Alcohol drinking cessation and its effect on esophageal and head and neck cancers: a pooled analysis. *International Journal of Cancer* **121**: 1132–1137.

Retterstøl, K., Svendsen, M., Narverud, I. and Holven, K.B. (2018). Effect of low carbohydrate high fat diet on LDL cholesterol and gene expression in normal-weight, young adults: A randomized controlled study. *Atherosclerosis* **279**: 52–61.

Ritchie, H. and Roser, M. (2019). Alcohol consumption. *Our World in Data* https://ourworldindata.org/alcohol-consumption (accessed 11 April 2021).

Roche, H.M., Phillips, C. and Gibney, M.J. (2005). The metabolic syndrome: the crossroads of diet and genetics. *Proceedings of the Nutrition Society* **64**: 371–377.

Rodriguez, J., Olivares, M. and Delzenne, N.M. (2021). Implication of the gut microbiota in metabolic inflammation associated with nutritional disorders and obesity. *Molecular Nutrition and Food Research* **65**: e1900481.

Sackner-Bernstein, J., Kanter, D. and Kaul, S. (2015). Dietary intervention for overweight and obese adults: comparison of low-carbohydrate and low-fat diets. a meta-analysis. *PLoS One* **10**: e0139817.

Sacks, F.M., Svetkey, L.P., Vollmer, W.M. *et al.* (2001). Effects on blood pressure of reduced dietary sodium and the Dietary Approaches to Stop Hypertension (DASH) diet. DASH-Sodium Collaborative Research Group. *New England Journal of Medicine* **344**: 3–10.

Schubert, J., Lindahl, B., Melhus, H. *et al.* (2020). Low-density lipoprotein cholesterol reduction and statin intensity in myocardial infarction patients and major adverse outcomes: a Swedish nationwide cohort study. *European Heart Journal* 42: 243–252.

Scientific Advisory Committee on Nutrition. (2015). *Carbohydrates and health*. London: Stationery Office.

Semlitsch, T., Jeitler, K., Berghold, A. *et al.* (2016). Long-term effects of weight-reducing diets in people with hypertension. *Cochrane Database of Systematic Reviews* (3): CD008274.

Sergentanis, T.N., Psaltopoulou, T., Ntanasis-Stathopoulos, I. *et al.* (2018). Consumption of fruits, vegetables, and risk of hematological malignancies: a systematic review and meta-analysis of prospective studies. *Leukemia and Lymphoma* **59**: 434–447.

Sesso, H.D., Buring, J.E., Christen, W.G. *et al.* (2008). Vitamins E and C in the prevention of cardiovascular disease in men: the Physicians' Health Study II randomized controlled trial. *JAMA* **300**: 2123–2133.

Sharp, L. and Little, J. (2004). Polymorphisms in genes involved in folate metabolism and colorectal neoplasia: a HuGE review. *American Journal of Epidemiology* **159**: 423–443.

Shaw, K., Gennat, H., O'Rourke, P. *et al.* (2006). Exercise for overweight or obesity. *Cochrane Database of Systematic Reviews* (4): CD003817.

Shi, H., Li, X.Y., Chen, Y. *et al.* (2020). Quercetin induces apoptosis via downregulation of vascular endothelial growth factor/akt signaling pathway in acute myeloid leukemia cells. *Frontiers in Pharmacology* **11**: 534171.

Shree, A., Islam, J. and Sultana, S. (2021). Quercetin ameliorates reactive oxygen species generation, inflammation, mucus depletion, goblet disintegration, and tumor multiplicity in colon cancer: Probable role of adenomatous polyposis coli, beta-catenin. *Phytotherapeutic Research* **35**: 2171–2184.

Siebenhofer, A., Jeitler, K., Berghold, A. *et al.* (2011). Long-term effects of weight-reducing diets in hypertensive patients. *Cochrane Database of Systematic Reviews* (9): CD008274.

Singh, B.M., Lamichhane, H.K., Srivatsa, S.S. *et al.* (2020). Role of statins in the primary prevention of atherosclerotic cardiovascular disease and mortality in the population with mean cholesterol in the near-optimal to borderline high range: a systematic review and meta-analysis. *Advances in Preventive Medicine* **2020**: 6617905.

Slavin, J. (2003). Why whole grains are protective: biological mechanisms. *Proceedings of the Nutrition Society* **62**: 129–134.

Smith-Warner, S.A., Spiegelman, D., Yaun, F. *et al.* (1998). Alcohol and breast cancer in women: a pooled analysis of cohort studies. *JAMA* **279**: 535–540.

Sneyd, M.J. and Cox, B. (2020). Do low-fat foods alter risk of colorectal cancer from processed meat? *Public Health* **183**: 138–145.

Stephens, N.G., Parsons, A., Schofield, P.M. *et al.* (1996). Randomised controlled trial of vitamin E in patients with coronary disease: Cambridge Heart Antioxidant Study (CHAOS). *Lancet* **347**: 781–786.

Sudlow, C., Gallacher, J., Allen, N. *et al.* (2015). UK biobank: an open access resource for identifying the causes of a wide range of complex diseases of middle and old age. *PLOS Medicine* **12**: e1001779.

Sun, L.P., Yan, L.B., Liu, Z.Z. *et al.* (2020). Dietary factors and risk of mortality among patients with esophageal cancer: a systematic review. *BMC Cancer* **20**: 287.

Tang, M., Wang, S.Q., Liu, B.J. *et al.* (2014). The methylenetetrahydrofolate reductase (MTHFR) C677T polymorphism and tumor risk: evidence from 134 case-control studies. *Molecular Biology Reports* **41**: 4659–4673.

Tantamango, Y.M., Knutsen, S.F., Beeson, W.L. *et al.* (2011). Foods and food groups associated with the incidence of colorectal polyps: the Adventist Health Study. *Nutrition and Cancer* **63**: 565–572.

Tantamango-Bartley, Y., Knutsen, S.F. *et al.* (2016). Are strict vegetarians protected against prostate cancer? *American Journal of Clinical Nutrition* **103**: 153–60.

Toomey, S., Roche, H., Fitzgerald, D. *et al.* (2003). Regression of pre-established atherosclerosis in the apoE-/-mouse by conjugated linoleic acid. *Biochemical Society Transactions* **31**: 1075–1079.

Tse, G. and Eslick, G.D. (2014). Cruciferous vegetables and risk of colorectal neoplasms: a systematic review and meta-analysis. *Nutrition and Cancer* **66**: 128–139.

Turner, P.C., Sylla, A., Gong, Y.Y. *et al.* (2005). Reduction in exposure to carcinogenic aflatoxins by postharvest intervention measures in West Africa: a community-based intervention study. *Lancet* **365**: 1950–1956.

UK Prospective Diabetes Study Group. (1998). Intensive blood-glucose control with sulphonylureas or insulin compared with conventional treatment and risk of complications in patients with type 2 diabetes (UKPDS 33). *Lancet* **352**: 837–853.

Ursell, L.K., Metcalf, J.L., Parfrey, L.W. and Knight, R. (2012). Defining the human microbiome. *Nutrition Reviews* **70**(Suppl 1): S38–S44.

US Department of Agriculture. (2005). MyPyramid. https://www.fns.usda.gov/mypyramid (accessed 11 April 2021).

van Dijk, S.C., Enneman, A.W., Swart, K.M. *et al.* (2015). Effects of 2-year vitamin B12 and folic acid supplementation in hyperhomocysteinemic elderly on arterial stiffness and cardiovascular outcomes within the B-PROOF trial. *Journal of Hypertension* **33**: 1897–906.

Varady, K.A. (2011). Intermittent versus daily calorie restriction: which diet regimen is more effective for weight loss? *Obesity Reviews* **12**: e593–e601.

Veldhorst, M.A., Westerterp-Plantenga, M.S. and Westerterp, K.R. (2009). Gluconeogenesis and energy expenditure after a high-protein, carbohydrate-free diet. *American Journal of Clinical Nutrition* **90**: 519–526.

VITATOPS Trial Study Group. (2010). B vitamins in patients with recent transient ischaemic attack or stroke in the VITAmins TO Prevent Stroke (VITATOPS) trial: a randomised, double-blind, parallel, placebo-controlled trial. *Lancet Neurology* **9**: 855–865.

Vogels, N. and Westerterp-Plantenga, M.S. (2007). Successful long-term weight maintenance: a 2-year follow-up. *Obesity* **15**: 1258–1266.

Wang, Y., Jin, Y., Wang, Y. *et al.* (2019). The effect of folic acid in patients with cardiovascular disease: A systematic review and meta-analysis. *Medicine* **98**: e17095.

Wark, P.A., Weijenberg, M.P., van't Veer, P. *et al.* (2005). Fruits, vegetables, and hMLH1 protein-deficient and -proficient colon cancer: the Netherlands cohort study. *Cancer Epidemiology, Biomarkers and Prevention* **14**: 1619–1625.

World Cancer Research Fund. (2020) *Diet, Nutrition, Physical Activity and Cancer: A Global Perspective. A Summary of the Third Expert Report*. London: WCRF.

World Cancer Research Fund. (2018a) *Diet, Nutrition, Physical Activity: Energy balance and body fatness*. London: WCRF.

World Cancer Research Fund. (2018b) *Diet, Nutrition, Physical Activity and Colorectal Cancer*. London: WCRF.

World Cancer Research Fund. (2018c) *Diet, Nutrition, Physical Activity and Stomach Cancer*. London: WCRF.

World Cancer Research Fund. (2018d) *Diet, Nutrition, Physical Activity and Lung Cancer*. London: WCRF.

World Cancer Research Fund. (2018e) *Diet, Nutrition, Physical Activity and Cancers of the Mouth, Pharynx and Larynx*. London: WCRF.

World Cancer Research Fund. (2018f) *Diet, Nutrition, Physical Activity and Breast Cancer*. London: WCRF.

World Cancer Research Fund. (2016) *Diet, Nutrition, Physical Activity and oesophageal cancer*. London: WCRF.

World Cancer Research Fund. (2015a) *Diet, Nutrition, Physical Activity and liver cancer*. London: WCRF.

World Cancer Research Fund. (2015b) *Diet, Nutrition, Physical Activity and kidney cancer*. London: WCRF.

World Cancer Research Fund. (2014) *Diet, Nutrition, Physical Activity and prostate cancer*. London: WCRF.

World Cancer Research Fund. (2008). Red and processed meat: finding the balance for cancer https://www.wcrf-uk.org/uk/preventing-cancer/what-can-increase-your-risk-cancer/red-and-processed-meat-and-cancer-risk (accessed 11 April 2021).

Weisell, R.C. (2002). Body mass index as an indicator of obesity. *Asia Pacific Journal of Clinical Nutrition* **11**: S681–S684.

Westerterp-Plantenga, M.S., Lemmens, S.G. and Westerterp, K.R. (2012). Dietary protein: its role in satiety, energetics, weight loss and health. *British Journal of Nutrition* **108**(Suppl 2): S105–S112.

Wilding, J.P.H., Batterham, R.L., Calanna, S. *et al.* (2021). Once-weekly semaglutide in adults with overweight or obesity. *New England Journal of Medicine* **384**: 989.

Willett, W.C. (1990). Epidemiologic studies of diet and cancer. *Progress in Clinical and Biological Research* **346**: 159–168.

Willett, W.C. (2001) Diet and breast cancer. *Journal of Internal Medicine* **249**: 395–411.

World Health Organization. (2020). Obesity and overweight. https://www.who.int/news-room/fact-sheets/detail/obesity-and-overweight (accessed 11 April 2021).

World Obesity Federation. (2021). Presentation maps. https://data.worldobesity.org/maps (accessed 11 April 2021).

Wright, M.E., Lawson, K.A., Weinstein, S.J. *et al.* (2006). Higher baseline serum concentrations of vitamin E are associated with lower total and cause-specific mortality in the Alpha-Tocopherol, Beta-Carotene Cancer Prevention Study. *American Journal of Clinical Nutrition* **84**: 1200–1207.

Wu, Q.J., Yang, Y., Wang, J. *et al.* (2013). Cruciferous vegetable consumption and gastric cancer risk: a meta-analysis of epidemiological studies. *Cancer Science* **104**: 1067–1073.

Xiang, Y., Zhao, J., Zhao, M. and Wang, K (2018). Allicin activates autophagic cell death to alleviate the malignant development of thyroid cancer. *Experimental Therapeutics and Medicine* **15**: 3537–3543.

Xue, K.S., Tang, L., Shen, C.L. *et al.* (2021). Increase in aflatoxin exposure in two populations residing in East and West Texas, United States. *International Journal of Hygiene and Environmental Health* **231**: 113662.

Yebyo, H.G., Aschmann, H.E., Kaufmann, M. and Puhan, M.A. (2019). Comparative effectiveness and safety of statins as a class and of specific statins for primary prevention of cardiovascular disease: a systematic review, meta-analysis, and network meta-analysis of randomized trials with 94,283 participants. *American Heart Journal* **210**: 18–28.

Zeng, J., Wang, K., Ye, F. *et al.* (2019). Folate intake and the risk of breast cancer: an up-to-date meta-analysis of prospective studies. *European Journal of Clinical Nutrition* **73**: 1657–1660.

Additional reading

If you would like to find out more about the material discussed in this chapter, the following sources may be of interest:

Haller, D. (2018). *The Gut Microbiome in Health and Disease*. Cham: Springer Nature.

Stanner, S. and Coe, S. (2019). *Cardiovascular Disease: Diet, Nutrition and Emerging Risk Factors. The report of the British Nutrition Foundation Rask Force*. 2nd ed. Oxford: Wiley Blackwell.

World Cancer Research Fund. (2020). *Food, Nutrition, Physical Activity, and the Prevention of Cancer: A global perspective. The third expert report*. London: World Cancer Research Fund.

CHAPTER 9

Nutrition, ageing and older adults

LEARNING OBJECTIVES

This chapter will enable the reader to:
- Show an awareness of the changing demographic profile of the population and the impact that the ageing population will have on global trends in health and disease.
- Describe the process of cellular ageing and how this contributes to physiological decline.
- Appreciate the differing theories that explain the mechanistic basis of cellular senescence.
- Describe how changes in nutrition, particularly caloric restriction, may impact upon ageing and longevity.

- Discuss the energy, macronutrient and micronutrient requirements of the elderly population and how these differ with the younger adult population.
- Show an appreciation of the fact that older adults are at significant risk of malnutrition and the factors that contribute to this risk.
- Describe the nutrition-related disorders of older adults and the interrelationship between malnutrition and chronic disease.
- Discuss the role of specific nutrients including vitamin D, calcium, folic acid and vitamin B12 in the aetiology and prevention of conditions including osteoporosis, anaemia and dementia.

9.1 Introduction

The elderly population is generally considered to be those individuals who are aged 65 and over. The elderly population is rapidly growing in almost all parts of the world and, with the increase in the numbers of older adults, the specific nutrition-related problems of the later years take on greater significance in terms of healthcare and health resources. It is important to avoid stereotypes of older people as being frail, mentally incapable, dependent on others and plagued by chronic disease. Although older patients will make up a high proportion of the population in hospital and receiving long-term medical care, the vast majority of older adults are healthy, free living and active. The later years are, however, inevitably the years of decline and ultimately ageing. The development of disease and the loss of physiological functions will lead to death. This chapter discusses the biological processes that are responsible for ageing and the degeneration of physiological systems associated with the later years. It considers the particular nutrient requirements that accompany this life stage and

describes some of the main nutrition-related problems of older people.

9.2 The ageing population

Average life expectancy has been increasing year on year since the early 1900s. There is major variation across the world, with the lowest life expectancy at birth noted in the Central African Republic (53.3 years) and the highest in Japan (84.6 years). In the UK, life expectancy at birth in 2019 was 83.1 years for women and 79.8 years for men (Roser *et al.*, 2019). In 2016, while 89.5% of Australian men and 93.6% of women were expected to survive until at least 65 years of age, in the Central African Republic only 41% of men and 46.9% of women were expected to do so. The huge inequality in life expectancy across the world strongly reflects childhood mortality rates. The UK has a longer documented record of life expectancy than any other nation. The current life expectancy represents a remarkable shift that accompanied economic and health transitions, typical of all developed countries

Nutrition, Health and Disease: A Lifespan Approach, Third Edition. Simon Langley-Evans.
© 2021 John Wiley & Sons Ltd. Published 2021 by John Wiley & Sons Ltd.
Companion website: www.wiley.com/go/langleyevans/lifespan3e

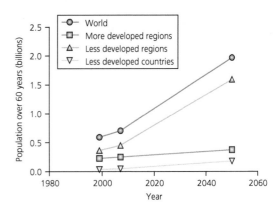

Figure 9.1 Global demographic trends show that the elderly population is rising. Increases in the proportion of the population over the age of 65 years in the developing world will drive a major demographic shift over the next four decades.

as, in 1900, life expectancy at birth was only 45.7 years for men and 49.6 years for women.

The number of older adults is increasing rapidly all over the world, and the United Nations estimates that almost two billion people will be aged over 60 by 2050 (Figure 9.1). These increases are most marked in the developing regions, but even in developed countries such as the UK, significant demographic shifts are taking place. While the proportion of the UK population aged 65–74 has not changed markedly since the mid-1940s (approximately 7.5% of the population), the overall proportion of older adults in the population has increased greatly, as more people are living on beyond 75 years. In 1948, 8.5% of the UK population was over 65. The 2011 Census indicated this had increased to 15.9%, and by 2036, this figure is expected to have risen to 24.1%, with almost 5% of the population being 85 years or over. Shifts in the balance between younger and older members of the population have important implications for health and health resources. While UK men and women live for three

decades longer than their counterparts 100 years ago, the extra life is not necessarily healthy life and for men, there are likely to be 14 years and for women, 17 years of chronic illness in the final years of life.

9.3 The ageing process

9.3.1 Impact on physiological systems

Ageing brings about a progressive decline in the functioning of all organs and systems (Table 9.1). The function of the gastrointestinal tract is particularly vulnerable to the negative effects of ageing. Loss of teeth throughout life means that many older adults will rely on dentures, which provide reduced power to masticate food. Periodontal disease afflicts many older adults and contributes to further tooth loss. Reductions in salivary flow impair the sense of taste and make it more difficult to swallow food. Production of stomach acid is reduced, and this impacts upon the bioavailability of several nutrients

Table 9.1 Age-related decline in physiological functions.

Organ or system	Degenerative characteristics
Skeletal muscle	Loss of muscle mass and neuromuscular tone
Adipose tissue	Increasing fat deposition
Upper gastrointestinal tract	Loss of teeth, periodontal disease, reduced saliva production, gastric atrophy
Lower gastrointestinal tract	Bacterial overgrowth, reduced absorption, reduced colon motility
Respiratory	Declining vital capacity
Cardiovascular	Increasing blood pressure, reduced elasticity of arteries, left ventricular hypertrophy
Renal	Loss of nephrons, slower responses to salt load or other challenges
Bone	Declining bone mass leading to osteoporosis
Immunity	Impairment of cellular and passive immunity

including folic acid, vitamin B6, vitamin B12 and iron. Lower down the tract, bacterial overgrowth of the small intestine limits nutrient uptake, and losses of colon motility lead to constipation and diverticular disease.

Some organs progressively lose function due to reductions in the numbers of functional units. For example, in the lungs, the alveolar numbers fall with ageing, and this reduces vital capacity and makes it harder for the elderly to partake in vigorous exercise. In the kidneys, loss of nephrons contributes to declining homeostatic functions, which can drive problems with fluid balance and lead to higher blood pressure. Skeletal mass is also lost with age, lean body mass declines and fat mass tends to increase. These changes in body composition can increase the propensity of older people to fall and sustain injury, as the loss of lean body mass is generally a product of sarcopenia. Loss of skeletal muscle is partly driven by physical inactivity and decreased use of muscles but may also be attributable to impairments of the central nervous system innervation of muscles, to declining concentrations of sex steroids and growth hormone and to reduction in muscle contractility.

Immune function also declines in older adults, with both cellular immunity and passive immunity (e.g. the skin barrier to infection) being compromised. The general level of chronic illness is also at its greatest within this group in the population, who are the most likely group in modern society to require long-term medication or to be hospitalized. In addition to these physical manifestations of ageing, there may also be psychological and cognitive changes, including depression and dementia. Sensory impairments also accumulate with ageing, including loss of taste, smell, sight and hearing.

9.3.2 Mechanisms of cellular senescence

The decline in physiological function and general degeneration of organs and systems that occurs during ageing is the physical manifestation of processes taking place at the cellular level. It is erroneous to believe that ageing is the product of programmed cell death (apoptosis), as in fact most cells enter a phase of senescence or quiescence and can remain in that state for a considerable period of time before their destruction via apoptotic pathways. The accumulation of senescent cells will impact upon the functions of organs and tissues with ageing, as generally these cells have altered phenotypes. Although they retain their differentiated state, they will tend to under- or overexpress the enzymes, receptors, cell signalling proteins and adhesion molecules necessary for their normal function (Campisi, 1997).

All tissues contain stem cells. These are undifferentiated cells that have the capacity to divide and replenish cells that have been destroyed or entered a state of senescence. With ageing, the capacity of the stem cells to regenerate tissues and restore tissue function becomes outstripped by the number of cells entering the senescent stage, and hence, functional capacity declines.

All mammalian cell types, like those of lower organisms, have the capacity to divide through the process of mitosis. Indeed, all cells will be at one of the stages in the cell cycle shown in Figure 9.2 and if they have sufficient energy and nutrients, they will continue to divide at varying rates until they reach the Hayflick limit. This limit is a set number of divisions, at which point the cell enters the senescent stage and is permanently arrested in the G1 phase of the cycle. With the exception of stem cells, tumour cells and the germ line cells that give rise to gametes, all mammalian cells will undergo senescence once they have completed their maximal number of cell divisions (Lee and Ong, 2021). All eukaryotic cells, with the exception of some single-celled organisms, appear to have this trait. It is now widely recognized that this control over cell division is essentially a tumour suppressor function and in fact the processes that lead to senescence and age-related degeneration are processes that prevent cancer formation (Lahalle *et al.*, 2021). Cellular senescence is promoted through activation of key proteins called p53, p16 and Ink4a, which are responsive to the number of prior cell divisions and the accumulation of damage by cells (Figure 9.3).

9.3.2.1 Oxidative senescence

As described in Chapter 8, DNA is highly vulnerable to damage through the actions of free radicals, reactive oxygen species (ROS), ionizing radiation and other environmental factors. While mutation and cancer is one possible outcome of this damage, ageing may also be driven by these oxidative processes. The production of ROS is continuous throughout the lifespan since the formation of superoxide radicals and subsequently hydrogen peroxide is a normal feature of aerobic respiration. However, the rates of ROS formation appear to increase with ageing, and this results in greater levels of damage to all macromolecules within the cell, including DNA (Sohal *et al.*, 2002). Increasing ROS formation may be a consequence of damage to the mitochondria, which are the main sources of the ROS. Some researchers argue that mutations of mitochondrial DNA may be mechanistically important in ageing, but it is unlikely that this plays more than a minor role in the process (Sohal *et al.*, 2006).

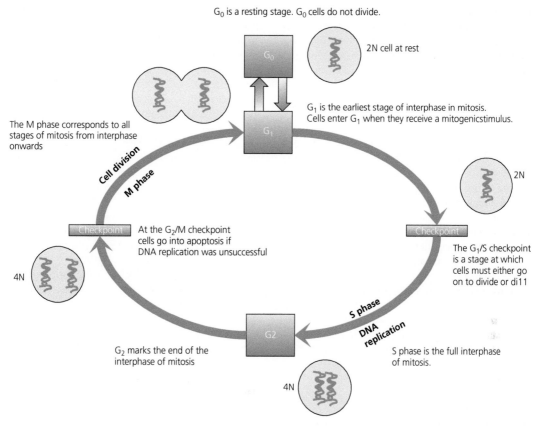

Figure 9.2 The mammalian cell cycle. A range of proteins, including the cyclins and tumour suppressors such as p53, are responsible for the regulation of cell division, ensuring that cells with damaged or incompletely replicated DNA are unable to pass through mitosis. 2N, diploid cell; 4N, tetraploid cell.

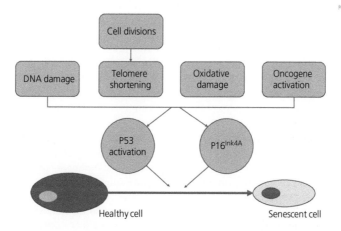

Figure 9.3 The drivers of cellular ageing. Accumulated DNA damage, including telomere shortening, activates senescence via the p53 tumour suppressor gene. The Ink4a/ARF axis also has the capacity to trigger senescence.

A role for oxidative processes in driving ageing has been demonstrated using transgenic mammalian and insect models. For example, Drosophila carrying extra copies of genes encoding antioxidant enzymes have a longer lifespan (Sohal *et al.*, 2002). Mice lacking superoxide dismutase-1 have reduced lifespan, and mice that overexpress catalase specifically within mitochondria have extended longevity

(Muller *et al.*, 2007). However, these animal studies do not correlate well with the normal in vivo situation, particularly in humans. Measurements of the levels of antioxidant protection in tissues of different species do not appear to relate to their lifespan or other markers of ageing. Importantly, interventions that extend longevity, such as caloric restriction (see Section 9.3.3), have no impact upon tissue antioxidant status.

Although antioxidant capacity is not a strong predictor of patterns of ageing, the oxidative damage theory is still considered to be of importance. Any ROS-mediated damage to DNA is likely to be repaired under normal conditions, and it is only in the older organism, where the capacity for repair is declining, that oxidative damage will begin to accumulate. It is clear that genomic instability (a loss or corruption of information carried in DNA) is a feature of ageing. There are a number of premature ageing syndromes, caused by rare mutations, that are associated with genomic instability, including xeroderma pigmentosa and ataxia telangiectasia. An imbalance between the level of oxidative damage to DNA and the capacity to repair that DNA might contribute to this instability (Muller *et al.*, 2007). The importance of these processes in individuals that do not have these rare mutations is unclear.

9.3.2.2 The role of p53 activation

The p53 protein is a transcription factor that regulates the cell cycle. During normal cellular function, it is in an inactive state, being bound to the protein product of the human double minute-2 oncogene. Cell cycle abnormalities, as seen in tumour cells or DNA damage, will result in the activation of p53, and this activation will result in one of two possible outcomes, senescence or cell death. In younger organisms, levels of p53 activation tend to be lower than in older organisms, and p53 essentially functions as a mechanism that allows damaged cells to be eliminated from healthy tissues and replaced by stem cells. In older animals, high levels of p53 activation mean that the capacity to replace and regenerate damaged tissue is insufficient to avoid loss of physiological function (Collado *et al.*, 2007).

Programmed cell death, or apoptosis, is driven by p53 through influences on the Bcl2 and Bax proteins. Bcl2 is anti-apoptotic and is down-regulated by p53, while the pro-apoptotic Bcl2-associated X protein (Bax) is up-regulated by p53. One of the actions of Bax is to increase the permeability of mitochondrial membranes. Leakage of material from the mitochondrial matrix results in the activation of the caspase system, which brings about cell death.

Senescence is driven by the activation of p53, as this protein is a key factor determining progress of

the cell from the G1 to the S phase of the cell cycle (Figure 9.2). If cells become arrested at this G1/S checkpoint, then division will not occur until the DNA damage that initially activated p53 is repaired. It appears reasonable to suggest that in the ageing organism, the capacity to repair DNA damage may be outstripped by the level of oxidative processes and hence the arrest of the cell cycle is permanent. However, a more important mechanism may ensure that p53-mediated cell cycle arrest cannot be overcome once the Hayflick limit has been reached. Cells have an inbuilt 'counter' or 'clock' that measures divisions, in the form of telomeres.

9.3.2.3 Telomere shortening

Telomeres are the regions of DNA that lie at the ends of the linear chromosomes in mammalian cells. They consist of long repeats of the base sequence TTAGGG and have important cellular functions, in that they prevent fusions between chromosomes, translocation of DNA from one chromosome to another and other harmful genetic defects. Telomere lengths vary widely within tissues and may be between 1.5 and 160 kilobases. Many studies have shown that the length of telomeres shortens with ageing, and there is a clear inverse association between age and telomere length in human and animal tissues.

Telomeres provide the principal ageing clock within cells as they shorten each time the cell divides (Figure 9.4). This is because the DNA polymerases that replicate DNA during the S phase of the cell cycle are unable to faithfully copy the ends of linear DNA. The enzyme telomerase can replace some of the lost length, but as most mammalian cells have only low telomerase activity, the 3' end of the telomeres is shortened with each replication (Collado *et al.*, 2007). Shortening of the telomeres to a critical length triggers p53 activation. This initiation of processes that result in cell cycle arrest or apoptosis most likely occurs as telomere shortening to critical levels is recognized as a form of DNA damage (Campisi, 1997). In addition to providing the equivalent of a countdown of the number of possible cell divisions remaining, telomere shortening may be a component of oxidative senescence. Experiments with cultured cells show that incubating them at low oxygen concentrations (3% O_2 instead of the usual atmospheric 21% O_2) increases the Hayflick limit and suppresses senescence. This suggests that under normal conditions, oxidative processes might cause damage to the telomeres and drive a more rapid shortening. There is some evidence that telomeric DNA is more vulnerable to oxidative damage than other regions of the chromosomes (Muller *et al.*, 2007).

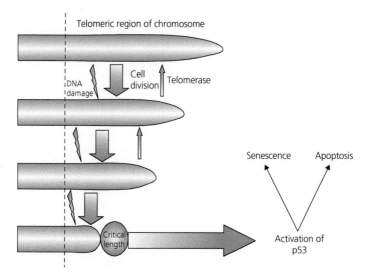

Figure 9.4 Telomere shortening is a key controller of cell division. Each mitotic division leads to loss of telomeric DNA. At critical shortening, this is recognized as DNA damage and leads to apoptosis or senescence through activation of p53. Telomeres consist of the repeated sequence TTAGGG and are between 300 and tens of thousands of bases long.

Leucocyte telomere length (LTL) is commonly reported as a biomarker of cellular ageing in human studies and has been shown to associate with age-related disease patterns. LTL has been shown in many studies to decrease with ageing, although in some longitudinal studies it has been observed to increase in some individuals. This may result from measurement artefacts (Hermann and Hermann, 2020). Analyses have indicated that shorter LTL is associated with greater all-cause mortality (Wang et al., 2018a). LTL is typically lower in subjects with diabetes or cardiovascular disease (Mather et al., 2011). Among 3316 participants in the LURIC study, longer LTL was associated with a lower hazard ratio (HR) for cardiovascular death (HR 0.84, 95% CI 0.72–0.97 comparing the shortest quartile of LTL to quartiles 2–4; Pusceddu et al., 2018). Zhao et al. (2014) reported that in a population of over 2300 Native Americans, individuals in the lowest quartile for LTL were 83% more likely to develop type 2 diabetes in the subsequent 5.5 years than those in the highest quartile. A meta-analysis (Zhao et al., 2013) confirmed this association, showing that shorter telomere length is significantly associated with type 2 diabetes (OR 1.29, 95% CI 1.11–1.49).

Absolute telomere length is not a factor determining ageing. Mice have significantly longer telomeres than humans but live for two to three years rather than the 80 of our species (Gomes et al., 2011). The rate at which telomeres erode is the key factor in triggering cellular senescence, and factors which limit oxidative damage or which increase telomere regeneration by telomerase are likely to have a positive impact upon cellular and physiological ageing. In an aged Italian population, high adherence to a Mediterranean dietary pattern was associated with better health longer, LTL and higher circulating telomerase activity (Boccardi and Poalisso, 2014). If telomerase is responsive to diet, then this may present a means by which prudent dietary patterns are beneficial for health and longevity.

9.3.2.4 The Ink4a/ARF axis

Ink4a and ARF are tumour suppressor proteins that are encoded by a single gene locus (p16^{Ink4}). Like other tumour suppressors, these proteins are known to have a pro-ageing influence by virtue of their ability to prevent cell division. Studies of cells in culture show that increased expression of the p16^{Ink4} locus will promote senescence, even if the cells have raised activities of telomerase and long telomeres (Collado et al., 2007). This indicates that the Ink4a/ARF axis can override the telomere clock, and it is suggested that these proteins provide a second form of counter that monitors the number of exposures a cell has to mitogenic agents.

Ink4a appears to contribute to the physiological signs of ageing by promoting the accumulation of senescent cells within tissues and by opposing regeneration of tissues by stem cells. Mice that lack p16^{Ink4} have been shown to possess an increased capacity for regeneration (Janzen et al., 2006). In tissues from aged rodents and humans, the expression of p16^{Ink4} can be shown to be related to age, which is in keeping with the suggestion that Ink4a/ARF somehow drives the ageing process. It is not clear why expression of p16^{Ink4} increases with age, but it may be that oxidative damage or age-dependent expression of transcriptional regulators is responsible (Collado et al., 2007).

9.3.3 Nutritional modulation of the ageing process

The long-lived nature of humans and the major difficulties of performing intervention studies that can go on for decades to assess the impact of nutritional factors upon the ageing process mean that most studies of nutrition and ageing have been performed using animal models. A wide variety of model systems are used including rats and mice and simpler organisms including the fruit fly *Drosophila melanogaster* and the nematode *Caenorhabditis elegans*.

9.3.3.1 Caloric restriction and lifespan

It was first reported in 1935 that feeding rats a diet of reduced caloric content throughout their lives significantly extended their lifespan. Generally speaking, in mammalian models, protocols that reduce caloric intake by 60% will increase lifespan by approximately 30–40%, although, in extreme cases, the extension of longevity is closer to 50%. The same effects on lifespan are reported in yeast cells, *Drosophila* and *C. elegans*. In rodents, in addition to the extension of lifespan, the caloric restriction protocol reduces the occurrence and extent of age-related diseases, including cancer, cardiovascular disease, diabetes, autoimmune disorders and neurodegenerative problems (Young and Kirkland, 2007). Some studies of non-human primates suggest that similar benefits are seen with caloric restriction in those species, and this raises the exciting possibility that human ageing might be countered by caloric restriction.

Two major studies spanning more than 20 years have examined the effects of caloric restriction in rhesus monkeys. Rhesus monkeys have a lifespan of approximately 27 years in captivity but in the wild are believed to live for up to 40 years. The Wisconsin National Primate Research Centre (WNPRC) study ran from 1989 to 2009, and the National Institute on Aging (NIA) study ran over a similar period. The WNPRC study reported a number of benefits of 30%, including delayed development of age-related changes in muscle associated with sarcopenia (McKiernan et al., 2012). The monkeys in the WNPRC study were less prone to age-related death than their control counterparts, with just 13% dying over the duration of the study compared with 27% of controls. The NIA study also used a 30%

caloric restriction protocol, but markers of ageing, such as telomere shortening (Smith et al., 2011), were not altered by caloric restriction and there was no significant difference in age-related death or disease between the caloric restriction and control monkeys (Mattison et al., 2012). The discrepancies between these studies could be argued equally strongly to indicate that genetic influences are more important than diet in ageing, or that diet has a major effect. In the WNPRC study, control monkeys were fed a relatively unhealthy diet containing less minerals and vitamins, more sucrose (28.5% of diet) and a single protein source compared with NIA controls (low sucrose, varied protein sources). This may indicate that caloric restriction is only an extension of current approaches to limiting weight gain and maintaining healthy dietary patterns as a means of preventing disease.

The mechanism through which caloric restriction extends lifespan is not fully understood, as animals undergoing caloric restriction protocols exhibit a wide range of metabolic, endocrine and physiological changes. In the early stages of caloric restriction, animals are in a state of negative energy balance and, in response, reduce their metabolic rate. Basal metabolic rates are rapidly reset, and energy balance is maintained largely through lower thermogenic capacity, resulting in a lower body temperature. Body mass is lost, and the animal maintained on caloric restriction has lower lean and fat mass. Although potentially of importance, the prevention of obesity is not, however, the sole mechanism through which health benefits and increased longevity accrue (Speakman and Hambly, 2007). Caloric restriction induces major changes in endocrine axes, upregulating the hypothalamic–pituitary–adrenal axis and suppressing the production of insulin, the thyroid hormones, the sex hormones and the somatotropic hormones (Dirks and Leeuwenburgh, 2006). At the cellular level, caloric restriction suppresses inflammatory processes and oxidative stressors while at the same time upregulating systems involved in repair and protein synthesis.

The extension of lifespan by caloric restriction in rodents is highly dependent upon the level of restriction and upon the timing of the introduction of the protocol. Maximal extension of lifespan is noted when rodents are fed only 35% of normal ad libitum intakes, and caloric restriction is most effective when introduced immediately after weaning. Rodent studies show that introducing caloric restriction later in life has a greatly attenuated effect or may not alter longevity at all. Speakman and Hambly (2007) used available data on rats and mice to model the anticipated benefits of caloric restriction in humans, making the assumption that humans and rodents would respond in a similar manner. On this basis, introducing a 30% caloric restriction at 16 years of age would add 11 years to life, while introducing caloric restriction at age 47 would extend life by less than 3 years (Figure 9.5). The studies of the effects of caloric restriction upon ageing in non-human primates in part support the view that following a lifelong caloric restriction in humans may be of minimal benefit in the absence of other forms of dietary change. Research Highlight 9.1 discusses some of the work with human volunteers that has sought to explore this further.

Despite these observations, which appear to lend support to the idea that human caloric restriction might be beneficial in ageing and avoidance of age-related disease, considerable caution is needed in translating the data from caloric restriction studies in animals into humans. Caloric restriction in humans could certainly have a number of adverse

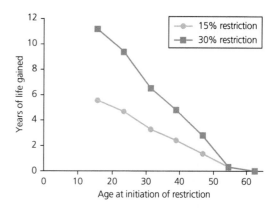

Figure 9.5 Estimated benefit of caloric restriction in humans. Adopting a more stringent reduction of energy intake at an earlier age is projected to give the optimal extension of longevity. *Source:* adapted from Banks (2010).

health effects that would offset many of the benefits. It is clear that caloric restriction would promote weight loss and excessive weight loss, and body

Research Highlight 9.1 Caloric restriction and human ageing.

The concept that restricting energy intake will extend lifespan is derived entirely from animal studies. Caloric restriction in invertebrate and rodents has a clear and robust effect on longevity, while studies of non-human primates have yielded conflicting findings. Until recently, there has been little robust research in humans that has evaluated the feasibility, safety and efficacy of caloric restriction protocols. Much has been assumed from studies of the population of Okinawa, Japan, which is renowned for its longevity, having remarkably low death rates among middle-aged men and women and the highest density of centenarians in the world. The Okinawan diet is believed to underlie this and is suggested to be similar to the calorie-restricted diet protocol used with rodents, being nutrient dense and lower in energy than the diet consumed elsewhere in Japan (Dirks and Leeuwenburgh, 2006).

Other studies have opportunistically explored the effects of caloric restriction among small numbers of participants who are members of the Caloric Restriction Optimal Nutrition Society (CRONies). While, for example, Fontana *et al.* (2004) reported that CRONies members who had restricted for 3–15 years had better cardiovascular health than age-matched controls, there was no assessment of markers of ageing per se and the study was purely cross-sectional in nature. It is not surprising that dietary change to induce weight loss will improve cardiometabolic indicators, even if the effect is short term.

The Comparative Assessment of Long-term effects of Reducing Intake of Energy (CALERIE) trials have advanced the human caloric restriction field by considering caloric restriction through a randomized controlled trial design. CALERIE phase 1 used caloric restriction protocols of 10% and 30% restriction of energy for 6–12 months (Dorling *et al.*, 2021). This study demonstrated that a caloric restriction of 10–15% was achievable and was associated with weight loss and reduced abdominal fat mass, even in those who were not obese (Racette *et al.*, 2006). After six months, the calorie-restricted participants had a lower core body temperature and fasting insulin concentrations, both of which are associated with attenuation of ageing (Heilbronn *et al.*, 2006). CALERIE phase 2 recruited 145 participants and 75 controls with baseline body mass index in the range 22–28 kg/m^2 (men 21–50 years; women 21–47 years), for a two-year randomized controlled trial of 25% caloric restriction compared with a normal ad libitum diet. The participants who were calorie restricted, on average, achieved a 12% energy restriction and this reduced body weight and fat mass and had cardiometabolic benefits including lower low-density lipoprotein-cholesterol and increased high-density lipoprotein-cholesterol concentrations (Ravussin *et al.*, 2015). Participants who restricted calories had lower concentrations of inflammatory markers (Meydani *et al.*, 2016). Belsky *et al.*, (2017) reported that following caloric restriction for two years markedly attenuated the age-related increase in a DNA-methylation-based biomarker of biological age. CALERIE has shown that modest caloric restriction is achievable, is largely safe and elicits favourable functional changes that might increase lifespan if maintained for a long period. However, there has yet to be a full demonstration that caloric restriction in humans would be as effective as in other mammalian species and it is not clear whether adverse effects might develop over longer periods. CALERIE 2 did observe a decrease in bone mineral density with caloric restriction (Ravussin *et al.*, 2015) and this may be a cause for concern in relation to longer-term bone health.

mass index (BMI) of less than 20 kg/m² is associated with menstrual irregularities and infertility, osteoporosis, poor wound healing and reduced capacity to metabolize drugs and toxins. Lower core temperature may be problematic in older individuals. Underweight is also associated with impaired immunity and hence excess levels of illness and reduced capacity for work. Mortality associated with all causes and in particular cardiovascular disease has been shown to increase when comparing BMI of less than 20 kg/m² with BMI in the optimal range (Romero-Corral *et al.*, 2006). Caloric restriction is also considered likely to result in depression and other psychological disorders (Dirks and Leeuwenburgh, 2006), despite some observations of improved mood in the Comparative Assessment of Long-term effects of Reducing Intake of Energy trial (Martin *et al.*, 2016).

9.3.3.2 Fetal programming of lifespan

In contrast to caloric restriction in postnatal life, manipulations of the diet during early development appear to programme shorter lifespan. The feeding of maternal low-protein diets, without caloric restriction, during rat pregnancy significantly reduced the lifespan of the offspring (Aihie-Sayer *et al.*, 2001; Figure 9.6), and similar observations in mice indicate that this programming of lifespan is exacerbated by feeding an obesity-inducing diet in postnatal life (Ozanne and Hales, 2004). The mechanism through which this programming occurs has not been fully elucidated but appears to involve both oxidative processes and more rapid telomere shortening in key tissues such as the liver (Langley-Evans and Sculley, 2006) and kidney (Jennings *et al.*, 1999).

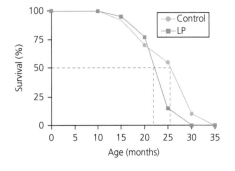

Figure 9.6 The effect of maternal protein restriction during pregnancy upon longevity in rats. Rats fed a low-protein (LP) diet were exposed to the diet in utero. Fetal undernutrition reduced average lifespan by 3.5 months (10% of lifespan). *Source:* adapted from Aihie-Sayer *et al.* (2001). With permission from Karger Publishers.

9.3.3.3 Supplementary antioxidants

Although it is well established that in cardiovascular disease and cancer (see Chapter 8), supplemental intakes of antioxidants are ineffective or even harmful to health, there is sufficient interest in the concept of oxidative senescence to merit experiments that consider the impact of increasing intakes of antioxidants on ageing processes. Analysis of human dietary patterns associated with longer life and healthier ageing shows that these diets are often rich in phytonutrients and antioxidants, in addition to unrefined carbohydrates, varied but not excessive sources of protein and low in saturated fat. This is true of the Okinawan diet, which is likely to play a role in the long average longevity of Okinawan islanders (Willcox *et al.*, 2014). Given the association between oxidative stress and telomere shortening, there has been considerable attention paid to the effects of antioxidants upon longevity in mammals.

Studies in which animals are supplemented with antioxidants yield variable results. Generally, there is good evidence that antioxidants reduce inflammation and oxidative injury in specific tissues. For example, Mosoni *et al.* (2010) found that a mixed antioxidant supplement (rutin, zinc, selenium, vitamin E and vitamin A) given to aged male rats for seven weeks, improved muscle metabolism and reduced oxidative damage in most major organs. Similarly 10 weeks of supplementation of resveratrol reduced inflammation, oxidative stress and apoptosis in the ageing rat heart (Torregrosa-Munumer *et al.*, 2021). Supplementation of rats with magnesium for two years reduced oxidative stress and was associated with reduced telomere shortening in rats (Martin *et al.*, 2008). Selman *et al.* (2008) reported that when mice were supplemented with vitamin E from four months of age for the rest of their lives, lifespan was extended by approximately 100 days (15% of full lifespan of control mice). This effect of vitamin E was shown to be unrelated to the antioxidant properties of vitamin E and was instead driven by the anti-cancer action of the supplement. A study in which rats were switched from a lifespan-extending dietary restriction protocol to ad libitum feeding with a supplement of α-lipoic acid, found that the antioxidant supplement maintained the lifespan-extending trajectory of the original dietary restriction (Merry *et al.*, 2008).

These experiments with rodents are largely inconclusive and have failed to establish a clear benefit of supplementary antioxidants. It is oversimplistic to assume that supplementing with a single nutrient could have any real benefit in extending lifespan, since cellular senescence and the associated tissue degeneration occur through multiple mechanisms and are the products of the balance between pro-ageing and anti-ageing processes and between cellular damage and repair. Selman *et al.* (2006) noted that supplementing mice with ascorbate apparently had no impact upon levels of oxidative injury within cells, but downregulated genes associated with ROS scavenging and repair processes. It seems likely that any benefit attained by providing greater antioxidant protection from the diet was offset by downregulation of endogenous systems. On this basis, antioxidant therapy to increase longevity appears unlikely to succeed in isolation.

9.4 Nutrient requirements of the elderly

9.4.1 Macronutrients and energy
The requirement for energy declines with ageing, reflecting typically lower levels of energy expenditure through physical activity and a fall in basal metabolic rate (Table 9.2). The latter is largely attributable to a loss of lean body tissue that is seen in most older adults. Generally, there are no other major changes in the macro- or micronutrient requirements of this population, and although protein requirements, for men at least, fall slightly with

Table 9.2 Dietary reference values (UK) for energy and protein.

	Years	EAR	RNI
		Energy (MJ/day)	Protein (g/day)
Males	19–29	11.0*	
	30–59	10.5*	
	60–64	9.93	
	65–75	9.71	
	75+	8.77	
	19–50		55.5
	50+		53.3
Females	19–29	9.1[†]	
	30–59	8.6[†]	
	60–64	7.99	
	65–75	7.96	
	75+	7.61	
	19–50		45.0
	50+		46.5

EAR, estimated average requirement; RNI, reference nutrient intake.
* Assumes physical activity level 1.5 and weight 70 kg.
[†] Assumes physical activity level 1.5 and weight 65 kg.

age, the percentage of energy derived from protein remains relatively unchanged with ageing. With a lower energy requirement and unchanged, or in some cases increased, requirements for other nutrients, the optimal diet for older adults needs to be nutrient dense.

9.4.2 Micronutrients
There are few micronutrients recognized within the dietary reference values of westernized countries as being required by the elderly at greater levels of intake (Department of Health, 1999). This is surprising, given the high levels of malnutrition and nutrient deficiency observed in this population and the high prevalence of chronic disease states that lead to micronutrient malabsorption. The assignment of dietary reference values that are similar to those for younger adults reflects the fact that dietary reference values are derived for healthy populations and that they were determined from relatively sparse data on the elderly.

There are a number of nutrients where, despite there being no special requirement set for the elderly, special care to maintain intake at an optimal level may be worthwhile. Vitamin B6, for example, has been set a reference nutrient intake (RNI) value of 15 µg/g protein per day for both men and women aged 19–50 and over 50 years. This reference value reflects requirements extrapolated from studies of younger people. However, in the elderly, vitamin B6 may be of additional importance in maintaining immune function, so demands may be greater than the dietary reference values suggest. Vitamin C (RNI 40 mg/day) intakes should be comfortably maintained by most elderly individuals and therefore positively contribute to absorption of iron. However, in institutionalized settings where bulk food preparation and delivery systems necessitate maintaining food at high temperatures for long periods of time, actual intakes of ascorbate may be suboptimal. Consideration of potential raw sources of this nutrient is therefore relevant.

9.4.3 Specific guidelines for the elderly
There are few specific guidelines for the nutrition of older adults, since in general this population is advised to follow a healthy balanced diet, as at earlier stages of adulthood. Mild to moderate physical activity is considered to be an important element of a healthy lifestyle for the elderly, since activities such as walking, climbing stairs and gardening are sufficient to increase appetite and contribute to maintenance of bone health.

In the UK and the United States, the few specific recommendations that have been made regarding intakes of older adults relate to a narrow range of nutrients. In both countries, it is recommended that the elderly increase intakes of vitamin D either through supplementation (10 μg/day) or by increasing intakes of fortified margarines and other sources. In the United States, it is recommended that the over-50s increase their intakes of vitamin B12 through supplementation with 2.4 μg/day to offset declining absorption of this micronutrient. The US, UK and Australian guidelines for the elderly stress the need to reduce salt intake, maintain intakes of micronutrients that promote bone health and consume water to maintain hydration. Dehydration is considered to be an important issue for the elderly as fluid intakes are often poor. This may not only be partly due to declining physiological control of the thirst centre and fluid homeostasis but can also come from concerns about urinary incontinence. Dehydration can contribute to mental confusion, headaches and irritability. Older adults are recommended to consume 1.5 litres of fluid per day (excluding alcoholic beverages).

Maintaining the desired nutrient density for this age group might best be achieved by encouraging a diet that is rich in whole grain and fortified breads, pasta and cereals. Using these foods to replace refined grains helps to maintain intakes of B vitamins. The elderly should favour deeply pigmented fruits and vegetables to maximize intakes of folate and antioxidant nutrients. In keeping with guidelines to prevent cardiovascular disease, choosing low-fat dairy options also maximizes intakes of calcium. Fibre is an important element of the diet to optimize bowel function. However, wheat bran should be avoided, owing to the presence of phytates that impede the absorption of iron, calcium and zinc.

Older adults tend to consume less food overall than the younger population. However, the burden of chronic diseases such as cardiovascular disease, osteoporosis and gastrointestinal disorders means that for some in this population, energy and protein requirements are actually increased. As individuals with these chronic diseases make up a high proportion of the population within long-term institutional care (e.g. nursing homes), there are major challenges in providing high-quality nutrition in these settings. As a diet rich in complex carbohydrate is bulky, attaining both the extra energy requirement and nutrient intake in frail elderly patients might best be achieved by increasing intakes of fat-rich foods.

9.5 Barriers to healthy nutrition in the elderly

9.5.1 Malnutrition and the elderly

Outside the developing countries where children are the main group at risk of malnutrition, older adults are the population group that are most likely to suffer significant protein–energy malnutrition. In the UK, it is estimated that 10% of those who are over the age of 65 and up to 19% of the over 85s are malnourished. The majority of the three million affected adults live in their own homes (BAPEN, 2020). The cost of managing and treating malnutrition in older adults is estimated at £4 billion per annum. Across Europe, malnutrition impacts upon 10% of independently living older people, but may be present in up to 50% of those in nursing homes, acute care hospitals and geriatric rehabilitation units (e.g for stroke treatment; Visser et al., 2017). The Tasmanian Government Department of Health (2020) estimated that 15% of elderly Australians are malnourished in community settings, and that this figure may rise to 60–70% in acute and long-term care settings. In addition to those who are malnourished, a high proportion of older adults are at risk of malnutrition.

Across cohorts studied in the UK, Europe and North America, 21.5% of independently living older people consumed protein at a below recommended levels (Hengeveld et al., 2020). In the Newcastle 85+ study, consumption of protein below recommendations was commonplace and was more likely in those who were frail due to age-related disease (Mendonca et al., 2019). Among older US adults, 46% were found to be consuming protein below recommendations in the 2005–2014 National Health and Nutrition Examination Surveys (Krok-Schoen et al., 2019).

When older people enter care settings their risk of malnutrition increases substantially, particularly if they are admitted to hospital to be treated for conditions that increase protein and energy demands (e.g. fractures and infections). Leistra et al. (2011) found that only one in four adults in hospital met requirements for energy and protein in the first four days of their admission, highlighting the need for early intervention to avoid a decline in patients who may enter hospital in an already undernourished state. Eastwood et al. (2002) reported that institutionalized elderly people had lower energy intakes than their independently living counterparts. Donini et al. (2012) found a greater prevalence of malnutrition among Italian nursing home residents than among independently living older adults.

The reasons why the elderly are so vulnerable to malnutrition are discussed in more detail in the following sections, including poverty, social isolation and ill health (Figure 9.5). The very high prevalence of malnutrition in institutionalized settings is both caused by, and is a contributor to, continuing health problems. Kiesswetter *et al.* (2014) followed older adults over one year following assessment of nutritional status using the Mini Nutritional Assessment tool. Subjects who were identified as at risk of malnutrition by the tool were more likely to die over the year of follow-up than those who were not (HR 2.21, 95% CI 1.02–4.75) and were more likely to develop functional deficits as assessed in terms of the activities of daily living scale (includes mobility, self-care, toileting, incontinence). An association between ill health and malnutrition is well established and many older adults who are admitted to hospital are already undernourished. However, up to 17% who enter hospital with adequate nutritional status develop hospital acquired malnutrition. The main risk factors for this are cognitive impairment (dementia), longer stays, development of pressure ulcers and transfer between units (Woodward *et al.*, 2020). Hospital-acquired malnutrition highlights a particular concern that nutritional status declines with long hospital stays. This is a state that can arise partly due to failures to apply nutrition screening tools and implement nutrition support interventions, including oral nutrition supplements, or simple measures such as helping patients to eat if they are unable to use cutlery or reach their meals.

The consequences of malnutrition are severe, as malnutrition is a cause as well as an outcome of major illness and trauma. Poor nutritional status resulting from a failure to balance supply and demand establishes a vicious cycle in the elderly (Figure 9.7). Malnutrition promotes infection, which itself drives and maintains malnutrition. Undernutrition is a predictor of morbidity and mortality among the elderly. It leads to longer stays in hospital and impaired ability to recover from infections, fractures and surgery and is ultimately a major contributor to death. Sund-Levander *et al.* (2007) reported that among women living in nursing homes, survival over a three-year period was very strongly related to nutritional status. Similarly, Gariballa and Forster (2007) found that lower serum albumin (a crude biochemical indicator of nutritional status) and lower mid-arm muscle circumference were predictors of increased risk of death over one year following admission to hospital for acute illness (e.g. stroke, falls and fractures, septicaemia and chest or urinary tract infections).

9.5.2 Poverty

Older adults are a group in the population for whom poverty is a major risk. The vast majority of older adults are retired from full- or part-time employment and are therefore dependent upon any pension provision built up during the working years or upon state benefits. In the United States, 9.2% of adults over the age of 65 years live below the poverty threshold (Li and Dalaker, 2019). Although this prevalence is lower than in many developed countries, this still constitutes close to five million people, and greater prevalence is noted among those over 80 years and in African Americans (21.5% of women and 16.1% of men). In the European Union, 14.2% of pensioners were living at risk of poverty in 2017 (Eurostat, 2019). Again, the risk was greater in women than men and the highest levels of poverty were seen in

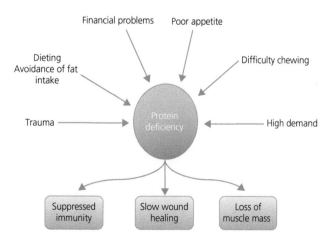

Figure 9.7 Factors leading to protein–energy malnutrition and its consequences in the elderly population.

Lithuania, Estonia, Latvia and Estonia. The Joseph Rowntree Foundation (2017) found that in the UK living alone was a major risk factor for poverty and that 22% of single women and 19% of single men were living below the poverty line. Risk was greatest among women of Asian ethnicity (48%).

Poverty may impact on the lives of older adults in multiple ways. Some will prioritize food over heating and light (greatly increasing risk of death in the winter months) and live in what is termed fuel poverty. Pirrie *et al.* (2020) found that among older adults living in social housing in Canada, 14.9% lived in poverty with 5.1% experiencing food insecurity. In countries such as the United States, where there is no welfare state to provide a safety net, the need to allocate pension income to cover medical expenses may exacerbate the impact of low income on food purchasing. Goldberg and Mawn (2015) found a strong relationship between poverty and food insecurity among older adults who required routine healthcare, but who lacked health insurance to cover the cost.

Poverty impacts upon nutritional status in a number of ways. Primarily, a lack of money will reduce the quantity of food consumed, but importantly, it also reduces the scope for choice and variety within the diet. A study of deprivation among the elderly population of Northern Ireland showed that low consumption of fruit and vegetables was a feature of poverty in this population (Appleton *et al.*, 2009). Modern shopping practices can also make it difficult to access food without transport, so poverty may disadvantage those unable to run a car or access public transport for shopping, which also reduces the range and quality of food available within limited budgets. Russell *et al.* (2016) reported that food insecurity was associated with worse mental and physical health and quality of life.

9.5.3 Social isolation

As many as one in seven older adults will live alone, and a high proportion of these will be widowed. The sense of grief, loneliness and isolation that accompanies widowhood can be particularly great in relation to food, as the purchase of food, the preparation of food and the sharing of food at mealtimes are especially important elements of a close relationship. Pantell *et al.* (2013) reported that social isolation is more strongly associated with mortality among the elderly than high blood pressure or elevated cholesterol concentrations. Isolation is commonly associated with poverty and loss of appetite (Ramic *et al.*, 2011). Many people living alone are reluctant to invest time in cooking and eating and as a result are vulnerable to malnutrition.

Social isolation and infirmity may also make shopping difficult. The SOLINUT study (Ferry *et al.*, 2005) found that in a population of 150 elderly men and women living alone, 44% could not lift a 5-kg shopping bag and therefore could not purchase adequate food supplies; 32% never shared a meal with family or friends and 43% consumed inadequate energy to meet their requirements. Living alone is a major negative influence on shopping, cooking and eating habits (Whitelock and Ensaff, 2018). Older men who have lost their life partner may be especially at risk of these negative influences of social isolation as they may never have been actively involved in decisions about food and have limited cooking skills (Thompson *et al.*, 2017). Shopping for a single person can be more challenging as food is often not sold in quantities suitable for one serving. A three-year follow-up of older Japanese adults found that in men, but not women, who lived with other people but ate alone, risk of death during the follow-up period was significantly increased (HR 1.48, 95% CI 1.01–1.41; Tani *et al.*, 2015).

For institutionalized older adults, the opportunities for social interaction around mealtimes can be an advantage over living alone in the home setting. However, there are still factors at work that are likely to reduce intakes. In an institutional setting, individuals are no longer preparing their own food or playing a role in the purchase of food items. Regimented mealtimes that may not correspond to peaks in appetite can detract from overall intakes. Odencrants *et al.* (2019) found that residents of nursing homes missed the opportunity to decide when and what to eat and who to share their meal time experience with.

9.5.4 Education

For many older adults, the knowledge of food and health and the cooking skills that they accrued in their younger years may be not be helpful in providing the balance of nutrients required to meet requirements. Favoured cooking and food preparation techniques may use excessive amounts of saturated fat, sugar and salt and also reduce the bioavailability of nutrients (e.g. boiling rather than steaming vegetables will reduce vitamin content). Contemporary foods (particularly foods from imported cuisines) may also be unfamiliar to some older adults, and this reduces the number of acceptable choices when shopping and can make the diet narrow in scope. Individuals who are advised to make adjustments to their diet to manage chronic health conditions may also struggle to meet nutrient demands due to lack of education and understanding.

9.5.5 Physical changes

Even in healthy individuals, physical changes associated with ageing will have a deleterious effect upon nutritional status. The reduced efficiency of the gastrointestinal tract leads to malabsorption and reduced bioavailability of micronutrients. Older adults may also develop a variety of conditions within the bowel that lead to discomfort and the avoidance of certain types of food. For example, the degeneration of the brush-border cells of the small intestine can limit the production of lactase, promoting lactose intolerance. Given the discomfort that will ensue with consumption of dairy products, these nutrient-rich sources will tend to be cut from the diet and not replaced with suitable alternatives. Within the mouth, periodontal disease and poorly fitted dentures can also result in avoidance of foods such as meat that require longer mastication.

The senses of taste and smell decline with age, and this can reduce enjoyment of food and impair appetite. The sense of taste can change quite abruptly. Often, it is the sensing of sweetness and saltiness that is initially lost, effectively making food seem more bitter (Omran and Morley, 2000). Around half of the 65–80 years age group report reductions in the sense of smell (Griep *et al.*, 1995). These changes may be partly age related but are also brought on by medication used to manage chronic disease (e.g. phenothiazines used in treatment of mental disorders).

Physical infirmity stemming from disability or disease will also contribute to the development of malnutrition. Major disease states such as cancer, cardiovascular disease, renal disease and diabetes are important comorbidities of malnutrition in the elderly. Chronic disease increases requirements for energy and protein and micronutrients such as zinc and can promote nutrient losses via the bowel and urine. In addition, these diseases and physical disability associated with musculoskeletal disorders will contribute to immobility and increase dependence upon carers. The ensuing impairment of the ability to shop, cook and self-feed and social isolation are obvious contributors to malnutrition.

9.5.6 Combating malnutrition in the elderly

The prevention and treatment of malnutrition among older adults have to be a major public health priority in all nations. Malnutrition is clearly more prevalent among individuals who are hospitalized or otherwise institutionalized for long periods of time but is not confined to that subgroup in the population. Malnutrition is also a problem for independently living elderly people, and this group perhaps provides the greater challenge in terms of intervention.

Most malnutrition goes unnoticed, particularly among the elderly living in nursing homes. This is because nutrition is often overlooked in the face of other care priorities such as managing dementia and other chronic conditions, overcoming mobility problems and personal care. There are a number of simple malnutrition screening tools that can be used by those who care for older adults, which enable interventions to prevent malnutrition to be applied at an early stage (see Research Highlight 9.2). In nursing home or hospital settings, these tools can be used for screening of the older adults on admission and for monitoring in the longer term.

Ideally, all staff working with elderly patients in care settings should be trained in nutritional screening, in taking responsibility for initiating nutritional support and in carrying out basic feeding and food-related support tasks. In addition to this, there are a number of steps that can be taken to promote food intake and boost nutritional status without the need for supplemental products or specialist intervention. It is important to target the quality of the food itself, ensuring that it is nutritious, varied and attractive. Appetite levels are low in a high proportion of older adults (van der Meij *et al.*, 2017), so exciting the appetite is of high importance. Large portion sizes suppress the appetite, so provision of smaller but more frequent meals helps to increase overall intake. However, for older adults in care settings, practical considerations often dictate meal frequency and menu formats, losing the opportunity to promote food intake through smaller but more frequent, attractive meals. Carrier *et al.* (2007) found that among Canadian nursing home residents, bulk-delivery food systems, repetitious menus and provision of meals in difficult-to-open packages and dishes all decreased food intake.

The environment provided for mealtimes is also of importance. All individuals involved with the feeding of dependent elderly people need to be aware of the fact that malnutrition has a multifaceted aetiology and stems not only from reduced food intake but also from all of the social, pharmacological and medical factors that contribute to reducing appetite. Eating is a social activity, so providing meals in a social, friendly and pleasant environment encourages greater intake. Mamhidir *et al.* (2007) showed that with a group of hospitalized patients with dementia, providing an intervention that made the ward seem more home-like and encouraging staff and caregivers to be more attentive and responsive at mealtimes prevented weight loss over a three-month period and in many cases promoted

Research Highlight 9.2 Nutrition screening tools for detection and management of malnutrition.

With more of the population living for longer and increasing prevalence of dementia and other chronic conditions, the number of older adults living with malnutrition is increasing. Malnutrition will be found in people living independently, particularly where individuals are living alone, but is more prevalent in care homes and in clinical settings. As malnutrition is both a consequence and a cause of significant ill-health, identifying those at risk and putting in place appropriate interventions and nutritional support is critical.

There are many nutritional screening tools available for use in detecting malnutrition and these should be used as a basic first step in nutritional management of vulnerable older people. Regular screening can track the nutritional status of older people over time and acts as a trigger for prompt intervention. The available tools use a variety of different criteria as described below.

- The Mini Nutritional Assessment (MNA; Vellas *et al.*, 1999) is a complex tool which evaluates meal consumption, body mass index (BMI), mid-arm circumference, polypharmacy, neuropsychological health and functional capacity (ability to walk, sit and self-care).
- The Nutrition Risk Screening 2002 tool (NRS2002; Kondrup *et al.*, 2003) calculates risk by evaluating current BMI and weight loss over the preceding three to six months, alongside the presence of disease effects on appetite.
- The Malnutrition Universal Screening Tool (Stratton *et al.*, 2004), like NRS2002, determines a malnutrition risk score by considering current BMI, recent weight loss and the impact of acute disease status.
- The Subjective Global Assessment tool (Fontes *et al.*, 2014) assesses malnutrition risk on the basis of weight change, food intake, disease symptoms and functional capacity.
- The Short Nutritional Assessment Questionnaire (SNAQ) has been modified specifically for use with older people (SNAQ65+; Borkent *et al.*, 2019). It evaluates risk on the basis of weight, mid-arm circumference, appetite and functional capacity.
- The Geriatric Nutritional Risk Index (GRNI; Bouillanne *et al.*, 2005) uses a calculation based on body weight and serum albumin concentration to determine nutritional risk.

With so many tools available, it is critical that the most appropriate is used for the individuals at risk. Tools must be evaluated for the population and, in this context, it is worth noting that MNA, GRNI and SNAQ65+ were developed specifically for use with older adults, while other tools have a more generalized application in clinical practice. Van Bokhurst-van der Schueren *et al.*, (2014) carried out a systematic review of tools and their predictive validity in hospital settings and found that MNA performed best among older patients. It was also concluded that not one tool was capable of both adequate nutrition screening and predicting poor nutrition-related outcomes.

Whichever tool is in use, it must be simple for staff involved in care of older adults to use and must not depend on specialist equipment, which might not be available in the care setting. Tools which depend on measures of BMI may be problematic in this regard, as older adults who are unable to stand can only have their height crudely estimated. Despite such concerns, the use of screening tools as a routine element of elderly care will at least raise awareness of the vulnerability of this population to malnutrition. This increases the likelihood that nutritional support will be a priority in the clinical or care community.

gains in weight. Assistance with feeding is also an essential element in the elderly care setting. This can range from physically feeding frail and dependent individuals to providing modified utensils that enable self-feeding. In all circumstances, encouragement, warmth and preservation of dignity are essential elements of maintaining a healthy intake.

In the independently living community, the challenges are different as the level of support that can be provided is often limited. There are schemes in place in many countries that are designed to prolong the period of time that frail older people can maintain independent living and reduce the risk of malnutrition (Diallo *et al.*, 2020). A range of solutions is available in developed countries, including meals on wheels, cook and eat classes and lunch clubs. The latter two are believed to promote eating and cooking skills by creating a social environment for eating, but there is no current evidence base to support the view that they reduce risk of malnutrition or reach

those most at need. Meals on wheels schemes are designed to provide meals to older adults in their own homes, ensuring food intake can be maintained among individuals who struggle to shop and cook. Most schemes provide one hot meal per day for five days per week. Extension of this scheme to include all meals and snacks for the full week can significantly improve nutritional intakes and promote weight gain among the malnourished (Kretser *et al.*, 2003), and the inclusion of breakfast in a two-meal scheme was shown to increase intakes of energy, protein, carbohydrate fibre and micronutrients; reduce depression scores; and increase enjoyment of food (Gollub and Weddle, 2004). Well-designed menus can have an enhanced impact upon nutritional status. An (2015) reported that use of a home-delivered meal service increased intake of protein, fibre, calcium, copper and other micronutrients, but had no impact on total energy intake. Despite observations of enhanced nutrient intake, the evidence that meals delivered to their homes reduces the prevalence of malnutrition among the frail elderly is relatively weak (Ijmker-Hemink *et al.*, 2020), and there are also concerns that these meals may increase the risk of food-borne disease (Roseman, 2007). Many recipients of delivered meals do not eat them immediately and then store the whole meal or leftovers in unsafe conditions (Almanza *et al.*, 2007).

9.6 Common nutrition-related health problems

9.6.1 Bone disorders

The degeneration of physiological function and physical wellbeing associated with ageing means that many chronic diseases first manifest in the later years of adulthood. While cardiovascular diseases and cancer are often first noted in older adults, they are clearly also a major problem in younger adults. In contrast, there are a number of diseases of bone that are almost exclusively seen in older adults.

9.6.1.1 Bone mineralization and remodelling

Bone has a complex structure and is a highly vascularized and innervated tissue. It essentially comprises a framework of collagen subtypes into which are deposited minerals to provide the hard, rigid structure. Most of the mineral in bone comprises calcium and phosphate, but there are many other minerals and trace elements present, including fluoride and sodium. Seventy to eighty per cent of the skeleton comprises cortical bone, which in section appears as concentric rings of bone in a bundled arrangement. The remaining bone is termed trabecular bone, which has a lattice structure, similar in nature to that of a sponge. The trabecular bone is found at the ends of the long bones, within the vertebrae and at the hips and wrist (Figure 9.8).

Bone mineralization is a process that essentially occurs during childhood and the pubertal growth spurt (Figure 9.8). As the body grows, the mass of mineral in the skeleton increases accordingly. At the end of the growth phase, coinciding with sexual maturity, there is no further net gain of mineral

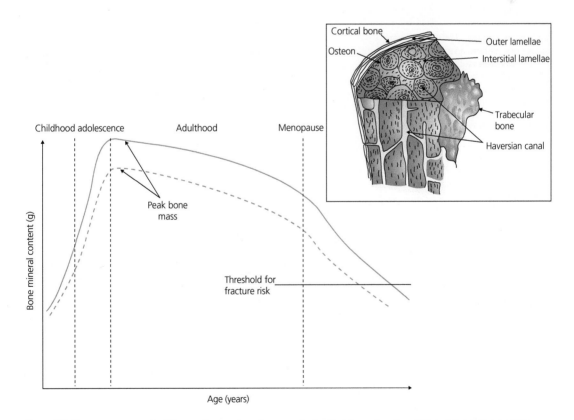

Figure 9.8 Bone mass across the lifespan. Bone mineral accrues in the first three decades of life but thereafter declines progressively. The rate of bone loss accelerates after the menopause. Inset: the structure of long bones. Spongy trabecular bone makes up the ends of the long bones, while compact cortical bone provides the main mass of the skeleton. Haversian canals contain blood vessels and nerves.

within the skeleton, and the individual is said to have achieved peak bone mass. Although there is now no further net gain of mineral, the skeleton is far from inert at this stage. There is a constant cycle of mineral loss and replacement taking place. This is essential not only to allow the skeleton to be repaired in the event of injury but also to allow the skeleton to be remodelled and maintained and for the release of minerals from bone to make up for any shortfall in supply for other critical processes.

The skeleton completely remodels itself every 7–10 years, and this process is driven by two cell types within the bone. Osteoclasts are cells that remove mineral from bone (Figure 9.9). They respond to hormonal signals including parathyroid hormone and vitamin D3 to release calcium from bone into the circulation. When bone is injured or fractured, they move into the damaged area to remove debris and begin the process of repair. In contrast, the osteoblasts bring about the remineralization of bone. During childhood and adolescence, osteoblast activity is in the ascendance as high concentrations of growth hormone stimulate osteoblast activity, and during puberty, rising sex steroid concentrations also promote bone mineralization. At the end of growth, the activities of osteoblasts and osteoclasts are in equilibrium, and the skeleton is maintained in a stable state through the continuing remodelling process. With ageing, however, osteoclast

activity tends to exceed the rates of remineralization and, hence, the bone mineral content and density begin to decline (Figure 9.8). In women, the rate of decline accelerates at the menopause as the loss of oestrogen production removes the stimulatory effect upon osteoblasts. Rates of bone remodelling are not even across the whole skeleton, and trabecular bone remodels around eight times faster than cortical bone. This means that with ageing, loss of bone density from the trabecular regions is much faster, declining by up to 2.5% every year.

9.6.1.2 Osteoporosis pathology and prevalence

Osteoporosis is one of the most common causes of hospitalization among the elderly. It is characterized by an increased susceptibility to bone fracture due to demineralization. While, at the present time, most osteoporosis is noted in the developed countries, the increasing lifespan of populations in developing countries means that the global prevalence of the condition will increase dramatically, possibly doubling over 50 years.

Osteoporosis is a serious condition and among older adults, one quarter of all individuals sustaining a fracture can be expected to die within one year. Often, the first indication of the condition comes when a person has a fall and fractures a bone at one of the main trabecular bone sites, such as the hip or wrist. Fractures to the vertebrae can often go

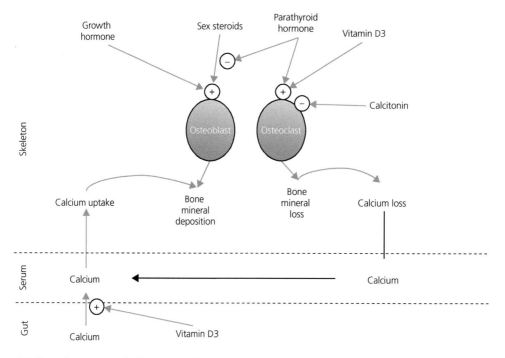

Figure 9.9 The endocrine control of bone mineralization.

unnoticed and manifest as a loss of height or the development of a humpbacked posture. Osteoporosis is generally diagnosed through x-ray, which shows the loss of mineral from affected regions, and is confirmed using the dual x-ray absorptiometry technique. This allows the determination of the total mineral present within the skeleton or specific bone regions (bone mineral content) and from this, the bone mineral density (BMD, mineral g/cm² bone) can be derived. BMD is the primary tool for diagnosis and monitoring of osteoporosis, with clearly characterized thresholds for defining the progression of the disease. Markers of bone degradation (e.g. N-telopeptide) or formation (e.g. alkaline phosphatase activity or procollagen 1 C-terminal peptide) can also be used to monitor the disease. Although osteoporosis is seen in both men and women, it is far more common in women due to the impact of the menopause on rates of bone loss. Kanis *et al.* (2002) reported that significant risk of osteoporosis begins at around the age of 50–55 years, when up to 10% of women meet the criteria for diagnosis. By the age of 80 years, osteoporosis was seen in 47% of women and 16% of men.

9.6.1.3 Risk factors for osteoporosis

The major non-modifiable risk factors for osteoporosis include female sex, early menopause and increasing age. There is believed to be a strong genetic component underlying the risk of osteoporosis, and some twin studies suggest that this may account for as much as 50% of risk. Polymorphisms in specific gene loci appear to impact differently on osteoporosis risk in populations of different ethnicity. These include variants of the oestrogen α and β receptors (Zhu *et al.*, 2018), vitamin D receptor (Wang *et al.*, 2018b) and insulin-like growth factor-1 (Chen *et al.*, 2017). A number of disease states will impact upon risk of osteoporosis, generally by virtue of the effects they have upon the endocrine regulation of bone turnover or the metabolism and transport of vitamin D and calcium. These include hyperthyroidism, hyperparathyroidism, cancer, rheumatoid arthritis, coeliac disease, inflammatory bowel disorders, renal failure and anorexia nervosa. Therapies that require administration of corticosteroids or disrupt the normal production of sex steroids will promote osteoporosis.

The level of peak bone mass attained at the end of the growth phase is considered to be an important determinant of the risk of osteoporosis later in life. Rates of bone loss are relatively constant among the population, so risk of BMD falling below the thresholds at which fractures become likely is increased in individuals for whom peak bone mass

was lower (Figure 9.8). For this reason, the optimal periods for targeting interventions to prevent osteoporosis may lie during childhood and adolescence, rather than in the adult years.

The main avoidable lifestyle risk factors for osteoporosis include smoking, physical inactivity and excessive consumption of alcohol and poor dietary intakes of calcium and vitamin D. The latter forms the main target for nutritional interventions. Physical activity is important as bone mineralization occurs at faster rates around lines of stress within bone. Low-to-moderate intakes of alcohol appear to be protective against osteoporosis, but with heavy use, any benefits are lost. Alcoholics typically develop an osteopenic skeleton and suffer high rates of falls and fractures. This is because alcohol specifically blocks bone formation, while having no effect on rates of resorption (Chakkalakal, 2005).

9.6.1.4 Dietary interventions for osteoporosis prevention

Once diagnosed, osteoporosis is generally treated using pharmacological agents. Rates of bone loss can be reduced by treating with bisphosphonates, which inhibit osteoclast activity. Calcitonin has a similar effect and can be administered as a nasal spray. Bone deposition can be increased through administration of drugs that boost hormone concentrations or mimic their actions. Raloxifene, for example, is a selective oestrogen receptor modulator, which mimics oestrogen activity and helps maintain bone mass in women after the menopause (Keen, 2007). Strontium ranelate is a drug that promotes bone deposition. In addition to these pharmacological approaches, older people with osteoporosis are advised to increase intakes of calcium and vitamin D to limit bone loss. However, this nutritional strategy is considered to be more important in the context of osteoporosis prevention and is the cornerstone of population-wide intervention strategies.

9.6.1.4.1 Calcium and vitamin D

Calcium has been shown to be effective in increasing bone mass in individuals at any stage of life, and most observational studies are generally supportive of a role for calcium supplementation as a means of preventing osteoporosis. Stear *et al.* (2003) showed that in 17-year-old girls with good baseline calcium intakes, a 1000 mg per day calcium supplement increased whole-body BMD over a two-year period, with particularly strong effects at the trochanter (5% increase in BMD). Among Chinese 12–15-year-olds, supplementation at a range of doses of calcium (230–966 mg/day) over 24 months increased lumbar spine and total body BMD but only in boys (Yin *et al.*, 2010).

The systematic review of Huncharek *et al.* (2008) found that supplemental calcium or increasing intake of dairy foods increased total body and lumbar spine BMD among children with low baseline calcium intakes. Studies of children generally show that initiating calcium supplementation during the pubertal growth spurt is particularly effective. Although this stage of life is well ahead of the appearance of any disease, boosting BMD at this time might enable the achievement of a greater peak bone mass.

In older adults, calcium intake and supplementation alone (i.e. without vitamin D) have limited effects and, surprisingly, most studies conclude that calcium is not beneficial for bone health. There is very little relationship between calcium intake and BMD. The Auckland Calcium Study reported that over a five-year follow-up of 570 women aged over 55 years, there was no association between intake and either bone loss or fracture risk (Reid *et al.*, 2015). Supplements have limited effects, but slow some aspects of bone turnover and increase BMD in women with very poor baseline calcium status (Rajatanavin *et al.*, 2013). There is some controversy as to whether supplements reduce fracture risk, with many studies finding no benefit. The RECORD trial, for example, found that calcium 1 g per day did not alter fracture risk in subjects aged over 70 (Grant *et al.*, 2005). Prince *et al.* (2006), however, found that calcium 1.2 g per day had a large impact on fracture risk (relative risk, RR, 0.66, 95% CI 0.45–0.97) and the meta-analysis of Tang *et al.* (2007) suggested a benefit of high doses.

Epidemiological studies are similarly equivocal regarding preventive strategies that use vitamin D alone. Most vitamin D is synthesized endogenously through the action of sunlight upon the skin and as a result, concentrations in circulation tend to vary with season, particularly among older adults in the northern hemisphere. As vitamin D3 concentrations fall in the winter months, the risk of fracture increases. Women with vitamin D insufficiency had lower BMD at the hip and femoral neck and were at greater risk of hip fracture (Zhu *et al.*, 2019). There is a significant relationship between serum 25-hydroxy vitamin D3 concentration and fracture risk (Wang *et al.*, 2020) but evaluation of the relationship between vitamin D3 supplementation and bone health suggests that in isolation there is little benefit. Supplements have a small effect on BMD at the femoral neck, but at no other sites (Reid *et al.*, 2014). Smith *et al.* (2018) evaluated a range of supplement doses between 400 and 4800 iu per day and found no effects of any dose on BMD in postmenopausal women. A randomized controlled trial of vitamin D3 400, 4000 and 10000 iu per day found

that compared with 400 iu per day, the higher doses actually reduced BMD at the wrist and the tibia (Burt *et al.*, 2019). Aspray *et al.* (2019) also found no benefits of high-dose supplementation. The meta-analysis of Hu *et al.* (2019) concluded that vitamin D alone did not reduce fracture risk in community dwelling older adults.

Most randomized controlled trials do not consider the effects of calcium and vitamin D in isolation and instead administer these two nutrients together. Combined supplements have been shown to increase BMD at the lumbar spine, wrist and femoral neck (Liu *et al.*, 2020) and this effect may be greatest with vitamin D doses of no less than 400 iu per day and in subjects who have low vitamin D status. Supplementing vitamin D deficient women with calcium 500 mg and vitamin D 400 iu per day decreased markers of bone remodelling and improved total body and vertebral BMD (Grados *et al.*, 2003). Boonen *et al.* (2007) performed a meta-analysis that showed that the observed benefits of vitamin D upon fracture risk were largely dependent upon the co-administration of calcium supplements. Comparing the relative risk of hip fracture associated with combined supplements with that associated with vitamin D alone, they reported a 25% decrease (RR 0.75, 95% CI 0.58–0.90). However, the more recent review by Hu *et al.* (2019) suggested that whether given alone or in combination, vitamin D and calcium supplements did not significantly reduce risk of fracture in independently living older people. The relationship between vitamin D and calcium and fracture risk may depend considerably on the baseline risk of the population under study. Vitamin D status is likely to be worse in nursing home residents than in independently living older people as the former are less likely to go outside in the sunshine as a result of reduced mobility, dementia and other chronic health problems (Bruyere *et al.*, 2009). As such, older adults in residential care are at much greater risk than individuals living independently. Avenell *et al.* (2014) suggested that while in low-risk community dwelling populations, supplementation might have limited effect on fractures, they would prevent 54 fractures per 1000 people among high-risk older adults. To simplify a complicated literature, it seems that for individuals with adequate calcium and/or vitamin D status there is no additional benefit associated with high-dose supplementation. Avoiding sub-optimal calcium and vitamin D status is important for older people and supplements may be a good strategy.

Falls are the main cause of fractures among older adults with osteoporosis. There is a growing body of evidence to suggest that calcium and vitamin D supplementation may contribute to reduced risk of fracture by preventing falls, in addition to increasing BMD. Falls are commonplace in some groups of older adults and among populations living in nursing homes may occur at least once per year per individual. Falls are more likely with cognitive impairment, cataracts, certain medication and cardiovascular disease (Karlsson *et al.*, 2013). Falls are the major cause of non-vertebral fractures among individuals with osteoporosis. There is evidence to suggest that individuals with higher circulating vitamin D3 concentrations suffer fewer falls (Stein *et al.*, 1999). Age at first fall tends to be earlier in those with lower vitamin D3 status (Rothenbacher *et al.*, 2014). Vitamin D increases the strength of the upper and lower limbs in the elderly (Boyé *et al.*, 2013; Sanders *et al.*, 2014). Bischoff-Ferrari *et al.* (2003) reported that administering cholecalciferol (vitamin D3) 800 iu per day with calcium 1200 mg per day to a population of 63–99-year-olds reduced risk of falling by 49%, while calcium alone increased risk. In contrast, Law *et al.* (2006) found no benefit of administering ergocalciferol (vitamin D2) 2.5 mg every two months, in terms of either fracture or falls risk. The meta-analysis of Cameron *et al.* (2018) concluded that vitamin D supplementation reduced the frequency of falls (RR 0.72, 95% CI 0.55–0.95) but made little difference to the overall risk of falling (RR 0.92, 95% CI 0.76–1.12). This was in contrast to earlier reviews which suggested that supplementation reduced risk of falls by around 22% in a dose-dependent manner (Broe *et al.*, 2007; Guo *et al.*, 2014). Benefits of vitamin D may be a result of enhanced neuromuscular tone.

With increasing emphasis upon increasing calcium intake to prevent age-related bone loss and fracture, concern has been raised about potentially negative consequences. Bolland *et al.* (2011) analysed data from the US Women's Health Initiative, a study of over 144 000 women (aged 50–79 at baseline) followed longitudinally from the 1990s to 2011. Women consuming supplements of calcium or calcium plus vitamin D were found to be at increased risk of myocardial infarction (hazard ratio, HR, 1.24. 95% CI 1.07–1.45). In contrast, in the EPIC-Norfolk prospective cohort (Pana *et al.*, 2021), consumption of calcium 1074–1254 mg per day was associated with lower cardiovascular mortality than consumption below 700 mg per day, although as there was no dose-dependent relationship this finding may be anomalous. Calcium supplements were not associated with cardiovascular events in either men or women. A meta-analysis of 26 prospective cohort studies and 16 randomized controlled trials found that dietary calcium intakes ranging from 200 to 1500 mg per day

were not associated with cardiovascular risk (Yang *et al.*, 2020), but there was a moderate increase in risk with calcium supplements (RR for CHD 1.08, 95% CI 1.02–1.22).

9.6.1.4.2 Minerals and protein

Other nutrients and dietary components may be influential in determining the risk of developing osteoporosis and fractures. Iron and magnesium have both been shown to contribute to bone mineralization. Serum magnesium concentrations are reported to be higher among older individuals with greater BMD. Iron, on the other hand, promotes bone loss but only when present in major excess, as is seen with the condition haemochromatosis. Neither of these minerals is likely to have a major influence on bone health within the normal range of dietary intakes.

Protein nutrition may also be a determinant of bone health. Availability of protein clearly plays a role in the formation of bone, and supplements are beneficial in the elderly following a fracture. Moreover, protein intake may be a determinant of muscle strength and may play a role in determining the risk of falling. Habitual protein intake may be a determinant of BMD. Rapuri *et al.* (2003) studied almost 500 older adults (aged 65–79) with protein intakes varying between 53 and 74 g per day. Over a three-year period, protein intake had no influence over rates of bone loss. A higher protein intake was associated with greater BMD at the spine and wrist, but only in the subjects whose calcium intake was adequate. In the Women's Health Initiative study, protein intake was not related to fracture risk at the hip, but risk of wrist fracture declined by 7% for every 20% increase in protein intake (Beasley *et al.*, 2014). Higher protein intake was also associated with total skeletal BMD and BMD at the hip. The meta-analysis of Groenendijk *et al.* (2019) concluded that higher protein intakes were associated with higher BMD at the hip and a significant reduction in hip fractures (HR 0.89, 95% CI 0.84–0.94).

9.6.1.4.3 Phytoestrogens

Phytoestrogens have been suggested as a safe alternative to hormone replacement therapy by virtue of their capacity to reduce bone loss after the menopause. However, their efficacy has not been firmly established, and they may only be useful as an adjunct to other therapies, such as the use of selective oestrogen receptor modulators. Some studies demonstrate benefits of isoflavones in terms of bone turnover markers (Sathyapalan *et al.*, 2017) or BMD. Lappe *et al.* (2013) reported that supplementation with genistein combined with vitamin D3, vitamin K, and n-3 fatty acids improved BMD at the hip. Other studies find that phytoestrogens have no positive impact. For example, a two-year study of isoflavone administration found that 300 mg per day did not attenuate the age-related decline in BMD among perimenopausal women. The general consensus is that the effects of isoflavones are insignificant at the important fracture-prone sites (Ricci *et al.*, 2010).

To some extent, the response to phytoestrogens may depend upon the composition of the gut microflora. Intestinal bacteria metabolize the soy isoflavone daidzein to O-desmethylangolensin (80–90% of population) or equol (20–30% of population). A trial of isoflavones 75 mg per day in postmenopausal women showed that bone loss was slowed significantly in equol producers, but less so among non-equol producers (Ishimi, 2010). In the placebo group, there was no difference in bone loss between equol producers and non-producers. Yoshikata *et al.* (2018) supplemented middle aged Japanese women with equol 10 mg per day directly and found that over one year this reduced bone fracture risk and improved other bone parameters.

9.6.1.4.4 Caffeine

Avoidance of caffeine might be advocated as a strategy to prevent bone loss in certain individuals, as there are numerous reports that high consumption interferes with calcium uptake from the gut and reduces bone mineralization (Barbour *et al.*, 2010). In a study of over 61 000 postmenopausal women in the Swedish Mammography Cohort, consumption of four or more cups of coffee per day was associated with a 2–4% lower BMD compared with women who consumed less than one cup per day (Hallström *et al.*, 2013). Coffee consumption was not related to fracture risk. The effects of caffeine upon bone health may also depend upon specific genotypes. Men with the rapid metabolizing variant of CYP1A2, the enzyme which metabolizes caffeine, showed a greater detriment of BMD when consuming more than four cups of coffee per day than those with the slow metabolizing variant (Hallström *et al.*, 2010). Rapuri *et al.* (2001) reported that bone loss over a three-year period was markedly greater among postmenopausal women consuming over 300 mg caffeine (10 cups of tea, 3–5 cups of coffee) per day compared with those consuming less than 300 mg per day. However, these effects were confined to the women who expressed the tt variant of the vitamin D receptor Taq1 polymorphism. This suggests that caffeine may interfere with vitamin D metabolism via its receptor.

9.6.1.5 Paget's disease of bone

Paget's disease of bone (osteitis deformans) is a disorder that is more common among the elderly population than in younger adults. It is characterized by the development of enlarged and deformed bone, particularly in the spine and any areas adjacent to joints. This is caused by excessive remodelling of bone, with high rates of breakdown and remineralization, and leads to malformations, including curvature of the spine, and weakness of bone that increases the likelihood of fracture. In contrast to osteoporosis, Paget's disease is more common in men than in women. It is treated using bisphosphonates to inhibit osteoclast activity, and patients taking these drugs are recommended to consume calcium supplements (1000–1500 mg/day) with vitamin D (400 iu/day).

9.6.2 Immunity and infection

Nutrition, infection and immunity are closely related (Figure 9.10). Nutrient deficits, particularly protein–energy malnutrition and deficits of the B vitamins, vitamin A and trace elements, impair both passive immunity and cellular immunity and therefore reduce the capacity to resist infection. Infection promotes malnutrition by activating the acute phase response to trauma. This response is characterized by an increase in demand for energy and protein, coupled with a decrease in appetite. Chronic or recurrent infections can therefore exacerbate the effects of continuing malnutrition. In the elderly, the relationship between nutritional status and immune function is of greater significance as the risk of malnutrition is heightened by other factors, and infection becomes more likely due to other medical conditions that either impair immune function or increased exposure to sources of infection, for example, following surgery. In developed countries, the elderly population are at two- to tenfold greater risk of death due to infectious diseases than younger adults (High, 2001). This population is also the major at-risk group for hospital-acquired infections such as multiple resistant *Staphylococcus aureus* or antibiotic-resistant strains of *Clostridium difficile* (Castle *et al.*, 2007).

While much of the increased infection risk seen among older adults might be attributed to nutritional status or comorbidities, it is important to appreciate that the immune system undergoes age-related changes in function that are probably greater than seen in any other tissue. Immune senescence is accompanied by complex changes to both innate and adaptive responses (Figure 9.11). Generally speaking, ageing is accompanied by a change in the profile of cytokines produced by immune cells, and increases in

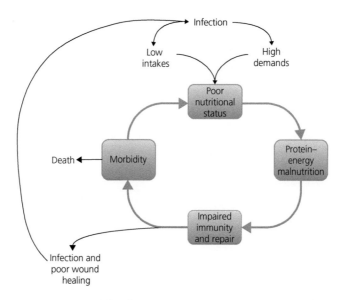

Figure 9.10 The vicious circle of malnutrition and disease.

baseline levels of secretion of interleukin-6 and interleukin-10 create an environment that is undergoing a chronic, low-grade inflammatory response (Castle *et al.*, 2007). The lymphocyte types that are present in circulation also undergo change with senescence, and the elderly possess more memory T cells. These cells are responsible for the recognition of pathogens that the body has previously encountered and orchestrate a stronger immune response than that at the first infection. This would appear to be a feature of a more robust immune response, but it appears that the predominance of memory T cells results in reduced numbers of other T cell types, including CD4+ helper cells (which activate cytotoxic T cells) and naïve T cells. This means that there are less effective responses to new pathogens. The senescent immune system is generally less responsive to stimuli, for example, producing less interleukin-1 with an antigen challenge. Vaccinations produce lower antibody responses and are therefore less helpful. Declining functions of phagocytic cells and the complement system make the response to bacterial and viral infections less effective. For these reasons older adults are at greater risk of severe consequences when infected with common seasonal pathogens such as influenza. The COVID-19 pandemic, in particular, had a devastating impact upon individuals aged over 70 (Figure 9.12). Reasons for this greater vulnerability are discussed in Research Highlight 9.3.

It is frequently stated that nutritional status and, in particular, micronutrient status plays a major role in determining immune function and capacity to resist

and fight infection. It is well established that providing nutritional support to patients in the postsurgical period can improve recovery rates, and that without such support, the elderly surgical patient might be expected to lose weight for around two months during their convalescence (High, 2001). However, the literature considering the impact of supplementation upon immune function in older adults is sparse and largely consists of animal and in vitro studies. Supplementation with vitamin D has been widely discussed and is suggested as a possible means of reducing the impact of infection with COVID-19 in the elderly (Shakoor *et al.*, 2021) but the underpinning evidence is weak. Costenbader *et al.* (2019) found that supplementation of older adults with n-3 fatty acids and vitamin D for one year had no effect on inflammation, and Goncalves-Mendes *et al.* (2019) reported that following supplementation with vitamin D, the antibody response of older adults to influenza vaccination was no different from that in placebo controls.

Pre- and probiotic supplements have also been investigated for their immunomodulatory benefits in older people, but with limited benefits reported. Consumption of *Bifidobacterium lactis* Bi-07 improved phagocytic and oxidative killing functions of immune cell populations (Maneerat *et al.*, 2014), but there is no strong evidence that supplementation increases resistance to infection or impacts on the response to vaccinations. Prebiotic supplementation did not improve immune function in the study of Wilms *et al.* (2021).

Any individual who is immobilized for a long period is susceptible to the development of pressure

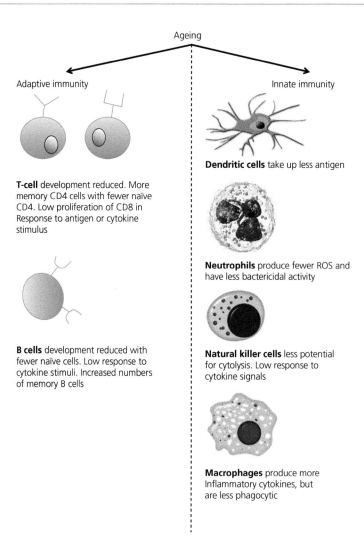

Figure 9.11 The impact of ageing on the cellular immune system.

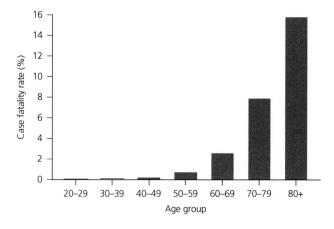

Figure 9.12 Mortality rates in the COVID-19 pandemic by age group.

Research Highlight 9.3 COVID-19 mortality in older adults: multiple risk factors.

In 2020 and 2021, the global economy and way of living was rocked by the pandemic of novel severe acute respiratory coronavirus 2 (SARS-CoV2), which became known as COVID-19. As of 12 April 2021, with no end in sight, this virus had infected more than 135 million people worldwide and had killed more than 2.9 million people (127 087 in the UK and 555 712 in the United States alone; World Health Organization, 2021). This is the worst global disease outbreak since the devastating 'Spanish' influenza pandemic that followed the First World War. In addition to high death rates, COVID-19 is associated with long hospital stays for patients, often with requirements for intensive care and longer-term debilitating conditions following recovery from the infection.

Although COVID-19 mortality was observed in people of all ages, the vast majority of deaths occurred in older people. For example, comparing people more than 80 years of age with those aged 40–49 reveals a mortality rate that was 50-fold higher among the older patients. In the UK and United States, older people in care homes represent the majority of deaths from COVID-19 that occurred in the early waves of the pandemic. The vulnerability of older people to COVID-19 death or severe infection can be explained by the presence of underlying health conditions, socioeconomic factors and living conditions, and immunosenescence (Crimmins, 2020).

The main risk factors for severe COVID-19 are male sex, non-white ethnicity, older age and the presence of chronic underlying health conditions. The latter group includes many conditions that are associated with nutritional status, including obesity, diabetes, hypertension and heart disease, together with chronic obstructive pulmonary disease and other lung conditions. Older adults are considerably more likely than their younger counterparts to suffer from these conditions. A study of New Yorkers showed that more than 80% of adults over the age of 70 years had at least one of five conditions: diabetes, stroke, hypertension, lung disease or heart disease (Crimmins, 2020).

Older adults are more likely to be of lower socioeconomic status and tend to live in smaller houses, with smaller and less well-ventilated rooms. They are also more dependent on others for care, cooking and shopping. At the height of the pandemic this meant that they were more likely to become infected by younger people carrying COVID-19 without symptoms, as their dependency necessitated less rigid social distancing and greater contact with people from outside their household. Care home settings, with communal areas and staff moving between closely grouped bedrooms, were particularly vulnerable to spread of COVID-19 once the infection had entered the building (Crimmins, 2020).

The most important factor associated with greater risk of severe COVID-19 in older people is the development of immunosenescence with age. Both passive and adaptive immunity are compromised in older people. B lymphocyte numbers are lower (Aiello et al., 2019) and T- cell numbers decline. This leaves older people less able to mount effective responses to novel pathogens such as COVID-19 (Mok et al., 2020). Macrophages have reduced phagocytic functions and produce lower levels of cytokines which orchestrate the immune response. Neutrophils similarly have impaired cytokine signalling and reduced killer activity (Mok et al., 2020). Ageing is therefore associated with major disruption of a normally well-integrated and controlled immune response. In older subjects with COVID-19 infection, levels of inflammatory cytokines are high compared with younger patients and this may increase the host cell damage and death associated with viral replication. Fever is another key element of the response to COVID-19 infection. Fever serves to shift metabolism towards antimicrobial activity (Kluger et al., 1998). In older people, the fever response is impaired (Norman, 2000). Taken together, the features of age-related immunosenescence make older people more likely to suffer severe COVID-19 infection as their bodies are less able to stop replication of the virus in host cells, eliminate the infection and to limit and repair viral damage (Mok et al., 2020).

The terrible impact of COVID-19 on the global population is therefore strongly associated with ageing and nutrition-related disease states. Although it is too soon to state with certainty, nutritional modulation of immune function may be an important element of how lifestyle factors determine which individuals are able to withstand infection and those who develop severe COVID-19 symptoms, complications and death.

sores or pressure ulcers. These are areas of deep damage to skin tissue caused by pressure and/or friction. Such lesions are seen in up to two thirds of all hospital inpatients and are most likely to occur in older individuals who are bedbound, often following other age-related injuries such as hip fracture or as a consequence of prolonged sitting and lack of physical activity (Stratton et al., 2005). Pressure ulcers carry considerable risk of further complications, extend periods of hospitalization associated with other medical problems, severely impair patients' quality of life and increase risk of death by fivefold. Malnutrition is a major risk factor for the development of pressure ulcers. This could be because there is reduced skin resistance and cushioning by body fat at areas of likely pressure in individuals of low BMI. In addition, malnutrition is associated with reduced availability of key nutrients for maintenance, repair and healing of the skin. The most effective nutritional support for those with pressure ulcers appears to be provision of oral supplements of protein and energy, which when given to at-risk patients without ulcers significantly reduce their occurrence (RR 0.75, 95% CI 0.62–0.89, Stratton et al., 2005). Among elderly patients, such supplements appear to reduce the stay in hospital associated with hip fractures, presumably by lessening occurrence of complications such as pressure ulcers (Delmi *et al.*, 1990). In addition to preventing pressure ulcers, nutritional status and nutritional support are important factors in determining rates of healing (Donini *et al.*, 2005).

9.6.3 Digestive tract disorders

As described earlier in this chapter, gastrointestinal tract problems are an important contributor to undernutrition in the older adult population. There is a wide variety of different disorders that impact upon gastrointestinal function, and these affect the whole length of the tract (D'Souza, 2007).

9.6.3.1 Mouth and oesophagus

Soreness of the mouth is a common problem among older people. This often stems from the reduced flow of saliva or poor fitting of dentures. Clearly, this will detract from the desire to eat and can impact upon nutritional status. However, factors impacting upon oesophageal function are of much greater significance and lead to dysphagia and malnutrition. Problems with swallowing fall into two categories. Inhibition of the swallowing reflex is usually an issue in individuals who are recovering from a stroke and therefore has a clear cause and generally an acute onset. Neuromuscular disorders affecting the oesophagus and chronic conditions such as Parkinson's disease can impact upon swallowing over a much longer period and have a greater impact on general health. These conditions, and age-related declines in the peristaltic functions of the oesophagus, can induce the feeling that food is becoming stuck in transit to the stomach, and this discourages swallowing. Swallowing can also become painful due to reduced production of mucous in the oesophagus (D'Souza, 2007). Age-related loss of function in the lower oesophageal sphincter can lead to gastric reflux and, over time, the exposure to gastric secretions can promote oesophagitis.

9.6.3.2 Stomach

The inflammation of the gastric mucosa and the formation of peptic ulcers are more common among the elderly than in the younger population. There are believed to be a number of physiological reasons for this, but it should also be borne in mind that infection with *Helicobacter pylori* is also more common in the elderly. *H. pylori* infests the mucous layer of the stomach wall and generates ammonia from urea that would normally buffer stomach acids. This ammonia causes damage to the gastric epithelium. Approximately 80% of the over-65s will have *H. pylori* within the stomach compared with 20–50% of younger adults (Marshall, 1994). Another cause

of peptic ulcers is irritation of the gastric mucosa by anti-inflammatory medications. In the elderly, gastrointestinal transit times are slower and gastric emptying is less frequent. Coupled with this, there is reduced production of mucous and gastric juices. As a result, irritants stay in the stomach for longer and undergo less dilution with stomach acid (D'Souza, 2007). With atrophy of the gastric mucosa, the capacity to repair any inflamed or damaged areas is reduced.

9.6.3.3 Small intestine

The functions of the small intestine are well preserved within the ageing gastrointestinal tract, and most of the small intestinal disorders reported in the elderly are secondary to other disease states (Hoffmann and Zeitz, 2002). Malabsorption of nutrients is a major problem in elderly patients and is driven by conditions such as pancreatitis, parasitic infections, inflammatory bowel disease (Crohn's disease) and coeliac disease. Bacterial overgrowth of the small intestine is another factor promoting malabsorption, which is not usually seen in younger individuals. McEvoy *et al.* (1983) reported that among a group of patients in an elderly care setting, 31% of those with malabsorption problems leading to malnutrition were showing evidence of bacterial overgrowth syndrome.

Bacterial overgrowth is most likely to occur in the elderly as a result of the other gastrointestinal and health problems that they develop. Immunosuppressive drugs, for example, will allow bacteria to resist the local immune system. The presence of blind loops formed during surgery to the small intestine, or diverticula (see following text), provides a foothold for bacterial colonization. As with all of the other causes of malabsorption, the condition is likely to manifest as abdominal pain, diarrhoea, bloating and flatulence but should be readily treatable with antibiotics.

9.6.3.4 Large intestine

Constipation is a commonly reported condition among the elderly population, with an estimated prevalence of 15–30% among the independently living older population, with a greater occurrence in women than in men (Schuster *et al.*, 2015). Blekker *et al.* (2016) found that among residents in Norwegian nursing homes 23.4% were constipated and 67% were regular users of laxatives. Similarly, in Swedish nursing home residents laxative use was reported by 40% of survey respondents (Gustafsson *et al.*, 2019). Constipation is a serious issue and the associated pain and occasional incontinence are associated with a decline in quality of life measures.

Constipation can impact upon psychological health and is noted to cause aggression and delirium in older adults. There are many factors that promote constipation in this group. Some are related to drug treatments or nutrient supplementation for other conditions. Iron and calcium supplements, for example, lead to constipation, as do diuretics, opiate-based painkillers, many antidepressant drugs and antihypertensive agents. Lifestyle is also a major issue, and gastrointestinal transit times are lengthened by physical inactivity, poor hydration and a lack of dietary fibre. It is often suggested that the latter is a major explanation of why the elderly are more prone to constipation. It is argued that the poor dentition of the elderly can discourage intakes of fibre-rich foods. The National Diet and Nutrition Survey rolling programme in the UK found that only 4% of women and 9% of men achieved the recommended fibre intake of 30 g per day (average of 19 g/day for men and 16.4 g/day for women; Roberts *et al.*, 2018).

Declining peristaltic function within the large intestine contributes to constipation in the elderly. With this loss of function, the pressures generated within the colon required to keep stools moving have to increase, and this is a cause of diverticular disease (Figure 9.13). Diverticula are sacs and pouches that form within the lining of the intestine. They are present in between 50% and 80% of older adults and in most cases are asymptomatic (in which case the condition is termed diverticulosis). In around 15–20% of cases, the condition progresses to diverticulitis, in which the pouches become blocked with faecal matter. Subsequent infection leads to abdominal pain, lower gastrointestinal bleeding and alternating diarrhoea and constipa-

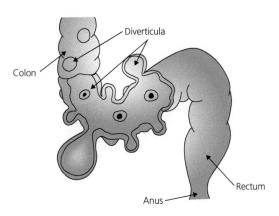

Figure 9.13 Low colonic mobility in the elderly leads to the development of diverticula, which are pockets in the colonic wall that act as a focus for the build-up of faecal material and infection.

tion. Infected diverticula can ulcerate or perforate, and this can become life threatening. Diverticular disease is best avoided by following a lifestyle that prevents constipation, including increased intake of non-starch polysaccharides, physical activity and maintaining adequate hydration (D'Souza, 2007).

9.6.4 Anaemia

Anaemia is a haematological condition characterized by abnormalities of the red blood cells. It is most simply defined on the basis of haemoglobin concentrations, and the World Health Organization sets cut-off values for adults at 13 g/dl for men and 12 g/dl for women. There are different forms of anaemia, and these require further examination of the red blood cells for diagnosis (Figure 9.14).

Anaemia, and in particular iron deficiency anaemia, is very common throughout the world, particularly among the female population. Older adults are especially at risk of anaemia, and many anaemias unrelated to iron deficiency are almost solely observed in older individuals. Steensma and Tefferi (2007) reported that the prevalence of anaemia in the US population was approximately 8% in the 65–74 age group (which is not significantly different to the prevalence in younger populations), 12% in the 75–84 age group and over 20% in the over-85s (26% in men, 20% in women). These figures are similar to those reported in other westernized countries, with 20.1% of elderly British men and 13.7% of elderly British women shown to be anaemic (Mukhopadhyay and Mohanaruban, 2002). A systematic review of elderly populations across the globe suggested an overall anaemia prevalence of 17%, with greater prevalence in men relative to women and Black relative to white populations (Gaskell *et al.*, 2008). Prevalence of anaemia increases with age and is more prevalent in nursing homes (47%) and hospital admissions (40%) than in the community (12%).

Anaemia in general is related to a number of poor health outcomes and reduced quality of life among the elderly. It is associated with reduced mobility, greater risk of falls and osteoporotic fractures, greater frailty and reduced cognitive function (Eisenstaedt *et al.*, 2006). Moreover, mortality rates are significantly greater among the anaemic population, either from specific causes such as cardiovascular disease or cancer or from all causes. The US Cardiovascular Health Study showed greater mortality over a 12-year period among elderly men and women in the lowest quintile of haemoglobin at baseline (Zakai *et al.*, 2005). Abrahamsen *et al.* (2016) followed older adults who had been discharged from hospital to nursing home care. Over the three years following discharge, those

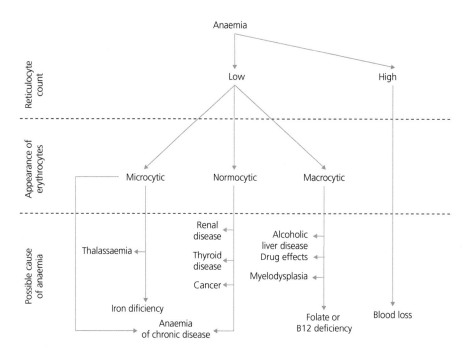

Figure 9.14 The diagnosis of nutritional and other causes of anaemia based upon histological examination of red blood cells. Reticulocytes are immature red cells.

with anaemia due to known causes were at greater risk of readmission to hospital and death than non-anaemic subjects. In anaemic individuals, concentrations of erythropoietin increase as part of the physiological response to maintain red cell function. In the Leiden 85-plus study, both cardiovascular and non-cardiovascular mortality over a two-year follow-up was greater among subjects in the highest tertile of erythropoietin concentration compared with the lowest (HR 1.73, 95% CI 1.32–2.26; den Elzen et al., 2010).

There are a wide range of different anaemias, with a range of different causes (Table 9.3), but those that are most commonly observed are iron deficiency anaemia, anaemia of chronic disease and the megaloblastic anaemias (Figure 9.15). These can be diagnosed using flow cytometry to determine the size of the red blood cells. Microcytic anaemia is diagnosed when the mean cell volume is low. This occurs when the haemoglobin concentration is low because of a failure to synthesize the protein, either due to iron deficiency or as a consequence of disordered erythropoiesis. Microcytic signs may also be noted with the anaemia of chronic disease, but this more usually manifests as a normocytic anaemia, in which the mean cell volume is in the normal range. Normocytic anaemia may also result from haemolytic anaemia in which the red cells are broken down at an abnormally high rate.

The anaemia of chronic disease is a product of inflammation and is seen commonly in patients with congestive heart failure and rheumatoid arthritis or after surgery. Approximately 65% of anaemia observed in older adults is likely to be chronic disease related. In these situations, there are high circulating concentrations of pro-inflammatory cytokines, such as tumour necrosis factor-α, interleukin-1 and interleukin-6, and these inhibit erythropoiesis. Moreover, the production of the iron transport inhibitor hepcidin increases during chronic inflammation, and this reduces the uptake of iron across the gut (Eisenstaedt et al., 2006). In chronic renal disease, the ability to produce erythropoietin is impaired, which can produce a microcytic anaemia of chronic disease.

The megaloblastic anaemias are characterized by the enlargement of red cells, which is related to the production of only immature and dysfunctional erythrocytes. The megaloblastic anaemias are the products of deficiencies of either vitamin B12 or folic acid. Megaloblastic anaemia due to vitamin B12 deficiency is often erroneously referred to as pernicious anaemia. Pernicious anaemia is a term that only applies to anaemia arising from B12 deficiency caused by atrophic gastritis or due to loss of the cells of the stomach lining, which secrete the intrinsic factor required for absorption of cobalamin. Pernicious anaemia is associated with severe neurological abnormalities that can result in sensory impairments, loss of appetite and cardiovascular and gastrointestinal problems.

9.6.4.1 Iron deficiency anaemia

Iron deficiency anaemia is relatively uncommon among the elderly populations of westernized countries, with prevalence estimated at 3–5%. Prevalence is higher in some groups with specific conditions such as heart disease. In developing countries, iron defi-

Table 9.3 Causes of anaemia in the elderly population.

Cause	Estimated % of cases
Iron deficiency	5–10
Anaemia of chronic disease	50–65
Acute haemorrhage	5–10
Vitamin B12 or folate deficiency	5–10
Myelodysplastic syndrome*	5
Leukaemia or lymphoma	5
Unknown causes	5–10

* A condition in which the bone marrow produces reduced numbers of red blood cells.

ciency is at a higher prevalence due to infection with malaria, hookworm, schistosomiasis and tuberculosis. In older adults, iron deficiency is most likely to be attributable to blood loss, and deficiency due to poor dietary intakes is rare (Lanier *et al.*, 2018). Occult bleeding can be the result of treatment with non-steroidal anti-inflammatory drugs, but it is more often the result of underlying gastrointestinal pathologies, including gastric cancers, peptic ulcers, colonic cancers and colonic polyps. Iron deficiency in older adults, as with younger groups, is most effectively treated through the administration of iron supplements, but given that it may indicate more sinister pathologies (Figure 9.14), this treatment should be accompanied by gastrointestinal investigations (Mukhopadhyay and Mohanaruban, 2002).

9.6.4.2 Vitamin B12 deficiency

Deficiency of vitamin B12 (cobalamin) is relatively common among the elderly population as a result of malabsorption. Most estimates (Andrès *et al.*, 2004) suggest that at least 20% of the over-65s are marginally deficient in cobalamin, with greater prevalence among institutionalized elderly (30–40%) than in the community (12%). In the UK National Diet and Nutrition Survey (Roberts *et al.*, 2018) 3–8% of older adults had serum B12 concentrations below the

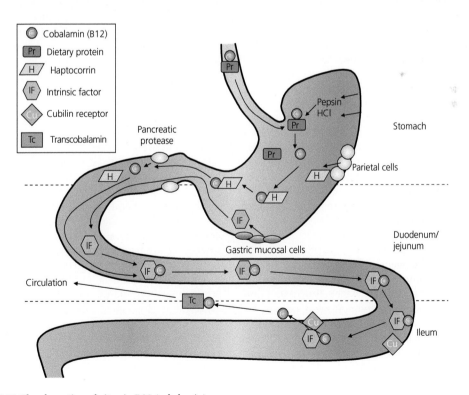

Figure 9.15 The absorption of vitamin B12 (cobalamin).

threshold for deficiency. The US National Health and Nutrition Examination Surveys reported a prevalence of 3.8% for deficiency and marginal deficiency in 20.9% among adults over 50 years (Qi *et al.*, 2014).

It is rare for vitamin B12 deficiency to arise through inadequate dietary intakes, which would only be a concern in individuals consuming a strict vegetarian diet or in very severely malnourished individuals. Kwok *et al.* (2002) reported that the prevalence of deficiency was up to 75% in a population of elderly vegetarians in Hong Kong. The major causes of deficiency relate to the function of the digestive tract, which is why the elderly are a high-risk group (Stabler and Allen 2004). Cobalamin is absorbed through a complex process involving actions of the stomach and the small intestine (Andrès *et al.* 2004). Cobalamin in the diet generally enters the stomach bound to animal proteins (Figure 9.15). Pepsin and the stomach acid release the free cobalamin, which is then bound by haptocorrin, a protein released in saliva. The haptocorrin–cobalamin complex passes into the duodenum, where it is degraded, again releasing free cobalamin. This is then bound by intrinsic factor, which is produced within the stomach by the gastric parietal cells. The intrinsic factor–cobalamin complex binds to cubilin receptors in the ileum, and the cobalamin is then taken up and transported around the body by the three transcobalamin transporter proteins.

In older adults, pernicious anaemia associated with loss of gastric parietal cells accounts for 15–20% of cases of cobalamin deficiency, while most other cases are the product of malabsorption due to atrophy of cells within the gastric mucosa, atrophy of the ileum or bacterial overgrowth of the small intestine. Infection with *H. pylori* can also contribute to cobalamin malabsorption. Cobalamin deficiency can be treated, with rapid improvements in associated symptoms. Treatment protocols seek to build up and maintain cobalamin reserves through repeated high-dose depot injections, as the underlying gastrointestinal causes of deficiency are unlikely to be resolved (Reynolds, 2006).

9.6.4.3 Folate deficiency

Folate deficiency is generally considered to be uncommon in westernized countries, although in some parts of the world, prevalence may be high and related to poverty. The most sensitive indicators of folate status are serum and red cell folate concentrations. Folate deficiency is defined as blood folate below 305 nmol/l, while concentrations below 550 nmol/l are indicative of high risk of insufficiency. In developed countries the preva-

lence of low folate status is highly dependent upon whether the diet includes fortified grains. The introduction of mandatory folate fortification in the United States and Australia has made folate deficiency extremely uncommon (Slagman *et al.*, 2019; Pfeiffer *et al.*, 2019). Gonzalez-Velez *et al.* (2020) reported deficiency in just 0.7% of a US population of older adults. This contrasts with the UK rolling National Diet and Nutrition Surveys (Bates *et al.*, 2017), which reported that 2% of men and 5% of women aged 65 and over were folate deficient and approximately one quarter had blood folate concentrations in the insufficient range. The contrasting prevalence in the UK compared with the United States is probably attributable solely to the lack of a fortification policy being in place. The Dutch Lifelines Micronutrients and Health Inequalities in Elderly study also reported high prevalence of deficiency (19.5%) and insufficiency (16.3%) among 60–75-year-olds. Lower socioeconomic status was a major risk factor for folate insufficiency, with the effect mediated through low dietary quality (Zhu *et al.*, 2020).

Any intervention to increase folic acid intakes in the elderly, whether through supplementation or fortification of staple foods, must be handled with caution. Folic acid repletion can have important consequences for the individuals in the population who are vitamin B12 deficient. B12 deficiency is often unrecognized as the clinical symptoms are often regarded as normal features of ageing. Most diagnosis is through the identification of megaloblastic anaemia in routine blood sampling, with follow-up measurements of methylmalonate, or cobalamin. Increased folic acid intakes can mask the haematological signs of vitamin B12 deficiency by resolving the megaloblastic anaemia, but do not remove the other consequences of B12 deficiency. Folic acid may also be toxic to individuals with B12 deficiency and accelerate neurological damage. For this reason, many people have expressed concerns about the general fortification of foods with folic acid, aimed at preventing spina bifida and improving population's cardiovascular health (Cuskelly *et al.*, 2007). However, evidence from the US post-introduction of folate fortification in 1998 suggests limited impact upon B12 status. Comparison of the US National Health and Nutrition Examination Surveys in 1994/1995 and 2001/2006 showed no change in the prevalence of low serum vitamin B12 among the population over 50 years of age and a decline in the prevalence of marginal deficiency post-fortification (Qi *et al.*, 2014).

9.6.4.4 Cognitive impairment and anaemia

Mild impairment of cognitive function, particularly memory, is a common feature of ageing, but in a substantial number of older adults the impairment is more serious. Dementia is a progressive and irreversible deterioration of memory, reasoning and mental acuity. The two major forms are Alzheimer's disease (AZD) and vascular dementia. AZD results from the formation of neuronal tangles and plaques of amyloid protein in the brain and, in particular, loss of neurons in the cerebral cortex and the temporal and parietal lobes. Vascular dementia is associated with impaired blood flow to the brain and neuronal death due to local hypoxia. This may occur due to atherosclerosis (and is hence subject to nutritional influences), major strokes and small strokes called transient ischaemic accidents. Some older people develop mixed dementia in which both vascular dementia and AZD are present.

With increasing lifespan, the numbers of people living with dementia are increasing rapidly and it is estimated that globally the numbers will double between 2020 and 2040 (Rizzi et al., 2014). It is estimated that over 11 million people in China, 9 million in Western Europe and 5 million in the United States are currently living with dementia; 80% of cases are AZD in developed countries, while in Asia and other regions vascular dementia is a little more common (30% of all cases; Wolters and Ikram, 2019). Prevalence in Europe is approximately 7% (Rizzi et al., 2014) and 11% in the United States (Hebert et al., 2013). Approximately one third of older people with dementia are unable to maintain independent living and two thirds of those living in institutional settings have dementia (Matthews and Dening, 2002). Many sufferers enter care settings because dementia increases the risk of falls and longer hospital stays that eventually lead to discharge to care rather than home (Bu and Rutherford, 2018).

Longer hospital stays are a factor which will promote poor nutritional status in dementia sufferers. Hospital-acquired malnutrition and the greater nutritional demands of healing, infection and pressure sores are drivers of poor nutrition. People with dementia are limited in terms of activities of daily living and will develop difficulties with simple tasks such as getting dressed, self-hygiene and, in more severe stages, communication and self-feeding (Prizer and Zimmerman, 2018). Tasks such as making and pouring drinks become challenging, leading to dehydration, while going shopping for food and cooking may be impossible.

A number of observations have suggested that long chain n-3 fatty acids may protect against cognitive decline. A 4.5-year follow-up of subjects aged 76 and over found that risk of dementia was lower in those in the highest tertile for docosahexaenoic acid (DHA) and eicosapentaenoic acid (EPA) intake (Gustafson et al., 2020). Higher concentrations of these fatty acids in circulation were associated with slower cognitive decline and lower risk of dementia in the study of Thomas et al. (2020). However, numerous studies have failed to show any benefit of supplementation in prevention of dementia. Andrieu et al. (2017) reported that DHA 800 mg per day and EPA 225 mg per day had no impact on cognitive decline over three years. The preDIVA study included n-3 fatty acids as part of a multidomain intervention for older adults but had no effect on development or progression of dementia over a six-year period (Moll van Charante et al., 2016). However, administration of very high dose n-3 fatty acids (DHA 1.7 g/day and EPA 0.6 g/day) over six months improved cognition in patients with mild to moderate AZD (Jernerén et al., 2019). This effect was greatest in subjects whose plasma homocysteine concentration was below 11.7 µmol/l, suggesting an interaction of n-3 fatty acids and B vitamins.

Homocysteine has been shown to cause neuronal death and promote formation of amyloid plaques in the brain and is seen as a risk factor for both AZD and vascular dementia (Perez et al., 2012; Gillette-Guyonnet et al., 2013). High circulating concentrations of homocysteine have been noted in patients with AZD and appear to precede the onset of any cognitive impairments. Hyperhomocysteinaemia was found to be a risk factor for cognitive decline (RR 1.53, 95% CI 1.23–1.91 when comparing subjects with hyperhomocysteinaemia with those in the normal range; Nie et al., 2014). The relative risk of AZD with hyperhomocysteinaemia is 2.5 (95% CI 1.38–4.56; Van Dam and Van Gool, 2009). The metabolism of homocysteine is closely associated with the dietary availability of folic acid, vitamin B12 and vitamin B6 (see Section 8.4.4.3.4) and, as such, these nutrients are of interest in this field.

Vitamin B12 deficiency has long been associated with cognitive problems. The deficiency manifests as both haematological and neuronal abnormalities, and a high prevalence of neuropsychiatric disorders and memory impairment is seen in patients with vitamin B12 deficiency (Malouf and Areosa Sastre, 2003). An extensive literature shows that low vitamin B12 and folate status are associated with dementia and cognitive decline. For example, in the study of Ma et al. (2017), patients with both AZD and mild cognitive impairment had elevated homocysteine and lower blood folate and vitamin B12 concentrations. Subjects in the lower tertile of folate concentration were at markedly greater risk of AZD (3.42, 95% CI 1.15–8.34). One of the major concerns about folic acid fortification on a population-wide scale is that it may mask haematological evidence of vitamin B12 deficiency and therefore increase risk of associated cognitive impairment. A cross-sectional evaluation of participants in the US National Health and Nutrition Examination Survey showed that low folate and vitamin B12 was associated with cognitive impairment, but that the combination of high folate and low vitamin B12 was also associated with worse cognitive function (Bailey et al., 2020). In contrast, the Irish Longitudinal Study on Ageing found that high folate, low vitamin B12 was not associated with cognitive deficit (O'Connor et al., 2020).

While homocysteine is a risk indicator for dementia, B vitamin supplementation strategies that aim to lower homocysteine are largely ineffective in reducing cognitive decline. The VITACOG study found that providing a supplement of folate 5 mg per day and vitamin B12 1 mg per day to patients with early-stage AZD over two years slowed cognitive decline and brain atrophy (de Jager et al., 2012). This study is the exception to a large body of evidence that suggests no cognitive benefits for older people. Kwok et al. (2020) randomized people over 65 years of age to placebo or cobalamin 500 µg/day and folic acid 400 µg/day for two years and found no cognitive benefit. A meta-analysis of 31 B vitamin supplementation trials found no evidence of significant benefits for dementia or mild cognitive impairment (Ford and Almeida, 2019). The discrepancy between observational studies and randomized controlled trials may arise because the trials recruit subjects at an age when it is too late to arrest the cognitive degeneration, because the trials are of too short a duration, or because they fail to control for the influence of factors such as genotype for enzymes in the methionine-homocysteine and folate cycles. It is also possible that the associations between the B vitamins, AZD and dementia may not be causal, despite the plausible mechanisms that have been advanced. Individuals with dementia are highly likely to become malnourished and hence develop anaemia as a result of their psychological difficulties. Dementia impacts upon all areas of self-care, and the ability to shop, cook and feed declines. It is therefore difficult to determine whether poor intakes and absorption of B vitamins associated with anaemia promote dementia, or vice versa.

SUMMARY

- On a global scale, numbers of older adults in the population are increasing rapidly. Greater lifespan means that nutrition-related health problems associated with ageing are set to become more prevalent.
- Ageing-related declines in physiological functions are a product of the accumulation of cells with a senescent phenotype within tissues. Cellular senescence may be driven by oxidative processes, but telomere shortening and activation of the Ink4a pathway also provide important mechanisms for limiting the normal lifespan of cellular functions.
- Caloric restriction may provide a means for extension of lifespan. However, this modulation of rates of ageing may be effective only when introduced early in life. The adverse impact of caloric restriction on human health and wellbeing may offset any benefit of a longer lifespan.
- Older adults have similar nutrient requirements to younger adults, but declining energy expenditure means that the optimal diet should be more nutrient dense.
- The elderly population are the main at-risk group for malnutrition in developed countries. Risk is associated with physical decline and chronic disease, with poverty, social isolation, institutionalization and a lack of knowledge of food and nutrition.
- Osteoporosis is a condition which primarily affects the elderly. Optimal intakes of vitamin D and calcium may reduce the risk of falls and fractures.
- Older adults are at high risk of gastrointestinal diseases, some of which will impact upon other aspects of health through impairment of the absorption of key micronutrients.
- There is a high prevalence of anaemia among the elderly population, with macrocytic anaemias associated with vitamin B12 and folate deficiencies predominating. Anaemia in the elderly is most commonly a product of chronic disease, but risk is also driven by malabsorption and other factors associated with malnutrition.
- The numbers of older adults living with dementia are increasing rapidly. Dementia impacts on capacity to acquire and prepare food and is a risk factor for malnutrition. Poor B vitamin status is a risk factor for dementia.

References

Abrahamsen, J.F., Monsen, A.L., Landi, F. et al. (2016). Readmission and mortality one year after acute hospitalization in older patients with explained and unexplained anemia: a prospective observational cohort study. BMC Geriatrics **16**: 109.

Aiello, A., Farzaneh, F., Candore, G. *et al.* (2019). Immunosenescence and its hallmarks: how to oppose aging strategically? a review of potential options for therapeutic intervention. *Frontiers in Immunology* **10**: 2247.

Aihie-Sayer, A., Dunn, R., Langley-Evans, S. *et al.* (2001). Prenatal exposure to a maternal low protein diet shortens life span in rats. *Gerontology* **47**: 9–14.

Almanza, B.A., Namkung, Y., Ismail, J.A. *et al.* (2007). Clients' safe food-handling knowledge and risk behavior in a home-delivered meal program. *Journal of the American Dietetic Association* **107**: 816–821.

An, R. (2015). Association of home-delivered meals on daily energy and nutrient intakes: findings from the national health and nutrition examination surveys. *Journal of Nutrition Gerontology and Geriatrics* **34**: 263–272.

Andrès, E., Loukili, N.H., Noel, E. *et al.* (2004). Vitamin B12 (cobalamin) deficiency in elderly patients. *Canadian Medical Association Journal* **171**: 251–259.

Andrieu, S., Guyonnet, S., Coley, N. *et al.* (2017). Effect of long-term omega 3 polyunsaturated fatty acid supplementation with or without multidomain intervention on cognitive function in elderly adults with memory complaints (MAPT): a randomised, placebo-controlled trial. *Lancet Neurology* **16**: 377–389.

Appleton, K.M., McGill, R. and Woodside, J.V. (2009). Fruit and vegetable consumption in older individuals in Northern Ireland: levels and patterns. *British Journal of Nutrition* **102**: 949–953.

Aspray, T.J., Chadwick, T., Francis, R.M. *et al.* (2019). Randomized controlled trial of vitamin D supplementation in older people to optimize bone health. *American Journal of Clinical Nutrition* **109**: 207–217.

Avenell, A., Mak, J.C. and O'Connell, D. (2014). Vitamin D and vitamin D analogues for preventing fractures in post-menopausal women and older men. *Cochrane Database of Systematic Reviews* (4): CD000227.

Bailey, R.L., Jun, S., Murphy, L. *et al.* (2020). High folic acid or folate combined with low vitamin B-12 status: potential but inconsistent association with cognitive function in a nationally representative cross-sectional sample of US older adults participating in the NHANES. *American Journal of Clinial Nutrition* **112**: 1547–1557

Banks, R., Speakman, J.R. and Selman, C. (2010). Vitamin E supplementation and mammalian lifespan. *Molecular Nutrition and Food Research* **54**: 719–725.

BAPEN. (2020). *National Survey of Malnutrition and Nutritional Care in Adults*. Redditch: BAPEN.

Barbour, K.E., Zmuda, J.M., Strotmeyer, E.S. *et al.* (2010). Correlates of trabecular and cortical volumetric bone mineral density of the radius and tibia in older men: the Osteoporotic Fractures in Men Study. *Journal of Bone and Mineral Research* **25**: 1017–1028.

Bates, B., Page, P., Cox, L. *et al.* (2017). *National Diet and Nutrition Survey Rolling Programme (NDNS RP) Supplementary report: blood folate results for the UK as a whole, Scotland, Northern Ireland (Years 1 to 4 combined) and Wales (Years 2 to 5 combined)*. London: Public Health England.

Beasley, J.M., Lacroix, A.Z., Larson, J.C. *et al.* (2014). Biomarker-calibrated protein intake and bone health in the Women's Health Initiative clinical trials and observational study. *American Journal of Clinical Nutrition* **99**: 934–940.

Belsky, D.W., Huffman, K.M., Pieper, C.F. *et al.* (2017). Change in the rate of biological aging in response to caloric restriction: CALERIE biobank analysis. *Journal of Gerontology A Biological Science and Medical Science* **73**: 4–10.

Bischoff-Ferrari, H.A., Stähelin, H.B., Dick, W. *et al.* (2003). Effects of vitamin D and calcium supplementation on falls: a randomized controlled trial. *Journal of Bone and Mineral Research* **18**: 343–351.

Blekken, L.E., Nakrem, S., Vinsnes, A.G. *et al.* (2016). Constipation and laxative use among nursing home patients: prevalence and associations derived from the residents assessment instrument for long-term care facilities (interRAI LTCF). *Gastroenterology Research and Practice* **2016**: 1215746.

Boccardi, V. and Poalisso, G. (2014). Telomerase activation: a potential key modulator for human healthspan and longevity. *Ageing Research Review* **15**: 1–5.

Bolland, M.J., Grey, A., Avenell, A. *et al.* (2011). Calcium supplements with or without vitamin D and risk of cardiovascular events: reanalysis of the Women's Health Initiative limited access dataset and meta-analysis. *BMJ* **342**: d2040.

Boonen, S., Lips, P., Bouillon, R. *et al.* (2007). Need for additional calcium to reduce the risk of hip fracture with vitamin D supplementation: evidence from a comparative metaanalysis of randomized controlled trials. *Journal of Clinical Endocrinology and Metabolism* **92**: 1415–1423.

Borkent, J.W., Naumann, E., Vasse, E. *et al.* (2019). Prevalence and determinants of undernutrition in a sample of Dutch community-dwelling older adults: results from two online screening tools. *International Journal of Environmental Research and Public Health* **16**: 1562.

Bouillanne, O., Morineau, G., Dupont, C. *et al.* (2005). Geriatric Nutritional Risk Index: a new index for evaluating at-risk elderly medical patients. *American Journal of Clinical Nutrition* **82**: 777–783.

Boyé, N.D., Oudshoorn, C., van der Velde, N. *et al.* (2013). Vitamin D and physical performance in older men and women visiting the emergency department because of a fall: data from the improving medication prescribing to reduce risk of falls (IMPROveFALL) study. *Journal of the American Geriatric Society* **61**: 1948–1952.

Broe, K.E., Chen, T.C., Weinberg, F. *et al.* (2007). A higher dose of vitamin D reduces the risk of falls in nursing home residents: a randomized, multiple-dose study. *Journal of the American Geriatric Society* **55**: 234–239.

Bruyere, O., Decock, C., Delhez, M. *et al.* (2009). Highest prevalence of vitamin D inadequacy in institutionalized women compared with noninstitutionalized women: a case-control study. *Womens Health* **5**: 49–54.

Bu, F., Rutherford, A. (2018). Dementia, home care and institutionalisation from hospitals in older people. *European Journal of Ageing* **16**: 283–291.

Burt, L.A., Billington, E.O., Rose, M.S. *et al.* (2020). Adverse effects of high-dose vitamin d supplementation on volumetric bone density are greater in females than males. *Journal of Bone and Mineral Research* **35**: 2404–2414.

Cameron, I.D., Dyer, S.M., Panagoda, C.E. *et al.* (2018). Interventions for preventing falls in older people in care facilities and hospitals. *Cochrane Database of Systematic Reviews* (9): CD005465.

Campisi, J. (1997). The biology of replicative senescence. *European Journal of Cancer* **33**: 703–709.

Carrier, N., Ouellet, D. and West, G.E. (2007). Nursing home food services linked with risk of malnutrition. *Canadian Journal of Dietetic Practice and Research* **68**: 14–20.

Castle, S.C., Uyemura, K., Fulop, T. *et al.* (2007). Host resistance and immune responses in advanced age. *Clinics in Geriatric Medicine* **23**: 463–479.

Chakkalakal, D.A. (2005). Alcohol-induced bone loss and deficient bone repair. *Alcoholism, Clinical and Experimental Research* **29**: 2077–2090.

Chen, Y.C., Zhang, L., Li, E.N. *et al.* (2017). Association of the insulin-like growth factor-1 single nucleotide polymorphisms rs35767, rs2288377, and rs5742612 with osteoporosis risk: a meta-analysis. *Medicine* **96**: e9231

Collado, M., Blasco, M.A. and Serrano, M. (2007). Cellular senescence in cancer and aging. *Cell* **130**: 223–233.

Costenbader, K.H., MacFarlane, L.A., Lee, I.M. *et al.* (2019). Effects of one year of vitamin d and marine omega-3 fatty acid supplementation on biomarkers of systemic inflammation in older US adults. *Clinical Chemistry* **65**: 1508–1521.

Crimmins, E.M. (2020). Age-related vulnerability to coronavirus disease 2019 (covid-19): biological, contextual, and policy-related factors. *Public Policy Aging Reports* **30**: 142–146.

Cuskelly, G.J., Mooney, K.M. and Young, I.S. (2007). Folate and vitamin B12: friendly or enemy nutrients for the elderly. *Proceedings of the Nutrition Society* **66**: 548–558.

D'Souza, A.L. (2007). Ageing and the gut. *Postgraduate Medical Journal* **83**: 44–53.

de Jager, C.A., Oulhaj, A., Jacoby, R. *et al.* (2012). Cognitive and clinical outcomes of homocysteine-lowering B-vitamin treatment in mild cognitive impairment: a randomized controlled trial. *International Journal of Geriatric Psychiatry* **27**: 592–600.

Delmi, M., Rapin, C.H., Bengoa, J.M. *et al.* (1990). Dietary supplementation in elderly patients with fractured neck of the femur. *Lancet* **335**: 1013–1016.

den Elzen, W.P., Willems, J.M., Westendorp, R.G. *et al.* (2010). Effect of erythropoietin levels on mortality in old age: the Leiden 85-plus Study. *Canadian Medical Association Journal* **182**: 1953–1958.

Department of Health. (1999). *Dietary Reference Values for Food Energy and Nutrients for the United Kingdom*. London: Stationery Office.

Diallo, A.F., Falls, K., Hicks, K. *et al.* (2020). The Healthy Meal Program: a food insecurity screening and referral program for urban dwelling older adults. *Public Health Nursing* **37**: 671–676.

Dirks, A.J. and Leeuwenburgh, C. (2006). Caloric restriction in humans: potential pitfalls and health concerns. *Mechanisms of Ageing and Development* **127**: 1–7.

Donini, L.M., De Felice, M.R., Tagliaccica, A. *et al.* (2005). Nutritional status and evolution of pressure sores in geriatric patients. *Journal of Nutrition, Health and Ageing* **9**: 446–454.

Donini, L.M., Scardella, P., Piombo, L. *et al.* (2012). Malnutrition in elderly: Social and economic determinants. *Journal of Nutrition, Health and Aging* **17**: 9–15.

Dorling, J.L., van Vliet, S., Huffman, K.M. *et al.* (2021). Effects of caloric restriction on human physiological, psychological, and behavioral outcomes: highlights from CALERIE phase 2. *Nutrition Reviews* **79**: 98–113.

Eastwood, C., Davies, G.J., Gardiner, F.K. *et al.* (2002). Energy intakes of institutionalised and free-living older people. *Journal of Nutrition, Health and Ageing* **6**: 91–92.

Eisenstaedt, R., Penninx, B.W. and Woodman, R.C. (2006). Anemia in the elderly: current understanding and emerging concepts. *Blood Reviews* **20**: 213–226.

Eurostat. (2019). One in seven pensioners at risk of poverty in the EU. https://ec.europa.eu/eurostat/web/products-eurostat-news/-/DDN-20190115-1 (accessed 13 April 2021).

Ferry, M., Sidobre, B., Lambertin, A. *et al.* (2005). The SOLINUT study: analysis of the interaction between nutrition and loneliness in persons aged over 70 years. *Journal of Nutrition Health and Ageing* **9**: 261–268.

Fontana, L., Meyer, T.E., Klein, S. *et al.* (2004). Long-term calorie restriction is highly effective in reducing the risk for atherosclerosis in humans. *Proceedings of the National Academy of Sciences of the United States of America* **101**: 6659–6663.

Fontes, D., Generoso Sde, V. and Toulson Davisson Correia, M.I. (2014). Subjective global assessment: a reliable nutritional assessment tool to predict outcomes in critically ill patients. *Clinical Nutrition* **33**: 291–295.

Ford, A.H. and Almeida, O.P. (2019). Effect of vitamin b supplementation on cognitive function in the elderly: a systematic review and meta-analysis. *Drugs and Aging* **36**: 419–434.

Gariballa, S. and Forster, S. (2007). Malnutrition is an independent predictor of 1-year mortality following acute illness. *British Journal of Nutrition* **98**: 332–336.

Gaskell, H., Derry, S., Andrew Moore, R. *et al.* (2008). Prevalence of anaemia in older persons: systematic review. *BMC Geriatrics* **8**: 1.

Gillette-Guyonnet, S., Secher, M. and Vellas, B. (2013). Nutrition and neurodegeneration: epidemiological evidence and challenges for future research. *British Journal of Clinical Pharmacology* **75**: 738–755.

Goldberg, S.L. and Mawn, B.E. (2015). Predictors of food insecurity among older adults in the United States. *Public Health Nursing* **32**: 397–407

Gollub, E.A. and Weddle, D.O. (2004). Improvements in nutritional intake and quality of life among frail homebound older adults receiving home-delivered breakfast and lunch. *Journal of the American Dietetic Association* **104**: 1227–1235.

Gomes, N.M., Ryder, O.A., Houck, M.L. *et al.* (2011). Comparative biology of mammalian telomeres: hypotheses on ancestral states and the roles of telomeres in longevity determination. *Aging Cell* **10**: 761–768.

Goncalves-Mendes, N., Talvas, J., Dualé, C. *et al.* (2019). Impact of vitamin D supplementation on influenza vaccine response and immune functions in deficient elderly persons: a randomized placebo-controlled trial. *Frontiers in Immunology* **10**: 65.

Gonzalez-Velez, M., Mead-Harvey, C., Kosiorek, H.E. *et al.* (2020). Racial/ethnic differences in patients with anemia and folate deficiency. *International Journal of Laboratory Hematology* **42**: 403–410.

Grados, F., Brazier, M., Kamel, S. *et al.* (2003). Effects on bone mineral density of calcium and vitamin D supplementation in elderly women with vitamin D deficiency. *Joint Bone and Spine* **70**: 203–208.,

Grant, A.M., Avenell, A., Campbell, M.K. *et al.* (2005). Oral vitamin D3 and calcium for secondary prevention of low-trauma fractures in elderly people (Randomised Evaluation of Calcium Or vitamin D, RECORD): a randomised placebo-controlled trial. *Lancet* **365**: 1621–1628.

Griep, M.I., Mets, T.F., Vercruysse, A. *et al.* (1995). Food odor thresholds in relation to age, nutritional, and health status. *Journal of Gerontology Series A: Biological Sciences and Medical Sciences* **50**: B407–B414.

Groenendijk, I., den Boeft, L., van Loon, L.J.C. and de Groot, L.C.P.G.M (2019). High versus low dietary protein intake and bone health in older adults: a systematic review and meta-analysis. *Computational and Structural Biotechnology Journal* **17**: 1101–1112.

Guo, J.L., Tsai, Y.Y., Liao, J.Y. *et al.* (2014). Interventions to reduce the number of falls among older adults with/without cognitive impairment: an exploratory meta-analysis. *International Journal of Geriatric Psychiatry* **29**: 661–669.

Gustafson, D.R., Bäckman, K., Scarmeas, N. *et al.* (2020). Dietary fatty acids and risk of Alzheimer's disease and related dementias: observations from the Washington Heights–Hamilton Heights–Inwood Columbia Aging Project (WHICAP). *Alzheimer's and Dementia* 16: 1638–1649.

Gustafsson, M., Lämås, K., Isaksson, U. *et al.* (2019). Constipation and laxative use among people living in nursing homes in 2007 and 2013. *BMC Geriatrics* **19**: 38.

Hallström, H., Melhus, H., Glynn, A. *et al.* (2010). Coffee consumption and CYP1A2 genotype in relation to bone mineral density of the proximal femur in elderly men and women: a cohort study. *Nutrition and Metabolism* **7**: 12.

Hallström, H., Byberg, L., Glynn, A. *et al.* (2013). Long-term coffee consumption in relation to fracture risk and bone mineral density in women. *American Journal of Epidemiology* **178**: 898–909.

Hebert, L.E., Weuve, J., Scherr, P.A. and Evans, D.A. (2013). Alzheimer disease in the United States (2010–2050) estimated using the 2010 census. *Neurology* **80**: 1778–1783.

Heilbronn, L.K., de Jonge, L., Frisard, M.I. *et al.* (2006). Effect of 6-month calorie restriction on biomarkers of longevity, metabolic adaptation, and oxidative stress in overweight individuals: a randomized controlled trial. *JAMA* **295**: 1539–1548.

Hengeveld, L.M., Boer, J.M.A., Gaudreau, P., *et al.* (2020). Prevalence of protein intake below recommended in community-dwelling older adults: a meta-analysis across cohorts from the PROMISS consortium. *Journal of Cachexia Sarcopenia and Muscle* **11**: 1212–1222.

Herrmann, W. and Herrmann, M. (2020). The importance of telomere shortening for atherosclerosis and mortality. *Journal of Cardiovascular Development and Disease* **7**: 29.

High, K.P. (2001). Nutritional strategies to boost immunity and prevent infection in elderly individuals. *Clinical Infectious Diseases* **33**: 1892–1900.

Hoffmann, J.C. and Zeitz, M. (2002). Small bowel disease in the elderly: diarrhoea and malabsorption. *Best Practice and Research. Clinical Gastroenterology* **16**: 17–36.

Hu, Z.C., Tang, Q., Sang, C.M. *et al.* (2019). Comparison of fracture risk using different supplemental doses of vitamin D, calcium or their combination: a network meta-analysis of randomised controlled trials. *BMJ Open* 9: e024595.

Huncharek, M., Muscat, J. and Kupelnick, B. (2008). Impact of dairy products and dietary calcium on bone-mineral content in children: results of a meta-analysis. *Bone* **43**: 312–321.

Ijmker-Hemink, V.E., Dijxhoorn, D.N., Briseno Ozumbilla, C.M. *et al.* (2020). Effective elements of home-delivered meal services to improve energy and protein intake: a systematic review. *Nutrition* **69**: 110537.

Ishimi, Y. (2010). Dietary equol and bone metabolism in postmenopausal Japanese women and osteoporotic mice. *Journal of Nutrition* **140**: 1373S–1376S.

Janzen, V., Forkert, R., Fleming, H.E. *et al.* (2006). Stem-cell ageing modified by the cyclin-dependent kinase inhibitor p16INK4a. *Nature* **443**: 421–426.

Jennings, B.J., Ozanne, S.E., Dorling, M.W. *et al.* (1999). Early growth determines longevity in male rats and may be related to telomere shortening in the kidney. *FEBS Letters* **448**: 4–8.

Jernerén, F., Cederholm, T., Refsum, H. *et al.* (2019). Homocysteine status modifies the treatment effect of omega-3 fatty acids on cognition in a randomized clinical trial in mild to moderate Alzheimer's disease: the OmegAD Study. *Journal of Alzheimers Disease* **69**: 189–197.

Joseph Rowntree Foundation. (2019). *Pensioner poverty*. https://www.jrf.org.uk/data/pensioner-poverty (accessed 13 April 2021).

Kanis, J.A., Johnell, O., Oden, A. *et al.* (2002). Ten-year risk of osteoporotic fracture and the effect of risk factors on screening strategies. *Bone* **30**: 251–258.

Karlsson, M.K., Vonschewelov, T., Karlsson, C. *et al.* (2013). Prevention of falls in the elderly: a review. *Scandinavian Journal of Public Health* **41**: 442–454.

Keen, R. (2007). Osteoporosis: strategies for prevention and management. *Best Practice and Research: Clinical Rheumatology* **21**: 109–122.

Kiesswetter, E., Pohlhausen, S., Uhlig, K. *et al.* (2014). Prognostic differences of the Mini Nutritional Assessment short form and long form in relation to 1-year functional decline and mortality in community-dwelling older adults receiving home care. *Journal of the American Geriatric Association* **62**: 512–517.

Kluger, M.J., Kozak, W., Conn, C.A. *et al.* (1998). Role of fever in disease. *Annals of the New York Academy of Science* **856**: 224–233.

Kondrup, J., Rasmussen, H.H., Hamberg, O. and Stanga, Z. (2003). Nutritional risk screening (NRS 2002): a new method based on an analysis of controlled clinical trials. *Clinical Nutrition* **22**: 321–336.

Kretser, A.J., Voss, T., Kerr, W.W. *et al.* (2003). Effects of two models of nutritional intervention on homebound older adults at nutritional risk. *Journal of the American Dietetic Association* **103**: 329–336.

Krok-Schoen, J.L., Archdeacon Price, A., Luo, M. *et al.* (2019). Low dietary protein intakes and associated dietary patterns and functional limitations in an aging population: A NHANES analysis. *Journal of Nutrition Health ad Aging* **23**: 338–347.

Kwok, T., Cheng, G., Woo, J. *et al.* (2002). Independent effect of vitamin B12 deficiency on hematological status in older Chinese vegetarian women. *American Journal of Hematology* **70**: 186–190.

Kwok, T., Wu, Y., Lee, J. *et al.* (2020). A randomized placebo-controlled trial of using B vitamins to prevent cognitive decline in older mild cognitive impairment patients. *Clinical Nutrition* **39**: 2399–2405.

Lahalle, A., Lacroix, M., De Blasio, C. *et al.* (2021). The p53 pathway and metabolism: the tree that hides the forest. *Cancers* **13**: 133.

Langley-Evans, S.C. and Sculley, D.V. (2006). The association between birthweight and longevity in the rat is complex and modulated by maternal protein intake during fetal life. *FEBS Letters* **580**: 4150–4153.

Lanier, J.B., Park, J.J. and Callahan, R.C. (2018). Anemia in older adults. *American Family Physician* **98**: 437–442.

Lappe, J., Kunz, I., Bendik, I. *et al.* (2013). Effect of a combination of genistein, polyunsaturated fatty acids and vitamins D3 and K1 on bone mineral density in postmenopausal women: a randomized, placebo-controlled, double-blind pilot study. *European Journal of Nutrition* **52**: 203–215.

Law, M., Withers, H., Morris, J. *et al.* (2006). Vitamin D supplementation and the prevention of fractures and falls: results of a randomised trial in older adults in residential accommodation. *Age and Ageing* **35**: 482–486.

Lee, J.W. and Ong, E.B.B. (2021). Genomic instability and cellular senescence: lessons from the budding yeast. *Frontiers in Cellular and Developmental Biology* **8**: 619126.

Leistra, E., Willeboordse, F., van Bokhorst-de van der Schueren, M.A. *et al.* (2011). Predictors for achieving protein and energy requirements in undernourished hospital patients. *Clinical Nutrition* **30**: 484–489.

Li, Z. and Dalaker, J. (2019). *Poverty among Americans aged 65 and older*. Washington, DC: Congressional Research Service.

Liu, C., Kuang, X., Li, K. *et al.* (2020). Effects of combined calcium and vitamin D supplementation on osteoporosis in postmenopausal women: a systematic review and meta-analysis of randomized controlled trials. *Food and Function* **11**: 10817–10827.

Luchsinger, J.A., Tang, M.X., Miller, J. *et al.* (2007). Relation of higher folate intake to lower risk of Alzheimer disease in the elderly. *Archives of Neurology* **64**: 86–92.

Ma, F., Wu, T., Zhao, J. *et al.* (2017). Plasma homocysteine and serum folate and vitamin b12 levels in mild cognitive impairment and Alzheimer's disease: a case–control study. *Nutrients* **9**: 725.

Malouf, R. and Areosa Sastre, A. (2003). Vitamin B12 for cognition. *Cochrane Database of Systematic Reviews* (3): CD004394.

Mamhidir, A.G., Karlsson, I., Norberg, A. *et al.* (2007) Weight increase in patients with dementia, and alteration in meal routines and meal environment after integrity promoting care. *Journal of Clinical Nursing* **16**: 987–996.

Maneerat, S., Lehtinen, M.J., Childs, C.E. *et al.* (2014). Consumption of *Bifidobacterium lactis* Bi-07 by healthy elderly adults enhances phagocytic activity of monocytes and granulocytes. *Journal of Nutrition Science* **2**: e44.

Marshall, B.J. (1994) Helicobacter pylori. *American Journal of Gastroenterology* **89**(8 Suppl): S116–S128.

Martin, C.K., Bhapkar, M., Pittas, A.G. *et al.* (2016). Effect of calorie restriction on mood, quality of life, sleep, and sexual function in healthy nonobese adults: the CALERIE 2 Randomized Clinical Trial. *JAMA Internal Medicine* **176**: 743–752.

Martin, H., Uring-Lambert, B., Adrian, M. *et al.* (2008). Effects of long-term dietary intake of magnesium on oxidative stress, apoptosis and ageing in rat liver. *Magnesium Research* **21**: 124–130.

Mather, K.A., Jorm, A.F., Parslow, R.A. *et al.* (2011) Is telomere length a biomarker of aging? A review. *Journal of Gerontology A. Biological Science and Medical Science*, **66**, 202–213.

Matthews, F.E., Dening, T. (2002). Prevalence of dementia in institutional care. *Lancet* **360**, 225–226.

Mattison, J.A., Roth, G.S., Beasley, T.M. *et al.* (2012) Impact of caloric restriction on health and survival in rhesus monkeys from the NIA study. *Nature*, **489**, 318–321.

McCaddon, A., Davies, G., Hudson, P. *et al.* (1998) Total serum homocysteine in senile dementia of Alzheimer type. *International Journal of Geriatric Psychiatry*, **13**, 235–239.

McEvoy, A., Dutton, J. and James, O.F. (1983). Bacterial contamination of the small intestine is an important cause of occult malabsorption in the elderly. *BMJ* **287**: 789–793.

McKiernan, S.H., Colman, R.J., Aiken, E. *et al.* (2012). Cellular adaptation contributes to calorie restriction-induced preservation of skeletal muscle in aged rhesus monkeys. *Experimental Gerontology* **47**: 229–236.

Mendonça, N., Kingston, A., Granic, A. and Jagger, C. (2019). Protein intake and transitions between frailty states and to death in very old adults: the Newcastle 85+ study. *Age and Ageing* **49**: 32–38.

Merry, B.J., Kirk, A.J. and Goyns, M.H. (2008). Dietary lipoic acid supplementation can mimic or block the effect of dietary restriction on life span. *Mechanisms of Ageing and Development* **129**: 341–348.

Meydani, S.N., Das, S.K., Pieper, C.F. *et al.* (2016). Long-term moderate calorie restriction inhibits inflammation without impairing cell-mediated immunity: a randomized controlled trial in non-obese humans. *Aging (Albany NY)* **8**: 1416–1431.

Mok, D.Z.L., Chan, C.Y.Y., Ooi, E.E. and Chan, K.R. (2020). The effects of aging on host resistance and disease tolerance to SARS-CoV-2 infection. *FEBS Journal* doi: 10.1111/ febs.15613.

Moll van Charante, E.P., Richard, E., Eurelings, L.S. *et al.* (2021). Effectiveness of a 6-year multidomain vascular care intervention to prevent dementia (preDIVA): a cluster-randomised controlled trial. *Lancet* **388**: 797–805

Mosoni, L., Balage, M., Vazeille, E. *et al.* (2010). Antioxidant supplementation had positive effects in old rat muscle, but through better oxidative status in other organs. *Nutrition* **26**: 1157–1162.

Mukhopadhyay, D. and Mohanaruban, K. (2002). Iron deficiency anaemia in older people: investigation, management and treatment. *Age and Ageing* **31**: 87–91.

Muller, F.L., Lustgarten, M.S., Jang, Y. *et al.* (2007). Trends in oxidative aging theories. *Free Radical Biology and Medicine* **43**: 477–503.

Nie, T., Lu, T., Xie, L. *et al.* (2014). Hyperhomocysteinemia and risk of cognitive decline: a meta-analysis of prospective cohort studies. *European Neurology* **72**: 241–248.

Norman, D.C. (2000). Fever in the elderly. *Clinics in Infectious Disease* **31**: 148–151.

O'Connor, D.M.A., Laird, E.J., Carey, D. *et al.* (2020). Plasma concentrations of vitamin B12 and folate and global cognitive function in an older population: cross-sectional findings from the Irish Longitudinal Study on Ageing (TILDA). *British Journal of Nutrition* **124**: 602–610.

Odencrants, S., Blomberg, K. and Wallin, A.M. (2019). 'The meal is an activity involving at least two people': Experiences of meals by older persons in need of elderly care. *Nursing Open* **7**: 265–273.

Omran, M.L. and Morley, J.E. (2000). Assessment of protein energy malnutrition in older persons, part I: history, examination, body composition, and screening tools. *Nutrition* **16**: 50–63.

Ozanne, S.E. and Hales, C.N. (2004). Lifespan: catch-up growth and obesity in male mice. *Nature* **427**: 411–412.

Pana, T.A., Dehghani, M., Baradaran, H.R. *et al.* (2021). Calcium intake, calcium supplementation and cardiovascular disease and mortality in the British population: EPIC-Norfolk prospective cohort study and meta-analysis. *European Journal of Epidemiology* doi: 10.1007/s10654-020-00710-8.

Pantell, M., Rehkopf, D., Jutte, D. *et al.* (2013) Social isolation: a predictor of mortality comparable to traditional clinical risk factors. *American Journal of Public Health* **103**: 2056–2062.

Perez, L., Heim, L., Sherzai, A. *et al.* (2012). Nutrition and vascular dementia. *Journal of Nutrition and Healthy Ageing* **16**: 319–324.

Pfeiffer, C.M., Sternberg, M.R., Zhang, M. *et al.* (2019). Folate status in the US population 20 y after the introduction of folic acid fortification. *American Journal of Clinical Nutrition* **110**: 1088–1097.

Pirrie, M., Harrison, L., Angeles, R. *et al.* (2020). Poverty and food insecurity of older adults living in social housing in Ontario: a cross-sectional study. *BMC Public Health* **20**: 1320.

Prince, R.L., Devine, A., Dhaliwal, S.S. and Dick, I.M. (2006). Effects of calcium supplementation on clinical fracture and bone structure: results of a 5-year, double-blind, placebo-controlled trial in elderly women. *Archives of Internal Medicine* **166**: 869–875.

Prizer, L.P., Zimmerman, S. (2018). Progressive support for activities of daily living for persons living with dementia. *Gerontologist* **58**(Suppl 1):, S74–S87.

Pusceddu, I., Kleber, M., Delgado, G. *et al.* (2018). Telomere length and mortality in the Ludwigshafen Risk and Cardiovascular Health study. *PLoS One* **13**: e0198373.

Qi, Y.P., Do, A.N., Hamner, H.C. *et al.* (2014). The prevalence of low serum vitamin B-12 status in the absence of anemia or macrocytosis did not increase among older U.S. adults after mandatory folic acid fortification. *Journal of Nutrition* **144**: 170–176.

Racette, S.B., Weiss, E.P., Villareal, D.T. *et al.* (2006). One year of caloric restriction in humans: feasibility and effects on body composition and abdominal adipose tissue. *Journal of Gerontology A Biological Science and Medical Science* **61**: 943–950.

Rajatanavin, R., Chailurkit, L., Saetung, S. *et al.* (2013). The efficacy of calcium supplementation alone in elderly Thai women over a 2-year period: a randomized controlled trial. *Osteoporosis International* **24**: 2871–2877.

Ramic, E., Pranjic, N., Batic-Mujanovic, O. *et al.* (2011). The effect of loneliness on malnutrition in elderly population. *Medical Archives* **65**: 92–95.

Rapuri, P.B., Gallagher, J.C., Kinyamu, H.K. *et al.* (2001). Caffeine intake increases the rate of bone loss in elderly women and interacts with vitamin D receptor genotypes. *American Journal of Clinical Nutrition* **74**: 694–700.

Rapuri, P.B., Gallagher, J.C. and Haynatzka, V. (2003). Protein intake: effects on bone mineral density and the rate of bone loss in elderly women. *American Journal of Clinical Nutrition* **77**: 1517–1525.

Ravussin, E., Redman, L.M., Rochon, J. *et al.* (2015). A 2-Year randomized controlled trial of human caloric restriction: feasibility and effects on predictors of health span and longevity. *Journal of Gerontology A Biological Science and Medical Science* **70**: 1097–1104.

Reid, I.R., Bolland, M.J. and Grey, A. (2014). Effects of vitamin D supplements on bone mineral density: a systematic review and meta-analysis. *Lancet* **383**: 146–155.

Reid, I.R., Bristow, S.M. and Bolland, M.J. (2015). Calcium supplements: benefits and risks. *Journal of Internal Medicine* **278**: 354–368.

Reynolds, E. (2006). Vitamin B12, folic acid, and the nervous system. *Lancet Neurology* **5**: 949–960.

Ricci, E., Cipriani, S., Chiaffarino, F. *et al.* (2010). Soy isoflavones and bone mineral density in perimenopausal and postmenopausal Western women: a systematic review and meta-analysis of randomized controlled trials. *Journal of Women's Health* **19**: 1609–1617.

Rizzi, L., Rosset, I. and Roriz-Cruz, M. (2014). Global epidemiology of dementia: Alzheimer's and vascular types. *Biomedical Research International* **2014**: 908915.

Roberts, C. Steer, T., Maplethorpe, N., *et al.* (2018). *National Diet and Nutrition Survey. Results from years 7 and 8 (combined) of the Rolling Programme*. London: Public Health England.

Romero-Corral, A., Montori, V.M., Somers, V.K. *et al.* (2006). Association of bodyweight with total mortality and with cardiovascular events in coronary artery disease: a systematic review of cohort studies. *Lancet* **368**: 666–678.

Roseman, M.G. (2007). Food safety perceptions and behaviors of participants in congregate-meal and home-delivered-meal programs. *Journal of Environmental Health* **70**: 13–21.

Roser, M., Ortiz-Ospina, E. and Ritchie, H. (2019). Life expectancy. *Our World in Data* https://ourworldindata.org/life-expectancy (accessed 13 April 2021).

Rothenbacher, D., Klenk, J., Denkinger, M.D. *et al.* (2014). Prospective evaluation of renal function, serum vitamin D level, and risk of fall and fracture in community-dwelling elderly subjects. *Osteoporosis International* **25**: 923–932.

Russell, J.C., Flood, V.M. and Yeatman, H. (2016). Food insecurity. *Australian Family Physician* **45**: 87.

Sanders, K.M., Scott, D. and Ebeling, P.R. (2014). Vitamin D deficiency and its role in muscle-bone interactions in the elderly. *Current Osteoporosis Reports* **12**: 74–81.

Sathyapalan, T., Aye, M., Rigby, A.S. *et al.* (2017). Soy reduces bone turnover markers in women during early menopause: a randomized controlled trial. *Journal of Bone and Mineral Research* **32**: 157–164.

Schuster, B.G., Kosar, L. and Kamrul, R. (2015). Constipation in older adults: stepwise approach to keep things moving. *Canadian Family Physician* **61**: 152–158.

Selman, C., McLaren, J.S., Meyer, C. *et al.* (2006). Life-long vitamin C supplementation in combination with cold exposure does not affect oxidative damage or lifespan in mice, but decreases expression of antioxidant protection genes. *Mechanisms of Ageing and Development* **127**: 897–904.

Selman, C., McLaren, J.S., Mayer, C. *et al.* (2008). Lifelong alpha-tocopherol supplementation increases the median life span of C57BL/6 mice in the cold but has only minor effects on oxidative damage. *Rejuvenation Research* **11**: 83–96.

Shakoor, H., Feehan, J., Al Dhaheri, A.S. *et al.* (2021). Immune-boosting role of vitamins D, C, E, zinc, selenium and omega-3 fatty acids: could they help against COVID-19? *Maturitas* **143**: 1–9.

Slagman, A., Harriss, L., Campbell, S. *et al.* (2019). Folic acid deficiency declined substantially after introduction of the mandatory fortification programme in Queensland, Australia: a secondary health data analysis. *Public Health Nutrition* **22**: 3426–3434.

Smith, D.L., Jr, Mattison, J.A., Desmond, R.A. *et al.* (2011). Telomere dynamics in rhesus monkeys: no apparent effect of caloric restriction. *Journal of Gerontology A: Biological Science and Medical Science* **66**: 1163–1168.

Smith, L.M., Gallagher, J.C., Kaufmann, M. and Jones, G. (2018). Effect of increasing doses of vitamin D on bone mineral density and serum N-terminal telopeptide in elderly women: a randomized controlled trial. *Journal of Internal Medicine* **284**: 685–693.

Sohal, R.S., Mockett, R.J. and Orr, W.C. (2002). Mechanisms of aging: an appraisal of the oxidative stress hypothesis. *Free Radical Biology and Medicine* **33**: 575–586.

Sohal, R.S., Kamzalov, S., Sumien, N. *et al.* (2006). Effect of coenzyme Q10 intake on endogenous coenzyme Q content, mitochondrial electron transport chain, antioxidative defenses, and life span of mice. *Free Radical Biology and Medicine* **40**: 480–487.

Speakman, J.R. and Hambly, C. (2007). Starving for life: what animal studies can and cannot tell us about the use of caloric restriction to prolong human lifespan. *Journal of Nutrition* **137**: 1078–1086.

Stabler, S.P. and Allen, R.H. (2004). Vitamin B12 deficiency as a worldwide problem. *Annual Review of Nutrition* **24**: 299–326.

Stear, S.J., Prentice, A., Jones, S.C. *et al.* (2003). Effect of a calcium and exercise intervention on the bone mineral status of 16-18-y-old adolescent girls. *American Journal of Clinical Nutrition* **77**: 985–992.

Steensma, D.P. and Tefferi, A. (2007). Anemia in the elderly: how should we define it, when does it matter, and what can be done? *Mayo Clinic Proceedings* **82**: 958–966.

Stein, M.S., Wark, J.D., Scherer, S.C. *et al.* (1999). Falls relate to vitamin D and parathyroid hormone in an Australian nursing home and hostel. *Journal of the American Geriatrics Society* **47**: 1195–1201.

Stratton, R.J., Hackston, A., Longmore, D. *et al.* (2004). Malnutrition in hospital outpatients and inpatients: prevalence, concurrent validity and ease of use of the 'malnutrition universal screening tool' ('MUST') for adults. *British Journal of Nutrition* **92**: 799–808.

Stratton, R.J., Ek, A.C., Engfer, M. *et al.* (2005). Enteral nutritional support in prevention and treatment of pressure ulcers: a systematic review and meta-analysis. *Ageing Research Reviews* **4**: 422–450.

Sund-Levander, M., Grodzinsky, E. and Wahren, L.K. (2007). Gender differences in predictors of survival in elderly nursing-home residents: a 3-year follow up. *Scandinavian Journal of Caring Sciences* **21**: 18–24.

Tang, B.M., Eslick, G.D., Nowson, C. *et al.* (2007). Use of calcium or calcium in combination with vitamin D supplementation to prevent fractures and bone loss in people aged 50 years and older: a meta-analysis. *Lancet* **370**: 657–666.

Tani, Y., Sasaki, Y., Haseda, M. *et al.* (2015). Eating alone and depression in older men and women by cohabitation status: the JAGES longitudinal survey. *Age and Ageing* **44**: 1019–1026.

Tasmanian Government Department of Health (2020). *Malnutrition.* https://www.dhhs.tas.gov.au/__data/assets/pdf_file/0004/343372/Malnutrition_background.pdf (accessed 13 April 2021).

Thomas, A., Baillet, M., Proust-Lima, C. *et al.* (2020). Blood polyunsaturated omega-3 fatty acids, brain atrophy, cognitive decline, and dementia risk. *Alzheimers and Dementia* doi: 10.1002/alz.12195.

Thompson, J. Tod, A., Bissell, P. and Bond, M. (2017). Understanding food vulnerability and health literacy in older bereaved men: A qualitative study. *Health Expectations* **2017**: 1–8.

Torregrosa-Muñumer, R., Vara, E., Fernández-Tresguerres, J.Á. and Gredilla, R. (2021). Resveratrol supplementation at old age reverts changes associated with aging in inflammatory, oxidative and apoptotic markers in rat heart. *European Journal of Nutrition* doi: 10.1007/s00394-020-02457-0.

van Bokhorst-de van der Schueren, M.A., Guaitoli, P.R., Jansma, E.P. and de Vet, H.C. (2014). Nutrition screening tools: does one size fit all? A systematic review of screening tools for the hospital setting. *Clinical Nutrition* **33**: 39–58.

Van Dam, F. and Van Gool, W.A. (2009). Hyperhomocysteinemia and Alzheimer's disease: a systematic review. *Archives of Gerontology and Geriatrics* **48**: 425–430.

van der Meij, B.S., Wijnhoven, H.A.H., Lee, J.S. *et al.* (2017). Poor Appetite and dietary intake in community-dwelling older adults. *Journal of the American Geriatric Society* **65**: 2190–2197.

Vellas, B., Guigoz, Y., Garry, P.J. *et al.* (1999). The Mini Nutritional Assessment (MNA) and its use in grading the nutritional state of elderly patients. *Nutrition* **15**: 116–122.

Visser, M., Volkert, D., Corish, C. *et al.* (2017). Tackling the increasing problem of malnutrition in older persons: The Malnutrition in the Elderly (MaNuEL) Knowledge Hub. *Nutrition Bulletin* **42**: 178–186.

Wang, Q., Zhan, Y., Pedersen, N.L. *et al.* (2018a). Telomere length and all-cause mortality: a meta-analysis. *Ageing Research Reviews* **48**: 11–20.

Wang, Q.X., Zhao, S.M., Zhou, Y.B. and Zhang, C. (2018b). Lack of association between vitamin D receptor genes BsmI as well as ApaI polymorphisms and osteoporosis risk: a pooled analysis on Chinese individuals. *International Journal of Rheumatic Disease* **21**: 967–974.

Wang, N., Chen, Y., Ji, J. *et al.* (2020). The relationship between serum vitamin D and fracture risk in the elderly: a meta-analysis. *Journal of Orthopedic Surgery Research* **15**: 81.

Whitelock, E., Ensaff, H. (2018). On your own: older adults' food choice and dietary habits. *Nutrients* **10**: 413.

Willcox, D.C., Scapagnini, G. and Willcox, B.J. (2014). Healthy aging diets other than the Mediterranean: a focus on the Okinawan diet. *Mechanisms of Ageing and Development* **136–137**: 148–162.

Wilms, E., An, R., Smolinska, A. *et al.* (2021). Galacto-oligosaccharides supplementation in prefrail older and healthy adults increased faecal bifidobacteria, but did not impact immune function and oxidative stress. *Clinical Nutrition* S0261-5614(21)00002-9. doi: 10.1016/j.clnu.2020.12.034.

Wolters, F.J., Ikram, M.A. (2019). Epidemiology of vascular dementia. *Arteriosclerosis Thrombosis and Vascular Biology* **39**: 1542–1549.

Woodward, T., Josephson, C., Ross, L. *et al.* (2020). A retrospective study of the incidence and characteristics of long-stay adult inpatients with hospital-acquired malnutrition across five Australian public hospitals. *European Journal of Clinical Nutrition* **74**: 1668–1676.

World Health Organization. (2021). WHO coronavirus (COVID-19) dashboard. https://covid19.who.int (accessed 13 April 2021).

Yang, C., Shi, X., Xia, H. *et al.* (2020). The evidence and controversy between dietary calcium intake and calcium supplementation and the risk of cardiovascular disease: a systematic review and meta-analysis of cohort studies and randomized controlled trials. *Journal of the American College of Nutrition* **39**: 352–370.

Yin, J., Zhang, Q., Liu, A. *et al.* (2010). Calcium supplementation for 2 years improves bone mineral accretion and lean body mass in Chinese adolescents. *Asia Pacific Journal of Clinical Nutrition* **19**: 152–160.

Yoshikata, R., Myint, K.Z.Y. and Ohta, H. (2018). Effects of equol supplement on bone and cardiovascular parameters in middle-aged Japanese women: a prospective observational study. *Journal of Alternative and Complementary Medicine* **24**: 701–708.

Young, G.S. and Kirkland, J.B. (2007). Rat models of caloric intake and activity: relationships to animal physiology and human health. *Applied Physiology, Nutrition, and Metabolism* **32**: 161–176.

Zakai, N.A., Katz, R., Hirsch, C. *et al.* (2005). A prospective study of anemia status, hemoglobin concentration, and mortality in an elderly cohort: the Cardiovascular Health Study. *Archives of Internal Medicine* **165**: 2214–2220.

Zhao, J., Miao, K., Wang, H. *et al.* (2013). Association between telomere length and type 2 diabetes mellitus: a meta-analysis. *PLoS ONE* **8**: e79993.

Zhao, J., Zhu, Y., Lin, J. *et al.* (2014). Short leukocyte telomere length predicts risk of diabetes in American Indians: the strong heart family study. *Diabetes* **63**: 354–362.

Zhu, H., Jiang, J., Wang, Q. *et al.* (2018). Associations between ERalpha/beta gene polymorphisms and osteoporosis susceptibility and bone mineral density in postmenopausal women: a systematic review and meta-analysis. *BMC Endocrine Disorders* **18**: 11.

Zhu, K., Lewis, J.R., Sim, M. and Prince, R.L. (2019). Low vitamin d status is associated with impaired bone quality and increased risk of fracture-related hospitalization in older Australian women. *Journal of Bone and Mineral Research* **34**: 2019–2027.

Zhu, Y., Minović, I., Dekker, L.H. *et al.* (2020). Vitamin status and diet in elderly with low and high socioeconomic status: the Lifelines-MINUTHE Study. *Nutrients* **12**: 2659.

Additional reading

If you would like to find out more about the material discussed in this chapter, the following sources may be of interest:

Bernstein, M. and Munoz, N. (2014). *Nutrition for the Older Adult*. Burlington, VA: Jones and Bartlett Learning.

Gasmi, A. (2020). *Nutrition for the Elderly: A clinical approach*. Orthodiet.

Stanner, S., Thompson, R. and Buttriss, J.L. (eds). (2013). *Healthy Ageing: The role of nutrition and lifestyle*. Chichester: Wiley-Blackwell.

World Health Organization. (2002). *Keep Fit for Life: Meeting the nutritional needs of older persons*. Geneva: WHO.

An introduction to the nutrients

The main body of this book focuses on the relationship between diet and health and how that relationship changes across the lifespan. As such, the text does not deal with some of the basic principles of nutrition or provide an overview of the biochemistry of the nutrients, the physiology of digestion or the main sources of nutrients. This Appendix is therefore intended as a very simple reference guide to the macro- and micronutrients.

A.1 Classification of nutrients

Nutrients are broadly classified into macro- and micronutrients, non-essential or essential categories. The concept of essentiality refers to the ability of the body to synthesize nutrients de novo. A nutrient that is essential has to be derived from the diet, either because there is no de novo synthesis within the human body or because the rate of synthesis is insufficient to meet requirements. Essential nutrients may also be referred to as indispensable. By contrast, non-essential nutrients are synthesized at a level in excess of that needed to meet requirements. Some nutrients (for example the amino acids glycine and taurine, and the monosaccharide ribose) may be considered conditionally essential, as they cannot be synthesized in sufficient amounts under certain circumstances, such as pregnancy or lactation. Macronutrient is the term used to refer to the nutrients that are consumed in large (tens of grammes per day) quantities. Generally speaking the macronutrients (carbohydrates, lipids, proteins) are required to meet energy requirements and provide the basic building blocks of molecules that are necessary to maintain life-critical metabolic and structural functions. Micronutrients are required in only small (micro- or milligrams per day) and include the vitamins and minerals. Some minerals such as calcium, sodium, chloride, magnesium and potassium are sometimes referred to as the macro-minerals, as they are required in considerably higher quantities than most other inorganic constituents in the diet. Other minerals required by the body in barely quantifiable amounts (chromium, boron, molybdenum) are referred to as trace elements.

A.2 Carbohydrates

A.2.1 Major roles

Within the human body carbohydrates are principally used in energy metabolism, providing around 50% of dietary energy. Glucose is the main energy substrate used for synthesis of adenosine triphosphate (ATP) via glycolysis and the citric acid cycle. Related to this function as an energy substrate, carbohydrates (specifically glycogen) are used as a mid-term (24-hour) energy store. Carbohydrates are important components and precursors of more complex molecules. The pentose sugar ribose, for example, is a component of coenzymes such as nicotinamide adenine dinucleotide and flavin adenine dinucleotide and is also incorporated into the structure of ATP. Ribose also makes up the backbone of RNA, and deoxyribose provides a key structural component of DNA. Other carbohydrates form glycoproteins and glycolipids, which are present on cell surfaces where they participate in intercellular signalling.

A.2.2 Structure and classification of carbohydrates

The basic structure of the carbohydrates is the monosaccharide unit. These five or six carbon units can polymerize via glycosidic bonds to form disaccharides

---

Nutrition, Health and Disease: A Lifespan Approach, Third Edition. Simon Langley-Evans.
© 2021 John Wiley & Sons Ltd. Published 2021 by John Wiley & Sons Ltd.
Companion website: www.wiley.com/go/langleyevans/lifespan3e

(e.g. maltose, sucrose and lactose), oligosaccharides (e.g. inulin and raffinose) or polysaccharides (e.g. starch and glycogen). Examples of mono-, di- and polysaccharide structures are shown in Figure A.1. The most important monosaccharides in mammalian biochemistry are glucose (the universal energy substrate), fructose, galactose and ribose.

Disaccharides are the main form in which sugars are consumed in the diet. What we describe as sugar is the disaccharide sucrose (glucose–fructose), while milk sugar is lactose (glucose–galactose). Increasingly, fructose is consumed directly in the diet as food manufacturers use it in food processing, particularly as the basis for soft drinks and any foods that require cheap sweeteners.

Carbohydrates comprising between three and nine monosaccharide units are referred to as oligosaccharides. Within the diet, these are plant-derived materials and are generally resistant to digestion. As a result, they pass through the upper digestive tract to the colon where they act as substrates for the growth of the colonic microflora. Prebiotics, which are designed to stimulate the microflora and which may improve gastrointestinal function, are generally based on oligosaccharides such as inulin. Carbohydrates with 10 or more monosaccharide units are described as polysaccharides. These may be further divided into digestible polysaccharides and non-starch polysaccharides (cellulose, hemicellulose, beta-glucans, pectins). The bulk of the digestible polysaccharides will be starches from plant sources. The non-starch polysaccharides, which are also referred to as dietary fibre, are resistant to digestion and pass through the

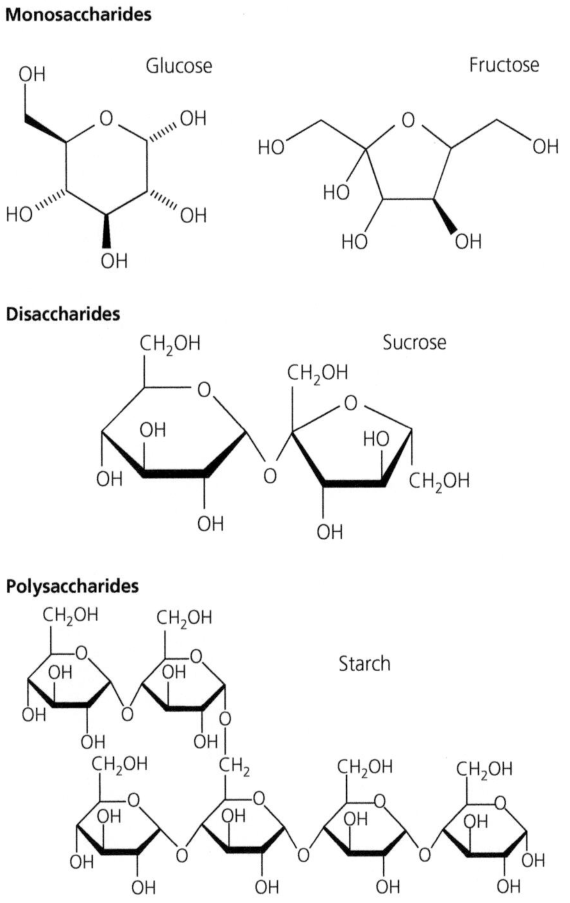

Figure A.1 The structures of the carbohydrates. Carbohydrates comprise monosaccharide units which are either hexose rings (e.g. glucose) or pentose rings (e.g. fructose). These can link through glycosidic bonds to form disaccharides (e.g. sucrose), oligosaccharides (3–9 units) or polysaccharides (10+ units).

gut largely unchanged. Like oligosaccharides they may be fermented by the colonic microflora, but they also make up a significant mass of faecal matter and contribute to healthy gastrointestinal function. Resistant starches, which are generally starches enclosed in indigestible structures (grain husk, unpolished rice), also contribute to the faecal bulk. Approximately 30% of ingested carbohydrate is likely to reach the colon unchanged and is available for bacterial fermentation.

A.2.3 Digestion and absorption of carbohydrates

Ingested carbohydrates undergo digestion, beginning in the mouth, where salivary amylase acts on starch molecules to release maltose and oligosaccharides. Amylase is also released in the small intestine, where hydrolysis of the polysaccharides generates disaccharides and oligosaccharides such as maltotriose and dextrins. The villi present in the small intestine express specific oligosaccharidases which hydrolyze these components to monosaccharides, which can be absorbed. Lactase, for example, breaks lactose down to glucose and galactose and sucrose is hydrolysed to glucose and fructose by sucrase-isomaltase. Monosaccharides are taken up by enterocytes by both active transport and facilitated diffusion. Glucose and galactose enter via sodium–potassium adenosine triphosphatase sodium/glucose cotransporter 1, while fructose is carried into the enterocyte by glucose transporter 5.

A.3 Lipids

A.3.1 Major roles

Lipids, derived from dietary fats, play a number of roles in cellular structure and metabolism, and have structural roles at the gross organ level. Lipids are a rich energy source (37 kJ/g fat) and are used in metabolic pathways that include hormone synthesis (from sterols) and phospholipid synthesis. The leucotrienes, eicosanoids and thromboxanes are derived from fatty acids and play important roles in inflammatory processes. Lipids are also to directly modulate the expression of genes through transcription factors such as the peroxisome-activated proliferator receptors. At the cellular level, lipids make up the bulk of the material that comprises cell and organelle membranes. Lipids are also present in a protective role (e.g. fat pads protect the kidneys from external injury) and provide insulation as a layer within the skin. Lipids have important transport functions and provide the vehicle for uptake of fat-soluble vitamins from the diet.

A.3.2 Structure and classification of lipids

From a nutritional perspective, the important lipids are the phospholipids, triacylglycerides, fatty acids and sterols. Structurally, the sterols (main representative is cholesterol) are distinct from the rest of the lipids as they comprise complex ring structures, which are the precursors for the synthesis of bile acids, vitamin D and steroid hormones. The sterols are not constructed from fatty acids.

A.3.2.1 Fatty acids

Fatty acids are the basic building blocks of triglycerides (triacylglycerides) and phospholipids. They comprise chains of 4–28 carbons and are classified on the basis of the number, location and type of double bonds present within their structure (Figure A.2). Saturated fatty acids have no double bonds and are solid at room temperature. They are generally derived from meat and milk within the human diet, but rich plant sources include palm and coconut oils. Monounsaturated fatty acids have a single double bond within their structure and tend to be oils rather than solid fats. Within the human diet most monounsaturated fatty acids are derived from rapeseed and olive oil. The polyunsaturated fatty acids have multiple double bonds and are all oils. The major dietary polyunsaturated fatty acids are in the series C18–C22 and are grouped into the n-3 and n-6 families (also referred to as omega-3 and omega-6). The nomenclature for fatty acids indicates their structure, following the format shown below:

$$Cx : y n - z$$

where x refers to the number of carbon atoms in the chain, y is the number of double bonds and z is the first carbon in the chain to be double bonded. Hence, C18:0 is the saturated fatty acid oleic acid, C18 : 1 n-9 is a monounsaturated fatty acid, with a double bond at carbon 9 (oleic acid) and C18 : 2 n-6 (linoleic acid) is a polyunsaturated fatty acid with the first double bond at carbon 6. Table A.1 gives the common name and nomenclature for some of the nutritionally important fatty acids. The fatty acid composition of commonly consumed fats and oils is shown in Table A.2.

There is a requirement for fatty acids within the diet and both n-6 (linoleic acid) and n-3 (alpha-linolenic acid) precursors of longer chain fatty acids are referred to as the essential fatty acids. The n-6 fatty acids are consumed in greater amounts than n-3 within the human diet (ratio of 20 : 1 within the western diet), and many studies have suggested that excessive n-6 consumption may have adverse health

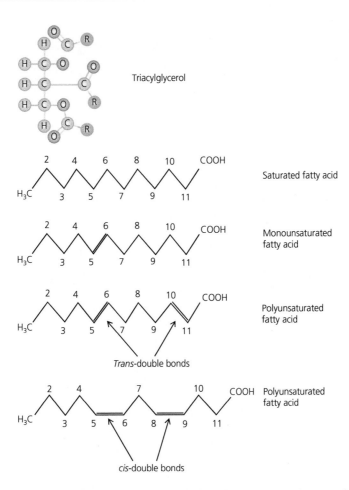

Figure A.2 The structure and classification of triacylglycerides (triglycerides) and fatty acids. A triacylglyceride comprises a glycerol backbone conjugated to three fatty acids, which are shown here as R groups. These fatty acids may be saturated (no double bonds), monounsaturated (one double bond) or polyunsaturated (multiple double bonds). When double bonds are in the trans-orientation, then the overall structure of unsaturated fatty acids and the biological behaviour of those fatty acids differ significantly to when the double bonds are in the cis orientation.

Table A.1 Common dietary fatty acids.

Saturated	Monounsaturated	Polyunsaturated
C12 : 0 lauric	C16 : 1 n-5 palmitoleic	C18 : 2 n-6 linoleic
C14 : 0 myristic	C18 : 1 n-9 oleic	C18 : 3 n-6 γ-linolenic
C16 : 0 palmitic	C18 : 1 n-7 vaccenic	C18 : 3 n-3 α-linolenic
C17 : 0 margeric	trans C18 : 1 n-9 elaidic	C20 : 4 n-6 arachadonic
C18 : 0 stearic		C20 : 5 n-3 eicosapentanoic
C20 : arachidic		C22 : 6 n-3 docosahexanoic

effects. Higher consumption of n-3, particularly derived from fish, has been associated with lower risk of coronary heart disease and cancer. This relationship with health outcomes is believed to derive from the contributions of these fatty acids to inflammatory processes. The n-6 and n-3 fatty acid precursors (linoleic acid and alpha-linolenic acid) give rise to different metabolites. The n-6 series are proinflammatory, while the n-3 have the opposite effect.

The unsaturated fatty acids are also classified according to their isomeric forms as double bonds may be in a cis- or trans-orientation. This changes the overall structure of the fatty acid and trans-fatty acids have a chemical structure more akin to

Table A.2 The fatty acid composition of commonly consumed fats and oils.

Cooking Oil	SFA							MUFA				PUFA		
	C6:0	C8:0	C10:0	C12:0	C14:0	C16:0	C18:0	C16:1 n-7	C18:1 n-9	C20:1	C22:1	C18:2 n-6	C18:3 n-3	Other
Canola (rape)						4.0	2.0		55.0		2.0	26.0	10.0	1
Soya bean					0.1	10.3	3.8	0.2	22.8	0.2		51.0	6.8	4.8
Corn						10.9	1.8		24.1			58.0	0.7	4.5
Olive						11.0	2.2	0.8	72.5	0.3		7.9	0.6	4.7
Safflower						4.8	1.3		75.3			14.2		4.4
Palm				0.1	1.0	43.5	4.3	0.3	36.6	0.1		9.1	0.2	4.8
Coconut	0.6	7.5	3.7	44.6	16.8	8.2	2.8		5.8			1.8		8.2
Peanut						9.5	2.2	0.1	44.8	1.3		32.0		10
Lard				1.7	0.1	26.0	16.5	2.3	36.6	0.8		11.3	0.7	4.1
Butter		0.5	2.5	3.9	12.9	31.4	12.1	2.0	30.2	1.6		2.1	0.8	

MUFA, monounsaturated fatty acids; PUFA, polyunsaturated fatty acids; SFA, saturated fatty acid.

saturated fatty acids (Figure A.2). Trans-fatty acids are present in the diet as naturally occurring components of dietary fat in milk and meat, and are also generated during processing of food oils. To make unsaturated fats solid, or into spreadable materials such as margarines, they undergo partial hydrogenation which converts cis bonds to trans. High intakes of trans-fatty acids produced by partial hydrogenation in industrial processing are associated with increased risk of cardiovascular disease.

A.3.2.2 Phospholipids and triglycerides

Within the body, most lipid that is present in structures such as membranes, is in the form of phospholipids. Most phospholipids comprise a glycerol backbone, which is bonded to two fatty acids (a diacylglyceride) and to a phosphate group and amino acids (e.g. phosphatidylserine), alcohols (phosphatidylinositol) or vitamins (phosphatidylcholine). The exception to this is sphingomyelin, where glycerol is replaced by sphingosine. Phospholipids all share the property of being amphipathic, meaning that have a hydrophilic polar head and hydrophobic tail. As such, they can form bilayers in cell membranes, which associate with sterols and proteins.

Fat stores within the body, lipids for transport and the vast majority of dietary fat are in the form of triglycerides. Triglycerides comprise a glycerol backbone bonded to three fatty acids (Figure A.2).

A.3.3 Digestion and absorption of lipids

Dietary fat is digested in the stomach, duodenum and ileum. Gastric processing involves the churning of food, which separates the fat from the aqueous portion of the food within chyme. Emulsified fats are released from the stomach into the duodenum, where they undergo lipolysis through the action of lipases (on triglycerides), phospholipase A2 (on phospholipids) and cholesterol ester hydrolase upon cholesterol esters. Lipase action yields glycerol, monoacylglycerides and free fatty acids. Shorter chain fatty acids (<12 carbon) are absorbed directly into the portal circulation, while longer chain fatty acids and cholesterol are bound to bile salts and taken up by enterocytes in the ileum. Following uptake of lipids into the hepatic portal circulation or enterocytes, they are packaged into lipoproteins for transport (Figure A.3).

A.4 Proteins

A.4.1 Major roles

Protein is a basic component of all cells and is incorporated into cellular structures (cell membranes, cytoskeleton, organelles). All metabolic, physiological and endocrine functions within the body are critically dependent on the synthesis of proteins from amino acids that are derived either from the diet or produced de novo. Enzymes, neurotransmitters, peptide hormones, cell surface markers, hormone receptors and membrane transporters are all proteins that undergo constant turnover (synthesis–degradation–synthesis) to maintain cellular functions.

Dietary protein plays a different role as it is broken down into constituent parts prior to absorption. As such, protein is required within the diet to meet the demands of the body for the amino acids that are required for protein synthesis, energy metabolism and other biochemical pathways. Not all dietary protein is the same, as proteins derived from some food sources contain an incomplete range of the amino acids required by humans. While animal derived protein is considered 'high quality', plant proteins may be low quality, as one or more amino acids are missing or present in low quantities. For example, many beans and peas lack the sulphur-amino acids cysteine and methionine, while maize lacks tryptophan and lysine.

A.4.2 Amino acids

The properties of proteins depend on the properties and interactions between the constituent amino acids which comprise the protein structure. There are 20 amino acids that are classically used in protein synthesis, with additional amino acids that are involved in intermediary metabolism but which do not appear in proteins (citrulline, ornithine, taurine). Amino acids have the structure shown in Figure A.4. Each comprises an amine group conjugated to a carbon that also bonds to an acid group and a side chain or 'R group'. These R groups may be simple carbon chains (e.g. glycine), branching carbon chains (leucine, valine, isoleucine) or ring structures (e.g. tyrosine, histidine, phenylalanine). The R groups present give each amino acid its specific biochemical properties, determine how they will contribute to protein structure and what other biochemical functions may be served (e.g. glycine is a donor in methylation reactions, leucine, aspartate and alanine are nitrogen donors). The amino acids are classified as essential, nonessential and conditionally essential (Table A.3).

A.4.3 Structure of proteins

Proteins have a complex structure that is primarily based on the formation of chains of amino acids (Figure A.4). Amino acids link together by virtue of peptide bonds that form between the amine group on one moiety and the acid moiety on another. The resulting peptide or polypeptide chains have more complex structures and functions by virtue of the properties of the R-group side chains on each amino acid. Some

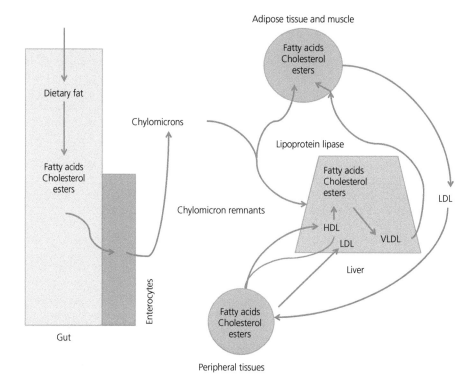

Figure A.3 The uptake and transport of fatty acids and cholesterol. Fatty acids and cholesterol esters are packaged into chylomicrons after uptake by enterocytes. Chylomicrons deliver fatty acids and cholesterol to adipose tissue and muscle with chylomicron remnants transported to the liver. Here, packaging into very low density lipoprotein (VLDL) allows further transport of cholesterol and triglycerides to adipose tissue and muscle, where low-density lipoprotein (LDL) picks up lipid for transport to the rest of the periphery. High-density lipoprotein (HDL) carries triglycerides and cholesterol back from the periphery to the liver.

short peptides may have important biological activity (e.g. the tripeptide antioxidant glutathione or the octapeptide hormone angiotensin II), but most proteins would comprise 50–1000 amino acid residues.

The sequence of amino acids in a polypeptide chain provides the primary structure of a protein. The formation of cross-links between R groups, either through covalent bonds or weak hydrogen bonds, enables the chains to coil and fold into the conformation that enables biological activity. This folding and cross-linking is referred to as the secondary and tertiary structure of the protein.

A.4.4 Digestion and absorption of proteins

Dietary protein is generally broken down to dipeptides or single amino acids during digestion in the alimentary canal. Proteins are relatively resistant to digestive enzymes when in their normal conformation, as the tertiary and secondary structure limits access to the peptide bonds. Acid action in the stomach denatures these structures allowing enzymes (endopeptidases, carboxypeptidases, trypsin, chymotrypsin) to break

peptide chains liberating amino acids for absorption by either passive diffusion or active transport. Small amounts of whole proteins may pass unchanged across the gut to the circulation through the process of paracellular uptake. This movement between the tight junctions of the epithelial layer of the gut plays an important role in priming the immune system.

A.5 Intermediary metabolism

Intermediary metabolism is the term used to describe the processes through which nutritive factors become incorporated into cellular components and functions. Metabolism comprises anabolism (the process through which complex macromolecules are synthesized from simple precursors) and catabolism (the degradation of macromolecules to simple products and waste). Intermediary metabolism covers the processes and intermediate forms of macromolecules that participate in metabolic pathways, and the mechanisms which regulate pathways to maintain cellular homeostasis. This

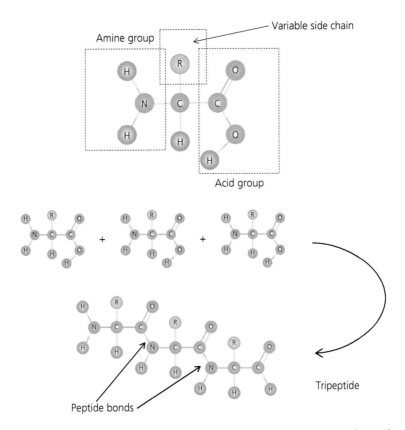

Figure A.4 The structure of amino acids and peptides. Amino acids comprise an amine group and an acid group bound to a single carbon which also bears a side chain (R). R groups may be carbon chains or ring structures. Amino acids form peptide bonds allowing them to form short chains (e.g. the tripeptide chain shown) or complex proteins with up to 1000 amino acid residues.

Table A.3 The essential and non-essential amino acids.

Essential	Conditionally essential	Non-essential
Isoleucine	Arginine	Alanine
Leucine	Cysteine	Aspartate
Lysine	Glycine	Asparagine
Methionine	Glutamine	Glutamate
Phenylalanine	Histidine	Serine
Threonine	Proline	
Tryptophan	Serine	
Valine	Tyrosine	

is critical as metabolism must run in a way that ensures a supply of ATP to drive essential processes; maintains cellular ion gradients and; eliminates potentially toxic waste products such as ammonia.

The macromolecules are central to metabolism, with most biochemical pathways driving towards synthesis of carbohydrates, lipids, proteins and nucleic acids and their breakdown for energy release or elimination. The macronutrients derived from the diet are required to ensure that there is

sufficient supply of simple substrates to maintain these functions. The micronutrients play a supporting role by acting as coenzymes and cofactors (e.g. folate) or as regulatory molecules which activate processes at the level of gene expression (e.g. vitamins A and D).

The macronutrients are interrelated from a metabolic perspective (Figure A.5). Glucose is the main energy source for metabolism, as it feeds into glycolysis and the citric acid cycle. Fatty acids, which

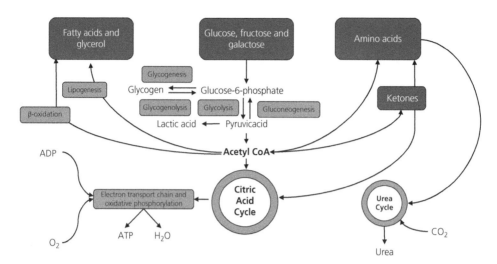

Figure A.5 Intermediary metabolism. Glucose, fatty acids and amino acids can all be used as energy sources through the citric acid cycle.

are the longer-term energy source for the body, also feed in to the citric acid cycle after being broken down to acetyl coenzyme A by the beta-oxidation pathway. Proteins can also feed into energy metabolism through amino acid degradation to alpha-ketoacids, which can enter the citric acid cycle directly or be metabolized to form glucose.

A.6 Micronutrients

A.6.1 Minerals

Minerals and trace elements are inorganic components of food and water intake which are required to maintain normal cellular and whole body physiological function. All the minerals can be accumulated in storage forms, either as components of structures (e.g. bone is a reservoir for calcium, phosphorus and magnesium) or bound to proteins in a storage form (e.g. ferritin binding of iron). Approximately 3% of the mass of the human body comprises these elements.

Uptake of the minerals from the diet tends to be low and their bioavailability will be dependent on person specific features such as age, life stage or disease, and the nature of the food matrix from which absorption occurs. The presence of inhibitors and enhancers of absorption from food and competition between minerals for gut transporters determines bioavailability. For example, approximately 14–18% of ingested iron will be absorbed from a mixed diet, and this falls to 5–12% from a vegetarian diet.

The functions of the minerals in the body are varied and specific, but in general terms they are critical for the formation of rigid structures such as teeth or bone; as catalytic centres for enzymes; as components of hormones; in regulation of fluid balance; in regulation of acid–base balance; and enabling muscle contraction and generating action potentials in the transmission of nervous impulses. Each mineral and trace element is associated with characteristic symptoms of deficiency as these associated functions become limited. Table A.4 lists the main minerals required within the diet, together with their main functions, dietary sources and the symptoms of deficiency. Table A.5 shows the minerals and trace metals which function as cofactors in mammalian biochemistry. Cofactors are non-protein components that are required by enzymes to enable catalysis to occur. Cofactors are chemically bound to the enzyme protein and many of them are metal ions. Other metal ions, for example sodium and potassium, are associated with cellular transport proteins, or have structural roles in cells and tissues.

A.6.2 Vitamins

The vitamins are organic molecules that are critical for biochemical functions by virtue of their specific characteristics as coenzymes. A number of the vitamins also have important regulatory functions, controlling gene expression (e.g. vitamin A), or regulating the uptake and excretion of minerals (e.g. vitamin D). Where vitamins are required as coenzymes, they are involved in a limited number of biochemical pathways. Thiamine, for example, is a coenzyme for just three enzymes (pyruvate dehydrogenase, alpha-ketoglutarate dehydrogenase and branched chain amino acid dehydrogenase), but this is sufficient to make it essential for normal energy

Table A.4 The minerals: sources, functions and deficiency symptoms.

Mineral	Main dietary sources	Principal functions	Deficiency symptoms
Sodium	Ubiquitous, but high in cheese, processed and preserved foods	Acid–base balance Fluid balance Nerve transmission Muscle function	Low appetite, nausea and fatigue
Potassium	Fruit and vegetables	Acid–base balance Fluid balance Nerve transmission Muscle function	Confusion, muscle weakness, cardiac arrest
Calcium	Dairy produce	Bones and teeth Muscle contraction Blood clotting Nerve transmission	Convulsions, stunted growth, rickets osteoporosis
Phosphorus	Meat and fish Wholegrains Dairy produce	Bones and teeth Acid–base balance	Bone demineralization
Iron	Meat Fortified cereals Dried fruits Green vegetables	Haemoglobin synthesis	Pallor, fatigue, breathlessness
Iodine	Seafoods Iodized salt Milk (some countries)	Synthesis of thyroid hormones	Enlarged thyroid (goitre), restricted growth, fetal abnormality
Magnesium	Wholegrains Nuts Green vegetables	Bone structure DNA and protein synthesis	Neuromuscular disorders
Zinc	Meat Eggs Pulses Wholegrains	Immune function DNA synthesis Enzyme cofactor	Growth failure, reduced immunity
Copper	Meat Vegetables	Ion absorption Enzyme cofactor	Reduced immunity
Fluorine	Seafood Tea Fortified water	Maintenance of tooth enamel	Tooth decay
Selenium	Brazil nuts Seafood Meat	Antioxidant functions Thyroid hormone synthesis Muscle function	Cardiomyopathy (with infection) Male infertility Hypothyroidism

Table A.5 Role of minerals as enzyme cofactors and metabolic function.

Mineral	Functional significance	Examples of enzymes with metal cofactor
Calcium	Cell signalling	Pyruvate kinase C
Copper	Red blood cell formation Antioxidant Connective tissue formation Energy metabolism	Aminolevulinic acid synthase Superoxide dismutase Lysyl oxidase Cytochrome oxidase
Iron	Energy metabolism Antioxidant Amino acid metabolism	NADH-ubiquinone reductase, succinate-ubiquinone reductase Catalase Phenylalanine hydroxylase
Magnesium	DNA repair Energy metabolism	DNA polymerase, helicase, nuclease Glucose-6-phosphatase, hexokinase, pyruvate dehydrogenase
Manganese	Gluconeogenesis Urea cycle	Pyruvate carboxylase, phosphoenolpyruvate carboxykinase Arginase
Molybdenum	Amino acid catabolism Purine nucleotide catabolism	Sulfite oxidase Xanthine oxidase
Selenium	Antioxidant	Glutathione peroxidases
Zinc	Regulation of gene expression Neurotransmitter synthesis DNA synthesis	Histone deacetylases Monoamine oxidase DNA polymerase, aspartate transcarbamoylase

Table A.6 The fat soluble vitamins: sources, functions and deficiency symptoms.

Vitamin	Main dietary sources	Principal functions	Deficiency symptoms
A: retinol/beta carotene	Liver and fish oils (retinol) Fruits and vegetables (carotene)	Cell differentiation Antioxidant (beta carotene) Visual function	Night blindness, keratinization of the skin
D: calciferol	Fish and fish oils Fortified cereals Fortified milk Margarine	Maintenance of calcium balance	Rickets, osteomalacia
E: tocopherols	Vegetable oils Nuts and nut oils	Antioxidant	Rare but serious neurological symptoms
K: phylloquinone	Green vegetables Cereals	Blood clotting	Impaired clotting

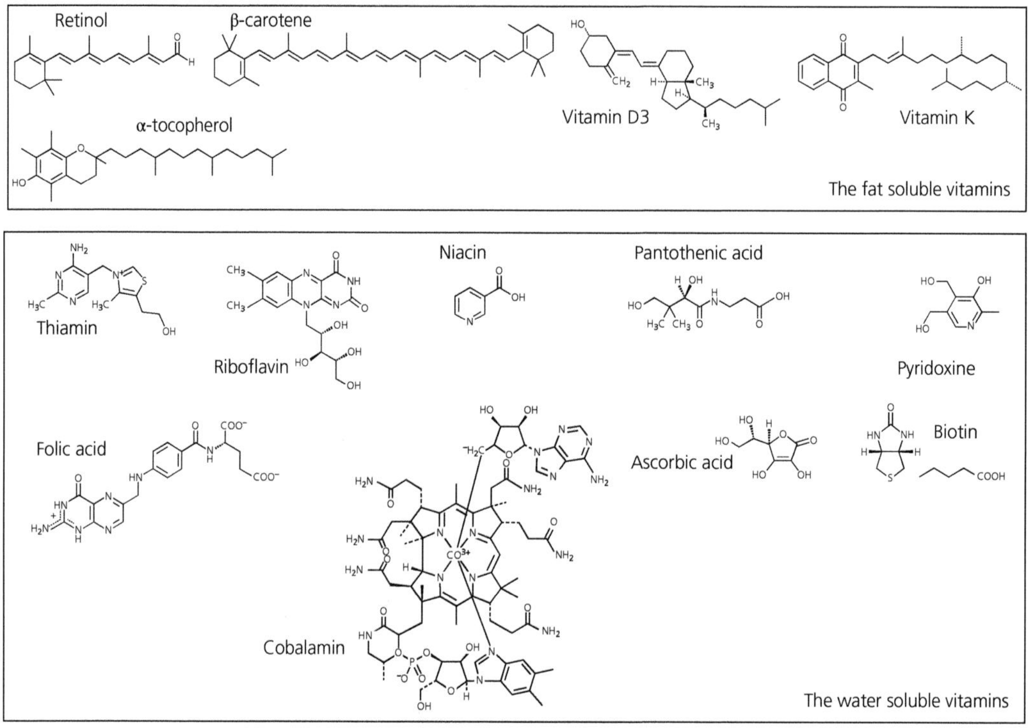

The fat soluble vitamins

The water soluble vitamins

Figure A.6 The structures of the vitamins.

and amino acid metabolism. Where the supply of vitamin is limiting the associated biochemical pathways will be affected and the resulting failure to synthesize products or the accumulation of precursors will be drivers of deficiency symptoms and diseases.

Most of the vitamins are essential nutrients, but some can be synthesized de novo, provided that there is sufficient precursor available. Niacin, for example, is synthesized from the amino acid tryptophan. In the case of vitamin D, this de novo synthesis is far in excess of dietary intake. Several of the B vitamins and vitamin K are also synthesized by the colonic microflora,

but it is believed that this bacterial synthesis is of little significance in human nutrition as there is limited uptake of these bacterial products from the gut.

The vitamins are classified according to solubility in fat or water. Several exist in multiple forms, so vitamin D, for example, comprises vitamin D2 and D3, each of which has five to six metabolites. Vitamin K has three vitamers (phylloquinone, menadione, menaquinone). Table A.6 summarizes the functions of the fat soluble vitamins and Table A.7 describes the water-soluble vitamins. Many of the vitamins have complex structures (Figure A.6).

Index

Nutrition, Health and Disease: A Lifespan Approach, Third Edition. Simon Langley-Evans.
© 2021 John Wiley & Sons Ltd. Published 2021 by John Wiley & Sons Ltd.
Companion website: www.wiley.com/go/langleyevans/lifespan3e